BLOOD:

PATHOPHYSIOLOGY

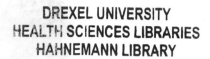
BLOOD:
PATHOPHYSIOLOGY

James H. Jandl, M.D.

George Richards Minot Professor of Medicine
Harvard Medical School

Physician
Beth Israel Hospital

Senior Consultant in Medicine
Brigham and Women's Hospital
Boston

☐

Boston

Blackwell Scientific Publications

Oxford   London   Edinburgh   Melbourne
Paris   Berlin   Vienna

Blackwell Scientific Publications

Editorial offices:
Three Cambridge Center, Cambridge, Massachusetts 02142, USA
Osney Mead, Oxford OX2 0EL, England
25 John Street, London, WC1N 2BL, England
23 Ainslie Place, Edinburgh, EH3 6AJ, Scotland
54 University Street, Carlton, Victoria 3053, Australia

Other Editorial Offices:
Arnette SA
2, rue Casimir-Delavigne, 75006 Paris, France
Blackwell Wissenschafts
Meinekestrasse 4, D-1000 Berlin 15, Germany
Blackwell MZV
Feldgasse 13, A-1238, Vienna, Austria

Distributors:
USA and Canada
  Mosby-Year Book, Inc.
  11830 Westline Industrial Drive
  St. Louis, Missouri 63146
  (Orders: Tel. 800-633-6699)

Australia
  Blackwell Scientific Publications (Australia) Pty Ltd
  54 University Street
  Carlton, Victoria 3053

Outside North America and Australia
  Blackwell Scientific Publications, Ltd.
  Osney Mead
  Oxford OX2 0EL England

Typeset by Huron Valley Graphics
Printed and bound by The Maple-Vail Book Manufacturing Group
Blackwell Scientific Publications, Inc.

© 1991 by James H. Jandl
Printed in the United States of America
91 92 93 94 5 4 3 2 1

Library of Congress Cataloging in Publication Data
Jandl, James H., 1925–
    Blood : pathophysiology / James H. Jandl.
        p.   cm.
    Includes bibliographical references.
    Includes index.
    ISBN 0-86542-122-6 :
    1. Blood—Pathophysiology.   2. Blood—Diseases.   I. Title.
    [DNLM: 1. Blood—physiology.   2. Hematologic Diseases-
    -physiopathology.   WH 100 J33ba]
    RC636.J35   1991
    616.1'507—dc20
    DNLM/DLC
    for Library of Congress   90-1160
                                                     CIP

Dedicated to

Dr. William B. Castle

1897–1990

Contents

Preface

◻

Hematology has long enjoyed an advantaged position in the study and teaching of disease mechanisms—pathophysiology—because of the accessibility of blood and marrow to examination and quantitation. Knowledge of hematologic disease mechanisms opens a window on the pathophysiology of nearly all cellular disorders. With the advent of molecular biology, it was no surprise that the foremost medical applications of this technical revolution emanated from hematology laboratories. These applications began with the cloning of globin genes and swiftly expanded to include discovery of leukemia-causing retroviruses, characterization of oncogenes and their products, and devising of gene-amplification techniques useful in pursuits ranging from criminal apprehension to prenatal testing for specific mutations in gene expression.

The very fecundity of hematology when wed to molecular biology has generated an intimidating body of principles and information that dismay student and physician alike. The teaching of pathophysiology of blood disorders, once a delight and a vanguard section of student and postgraduate coursework, is now as treacherous as it was treasured. Even the best of many brief written surveys or introductions to hematology don't say enough, and the several ponderous textbooks in vogue are too much for those with a vigorous but not obsessive interest in the subject. The embattled, overtaught medical students are needful of the curricular refuge of tutorial self-instruction; for them, this cafeteria of hematologic information is offered as a sourcebook. Written with well-founded humility, this book represents an adjustment in scope and scale to encompass as gracefully as possible what we know of the fundamental mechanisms of blood disorders.

For students or physicians who do not yet have a deep background in the techniques and terms of cellular and molecular biology, the first three chapters provide a modest review, which also includes coverage of cytogenetics, cytokinetics, and mechanisms of neoplasia. For the cognoscenti these opening chapters can be bypassed to concentrate on the mechanisms and perversions responsible for hematologic disorders. Medically oriented readers feel let down and unrequited if not given some inkling as to how to combat the cruel consequences of disease; where unique biologic insights are provided by therapy itself, as is spectacularly the case in marrow transplantation, treatment is described in specific terms.

This exposition could not possibly have come to fruition without the remarkable industry, technology, and editorial talents of Mr. Ronald Rouse. The quality of the photographic illustrations reflects the artistry of Mr. Kenneth L. Bates, and one can only marvel at Ms. Carola Kapff's ability to capture morphologic definition so luminously without benefit of color. As in a prior work, the author is deeply indebted to Dr. John W. Harris, whose assiduous editing has exorcized many mistakes and improved this presentation immensely.

NOTICE

The indications and dosages of all drugs in this book have been recommended in the medical literature and conform to the practices of the general medical community. The medications described do not necessarily have specific approval by the Food and Drug Administration for use in the diseases and dosages for which they are recommended. The package insert for each drug should be consulted for use and dosage as approved by the FDA. Because standards for usage change, it is advisable to keep abreast of revised recommendations, particularly those concerning new drugs.

BLOOD:
PATHOPHYSIOLOGY

1

Blood Cell Formation

□

Blood is a complex suspension in plasma of nondividing differentiated cells which continuously perfuses the vasculature. It contains a mixture of several very different kinds of cells, all of which stem from an oligarchy of progenitors that originate in marrow or lymph follicles.

Blood cells are deciduous Blood cells, like cut flowers, do not last. It is a tribute to nature's recondite harmony that the primitive progenitor populations—known collectively as stem cells—are so organized and responsive to feedback signals that blood cell levels normally are maintained within narrow limits despite life's perturbations. The logistic demands on marrow hematopoietic (blood-creating) cells are numerically numbing. The bloodstream of an adult contains 24 trillion (24×10^{12}) red cells, roughly one-third the number of cells in the entire body. As the actuarial expectation of each individual red cell is 4 months, the daily death rate is 2×10^{11} cells, ensuring destruction of about 400 trillion (400×10^{12}) colorful molecules of hemoglobin every second. The concentration of other kinds of blood cells in circulation is much smaller, but their lifespans are proportionately briefer: platelets survive 10 days and suffer a mortality of 1.2×10^{11} cells per day; the valiant granulocytes, which roam for but a few hours, have a similar attrition rate. Altogether, the quotidian drain of spent blood cells including lymphocytes totals about 5×10^{11} cells (500,000 million), a magnitude of exfoliation not even rivaled by the mucosal cells of the intestine. Most mature blood cells were programmed not to proliferate or regenerate, but to differentiate. Differentiation to maturity is inescapably a step toward cell death ("suicidal maturation"), an outcome guaranteed in nucleated red cells (erythroblasts) by nuclear expulsion.

Prerequisites of Stemhood

If the rate of cell death through suicidal maturation were constant, the proliferative demand would be constant and could be met by a cytokinetic organization having the inflexible pyramidal structure characteristic of most governments or companies: in steady-state biological systems a conventional corporate organizational chart would suffice to describe the numbers and levels of authority involved. As a true steady state rarely exists, the stem cell oligarchy must act collectively to assure its own numerical preservation ("self-renewal") while responding to varying losses through differentiation. Self-renewal is not simply the division of one precursive cell into two precursive cells. If too many stem cells differentiated, marrow renewal would cease [1]. If too many stem cells replicated, production of differentiated cells would plummet to life-threatening levels. Hence by definition stem cells as a class must have two capabilities: replicating themselves and generating more-differentiated daughter cells [2, 3, 4]. As vacancies arise, how do stem cells decide which to do? Do they go through a phase of repeated replications first (set up assembly lines), and then undergo regulated maturation-division (mass production)? Or when summoned by demand do stem cells respond by asymmetric division, yielding one self-renewing cell and one differentiating cell? Finally, is there a depot of precursive cells that respond to on-call signals in a random (stochastic) manner, or is there an ordered hierarchy of primitive cells whose destiny is assigned during embryogenesis? Are some normal stem cells immortal?

At present there are no settled or unanimous answers to the questions just posed, but the following generalizations may help the reader to handle what follows. (1) In marrow there is a hierarchy of hematopoietic stem cells, the most senior of which is termed the multipotential stem cell. (2) Differentiation of stem cells is unidirectional and is associated with restriction of cell renewal capacity. (3) Stem cell proliferation depends upon contact with stromal cells of marrow. (4) Stem cell proliferation and differentiation are regulated by local and systemic growth factors and their inhibitors.

THE STEM CELL HIERARCHY

The Necessity for a Multipotential Stem Cell

Stem cell terminology is befuddled by redundant dependence on the term "stem" to define precursive cells regardless of rank. To preserve a larger perspective it should be borne in mind that the only true stem cell is the issue formed by fusion of two gametes at the time of conception. During early embryogenesis no participant cell emerges unchanged. At each cell doubling the component embryonal cells forfeit some of their potential, and the prevalent use of the term "totipotential" for even the founder of all hematopoietic cells smacks of hyperbole. In this presentation the ancestor of all blood cells is granted the hereditary title of multipotential hematopoietic stem cell. Its existence has been a theoretical necessity; identification was possible only after phenomenologic characterization of its progeny.

Pluripotential and Unipotential Stem Cells

The existence of an intermediate echelon of precursive cells, best termed pluripotential stem cells, was demonstrated by Till and McCulloch. When infused into irradiated syngeneic mice, marrow cells from normal donors formed discrete clonal colonies which at 7 days were composed of cells derived from multiple unipotential committed progenitors (Figure 1-1). Later it was established by use of cell culture in semisolid media that each discrete colony— colony-forming unit, spleen, alias CFU-S— represents a clone capable under various conditions of generating granulocyte-macrophage colony-forming units (CFU-GM), erythroid colony-forming units (CFU-E), and megakaryocyte colony-forming units (CFU-M or CFU-Meg), or partial combinations thereof. Analogous studies revealed the existence of erythroid burst-forming units (BFU-E), a picturesque term descriptive of the rocketlike growth pattern in culture of a midechelon stem cell precursive to CFU-Es. Some CFU-GMs from marrow cultures in viscous media contain discrete colonies of neutrophils, eosinophils, and basophils, whereas others grow into large CFU-S–like multilineage colonies (CFU-Mix) in

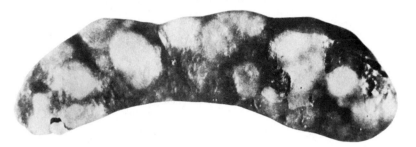

FIGURE 1-1

Macroscopic surface view of the spleen of an
irradiated mouse 7 days after infusion of syngeneic donor marrow cells. The spleen colonies
(CFU-Ss) are heterogeneous, but each individual
colony is a clone derived from a single sequestered stem cell. (Courtesy of Dr. AJ Erslev.)

which all committed "myeloid" progenitors are
represented (CFU-GEMM). Together, spleen
colony and cell culture studies have revealed a
cadre of pluripotential cells (the "mixed myeloid progenitor") that is capable of begetting
unipotential, bipotential, and tripotential cells.
Independent studies have revealed the existence
of analogous pluripotential ancestors of the
several lymphocyte lineages: B lymphocytes (B
cells), T lymphocytes (T cells), and natural killer
(NK) lymphocytes. From these observations in
vitro a cell hierarchy can be inferred, having the
mathematical potential for both replication and
proliferative amplification (Figure 1-2). Figure
1-2 portrays in simplified format a branching
hierarchy in keeping with stochastic models of

FIGURE 1-2

Proposed genealogy of blood cells. Acronyms
are defined in the text. Serial amplification of
each committed cell line is not shown to avoid
clutter.

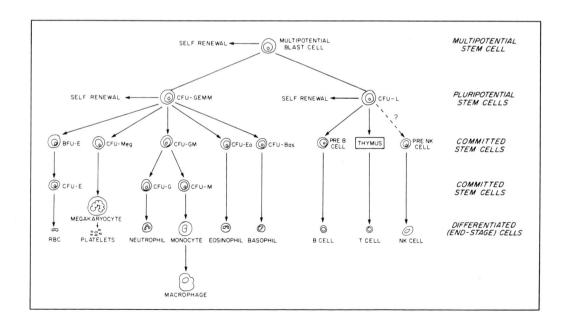

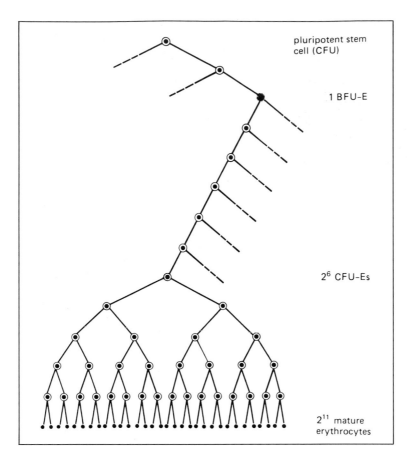

pluripotent stem
cell (CFU)

1 BFU-E

2^6 CFU-Es

2^{11} mature
erythrocytes

FIGURE 1-3

Erythroid pedigree ex-
emplifies the astounding
amplification possible
when self-renewing cells
(pluripotential cells and
BFU-Es) act in series to
generate teeming colo-
nies of CFU-Es, each of
which undergoes several
terminal steps of
maturation-division.
The sweet simplicity of
binary division accounts
for the bountiful re-
sponse to red cell attri-
tion. (From Alberts B et
al: Molecular Biology
of the Cell. New York,
Garland Publishing,
Inc.,1983.)

ordered commitment. The generous fertility of such a system in restocking end-stage cells such as mature red cells (erythrocytes) can be appreciated by examining Figure 1-3.

Multipotential Stem Cells

Multipotential stem cells, which bear the heavy burden of sustaining and regulating all hematopoiesis, are morphologically and antigenically anonymous, and their numbers, back-calculated from studies of multilineage colony growth and radioprotective ability, are very small. As only 10 to 50 hematopoietic stem cells are sufficient to rescue lethally irradiated mice [5, 6], it is possible that human hematopoiesis can be maintained by as few as several thousand multipotential cells [7]. If multilineage human hematopoietic colonies are cultured beyond about 16 days the pluripotential GEMM colonies begin to die off, leaving

macrophages, megakaryocytes, and an immortal population of blast cells that can be replated repeatedly without undergoing terminal differentiation (Figure 1-4). These multipotential blast cell progenitors have been isolated from culture by micromanipulation and have been observed to undergo division within 15 hours into two identical-appearing daughter cells having translucent, refractile cytoplasm and possessing lamellipodal processes, connoting locomotor capability (Figure 1-5) [8]. The multipotentiality of the blast cells shown in Figures 1-4 and 1-5 was affirmed by replating experiments. The functional reality of a high-echelon myeloid-lymphoid stem cell has been confirmed by marking candidate cells by retrovirus-mediated gene transfer and then tracking the labeled cells after transplantation into lethally irradiated recipients [9]: in these experiments as few as one or two stem cell clones have been shown to account for all hematopoiesis.

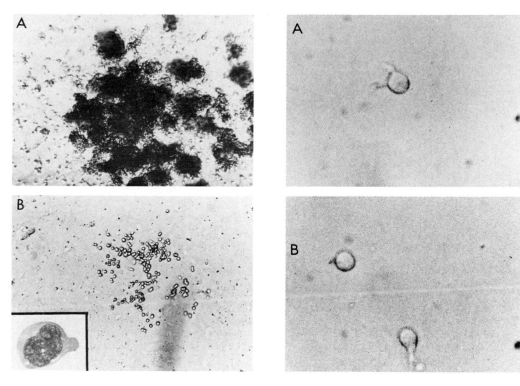

FIGURE 1-4

(A) Macroscopic GEMM colony grown in methylcellulose culture medium for 16 days showed terminal differentiation. (B) At 25 days differentiated myeloid cells had disintegrated and were replaced by colonies of rounded, translucent cells. After Giemsa staining, these survivors (inset) displayed the undifferentiated appearance of blast cells, many of which were equipped with a blunt lamellipod. (Courtesy of M. Ogawa. From Nakahata T and Ogawa M: Hemopoietic colony-forming cells in umbilical cord blood with extensive capability to generate mono- and multipotential hemopoietic progenitors. Reproduced from the *Journal of Clinical Investigation,* 1982, 70:1324, by copyright permission of the American Society for Clinical Investigation.)

FIGURE 1-5

(A) Hematopoietic progenitor cell isolated from primary culture in a viscous medium and examined with an inverted microscope. (B) Appearance 15 house later of two daughter cells (both in locomotor mode), products of a witnessed division of the cell shown in (A). (From Nakahata T et al: Single-cell origin of human mixed hemopoietic colonies expressing various combinations of cell lineages. Blood 65:1010,1985.)

Most stem cells are held in reserve Normally hematopoiesis is sustained through sequential activation of different stem cell clones rather than from the averaged contribution of the entire stem cell pool. Implicit in this generalization is that progenitor cells spend most of their time at rest, in an out-of-cycle G_0 phase (Chapter 2), during which they are preoccupied with DNA repair and other forms of genetic housekeeping. During this stately quiescence stem cells are less vulnerable to genetic damage by cycle-dependent agents such as ionizing radiation, alkylators, or viruses. As they accumulate at the end of the G_1 phase of cell cycle, stem cells are poised and equipped to respond within about 30 minutes to stimulatory factors that reach them from the circulation or are produced within marrow-support cells known as stromal or matrix cells. The importance of stromal cells upon which most hematopoietic cells are perched or embedded is borne out by the fact that only in the vicinity of endosteum do hematopoietic cells proliferate at full capacity. Pluripotential stem cells highly purified by fluorescence-activated cell sorting gradually flag and lose their capacity for self-renewal in even the most nutritious media. Longterm survival of stem cells in vitro and in vivo requires either actual contact with certain kinds of marrow stromal cells or the continued presence of growth promoters, known generically as colony stimulating factors, some of which are secreted by cellular components of the stromal microenvironment itself. Biological interdependence mandates that the mercurial capability of stem cells must submit to local regulation, a vital function prudently remanded to the resident population of stromal support cells.

STROMA, MATRIX, AND GROWTH FACTORS: NECESSITIES OF HEMATOPOIETIC LIFE

Hematopoietic cells are intimately associated with a complex interdigitating stromal cell network. This is composed of: an endothelial "pavement"; fibroblasts and reticular cells, which construct a three-dimensional spongiform matrix; energy-rich fat cells; and macro-

phages, which worm their way beneath the reticular and endothelial cells [10, 11]. An imitation of life can be observed within a few weeks in longterm marrow cultures, in which intimate contact between surface-adherent endothelial cells and macrophages engenders the local release of hematopoietic growth factors. The characteristic physics of an adherent multilayer complex capable of providing a fertile microenvironment for stem cells is shown in Figure 1-6 [12]. Hematopoietic cells lodge within this matrix and undergo both self-renewal and development. Stem cells con-

FIGURE 1-6

(a) Scanning electron micrograph (SEM) of a longterm marrow culture, showing an adherent layer two to four cells deep. Most macrophages (M) lurk beneath the sheet of endothelial-derived cells (E). (b) Transmission electron micrograph (TEM) cross-secting the adherent culture exposes a monocyte (M) treading with fat foot processes upon the upper surface of a flattened endothelial cell (E). The endothelial blanket is draped over adherent macrophages (M), some of which are fat-laden (MF), and immature granulocytes (IG). (From Chervenick PA and Zucker-Franklin D: Chapt 2, in Atlas of Blood Cells. Function and Pathology, vol. 1. Zucker-Franklin D et al, Eds. Milan, Edi. Ermes, s.r.l.,1981.)

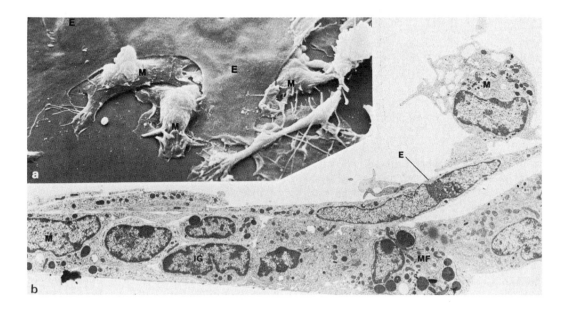

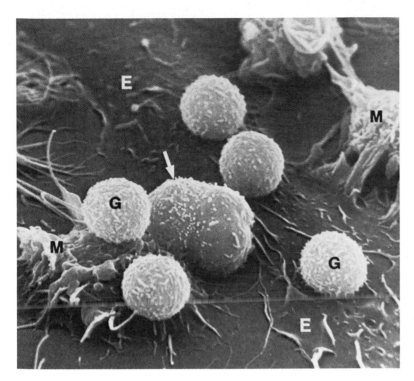

FIGURE 1-7

SEM of marrow culture displaying the endothelial pavement (E), spherical granulocytes (G), and medusalike macrophages (M). A dividing granulocyte is seen at center (arrow). (From Chervenick PA and Zucker-Franklin D: Chapt 2, in Atlas of Blood Cells. Function and Pathology, vol. 1. Zucker-Franklin D et al, Eds. Milan, Edi. Ermes, s.r.l.,1981.)

tinue to replicate, and their progeny are released into the overlying growth medium. Hence stroma provides the site for both stem cell renewal and blood cell release. The division and launching of granulocytes from adherent endothelium is evident in Figure 1-7 [12]. Immature blood cells remain attached to stroma by the adhesive surface proteins, fibronectin and laminin, and are released only when membrane receptors for these adhesives are downregulated by the matured cell.

CYTOKINES: HORMONES OF HEMATOPOIESIS

Proliferation of hematopoietic cells and the comportment of their progeny are governed by a complex hierarchy of growth factors and their inhibitors. These are elaborated largely by vascular stromal cells and by differentiated blood cells themselves, and coordination is achieved through transmission of hormonal signals: when received by specific cell receptor molecules, target cell behavior is modified by receptor-mediated transduction that communi-cates instructions to the cell nucleus. Cytokine terminology is confusing and overlapping, its origins being partly operational and partly conceptual. By convention hormones that regulate myeloid and erythroid growth and differentiation are named colony stimulating factors (CSFs), and those concerned with immunity are called lymphokines; both (once their amino acid sequences are established) are then assigned interleukin numbers.

Myeloid CSFs

Myeloid growth factors are termed CSFs, their primary target cells are identified by prefixed initialisms (e.g., GM-CSF), and (in waning usage) their activities are denoted as CFAs. The four myeloid CSFs are GM-CSF, G-CSF, M-CSF, and multi-CSF; the last is a sovereign factor better known as interleukin-3 (IL-3). Both the IL-3 and GM-CSF genes have been mapped to band 32 on the long arm of chromosome 5; this region (5q32) also contains the genes for M-CSF and its receptor, the proto-oncogene, c-*fms*, plus several other growth factors and their receptors. All myeloid growth factors are small acidic glycoproteins with M_rs ranging from 14,000 to 45,000, depending on the level of glycosylation; three CSF molecules are of solitary habit, but M-CSF proteins are homodimers of two different subunit sizes. CSF complementary DNAs (cDNAs) have been cloned, expressed in mammalian cells, and sequenced, and the mRNAs and their functional protein products are fully characterized (Table 1-1) [13, 14].

Recombinant CSFs are capable of multiple levels of overlapping biologic activity, depending on concentration. The potential risk of chaotic growth responses is curbed by a class structure governing these factors that mirrors the rank order of the stem cell hierarchy itself. IL-3, the master control molecule, and its subordinate, CFU-GM, regulate growth of pluripotential and immature progenitor cells: these high-level mitogenic hormones are not lineage specific and possess broad and pervasive powers over the rates of self-renewal, proliferation, and differentiation. G-CSF, M-CSF, and erythropoietin (EP, Ep, or Epo) are lower-echelon factors of lesser scope: they act on more mature progenitors, motivating them to differentiate and become functional. The complex synergies characterizing the CSF hierarchy are portrayed simplistically in Figure 1-8.

Erythropoietin

Erythropoietin (EP) is the erythroid colony stimulating factor responsible for the feedback regulation of erythropoiesis. EP is a highly glycosylated hormone (M_r: about 34,000) synthesized by peritubular endothelial cells of the kidney [15] in response to an ill-defined renal mechanism (probably involving a heme protein) that senses tissue hypoxia (Figure 1-9). EP

TABLE 1-1

Myeloid CSFs

Factor (Synonym)	Chromosomal location	mRNA size (kb)	Protein size ($M_r \times 10^3$)	Cellular sources	Target cells	Cell types found in colonies
G-CSF	17q	2.0	18–22	Monocytes, fibroblasts	CFU-G	Neutrophils
GM-CSF	5q	1.0	14–35	T cells, endothelial cells, fibroblasts, macrophages	CFU-GM, BFU-GM, CFU-MIX, CFU-E$_0$, CFU-Meg	Neutrophils, monocytes, macrophages, eosinophils, red cells, megakaryocytes
IL-3 (multi-CSF)	5q	1.0	14–28	T cells	CFU-MIX, BFU-E, CFU-GM, CFU-G, CFU-M, CFU-E$_0$, CFU-Meg	Neutrophils, monocytes, macrophages, eosinophils, basophils, monocytes, red cells, megakaryocytes
M-CSF (CSF-1)	5q	4.0, 1.8	35–45 ($\times 2$), 18–26 ($\times 2$)	Macrophages, endothelial cells	CFU-M	Monocytes, macrophages

Source: Amended from Clark SC and Kamen R: The human hematopoietic colony-stimulating factors. Science 236:1229,1987 and Nathan DG and Sieff CA: The biological activities and uses of recombinant granulocyte-macrophage and multi-colony stimulating factors. Prog Hematol 15:1,1987.

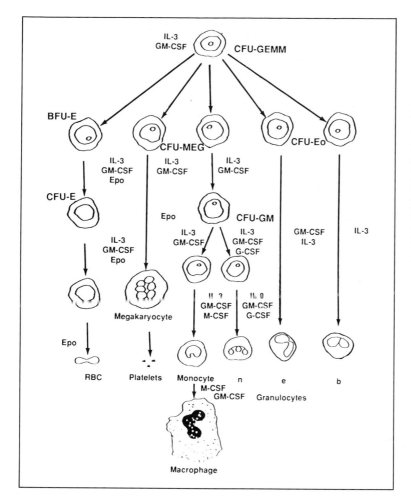

FIGURE 1-8

Lineage diagram show-
ing the overlapping and
collusive activities of
myeloid and erythroid
growth factors. Note
the pervasive participa-
tion of IL-3. Most acro-
nyms and abbreviations
are defined in the text.
The others are as fol-
lows: n, neutrophil; e,
eosinophil; and b,
basophil. (From Clark
SC and Kamen R: The
human hematopoietic
colony-stimulating fac-
tors. Science 236:
1229,1987. Copyright
1987 by the AAAS.)

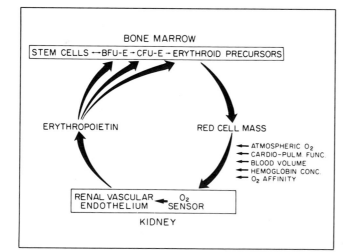

FIGURE 1-9

Feedback circuit regulating
erythropoiesis. Hypoxia stimulates
renal vascular synthesis of EP, molecules of which upregulate and then
bind to receptors on erythroid cells
and their precursors. The resultant
acceleration of erythropoiesis ceases
when normal O_2 transport is restored; EP production then declines
and receptors are down-modulated.
Continual servo regulation is responsible for the constancy of red cell
concentrations in the blood stream.
(Modified from Erslev AJ and
Gabuzda TG: Pathophysiology of
Blood, 3rd ed. Philadelphia, WB
Saunders,1985.)

mRNA in renal vascular cells is encoded by a 5-exon gene that has been localized to chromosome 7q11-22.

Recombinant EP binds to receptors on the surfaces of CFU-Es (and of their precursors, the BFU-Es) while these are resting in the G_1 phase of cell cycle, spurring immature erythroid elements to complete their maturation to erythroblasts and to inaugurate the highly amplifying succession of maturation-divisions depicted in Figure 1-3. There exists a continuum of erythroid precursors varying in their degree of commitment and sensitivity to EP. As the precursive cells that comprise BFU-Es mature to form CFU-Es they become increasingly responsive to EP, a sensitivity that accounts for the remarkable stability of red cell homeostasis. During episodes of severe hypoxic stress, unusually high levels of EP are secreted by renal endothelium, accounting for the explosive growth of BFU-Es; under extreme duress, a subset of those burst-forming progenitors grow in response to microvesicular bombardment by macrophages, a backup mechanism of erythroid excitation known as burst-promoting activity (BPA). Ordinarily, however, erythropoiesis adjusts to demand more smoothly through the growth factor-receptor-transducer signal sequence common to proliferating cellular societies.

Lymphokines

Lymphocytes are responsible for immunity (Chapter 12). The difficult task of controlling these excitable cells is made possible through a bewildering network of regulatory proteins known as lymphokines. Lymphokines are intercellular (hormonal) signals that adjust cell proliferations and functions during the upheavals provoked by immune or inflammatory reactions. The term "lymphokine" understates the catholicity of these proteins, for lymphokines are produced throughout the body and control cooperative interactions involving many cell lines. Among the major lymphokines are interleukins, interferons, tumor necrosis factors, and transforming growth factors (Table 1-2) [16, 17, 18]. Unlike antigens, which only trigger activation of selected T cells and B cells bearing specific receptors in the form of T cell antigen receptors and surface immunoglobulin (sIg), lymphokines function to amplify or suppress the response to antigen in a nonspecific or generic fashion.

Interleukin 1 and tumor necrosis factors   The 18,000 M_r interleukin, IL-1, is produced by macrophages, activated lymphocytes, and vascular cells, in response to antigens, toxins, injury, and inflammation. IL-1 is a multifunctional mediator of acute phase responses and commands the familiar set of reactions characteristic of inflammation: fever, slow-wave sleep, neutrophilia, and activation of T cells and other macrophages. IL-1 has influence in high places. In the presence of M-CSF, IL-1 stimulates multipotential stem cells to propagate colonies that manufacture mature macrophages [1]. Working in league with tumor necrosis factor (TNF), IL-1 also stimulates vascular endothelium to release GM-CSF and G-CSF [19]. Indeed, IL-1 and tumor necrosis factor alpha (TNFα), alias cachectin, act synergistically in causing tumor necrosis, fibrosis, the local Shwartzman reaction, and hypotension [20]. Although both TNFα and TNFβ (lymphotoxin) are members of a family of proteins that activate neutrophils and cause hemorrhagic necrosis of certain tumors, an activity simulated by recombinant TNFs, recombinant IL-1 alone does not induce tumor necrosis in vivo. When prompted by receptor-motivated macrophages, secretion of IL-1 and TNF engenders a gentler collaboration in ridding the body of advanced glycosylated end product proteins (dubbed "AGE proteins"); even this housekeeping activity has its risks, however, for reaction in the vasculature may progress to fibrosis and atherosclerotic degeneration.

Interleukin 2   Interleukin 2 (IL-2) is a 15,000 M_r protein dimer encoded by a locus on chromosome 4q and produced by activated T cells. Mitosis of T cells depends upon interaction of IL-2 with high-affinity membrane receptors, 55,000 M_r proteins formerly called Tac antigens. IL-2 receptors are absent on resting T cells, but within hours of antigenic activation IL-2 itself upregulates expression of these receptors. Hence, the IL-2 T cell system, which gives rise to clonal expansion of T cells and induces the synthesis of IL-1, represents an autocrine growth cycle self-governed in its progression by the IL-2 concentration, IL-2 receptor density, and the duration of IL-2 production.

TABLE 1-2

Biologic properties of human lymphokines

Name	Principal aliases	Function
Interleukin 1 (alpha and beta)	Lymphocyte activating factor (LAF)	Activates resting T cells; is cofactor for hematopoietic growth factors; induces fever, sleep, ACTH release, neutrophilia, and other systemic acute-phase responses; stimulates synthesis of lymphokines, collagen, and collagenases; activates endothelial cells and macrophages; mediates inflammation, catabolic processes, and nonspecific resistance to infection
Interleukin 2	T cell growth factor (TCGF)	Is growth factor for activated T cells expressing IL-2 receptors; induces synthesis of other lymphokines; activates cytotoxic T cells, natural killer cells, and activated B cells
Interleukin 3	Multi-CSF	Supports the growth of multipotent marrow stem cells; is growth factor for mast cells
Interleukin 4	B cell growth factor 1 (BCGF-1) and B cell stimulating factor 1 (BCSF-1)	Is growth factor for activated B cells; induces DR antigen expression on B cells; is also growth factor for resting T cells and enhances cytolytic activity of cytotoxic T cells; is mast cell growth factor
Interleukin 5	B cell growth factor 2 (BCGF-2) and B cell differentiation factor (BCDF)	Induces the differentiation of activated B cells into immunoglobulin-secreting plasma cells; is also eosinophil differentiation factor
Interleukin 6	B cell stimulating factor 2 (BCSF-2) and β_2 interferon	Enhances immunoglobulin secretion by B cells; acts in synergy with IL-3 to trigger multipotent stem cells into cell cycle; second signal in T cell activation; inhibits fibroblast growth
Interleukin 7	Lymphopoietin 1	Stimulates growth and maturation of primitive (pre B) B cells
Interleukin 8	Neutrophil activating peptide 1 (NAP-1)	Stimulates neutrophils to move directionally (chemotaxis), express surface adhesion molecules, and produce reactive O_2 metabolites
Gamma interferon	INFγ	Induces Class I, Class II (DR), and other surface antigens on a variety of cells; activates macrophages and endothelial cells; augments or inhibits other lymphokine activities; augments natural killer cell activity; exerts antiviral activity
Alpha interferon	INFα	Exerts antiviral activity; induces Class I antigen expression; augments natural killer cell activity; has fever-inducing and antiproliferative properties
Tumor necrosis factor alpha	TNFα and cachectin	Is direct cytotoxin for some tumor cells; induces fever, sleep, and other systemic acute-phase responses; stimulates the synthesis of lymphokines, collagen, and collagenases; activates endothelial and macrophagic cells; mediates inflammation, catabolic processes, and septic shock
Transforming growth factors (alpha and beta)	TGFα and TGFβ	TGFβ_2 causes immunosuppression by inhibiting the proliferation of T cells exposed to activating agents such as interleukin 2

Source: From Dinarello CA and Mier JW: Lymphokines. N Engl J Med 317:940,1987; Massague J: The TGF-β family of growth and differentiation factors. Cell 49:437,1987; and Baggiolini M et al: Neutrophil-activating peptide-1/interleukin 8, a novel cytokine that activates neutrophils. J Clin Invest 84:1045,1989.

Withdrawal or elimination of the activating antigen leads to involution of IL-2 receptors and cessation of further T cell proliferation. Recombinant IL-2 spurs the cytolytic activity of receptor-armed natural killer cells, a property that has therapeutic use in shrinking certain solid tumors.

Interleukin 4   Interleukin 4 (IL-4) is a 20,000 M_r glycoprotein secreted by activated T cells. IL-4 binds with high affinity ($K = 2 \times 10^{10}$ M^{-1}) to receptors on most hematopoietic cells and is particularly important as a growth factor for B cells. IL-4 also collaborates with IL-3 in driving mast cell division and can act as an alternative to IL-3 in cooperating with EP to foment growth of BFU-Es [21].

Interferons   Interferons were first recognized by their ability to interfere with viral replication in infected cells. Alpha (leukocyte) interferon, beta (fibroblast) interferon, and gamma (immune) interferon are structurally related glycoproteins having antiviral, immunoregulatory, and antiproliferative functions. Gamma interferon (IFNγ or γIFN) induces class I and class II histocompatibility molecules and is a

potent activator of macrophages. Activation by this lymphokine is mediated by specific receptors on macrophage membranes, and receptor occupancy is a prerequisite for induction of full-throttle tumoricidal and microbicidal activity, as well as for HLA-DR antigen display. Gamma interferon acts in concert with interleukins 4 and 5 in compelling proliferating B cells to transform into antibody-secreting plasma cells.

The busy network of intercellular signals conveyed by lymphokines is depicted cartoon-fashion in Figure 1-10.

Transforming growth factors   Transforming growth factors (TGFs) are a heterogeneous family of polypeptides that induce anchorage-independent growth in otherwise anchorage-dependent cells. TGFα competes with epidermal growth factor (EGF) for binding to the same receptors in longterm marrow cultures and shares with EGF the capacity to stimulate growth of multinucleated osteoclasts. The prototype of the TGF family is TGFβ, a 25,000 M_r homodimer that actually inhibits hematopoiesis and adipogenesis by forcing immature cells to differentiate. $TGF\beta_1$ causes mesenchymal cells

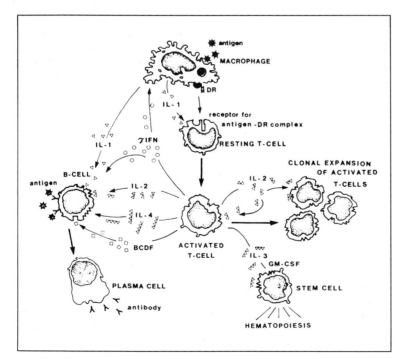

FIGURE 1-10

Intercellular signals transmitted by soluble lymphokines (white triangles, circles, and boxes) in response to challenge by antigen. Antigens (black burrs) are ingested by a macrophage and, after processing (black circle), are presented to a T cell possessing receptors for both antigen and a matching histocompatibility (DR) antigen. This activates the T cell which, among other things, prods a B cell exposed to the same antigens to differentiate and produce antibody. (From Dinarello CA and Mier JW: Lymphokines. Reprinted, by permission of the New England Journal of Medicine, 317:940,1987.)

to cease proliferating and instead to express fibronectin, collagen, proteoglycans, and other adhesive molecules essential to cell movement and morphogenesis [17]. The TGFβ_2 variant inhibits the proliferative response of T cells to IL-2, thus dampening immune responsiveness.

Oncogene-Encoded Growth Factors: A Faustian Compact

Cellular oncogenes (proto-oncogenes or c-oncogenes) are components of the normal genome. They are critical to regulation of gene expression, cell division, and differentiation. Human c-oncogenes are homologous to viral oncogenes (v-oncogenes) found in animal RNA tumor viruses; in cell culture systems, v-oncogenes are capable of transforming eukaryotic cells from benign to malignant phenotype. When moved out of position in vivo, especially if placed falsely in proximity to structural gene coding regions during chromosomal translocation, oncogenes can cause proliferative mistakes eventuating in cancer. This errant behavior has earned oncogenes undeserved notoriety; that oncogenes have been highly conserved in vertebrate evolution signifies that their importance in normal cell growth outweighs the risk of malfunction. Nevertheless, employment of proto-oncogenes as growth factors requires their supervision by allelic tumor-suppressing genes called anti-oncogenes (Chapter 13).

Many Oncogenes Code for Growth Factors or Growth Factor Receptors

Some of the 40 known oncogenes code directly for growth factors: an example of this is the c-sis oncogene located on the long (q) arm of chromosome 22. The c-sis encoded protein, the β chain of platelet-derived growth factor (PDGF), is the cellular homolog of p28 v-sis, the retroviral transforming protein product of simian sarcoma virus (SSV). PDGF, a 30,000 M_r peptide, binds with high affinity to specific surface receptors on cells of mesenchymal origin, thereby activating the receptor's tyrosine kinase domains. This causes phosphorylation of the receptor itself as well as of other cellular substrates. Hence PDGF binding provides both autocrine and paracrine growth stimulation by acting as a potent mitogen for immature

fibroblasts, endothelium, smooth muscle cells, monocytes, and neutrophils, the agents of acute inflammation. PDGF and other growth factor peptides also elicit receptor-mediated activation of mature white blood cells, exciting monocytes and neutrophils to move (chemotaxis) and to disgorge cytocidal free radicals such as the superoxide anion [22].

Several oncogenes encode the receptors for growth factors; without receptors all growth factors would ineffectually bounce off cell membranes. The oncogene erb B encodes the receptors for epidermal growth factor (EGF), and c-fms encodes high-affinity macrophage receptors. In a tidy arrangement stipulated by neighboring genes on the q arm of chromosome 5, M-CSF produced by marrow stromal cells ligates to macrophage receptors encoded by c-fms. Most oncogenes, including c-fms, possess either tyrosine kinase or threonine (or serine) kinase activity: receptor occupancy acts as a first messenger by phosphorylating the receptor, activating it to transmit signals to the cell interior. Certain membrane-bound oncogene products, such as ras proteins, activate the guanosine triphosphate–binding G protein (GTP) transduction pathway by which extracellular signals are transmitted to target enzymes. Several other c-oncogene products appear to bind directly to specific regions on DNA, promoting transcription of growth factors. The identities and properties of oncogenes and their products are only partially understood. The best-known are listed in Table 1-3 [23].

Growth Factors and Receptors: Yang and Yin

The recurring theme of organized cell growth is that growth factors and other hormones exert their effect on target cells by binding to receptors: it is the occupied receptors that induce nuclear and cytoplasmic activation. Stimuli for hematopoietic cell growth or growth inhibition come from outside the cell. Growth factors can arouse attention only if their messages are received. This crucial role is played by membrane-spanning proteins which undergo deformation when the external receptor portion binds to the growth-affecting ligand. The allosteric reaction to external ligand occupancy is activation of the enzymatic

TABLE 1-3

Functional properties of retrovirus-associated oncogene products

Oncogene	Cellular location	Chromosome location	Protein product	Function of protein
abl	Plasma membrane	9q34	p150	Tyrosine kinase
erb A	. . .	17q21–22	. . .	Thyroid hormone receptor
erb B	Plasma membrane	7p11–13	EGF receptor	Binding of epidermal growth factor
ets-1	. . .	11q23–24	. . .	. . .
fes/fps	Cytoplasm; plasma membrane	15q25	p92/p98	Tyrosine kinase
fgr	. . .	. . .	. . .	Tyrosine kinase
fms	Plasma membrane	5q32	CSF-M receptor	Binding of CSF-M
fos	Nucleus	14q21–31	p55	. . .
mos	Cytoplasm	8q22	. . .	Threonine kinase
myb	Nucleus	6q22–24	p75	DNA binding, transcriptional activation
myc	Nucleus	8q24	p58	DNA binding, transcriptional activation
raf/mil	Cytoplasm	3p25	. . .	Threonine kinase
H-*ras/bas*	Plasma membrane	11p14–15	p21	Threonine kinase; GTP-GDP binding*
K-*ras-1*	Plasma membrane	6p11/12	p21	Threonine kinase; GTP-GDP binding*
K-*ras-2*	Plasma membrane	12p12	. . .	Threonine kinase; GTP-GDP binding*
N-*ras*	. . .	1p11–13	. . .	Threonine kinase; GTP-GDP binding*

Oncogene	Cellular location	Chromosome location	Protein product	Function of protein
rel	. . .	2p	. . .	. . .
ros	Cytoplasm; plasma membrane	6q16–22	. . .	Tyrosine kinase
sis	Cytoplasm	22q13	PDGF β chain	Mesenchymal growth factor
src-1	Plasma membrane	20q12–13	pp60	Tyrosine kinase
src-2	Plasma membrane	1p34–36	pp60	Tyrosine kinase
yes	. . .	18q21	. . .	Tyrosine kinase

*Guanosine triphosphate; guanosine diphosphate.

Source: With amendments, from Woloschak GE: Association of oncogene activity and hematologic malignancy. Curr Hematol Oncol 5:171,1987.

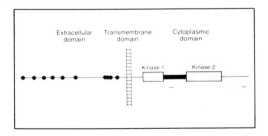

FIGURE 1-11

Representation of PDGF receptor domains. Black circles indicate cysteine residues, which when paired off by disulfide bonding form five looped immunoglobulinlike domains; the thick black line denotes a 107–amino acid inserted sequence that separates two tyrosine kinase domains. (From Williams LT: The stimulation of paracrine and autocrine mitogenic pathways by the platelet-derived growth factor receptor. J Cell Physiol [Suppl] 5:27,1987.)

kinase domain or domains located at the interior end of the receptor molecule (Figure 1-11) [24].

Signal Transduction: G Proteins and Protein Kinase C

In most blood cells, hormone occupancy stimulates surface receptors to initiate signals that are transmitted to target enzymes (effectors) via guanyl nucleotide–binding G proteins. Allosteric changes induced in integral membrane receptors activate G proteins bound to the cytosolic face of the cell membrane. All G proteins have a common design. They consist of three unlike polypeptides: a guanyl nucleotide–binding α chain plus a β and γ chain. G proteins cycle between an inactive G·GDP complex that is bound to the membrane and an active effector state in which the Gα·GTP subunit is released from the β and γ chains to react with its target enzyme or ion channel. The role of the G$\beta\gamma$ part of the complex is to present Gα·GDP to the activated receptor for phosphorylation back to G·GTP by receptor kinase action, demonstrating the intrinsic GTPase activity of the reaction cycle [25].

The object of signal transduction by GTP-binding G proteins is to launch the phosphoinositol cascade, a sequence of reactions eventuating in activation of the intracellular regulator, protein kinase C. Hydrolysis of phosphatidylinositol 4,5-biphosphate (Pi-P$_2$, or PIP$_2$) by a specific membrane-bound phosphodiesterase—phospholipase C, alias phosphoinositide phosphodiesterase (PPDE)—generates two intracellular second messenger molecules, diacylglycerol (DG or DAG) and inositol 1,4,5-triphosphate (IP$_3$). DG activates protein kinase C, and IP$_3$ triggers release of intracellular Ca^{2+} into the cytosol. The rational but intricate transduction pathway by which receptor binding of growth factors generates cellular responses is depicted schematically in Figure 1-12 [26].

Protein kinase C   Protein kinase C is a multifunctional 80,000 M_r phosphoprotein that is specific for phosphorylation of tyrosine, serine, and threonine residues. Activity of this normally inert oncogenelike molecule is dependent on both Ca^{2+} and phospholipid; the affinity for these activators is heightened critically by DG, which regulates this growth-promoting

enzyme [27, 28]. Protein kinase C appears to be the effector enzyme that is activated when certain oncogene growth products bind to appropriate receptors. The entire cast of participants involved in the response to the oncogene encoded protein PDGF is reprised schematically in Figure 1-13 [29].

Growth responses require good timing   The ultimate intent of effector enzymes such as protein kinase C and of other growth factors including nucleophilic oncogenes is to activate genes which then produce mRNAs and proteins that are required for cellular escape from quiescence and for entry into the S phase of cell cycle (Chapter 2). Commitment to cell growth is dependent upon two yes/no switches. The first switch makes the decision between quiescence (G$_0$ or G$_1$ phase of cell cycle) and proliferative competence under the influence of factors such as PDGF. Under the spell of other factors such as EGF or TGFβ, cells will either progress toward DNA synthesis or become dormant. This second switching decision is made at the restriction point terminating G$_1$ phase, occurring about 2 hours before onset of DNA synthesis. After this magic moment, cells are no longer influenced by growth factors. The general relationship between growth factor stimulation and cell cycling (proliferation) is diagrammed in Figure 1-14 [30].

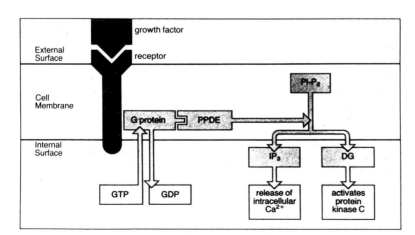

FIGURE 1-12

Pathway by which the signal generated by binding of growth factor to receptor is transduced, resulting in release of two second messengers: IP$_3$ and diacylglycerol (DG). (From Hoffbrand AV and Pettit JE: Clinical Hematology Illustrated. An Integrated Text and Color Atlas. Philadelphia, WB Saunders Company, 1987.)

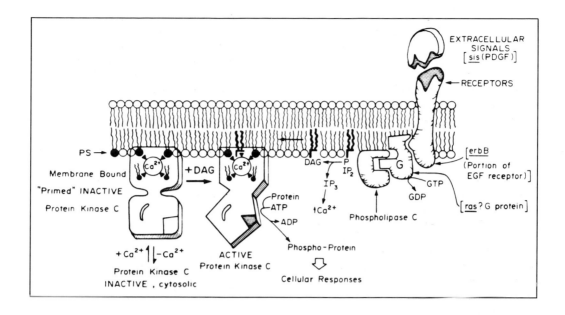

FIGURE 1-13

Mechanism of protein kinase C activation by second messengers generated in response to binding of PDGF to its receptor. (DAG = DG.) (From Bell RM: Protein kinase C activation by diacylglycerol second messengers. Cell 45:631,1986. © Cell Press.)

MARROW ORGANIZATION AND FUNCTION

Ontogeny and Cellularity

In the initial month or two of fetal life the first, pioneering hematopoietic stem cells arise from the mesoderm of the yolk sac. From the second to the seventh month of life the liver is the primary blood-forming organ, but as bone cavities develop during the fifth fetal month,

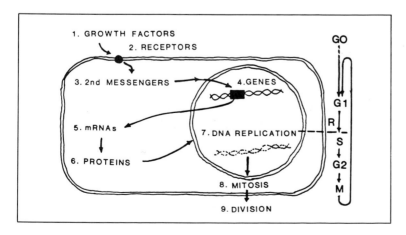

FIGURE 1-14

Major events of cell proliferation as related to phases of the cell cycle. (R represents point at which responsiveness to growth factor stimulation is restricted.) (From Pardee AB: The yang and yin of cell proliferation: an overview. J Cell Physiol [Suppl] 5:107,1987.)

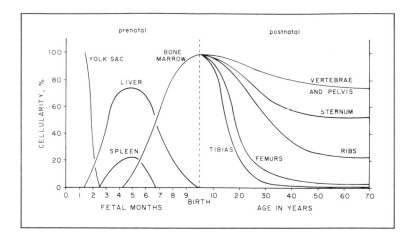

FIGURE 1-15

Shifts in deployment of
hematopoietic tissue be-
fore and after birth. Following birth over 90%
of hematopoiesis is
maintained by marrow
of the central skeleton.
(Modified from Erslev
AJ and Gabuzda TG:
Pathophysiology of
Blood, 3rd ed. Philadel-
phia, WB Saunders
Company,1985.)

multipotential stem cells migrate to colonize
permanently the sheltered colony-forming environment provided by marrow stroma. In people the hematopoietic hospitality of marrow is
so superior to that of other sinusoidal tissues
that only medullary invasion or cruel demands
on marrow productivity cause stem cells to
seek lodgings in the liver or spleen. During
childhood, as growth of bone cavities outstrips
the housing requirements of blood-forming
cells, fatty replacement of unoccupied marrow
space commences, beginning in the peripheral
diaphyses of long bones, and slowly creeping
centripetally until the majority of centrifugal
space is filled with adipose. Deployment of
marrow parenchyma is largely consummated
by early adulthood (Figure 1-15).

In the steady state, the adult skeleton houses
about 600 g of hematopoietic marrow, over
70% of which is located in the pelvis, vertebrae, and sternum—sites readily accessible for
sampling by means of needle aspiration or
biopsy. Quantitative distribution and volume
of erythropoietic marrow can be assessed
noninvasively by radionuclide imaging (Figure
1-16). Direct examination of marrow cellularity is perforce invasive. Spread films of
marrow aspirates stained with Wright-Giemsa
are most suitable for determining cytologic
detail and the proportion of myeloid to
erythroid elements (the M:E ratio). In core
samples secured by needle or trephine biopsies
the compact cell populations are less amenable
to refined scrutiny, but the specimens are
geographically intact, enabling evaluation of

FIGURE 1-16

Radionuclide imaging of erythropoietic marrow
in a normal adult, as revealed by ^{52}Fe and a
positron camera. Most radioiron is localized in
the centroidal marrow, with traces of uptake in
the proximal heads of long bones and some
"spillage" of the isotope into macrophages
(Kupffer cells) of the liver. (From Fordham EW
and Amjad A: Radionuclide imaging of bone
marrow. Semin Hematol 18:222,1981.)

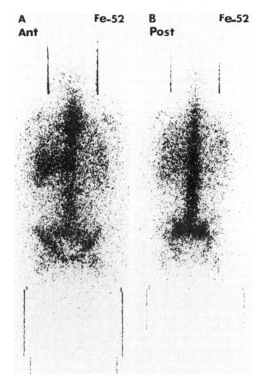

marrow cellularity and architecture. Values for normal differential cell counts of marrow aspirates are given in Table 1-4.

Marrow Histology

Examined by routine histologic means, or even by scanning electron microscopy (SEM), marrow appears at first glance to be a disorderly farrago lacking compartmental design (Figure 1-17). Rigorous three-dimensional mapping of marrow structures has revealed blood cells to be arranged in colonial compartments, packed so tightly against the spokelike collecting veins that neighboring cells become faceted from mutual compression. Retention of morular clusters of dividing blood cells is partly accomplished by simple physical factors. The marrow sinus wall has three layers: a simple luminal monolayer of endothelium; a discontinuous basement membrane riddled with perforations; and an outer (adventitial)

TABLE 1-4

Differential counts of marrow aspirates from 20 normal adults

Cell type	Mean (%)	Range (%)
Neutrophil series	56.0	45.1–66.5
Myeloblasts	1.0	0.5–1.8
Promyelocytes	3.4	2.6–4.6
Myelocytes	11.9	8.1–16.9
Metamyelocytes	18.0	9.8–25.3
Band forms	11.0	8.5–20.8
Segmented forms	10.7	8.0–16.0
Eosinophil series	3.2	1.2–6.2
Myelocytes	0.9	0.3–1.9
Metamyelocytes	1.4	0.5–2.3
Band forms	1.0	0.3–2.7
Segmented forms	0.9	1.1–1.7
Basophil series	<0.1	0.0–0.2
Erythroid series	21.5	14.2–30.4
Proerythroblasts	0.6	0.2–1.4
Basophilic erythroblasts	2.0	0.7–3.7
Polychromatophilic erythroblasts	12.4	12.2–24.2
Orthochromatic erythroblasts	6.5	2.0–22.7
Lymphocytes	15.8	10.8–22.7
Monocytes	1.8	0.2–2.8
Plasma cells	1.8	0.2–2.2
Macrophages (reticular cells)	0.3	0.0–0.5
Megakaryocytes	<0.1	0.0–0.2

Source: From Jandl JH: Chapt 1, in Blood: Textbook of Hematology. Boston, Little, Brown and Company, 1987.

FIGURE 1-17

SEM of the cut surfaces of marrow, showing spongy clusters of hematopoietic cells crowding around a drainage system of vascular sinuses. The collecting sinuses form a confluent fernlike pattern of tributaries originating at the periphery of the parenchyma (below) and emptying into a large vein (upper right). Apertures in the wall of the large vein represent other sinus outlets. (From Weiss L: The hematopoietic microenvironment of the bone marrow: an ultrastructural study of the stroma in rats. Anat Rec 186:161,1976.)

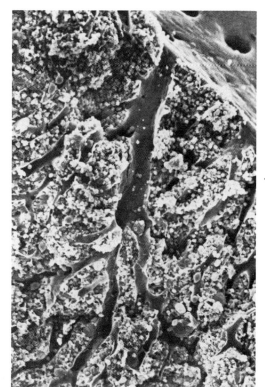

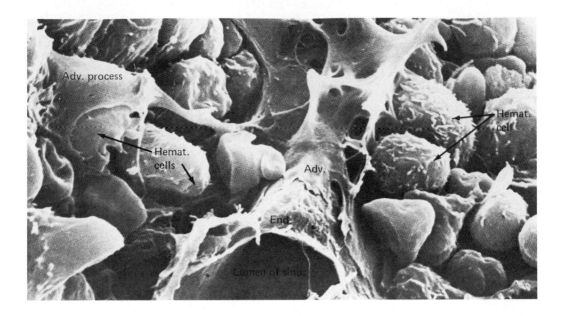

FIGURE 1-18

SEM view of a vascular sinus, with its discharging lumen (below) open to the viewer. Sinus endothelium (End.) is clothed by reticular cells in adventitial (Adv.) position. On the left an elaborate flattened reticular cell embraces hematopoietic cells (Hemat. cells) and insinuates complex processes deeply into surrounding parenchyma. On the right, two ruffled young granulocytes (Hemat. cell) appear to be attempting an escape. Most unlabeled cells are red cells. (From Weiss L: The hematopoietic microenvironment of the bone marrow: an ultrastructural study of the stroma in rats. Anat Rec 186:161,1976.)

layer of specialized sinus macrophages (reticular cells). Elaborate arborizing projections and fibrils from the reticular cells (macrophages) divide and subdivide the cordal compartments into hospitable chambers that temporarily imprison and segregate colonies of differentiating cells (Figure 1-18).

Colonies of dividing and maturing blood cells are not distributed randomly through the "red marrow" of the central skeleton. Lymphocytes lie in compact clusters surrounding small radial arteries that eventually feed into the sinuses. Granulocyte precursors are situated deep in the axial marrow parenchyma and do not emigrate toward effluent sinuses until they mature to a stage as metamyelocytes when they acquire the motor and sensory capability to crawl toward gaps in the sinus wall. Sinus lining endothelium is not tightly knit and is sufficiently lax to part as the agile, deformable mature granulocytes worm their way through or between endothelial shingles. Islands of erythroblasts form in close proximity to the abluminal sinus wall. Through a marvel of evolved expertise, late erythroblasts are empowered to expel their spent pyknotic nucleus, subtracting thereby one-third of the cell weight, and freeing up the anucleate red cell for release and service as an O_2 transport vehicle. The terminal "asymmetric division" responsible for the Venuslike birth of naked red cells is shown in Figure 1-19. Reticulocytes relieved of nuclei slip away from their adhesive moorings and bore their way through thinned-out patches of overlying endothelium. Megakaryocytes bind tightly to the adventitial surfaces of vascular sinuses, pressing their vast bellies over endothelial apertures. Megakaryocytes are sessile residents of marrow, too large to circulate; to avoid the dimensional hazards of cell division, they multiply their complement of DNA by endoreduplication (endomitosis).

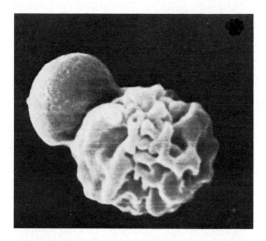

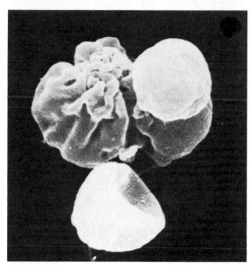

FIGURE 1-19

Nuclear extrusion by erythroblasts. (Above) A mature (late) erythroblast displaying coarse gyri and sulci is in the act of expelling its thinly cloaked, pyknotic nucleus. (Below) An erythroblast engaged in denucleation is seen adjacent to a recently denucleated, cup-shaped reticulocyte. (From Tsai S et al: Differential binding of erythroid and myeloid progenitors to fibroblasts and fibronectin. Blood 69:1587,1987.)

When the cytoplasm of these multilobate (not multinucleate) monsters is demarcated and partitioned into platelet territories, the ripened cell abruptly reels out streamers of entrained platelets directly into the sinus.

For each blood cell line release of mature cells across the marrow:blood barrier requires peculiar physical mechanisms, including changes in blood cell size, deformability, stretch, and locomotor capability. The exquisite control regulating cell release by marrow cannot be explained by changes in mechanical compliance alone. Release of matured cells from their tender traps in the marrow is governed by refined adjustments in the adhesion between cells and matrix.

Adhesive Proteins and Timely Release of Mature Blood Cells from Marrow

Attachment to stromal cells and the reticular matrix is important for retention of immature blood cells and their progenitors and is a requirement for their maturation and development. Attachment to extracellular matrices is mediated by a family of adhesive proteins which act as biological organizers by holding cells in position and guiding their migration. The principal adhesive proteins are fibronectin, vitronectin, collagen, thrombospondin, fibrinogen, and von Willebrand factor. Each of these fibrillar molecules possesses a recognition site containing the tripeptide arginine-glycine-aspartic acid (RGD), and some have in addition a serine residue. These sites are recognized by specific membrane-spanning receptors in parenchymal cells such as immature blood cells and platelets [31, 32]. The prototype adhesive molecule is fibronectin, an elongated dimer $(M_r: 250,000 \times 2)$ that is 2 to 3 nm thick and 60 to 70 nm long. This multifunctional molecular organizer is subdivided into a train of tightly folded domains containing numerous repeating structures. The Arg-Gly-Asp-Ser repeat distinguishes the cell binding domain from domains recognized by sites on collagen, fibrin, and heparin. When fibronectin of matrix and fibronectin receptors of blood cells are in full display, the blood cells are anchored to the marrow. When receptors for adhesive molecules are partially downregulated, the level of surface stickiness is intermediate, providing the possibility of traction and accordingly subserving locomotion. Receptor expression of granulocytes is regulated by the level of GM-CSF: if upregulated, the cells are

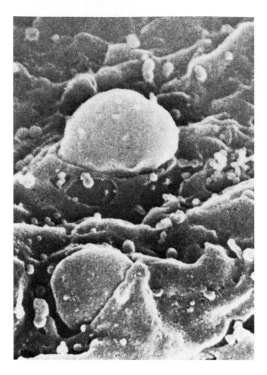

FIGURE 1-20

SEM view of the luminal surface of a marrow sinus showing two blood cells beginning to surface, prepared for circulation. (From Weiss L and Chen L-T: The organization of hematopoietic cords and vascular sinuses in bone marrow. Blood Cells 1:617,1975.)

immobilized by leukocyte adhesion molecules; if downregulated, cells are capable of movement [33]. Primitive erythroid stem cells such as BFU-Es are glued to the matrix latticework by fibronectin-receptor bonding. As the full sequence of maturation-division progresses, erythroid progenitors gradually differentiate: as they do so, they lose affinity for fibronectin and are set free to traverse the endothelial layer and then to circulate [34, 35]. The emergence of nonadherent blood cells through endothelium (Figure 1-20) is the start of their long trek through the bloodstream.

REFERENCES

1. Dexter TM: Stem cells in normal growth and disease. Br Med J 295:1192,1987

2. Sieff CA: Membrane antigen expression during hemopoietic differentiation. CRC Crit Rev Oncol Hematol 5:1,1986

3. Ogawa M et al: Renewal and commitment to differentiation of hemopoietic stem cells (an interpretive review). Blood 61:832,1983

4. Leary AG and Ogawa M: Blast cell colony assay for umbilical cord blood and adult bone marrow progenitors. Blood 69:953,1987

5. Messner HA: Human stem cells in culture. Clin Haematol 13:393,1984

6. Ploemacher RE and Brons HC: Isolation of hemopoietic stem cell subsets from murine bone marrow: I. Radioprotective ability of purified cell suspensions differing in the proportion of day-7 and day-12 CFU-S. Exp Hematol 16:21,1988

7. Gorin NC: Collection, manipulation and freezing of haemopoietic stem cells. Clin Haematol 16:19,1986

8. Nakahata T et al: Single-cell origin of human mixed hemopoietic colonies expressing various combinations of cell lineages. Blood 65:1010,1985

9. Lemischka IR et al: Developmental potential and dynamic behavior of hematopoietic stem cells. Cell 45:917,1986

10. Dexter MT et al: Haemopoietic stem cells and the problem of self-renewal. Blood Cells 10:315,1984

11. Eaves AC et al: Clinical significance of long-term cultures of myeloid blood cells. CRC Crit Rev Oncol Hematol 7:125,1987

12. Chervenick PA and Zucker-Franklin D: Chapt 2, in Atlas of Blood Cells. Function and Pathology, vol. 1, Zucker-Franklin D et al, Eds. Milan, Edi. Ermes s.r.l.,1981

13. Clark SC and Kamen R: The human hematopoietic colony-stimulating factors. Science 236:1229,1987

14. Nathan DG and Sieff CA: The biological activities and uses of recombinant granulocyte-macrophage and multi-colony stimulating factors. Prog Hematol 15:1,1987

15. Lacombe C et al: Peritubular cells are the site of erythropoietin synthesis in the murine hypoxic kidney. J Clin Invest 81:620,1988

16. Dinarello CA and Mier JW: Lymphokines. N Engl J Med 317:940,1987

17. Massague J: The TGF-β family of growth and differentiation factors. Cell 49:437,1987

18. Baggiolini M et al: Neutrophil-activating peptide-1/interleukin 8, a novel cytokine that activates neutrophils. J Clin Invest 84:1045, 1989

19. Zsebo KM et al: Vascular endothelial cells and granulopoiesis: interleukin-1 stimulates release of G-CSF and GM-CSF. Blood 71:99,1988

20. Vilcek J et al: Tumor necrosis factor: receptor binding and mitogenic action in fibroblasts. J Cell Physiol [Suppl] 5:57,1987

21. Paul WE: Interleukin 4/B cell stimulatory factor 1: one lymphokine, many functions. FASEB J 1:456,1987

22. Deuel TF: Platelet-derived growth factor/sis in normal and neoplastic cell growth. J Cell Physiol [Suppl] 5:95,1987

23. Woloschak GE: Association of oncogene activity and hematologic malignancy. Curr Hematol Oncol 5:171,1987

24. Williams LT: The stimulation of paracrine and autocrine mitogenic pathways by the platelet-derived growth factor receptor. J Cell Physiol [Suppl] 5:27,1987

25. Stryer L: G Proteins: A family of signal transducers. Annu Rev Cell Biol 2:391,1986

26. Hoffbrand AV and Pettit JE: Clinical Hematology Illustrated. An Integrated Text and Color Atlas. Philadelphia, WB Saunders Company,1987

27. Parker PJ and Ullrich A: Protein kinase C. J Cell Physiol [Suppl] 5:53,1987

28. Normura H et al: Inositol phospholipid turnover in stimulus-response coupling. Prog Hemost Thromb 8:143,1986

29. Bell RM: Protein kinase C activation by diacylglycerol second messengers. Cell 45: 631,1986

30. Pardee AB: The yang and yin of cell proliferation: an overview. J Cell Physiol [Suppl] 5:107,1987

31. Ruoslahti E and Pierschbacher MD: New perspectives in cell adhesion: RGD and integrins. Science 238:491,1987

32. Hynes RO: Fibronectins. Sci Am 254(6):42, 1986

33. Arnaout MA et al: Human recombinant granulocyte-macrophage colony-stimulating factor increases cell-to-cell adhesion and surface expression of adhesion-promoting surface glycoproteins on mature granulocytes. J Clin Invest 78:597,1986

34. Patel VP et al: Mammalian reticulocytes lose adhesion to fibronectin during maturation to erythrocytes. Proc Natl Acad Sci USA 82:440,1985

35. Tsai S et al: Differential binding of erythroid and myeloid progenitors to fibroblasts and fibronectin. Blood 69:1587,1987

2

Chromosomes, Cytogenetics, and the Kinetics of Malignancy

☐

To generate faithful copies of genomic DNA, all growing cells undergo a cell cycle. This consists of two periods: cell division, a conspicuous but brief process leading to separation of replicate daughter cells, and interphase, an understated but prolonged period during which all the elaborate preparations for cell replication are carried out. As survival of all cell lines comprising the organism is paramount, the 10^{14} cells making up the human body divide at different rates according to their different roles and destinies. Most committed stem cells and their dividing progeny are required to cycle continuously to offset suicidal maturation (Chapter 1). High-echelon stem cells (and some longlived subsets of lymphocytes and macrophages) repose for the most part out of cycle. Resting stem cells, denoted G_0, are actually in reserve status, preparing themselves for active duty if the marrow compartment requires expansion or replenishment. A third cadre of cells, such as mature granulocytes, have completed differentiation, are in the "postmitotic pool," and are not programmed to divide; in mature red cells all risk of returning to cycle is precluded by extrusion of the nuclear material.

THE GENERATIVE CYCLE

In cytokinetic jargon, proliferating cells are said to enter cell cycle, or the generative cycle, and dividing cells are characterized as "cycling cells." Dividing cells do not cycle in circles but undergo consecutive binary divisions ($\log_2$ growth). The duration of cell cycle varies among proliferating cell lines. During full-throttle replication under intense stimulation by growth factors, some cells divide every 8 to 12 h. During steady-state replacement of cells lost to attrition, division occurs every 16 to 24 h, the intermitotic intervals becoming less hurried (48 h) as level of differentiation increases.

Phases of Cell Cycle

Cycling cells pass through four major phases or periods (Figure 2-1) [1]. Interphase commences with the G_1 phase (G is for gap), during which metabolic and biosynthetic preparations are made for the S phase. Differences in cell cycle times are due mainly to variations in the duration of G_1. Cells unstimulated by cytokines repose in early G_1; those passing the restriction (R) point of cell cycle late in G_1 are compelled to complete the rest of the cycle and to divide.

S phase begins with synthesis of DNA and ends when the DNA content of the nucleus has doubled and each chromosome of the 23 pairs of chromosomes has been reduplicated into two identical spiral filaments called sister chromatids; in reduplication the diploid cell with a DNA complement of $2n$ is converted to a tetraploid cell with a complement of $4n$ (Figure 2-2) [2].

Cell Division

The two consecutive processes of cell division—nuclear division and cytoplasmic division—are conventionally conflated as mitosis. The purpose of mitosis is to bequeath to each of two daughter products of division an identical version of the DNA code. The nucleus of an average blood cell is about 10 μm across, but contains roughly 3 meters of double-stranded DNA [3]. This length of DNA is made of 3×10^9 nucleotide base pairs (bps), divided and packed into 23 pairs of chromosomes. Every chromosome represents a single long molecule of DNA, and the DNA content of each human chromosome varies between 10^8 and 3×10^8 base pairs. As such DNA molecules are between 5 and 10 cm long, the importance to mitosis of preparatory folding of chromosomes into small casettes and solenoids is fundamental to the packaging miracle culminating in mitosis.

Packing for Mitosis: Solenoids and Loops

The enormous length of DNA is prepacked during interphase and prevented from extending or snarling by several orders of binding to basic proteins called histones. The union of coils of DNA with basophilic histones creates the basic unit of nuclear chromatin known as the nucleosome. Artificially stretched-out

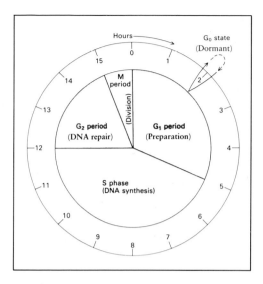

FIGURE 2-1

Cell cycle having a generation time of 16 h. During about 15 h of this cycle clock, the cell is preparing for division. The complex sequential processes of nuclear division (mitosis) and cytoplasmic division (cytokinesis) embodied in the M period are consummated within 1 h. The S, G_2, and M periods are constant: about 7 h, 3 h, and 1 h, respectively. The G_1 phase shown here is 5 h but may range from 2 h to many days. In the absence of growth promoters, cells become dormant (G_0 state). (Modified from Darnell J et al: Chapt 5, in Molecular Cell Biology. New York, Scientific American Books,1986.)

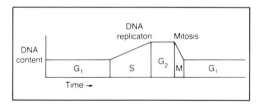

FIGURE 2-2

Sequences in the cell generative cycle. DNA doubling occurs only during the S phase. The cell then enters the postsynthetic G_2 phase during which imperfections in the duplicated DNA are remedied by repair enzymes and the newly formed DNA strands become coated with nuclear histones. The M phase begins when replicated chromosomes begin to thicken, the prelude to mitosis, and ends with overt cell division (cytokinesis). (From Weiss L: Chapt 1, in Histology. Cell and Tissue Biology, 5th ed., Weiss L, Ed. New York, Elsevier Science Publishing Co., Inc.,1983.)

nucleosomes can be seen by electron microscopy (EM) to be arranged as beads on a
string. Each nucleosome bead contains a set
(octamer) of eight nuclear histones, and each
bead is connected to the next by "linker
DNA." In interphase nuclei examined gently
the nucleosomes are found to be packed
together to form 30-nm-thick highly ordered
structures known as chromatin fibers. The
coiling up of DNA strands into beads and
then into beaded spools is made possible
because DNA winds around the disc-shaped
histone octamers, solenoid fashion, in an orderly cooperative sequence, with about 200
bps per nucleosome. The internal arrangement
of a solenoid is a chromatin fiber coiled into a
helix containing six nucleosomes per turn [1].
As chromatids prepare for metaphase, solenoids are organized further by forming giant
supercoiled loops. The sequential coiling by
which 5 or 10 cm of DNA is systematically
packed into chromosomes a few μm long is
rendered schematically in Figure 2-3.

The chromosome scaffold   The several meters
of DNA of each nucleus would become hope-
lessly entangled in a world-class Gordian knot
during the chromosomal movements of cell

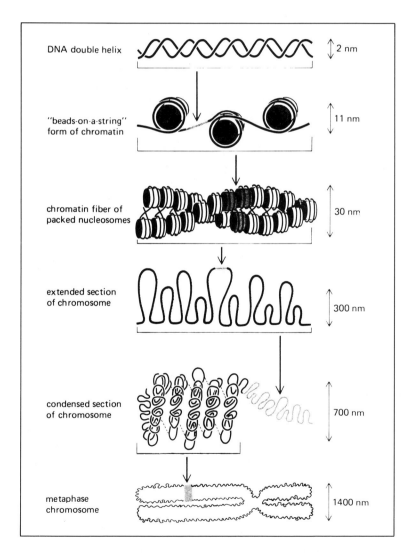

DNA double helix — 2 nm

"beads-on-a-string" form of chromatin — 11 nm

chromatin fiber of packed nucleosomes — 30 nm

extended section of chromosome — 300 nm

condensed section of chromosome — 700 nm

metaphase chromosome — 1400 nm

FIGURE 2-3

Schematic depiction of the many orders of chromatin packing postulated to yield the highly condensed metaphase chromosome. (From Alberts B et al: Chapt 8, in Molecular Biology of the Cell. New York, Garland Publishing Inc.,1983.)

(a)   (b)

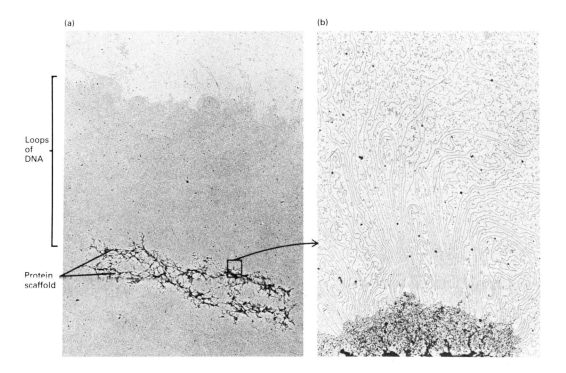

Loops
of
DNA

Protein
scaffold

FIGURE 2-4

EM of a histone-disrobed metaphase chromosome, exposing the underlying protein scaffold. (a) The heavy protein trelliswork, which confers an elongate shape to the chromosome and anchors its intricate, lacy loops of DNA. (b) The delicate but unsnarled arrangement of extended loops of DNA is revealed at higher power. (Adapted from Paulson JR and Laemmli UK: The structure of histone-depleted metaphase chromosomes. Cell 12:817,1977 by Darnell J et al: Chapt 10, in Molecular Cell Biology. New York, Scientific American Books,1986.)

cycling were it not for the network of anchoring proteins at the core of each individual chromosome. During metaphase the long looped domains of chromatin are attached to this scaffolding, forming plumed patterns of elegant order (Figure 2-4).

Mitosis

The complex machinery responsible for separating the original and replicated molecules of DNA is called the mitotic apparatus. This miraculously accurate movement of genetic material ensures that duplicated homologous pairs of chromosomes are separated from one another and distributed equitably between two nuclei. Despite all its baroque complexity, mitosis is consummated and the large tetraploid cell of G_2 is transformed into two identical diploid daughters within less than 1 h. Mitosis has been partitioned into six stages (including cytokinesis). In prophase, chromatin is condensed into homologous pairs of chromosomes known as sister chromatids, which are joined at the centromere (kinetochore) after having divided during late S phase; as the chromosomes shorten and thicken they first become visible as extended duplicate structures. Mitosis becomes dominated by the formation of highly ordered spindles composed of microtubules and associated proteins that emanate from two mitotic centers located at opposite poles of the cell. Softening and dissolution of the nuclear membrane marks the end of prophase. In early prometaphase the fibers of this bipolar spindle link up with kinetochore microtubules extending out from the chromosomes. During metaphase, kinetochore fibers align the chromosomes halfway between the spindle poles, forming the equatorial metaphase plate. The chromosomal complement visualized at metaphase is called its karyotype. Anaphase begins with abrupt separation of the paired kinetochores from their apposed chromosomes. Both pushing and pulling forces act at anaphase to separate sister chromatids: elongation and sliding of the polar microtubules pushes the two poles apart; forces acting on the shorter kinetochore fibers pull the detached chromatids toward opposite poles at a rate of 1 μm/min. Telophase marks the arrival of the full complement of daughter chromatids at the opposite poles (Figure 2-5). During telophase a new nuclear envelope forms around each group of daughter chromatids, nucleoli reappear, and mitosis is complete. An actin-operated contractile ring clamps off the bridge connecting tandem cells, and the cytoplasm divides by cleavage during cytokinesis. Each daughter cell released by cytokinesis begins life fully equipped with two copies of each chromosome, the chromosomes decondense, and RNA synthesis is resumed.

Meiosis: A Mechanism for Recombinant Diversity

Meiosis is a complex form of nuclear division restricted to gametes. Meiosis confers genetic individuality through the exchange of segments of DNA between homologous chromosomes and by random selection of one of the two homologs prefatory to fusion of sperm and egg. Meiosis involves two separate cell divisions, I and II, that yield four haploid gametes from a single diploid cell. The first

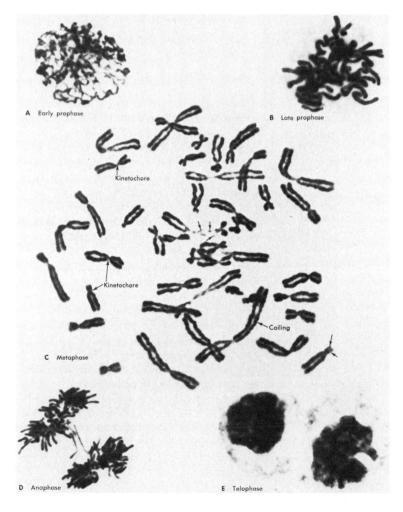

A Early prophase
B Late prophase
Kinetochore
Kinetochore
Coiling
C Metaphase
D Anaphase
E Telophase

FIGURE 2-5

Patterns of stained chromosomes witnessed during the five sequential phases of mitosis, A through E, preparatory to division. The structure of condensed chromosome pairs is exposed during early metaphase, revealing among other things chromatid coiling, the kinetochores (centromeres), and terminal constrictions or "satellites." (From Weiss L: Chapt 1, in Histology: Cell and Tissue Biology, 5th ed., Weiss L, Ed. New York, Elsevier Science Publishing Co., Inc.,1983.)

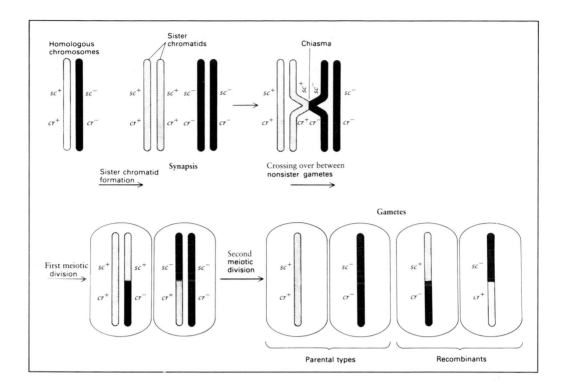

FIGURE 2-6

Diagram of crossover at meiosis. When cross-over occurs between nonsister chromatids, genetic recombination leads to altered expression of the genome. The meiotic divisions yield two parental and two recombinant gametes. (Modified from Darnell J et al: Chapt 10, in Molecular Cell Biology. New York, Scientific American Books, 1986.)

meiotic division is characterized by a protracted prophase during which homologous chromosomes undergo duplication before they pair off (synapse) and form a synaptonemal complex. The homologous paired chromosomes, termed a bivalent or tetrad, are intimately matched up by complementarity, a snug alignment that predisposes to chromosomal crossing over, in which parts of neighboring homologous chromosomes are exchanged. Ordinarily, two or three such crossover events occur on each pair of chromosomes. When crossover is between sister chromatids no genetic effect is discernable, but when a crossover occurs between nonsister chromatids genetic recombination results (Figure 2-6).

Normally division I of meiosis yields two sorts of diversity that account for the fact that no two offspring (barring monozygotic twins) of the same parents are exactly alike. First, the number of different kinds of cells generated by the first meiotic division of a diploid cell having $2n$ chromosomes is 2^n. Second, chromosomal crossovers occur during prophase I when each pair of homologous chromosomes is held in register by synaptonemal complexes, each of which is marked by formation of a chiasma. Meiotic division II follows without further replication, and chromatids separate more formally into individual daughter cells. The net result of meiosis is to divide the starting number of $4n$ chromosomes into four haploid cells (gametes), in which the pairs of parental and recombinant homologs are kept separate. Fusion of sperm and egg generates a new diploid cell having an individual biological soul.

Nonhomologous crossing over   If the crossing over occurs between nonhomologous chromosome loci, misalignment may result in improper pairing and fusion of unrelated gene regions, which then code for a defective protein. Hemoglobin Lepore, for example, is the pathologic product caused by nonhomologous crossing over between part of the δ chain locus on one chromosome 11 and part of the β chain locus on the complementary chromosome, creating a fused and functionally defective δβ "Lepore gene" [4].

Sister chromatid exchanges may repair DNA
Agents such as irradiation are known to create nicks (cuts) in DNA strands. This can trigger an act of recombinant repair through sister chromatid exchange. A nick in a single DNA strand frees the dangling end which then invades the second complementary helix to form a short pairing region, thereby initiating a general recombination event and DNA renaturation. DNA nicking agents induce reparative exchanges between sister chromatids during the S and G_2 phases of cell cycle. As these exchanges do not alter the genomic structure they cannot be detected by genetic means but may display striking harlequin patterns by autoradiography or after special staining procedures (Figure 2-7).

DNA repair   Sister chromatid exchange is only one of a battery of mechanisms designed to safeguard or repair DNA. The most celebrated example of DNA repair is the process called photoreactivation, a light-dependent enzyme mechanism that expunges intrastrand thymine

dimers caused by UV light. Damaged segments of DNA may be replaced by means of an excision-repair system, involving: activation of an endonuclease that cleaves the DNA strand on both sides of the damage; activation of a $5' \rightarrow 3'$ exonuclease that excises the damaged segment; a repair step in which a replacement patch is synthesized by DNA polymerase; and finally a DNA ligase comes forward to covalently link the patch to the wounded strand [5]. These repair and retrieval systems are similar to those involved in genetic recombination. Genetic deficiencies in DNA repair enzymes are responsible for a group of deadly maladies, many of which predispose to malignancies: among these are xeroderma pigmentosum, Bloom's syndrome, and Fanconi's anemia.

CHROMOSOMES AND CYTOGENETICS

The vague abstractions of formal genetics held little interest for the visually oriented medical world until a serendipitous discovery launched the era of human cytogenetics in 1956. Using hypotonic media and the practiced pressure of thumb-on-coverslip, nuclear chromosomes in prophase or metaphase can be spread out, enumerated, profiled, and photographed. Beginning with Caspersson's work in the late 1960s, selective "banding" methods have been developed that make possible the unambiguous

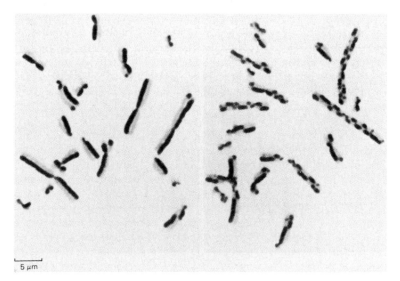

5 µm

FIGURE 2-7

Sister chromatid exchanges visualized in metaphase by differential staining with Giemsa and a fluorescent dye. In chromosomes treated to induce nicks in the DNA, numerous chromatid exchanges are visible (right), as compared with the control (left). (From Alberts B et al: Chapt 5, in Molecular Biology of the Cell. New York, Garland Publishing, Inc.,1983.)

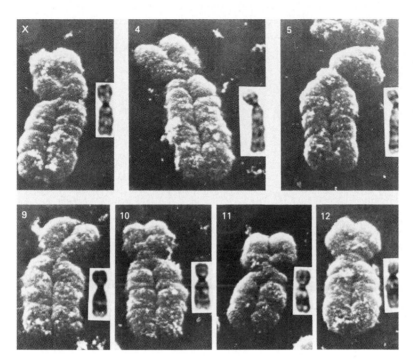

FIGURE 2-8

Appearance of seven different chromosomes after G banding. The light micrographs (insets) show the bands at low resolution. The SEM views reveal constrictions and creases at the sites where the dark-stained depressed bands were exposed. (From Harrison CJ et al: Scanning electron microscopy of the G-banded human karyocyte. Exp Cell Res 134:141,1981.)

identification of each of the 46 chromosomes and their parts. By examining partially condensed chromosomes very early in mitosis it is possible to visualize over 2,000 distinct bands of adenine:thymine (A-T) base pair–rich DNA per haploid set. Identification of chromosome segments and the tracking of chromosomal rearrangements in disease has been facilitated by introduction of high-resolution cytogenetic technology. It is likely that early prophase chromosomes soon will achieve a resolution comparable to the 5,000 bands of *Drosophila* polytene chromosomes. With such refinement each band would represent only a few dozen genes, helping to bridge the gap between genes and chromosomes. The use of high-resolution techniques in conjunction with gene mapping by in situ hybridization and recombinant DNA technology should enable molecular characterization of most genomic defects before the year 2000.

Chromosome Banding and Band Nomenclature

Cytogenetics, the art of chromosome analysis, has contributed so much to our understanding of blood cell disorders, particularly malignancies, that its methodology warrants expatiation. When metaphase preparations are viewed by UV optics after staining with fluorescent dyes such as quinacrine and acridine adducts, which intercalate into the grooves in the DNA helix, glowing "Q" bands emerge that denote the presence of DNA regions rich in A-T base pairs. Giemsa (G) bands appear when air-dried chromosomes are pretreated with trypsin. The bold but decorative striations produced by quinacrine and by Giemsa techniques are nearly superimposable, differing only in the uniquely intense quinacrine staining of the distal part of the long (q) arm of the Y chromosome and the dark staining of centromeric heterochromatin by Giemsa. R (reverse) bands are brought out by hot-alkaline denaturation of metaphase preparations; R banding simulates a photographic negative of G banding. Because of its simplicity and permanence, Giemsa banding after proteolytic treatment has become the standard methodology. The appearance of several chromosomes after exposure to trypsin and Giemsa is shown in Figure 2-8 [6]. Additional measures by which normal chromosomes can be characterized in-

FIGURE 2-9

Schematic representation of chromosome 14 at the 400 (left), 550 (center), and 850 (right) band levels. (From Yunis JJ and Lewandowsky RC: High-resolution cytogenetics. In Finley SC, Finley WH, and Flowers CE, Jr. (eds.): Birth Defects: Clinical and Ethical Considerations. New York: Alan R. Liss, BD:OAS XIX(5):12,1983, with permission of the copyright holder, the March of Dimes Birth Defects Foundation.)

FIGURE 2-10

Schematic representations and band identification of chromosomes at the 1,000 band stage per haploid set. For expository purposes, both sex chromosomes are shown. Differences in shading represent varying color saturation of bands after G banding (From Yunis JJ: Midprophase human chromosomes. The attainment of 2,000 bands. Hum Genet 56:293,1981.)

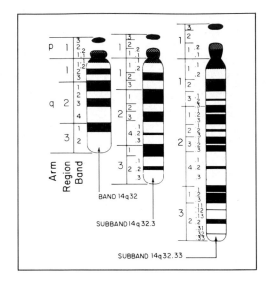

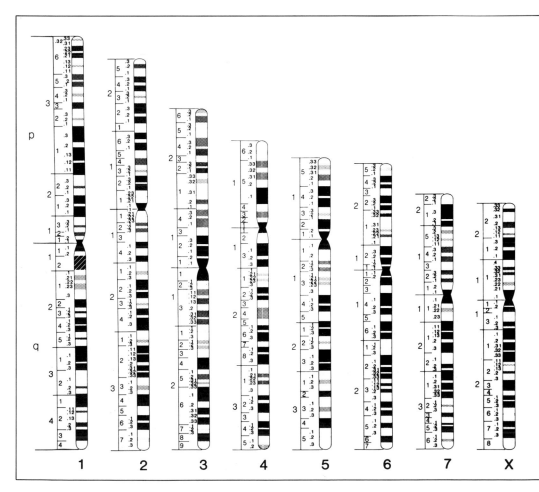

clude: "C banding" of the pericentromeric region, silver staining for nucleolus organizer regions, and a search for satellites. Satellites are small outward projections of chromatin affixed by short stalks to the short (p) arms of the "acrocentric" chromosomes: 13, 14, 15, 21, and 22.

The Normal Karyotype

The chromosomal constitution, or karyotype, of cells can be ascertained by photographing a metaphase plate, cutting out the images, and arranging these in homologous pairs. The normal female diploid karyotype is denoted 46,XX; the normal for males is 46,XY. A schematic representation of a karyotype in which images of chromosomes are arranged systematically according to length and centromeric position is an ideogram. Expansion of the 1971 Paris Conference nomenclature has been adopted to specify chromosome arms, regions, bands, and subbands. To specify a subband, a decimal point placed after the band designation is followed by an identifying number; if the subband is divided, an appropriate second-place digit is added. Thus, for region 3, band 2, of the long (q) arm of chromosome 14, the band is designated 14q32, the subband farthest from the centromere is denoted 14q32.3, and the most distal (third) sub-subband is labeled 14q32.33 (Figure 2-9) [7]. The normal haploid ideogram is a packet of 22 somatic chromosomes plus one of the two sex chromosomes. An amended haplotype is portrayed in Figure 2-10 [8].

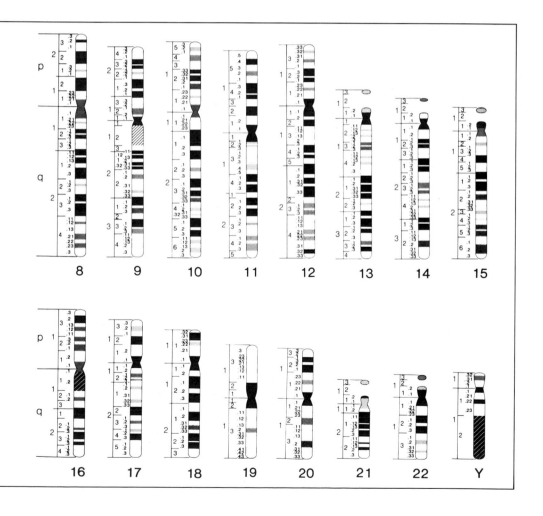

The Clinical Place of Cytogenetics

The principal contribution of cytogenetics to pathophysiologic understanding of genetic problems, inborn or acquired, is to provide a low-power screening method for detecting dislocated or missing chunks of chromosomes. To place present limits of resolution in perspective it should be borne in mind that the human genome consists of approximately 3×10^9 base pairs of DNA distributed among 46 chromosomes. It is likely that there are between 100,000 and 200,000 genes in this genome, with gene sizes ranging from a few thousand to several hundred thousand base pairs. (In addition there are large families of repeat sequences scattered throughout the genome, and the number of rearrangements of B cell immunoglobulin and T cell antigen receptor genes runs in the millions.) Currently the resolution limit of cytogenetics precludes microscopic recognition of genome regions smaller than 2 to 5 million base pairs, stretches sufficient to accommodate an average of about 50 to 100 genes. In contrast, gene mapping procedures are capable of focusing down to the level of several hundred base pairs, a very manageable fragment from the sequencing viewpoint. The strength of cytogenetics is its capability for locating major rearrangements, which can then be characterized at the gene level by methods for DNA analysis (Chapter 3).

Chromosome Rearrangements, Structural and Numerical

Genes are moved around during cell cycle: for genes to be expressed their component coding sequences, which exist as pieces (exons) broken up along the DNA strand and interrupted by noncoding intervening sequences (introns), must be assembled and then spliced into functional units. Mobility of gene pieces is fundamental to the multitudinous rearrangements that are required for widely separated regions of immunoglobulin (Ig) genes on the long arm of chromosome 14, which codes for heavy chains, and regions of the q arms of chromosomes 2 and 22, which code for the κ and λ light chains, respectively. Similar rearrangements involving chromosomes 7 and 14 are required for assembly of coding regions for the T cell antigen receptor. The gathering of exons required for gene assembly is carefully regulated, as described in Chapter 3, but with every movement there is an inevitable risk of error. Risk is compounded by the fact that the genome is mysteriously flawed by over 100 hereditary fragile sites, transmitted in a mendelian codominant pattern. Nature's purpose in conserving fragile sites is unexplained, but the potential for genetic havoc is apparent when one considers that the genome is studded with promoters, amplifiers, oncogenes, genes for growth factors, and genes for growth factor receptors. That most individuals are not victimized by chromosomal fragility attests to the efficiency of DNA repair mechanisms described above and possibly to custodial alleles known popularly as anti-oncogenes or tumor-suppressing genes.

Symbols for chromosome rearrangements   In shorthand, gains, losses, and transpositions of chromosomes are denoted by citing the nature of the aberration with a lowercase prefix, followed by the number, arm, and band of the chromosome affected.

Translocations   Translocations are identified by t, and the chromosomes involved are indicated within the first set of parentheses; chromosome arms and bands in which breakpoints have occurred are denoted within a second set. For example, the reciprocal translocation most characteristic of the high-grade malignancy Burkitt's lymphoma involves breakpoints in subband q24.13 of chromosome 8 and subband q32.33 of chromosome 14. When the detached terminal pieces are set free by these breakages, the pieces may be exchanged and become annealed to the open stumps of the other defective chromosome. In this unequal reciprocal translocation, t(8;14)(q24.13;q32.33), the oncogene, c-*myc*, of chromosome 8 becomes joined to the heavy chain coding region of chromosome 14, and the Ig variable coding region of chromosome 14 fuses to the broken tip of 8q (Figure 2-11). Fusion of c-*myc* genes to the unstable switch region of the Ig genes on chromosome 14 dislocates c-*myc* from trans control by the allelic normal gene. The inappropriate intrusion of an oncogene growth factor into the highly mutable Ig gene region of 14q somehow

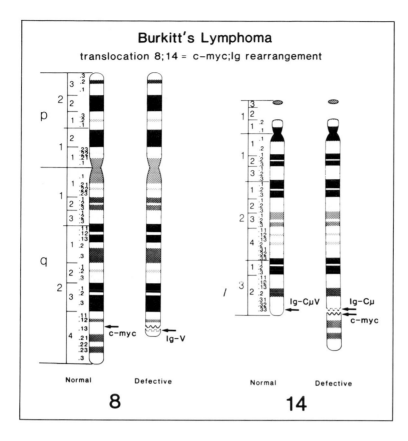

Burkitt's Lymphoma

translocation 8;14 = c–myc;Ig rearrangement

c–myc

Ig-V

Normal   Defective

8

Ig-CμV   Ig-Cμ

c–myc

Normal   Defective

14

FIGURE 2-11

Schematic representation of the t(8;14) translocation in Burkitt's lymphoma. Jagged gaps in the defective chromosomes indicate breakpoint sites. Arrows point to the location of the c-*myc* oncogene and heavy chain variable (Ig-V) and constant (Ig-Cμ) genes on normal and defective chromosomes 8 and 14. Defective chromosome 8 donates c-*myc* in exchange for Ig-V from chromosome 14. (Courtesy of Dr. JJ Yunis. From Jandl J: Chapt 20, in Blood: Textbook of Hematology. Boston, Little, Brown and Company, 1987.)

accounts for generation of the malignant B cells characteristic of Burkitt's lymphoma.

Trisomies and deletions   Gain (trisomy) or loss (deletion) of an entire chromosome is signified by a plus or minus sign before the chromosome number. Gain or loss of part of a chromosome is indicated by a plus or minus after the stipulated chromosome arm.

The most notorious trisomy (+21) is associated with Down's syndrome. Trisomy is the consequence of nondisjunction, which is either failure of sister chromatids to separate during the second meiotic division or failure of homologous chromosomes to separate during the first meiotic division. Trisomy 21 is the most common serious chromosomal defect, and 95% of cases result from nondisjunction. For reasons unknown, addition of a third chromosome to the genome profoundly deranges somatic and cerebral development and increases sharply the risk of leukemia.

Deletion (del) of chromosome 7 (−7) or of its long arm (7q−) and partial deletions of chromosome 5 (5q−) are characteristic of acute myelogenous leukemia (AML) secondary to alkylator chemotherapy or X-irradiation. Subtractions affecting the long arms of chromosomes 7 and 5 imperil hematopoietic activity and regulation. The long arm of 7 contains coding regions for the β chain of the T cell antigen receptor (q32–35) and for erythropoietin (q11–22). Interstitial deletions confined to 5q32 alone rob the genome of an entire cluster of genes that code for IL-3, GM-CSF, M-CSF, and for the M-CSF receptor (c-*fms*). It is no surprise that the "5q− syndrome" is associated with dysplasia of all marrow precursors and entails a high risk of transformation to AML. Abbreviations for other anomalies less regularly associated with leukemia or lymphoma include the following: ins, insertion; i, isochrome; r, ring chromosome; ter, terminal deletion; der, derivative chromosome; inv ins, inverted insertion; and rec, recombinant chromosome.

Most critical genomic errors found by cytogenetic studies to be associated with neoplasia involve translocations, deletions, and amplified repeats, rather than point mutations [9].

Lyonization   The "Barr body," first discovered by Barr and Bertram, is a heterochromatic mass about 1 μm across that usually is located at the periphery of interphase cells in females. The Barr body (X body, sex chromatin body) is the pyknotic inactivated remains of one of the two X chromosomes found in cells of normal women. Corresponding bodies are found in 2 to 3% of the neutrophils of women and appear as heterochromatic drumstick-shaped appendages connected to a terminal lobe of the nucleus (Figure 2-12). The process of X chromosome inactivation is named lyonization after the British cytogeneticist Mary Lyon, who recognized that inactivation of the redundant X chromosomes is a random process occurring

FIGURE 2-12

A characteristic drumstick or Barr body in a neutrophil from a normal woman is seen as a bulbous projection extending from the inner aspect of the terminal lobe on the right. True drumsticks, containing a pyknotic inactivated X chromosome, are rounded bodies attached to a terminal lobe by a thin chromatin strand. In normal women 2 to 3% of neutrophils contain a single drumstick, which must be distinguished from the "pseudodrumsticks" found in about 20% of neutrophils of both sexes; the small projection from the inner aspect of the left terminal lobe of this neutrophil can be differentiated from the true thing by its smaller size and atypical shape. (Photo by CT Kapff.)

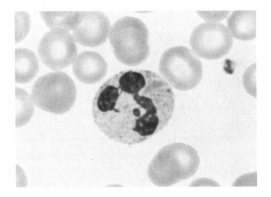

early in embryonic life, probably at the trilaminar blastodermal stage, when the number of multipotential hematopoietic stem cells is only eight [10].

Each cell in females has two X chromosomes, one of maternal origin (X_m) and one of paternal provenance (X_p). After lyonization the embryo becomes a mosaic of cells in which about half have an inactive X_m and the rest have an inactive X_p. Genetic polyclonal diversity conferred by random X inactivation affects all cell lines arising from stem cells that differentiate before inactivation takes place; with regard to X chromosome expression, most females are a patchwork of clones. Inactivation is caused by regulated methylation which inactivates nearly all genetic elements of the "surplus" X chromosomes. Inactivation is random and permanent in nature, and so sturdy a feature of descendent cells that even anaplastic cancer cells retain the inactivation mechanism. The process is not perfect, however, sparing some X-linked genes, and the percentage of cells evading inactivation during blastocyst development can depart from 50%. Cell lines in which more or less than half of the X chromosomes have been inactivated are said to reflect "extreme lyonization."

Lyon's law and cellular mosaicism   In the words of geneticists Race and Sanger, the essential "truth of the theory is now triumphantly established." It is time to recognize that lyonization is no longer hypothetical and to elevate Lyon's hypothesis to Lyon's law. The mosaicism predicted by Lyon's law has been proved out in scores of X-borne anomalies and explains countless genetic puzzles such as gene dosage compensation: women, for example, do not have twice the amount of factor VIII (antihemophilic factor) as men; factor VIII levels are similar in both sexes, unless extreme lyonization shifts the level in women below or above that in men. X inactivation accounts for the dual cell populations in retinal mosaicism, X-linked ocular albinism, and chronic granulomatous disease.

Clonal Growth and the Definition of Cancer

A clone is defined as a group of identical cells descended from a common ancestor. Each committed stem cell, such as a CFU-E, will generate a clone of erythroid descendants, but the marrow manufactures many millions of CFU-Es daily and the derived red cell populations are, accordingly, polyclonal. The probability (P) that all red cells would descend from CFU-Es possessing only X_m or X_p in their karyotype would be 0.5 (50%) × the number of CFU-Es, or $0.5^{\text{many millionths}}$; P values would be ludicrously small. Normal cell populations are polyclonal with respect to their observable markers, their phenotypes.

G6PD as a marker of clonal growth   Glucose 6-phosphate dehydrogenase (G6PD) is one of many proteins encoded by alleles on the X chromosomes. The G6PD gene is polymorphic in black populations, with 30 to 40% of black women being heterozygous for the B isozyme variant (Gd^B), and for either Gd^A or Gd^{A-}. In G6PD heterozygous women somatic cells, including hematopoietic cells, are a mosaic mixture of cells, about half containing the Gd^B isozyme and half one of the Gd^A variants. In such women with multiple uterine fibroids (leiomyomas), it has been found that individual fibroid tumors contain either Gd^B or Gd^A variants, but never both, whereas intervening uterine cells display a mix of isozymes. This finding indicates beyond mathematical dispute that each of these benign tumors originated from a single mutant cell. In all patients with leukemias, lymphomas, and other hematologic malignancies who have been studied by isozyme analysis, all malignant cells have displayed a single G6PD phenotype. The simplest if not the sole explanation is that the abnormal cells comprise a clonal population descended from a single founder cell (phenotypic monoclonality). That monoclonality is a fixture of malignancy has been confirmed by studies of other X chromosome markers, and by the revelation that B cell malignancies are associated with monoclonal immunoglobulin gene rearrangements and T cell tumors are characterized by singular homogeneous rearrangements of the T cell antigen receptor genes (genotypic monoclonality). Indeed, most hematologic malignancies are associated with recurrent nonrandom (clonal) chromosomal rearrangements. During therapy-induced remission and during relapse of these malignancies, how-

ever, phenotypic monoclonality is a more durable feature than chromosomal abnormalities; the finding of recurrent chromosomal aberrations lacks the finality of isozyme analysis. At present, phenotypic clonality is not the only, but remains the best, definition of malignancy. Exceptions to the rule that single-enzyme clones are the hallmark of neoplasia exist among certain genetically determined neoplasms such as hereditary multiple neurofibromatosis and hereditary multiple trichoepitheliomas, in which each individual cell harbors its own unique demons of transformation.

Cytokinetics of Malignancy

Monoclonal cell populations are defective in their maturation   Monoclonal populations of cells, as identified by isozyme analysis, cell surface markers, or monotonous gene rearrangements, are defective but not necessarily antisocial. Most neoplastic populations are not programmed to complete a normal maturation and accordingly accumulate in unfinished form. Usually failure of maturation means failure of growth and the cells die off. It is estimated that in a normal lifetime each separate gene sustains about 10^{10} mutagenic insults, most of which are corrected by DNA repair enzymes. Stem cells that survive multiple chromosome mutations become kinetically faulty. Their pointless growth is slow, their cell cycle is prolonged, and the death rate is high. Happily, most monoclonal cell populations fail to flourish.

Clonal overgrowth is faulty but ceaseless: doubling time versus cell cycle time   Among normally dividing hematopoietic cells, the rate of cell loss (Θ) is only 5 to 10%. If proliferation were a perfect process, the time required to double the mass of cells (Td) would equal the potential doubling time, T, of the cell cycle. As normal proliferation is slightly imperfect, normal cells with a potential doubling time of 18 h and an error rate (Θ) of 10% (0.10) will require longer to double their numbers in accordance with the expression

$$Td = \frac{T}{1 - \theta} :$$

$$Td = \frac{18}{1 - 0.10} = 20 \text{ h}$$

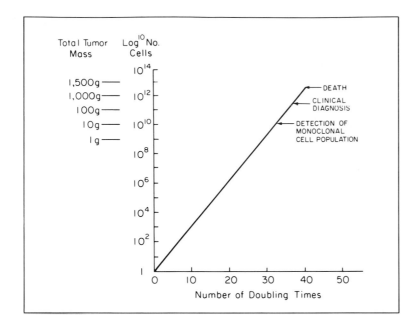

FIGURE 2-13

Relation of total tumor weight and number of tumor cells to the number of times the tumor mass has doubled. Tumor doubling time is not constant, as implied in this figure, but varies directly as a function of proliferative rate and indirectly in proportion to cell death rate. The seemingly explosive clinical emergence of leukemias or lymphomas is simply the arithmetic finale to a protracted period of latent cell growth. Commonly (not shown here) the doubling rate slows down as tumor cell infiltrates choke off their own blood supply.

In acute myelogenous leukemia, the value for T averages 80 to 84 h, as compared with the cell cycle time for normal myeloblasts of 18 h [11, 12]. In animal leukemias the value for Θ often exceeds 0.50. Combining these estimates, it is clear that the doubling time of a monoclonal cell mass may be very slow, namely: $\frac{84\,h}{1-0.50}$ or 168 h (7 days). In human leukemias and lymphomas, accumulation of a lethal burden of tumor cells (about 5×10^{12}, or 1.5 kg) usually occurs within 40 to 60 doubling times over a period ranging from 2 to 8 years (Figure 2-13). Growth of functionless tumor cells is dangerous not because new cells are produced rapidly but because they are generated constantly, indifferent to cytokine signals. Severe cytokinetic retardation gives rise to slow but remorseless displacement from marrow of normal functioning residents by the teeming hordes of inert tumor cells.

REFERENCES

1. Darnell J et al: Molecular Cell Biology. New York, Scientific American Books,1986

2. Weiss L: Chapt 1, in Histology. Cell and Tissue Biology, Weiss L, Ed. New York, Elsevier Science Publishing Company,1983

3. Watson JE et al: Molecular Biology of the Gene, vol. 1, 4th ed. Menlo Park, The Benjamin/Cummings Publishing Company, Inc.,1987

4. Bunn HF and Forget GB: Hemoglobin: Molecular, Genetic and Clinical Aspects. Philadelphia, WB Saunders Company,1986

5. Lewin B: Chapt 15, in Genes, 3rd ed. New York, John Wiley & Sons, Inc.,1987

6. Harrison CJ et al: Scanning electron microscopy of the G-banded human karyocyte. Exp Cell Res 134:141,1981

7. Yunis JJ and Lewandowsky RC: High-resolution cytogenetics. Birth Defects OAS XIX(5):12, 1983

8. Yunis JJ: Mid-prophase human chromosomes. The attainment of 2,000 bands. Hum Genet 56:293,1981

9. Yunis JJ: Multiple recurrent genomic rearrangements and fragile sites in human cancer. Somatic Cell and Molecular Genetics 13:397,1987

10. Buescher ED et al: Use of an X-linked human neutrophil marker to estimate timing of lyonization and size of the dividing stem cell pool. J Clin Invest 76:1581,1985

11. Baserga R: Multiplication and Division in Mammalian Cells. New York, Marcel Dekker, Inc., 1976

12. Andreeff M: Cell kinetics of leukemia. Semin Hematol 23:300,1986

3

Molecular Genetics and Hemoglobin Synthesis

□

In nuclear chromosomes DNA is tightly complexed with basic proteins, histones, that package it in elaborate chromosomal spools to prevent snarling and facilitate its orderly unwinding during interphase (Chapter 2). Each diploid nucleus houses 46 chromosomes that contain collectively a constant amount of DNA ($\sim 10^{-12}$ g/nucleus) that is replicated faithfully during each cell division. Operationally DNA itself may be considered a stationary library, one of enormous complexity and capacity but nearly incapable of change: it is the apotheosis of mainframe technology, for in its 3 m of linear DNA is stored the archive of the genome. In this archive are 10 trillion triplet symbols and over 100,000 germline genes, each of which contains all the blueprints necessary to produce peptides. The cell's complement of DNA is kept apart from the cytoplasm by a double membrane called the nuclear envelope. This envelope isolates the central genetic processes of DNA replication (duplication) and RNA transcription (copying) and processing (copyediting) from the frenetic activities of protein synthesis in the cytoplasm. In the hard cover editions characteristic of eukaryotic cells, the amount of information stored and available for retrieval in the membrane-bound nucleus rivals that of the Library of Congress.

THE FLOW OF INFORMATION: DNA→RNA→PROTEIN

The central theme of molecular genetics is the stepwise flow of information from DNA to RNA to protein (Figure 3-1) [1]. As DNA is the repository of all hereditary information, review of its structure and the processes of replication and transcription are essential to understanding the chemical basis of heredity and the techniques of molecular genetics.

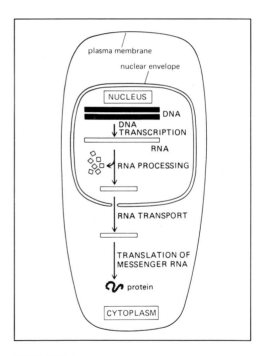

F I G U R E 3-1

Schematic view of the DNA → RNA → protein sequence. Because of the nuclear envelope, the steps of RNA processing in the nucleus and RNA transport to the cytoplasm are interposed between transcription of DNA into RNA and translation of messenger RNA into protein. (From Alberts B: Chapt 8, in Molecular Biology of the Cell. New York, Garland Publishing, Inc.,1983.)

DNA Structure and Replication

The exterior of the DNA double helix, or duplex, is dominated by the backbones of two polymeric chains that are twisted about each other like two vines. Human DNA is almost entirely in the right-handed *B* configuration having about 10 base pairs per twist, as discovered by Watson and Crick; there also is a more squat *A* form having a different tilt and a

FIGURE 3-2

The two intertwined strands of DNA in its native state. The chains are in antiparallel orientation, one running 5′→3′, the other 3′→5′. Bases on opposite strands are kept in longitudinal register by A:T and G:C bonding. (From Watson JD et al: Chapt 9, in Molecular Biology of the Gene, vol.1, 4th ed. Menlo Park, The Benjamin/Cummings Publishing Company, Inc.,1987.)

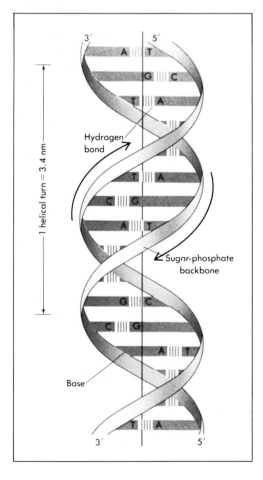

zigzag (Z) left-handed helix of uncertain physiologic importance. Each strand of right-handed ("ordinary") DNA is a long polymer of nucleotides in which the sugar (deoxyribose) of each nucleotide is covalently linked by a phosphate group (3′–5′ phosphodiester linkages) to the sugar of the adjacent nucleotide. There are four nucleotides each containing a deoxyribose residue, a phosphate group, and a purine or pyrimidine base: the two single-ringed pyrimidines are thymine (T) and cytosine (C), and the two double-ringed purines are adenine (A) and guanine (G). The two chains are joined by hydrogen bonding of opposing base pairs in an invariable coupling in which adenine is always paired to thymine (A to T) and cytosine to guanine (C to G). For example, if one chain has a 5′-ATGTC-3′ sequence, the opposite chain must have the sequence of 3′-TACAG-5′. The stringency of these pairing rules confers a complementarity between the base sequences of the intertwined chains. A steric consequence of the AT and GC rung arrangement is that the two polynucleotide chains have polarity, or direction: in the duplex they run in parallel but opposite (antiparallel) direction [2], as can be seen by examining Figure 3-2 before and after inverting it 180° [3]. The two sugar-phosphate backbones of the duplex are not spaced equally along the DNA axis, creating alternating major and minor screwlike grooves. The deep major grooves provide sites for attachment of sequence-specific regulatory proteins. Proteins that modulate or mask coding sequences, and the several DNases and polymerases that participate in slicing or replicating DNA, are all coded for by DNA, attesting to the absolute sovereignty of this majestic molecule.

DNA Even Codes Itself: Replication

The reason the genetic code issues faithful copy is that DNA is locked into a processing loop. DNA not only codes its decoders (RNAs), it also codes itself and thus duplicates the original template. Despite their coiled intimacy, the parental template and its complementary replica are held together by weak bonds, and the two strands can readily be untwisted by rotating about the axis of the unreplicated DNA double helix. To facilitate strand separation as

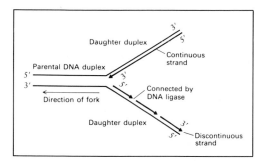

FIGURE 3-3

Replication of DNA. Nucleic acid chains grow only in the 5' → 3' direction. Hence one of the two copies of the parental DNA must be replicated in separate fragments, which then are turned around and connected by DNA ligase. The entire structure shown schematically here is called a growing fork. (Modified from Darnell J et al: Chapt 4, in Molecular Cell Biology. New York, Scientific American Books,1986.)

the prelude to replication, specific DNA-binding ATP-activated proteins called helicases unwind the double helix (Figure 3-3) [4]. Enzymes that copy DNA to make more DNA are called DNA polymerases.

Natures abhors single-stranded DNA   The very existence of single-stranded DNA, or exposed areas of unpaired DNA, appears to invite activation of DNA and RNA polymerases. DNA polymerases act processively; while adding nucleotides to a nascent strand, DNA polymerases remain attached until a stop signal is reached causing them to detach. The best characterized of these enzymes, which proceeds 5' → 3' during polymerization, is DNA polymerase I. Polymerase I has a major domain shaped like a hollow spindle or bobbin through which the growing end of replicating DNA is fed. In addition DNA polymerase I possesses a small region having 3' → 5' exonuclease activity that proofreads and edits out mismatched nucleotides [3]. Mechanisms causing initiation of DNA replication are less well understood than events occurring at the growing fork. It is probable that DNA polymerase is guided in the recognition of the initiating base by complementary pairing, for complemen-

tarity is the recurring motif causing single strands to seek partnership.

RNA Structure and Transcription

The decoding of DNA is called transcription, and the transcript is embodied in the structure of RNA. Synthesis of RNA on DNA templates is very similar to the process by which DNA replicates itself. Transcription involves formation of complementary base pairs under the guidance of RNA polymerase II, which links together the ribonucleoside triphosphates. RNA polymerase II is composed of five polypeptide chains, one of which, σ, functions only to recognize the "start transcribing" command on the upstream initiating region of DNA known as the promoter. This polypeptide then falls off, leaving the core enzyme which zips together the phosphoester linkages to form the mRNA transcript or track. Only RNA polymerase II transcribes the genes that will be translated into proteins. The other two polymerases synthesize RNAs that engage in protein synthesis: polymerase I generates ribosomal RNAs, and polymerase III makes a variety of small but essential and stable RNAs, including transfer RNAs (tRNAs) and the small 5S RNA of the ribosome.

Transcription begins when polymerase II binds to the DNA promoter sequence. The enzyme unwinds part of the double helix, exposing two single strands of DNA, one of which is then transcribed into RNA. As polymerase II travels along the DNA strand in a 5' → 3' direction, the 5' end of RNA transcript is capped by a basic 7-methylguanosine residue; this 5' cap confers a positive charge that later mediates binding of RNA to a ribosome. RNA is transcribed from DNA at a rate of 30 nucleotides per second until it reaches the termination signal in chromatin, which indicates "caboosehood" and halts transcription. In transcripts destined to become messengers conveying instructions from DNA to the protein synthetic apparatus (hence the term "messenger RNA," or mRNA), a poly-A-polymerase adds 100 to 200 residues of adenylic acid to the 3' end of the RNA chain to complete primary mRNA transcripts of various lengths, known as heterogeneous nuclear RNA (hnRNA). It should be emphasized that RNA does not readily form a double helical structure, because

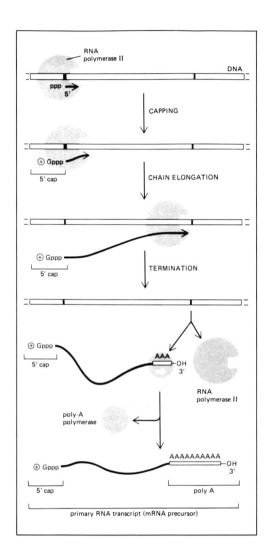

FIGURE 3-4

Sequential steps in transcribing primary mRNA from DNA, with RNA polymerase II functioning as word processor. ppp = 5' to 5' triphosphate. Gppp = 7-methylguanosine triphosphate. (From Alberts B et al: Chapt 8, in Molecular Biology of the Cell. New York, Garland Publishing, Inc.,1983.)

in RNA synthesis uridine (U) is substituted for thymidine, and the bulkier A and U pairs of RNA do not fit together as closely as do the A and T pairs of DNA. The sequence leading to formation of the primary (pre-mRNA) transcript is shown in Figure 3-4. The ultrastructural appearance of chromatin during active transcription is shown in Figure 3-5 [5].

Genes and Transcripts Are Made in Pieces: Exons and Introns

Genes of mammals are discontinuous, and component pieces are deployed along DNA strands into regions widely separated by noncoding DNA. Indeed, only about 1% of DNA is utilized for eventual translation. Not only are genes separated from each other by noncoding DNA, but the coding regions themselves are interrupted by intervening sequences (IVSs). When the DNA code is transcribed, the mRNA transcript contains copies of all coding regions (called exons) and of all IVSs (called introns). These intron sequences must be cut out of each transcript to convert the transcript into an uncluttered exon continuum, mature mRNA, that

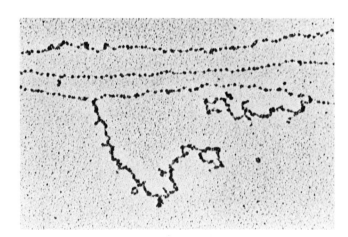

FIGURE 3-5

Three beaded strands of DNA cross the field horizontally: each bead is a nucleosome containing components of activatable genes. From the bottom strand of DNA, two nascent mRNA molecules dangle downward, caught in the process of active transcription. RNA polymerase is situated at the junction between the chromatin strand and the coarsely angulated pre-mRNA. (From Nienhuis WE and Maniatis T: Chapt 2, in The Molecular Basis of Blood Diseases, Stamatoyannopoulos G et al, Eds. Philadelphia, WB Saunders Company,1987.)

is small enough to escape through pores in the nuclear membrane and then to code for synthesis of protein. Most genes are more intron than exon: hence the full primary transcript must be processed and abridged extensively before the mature transcript can be exported safely into the cytoplasm. Errors in copyediting (RNA processing) are responsible for many hereditary blood disorders, but even these errors (as in β thalassemia) are traceable to DNA malfunction, for DNA encodes the decoders.

Splicing, Spliceosomes, Lariats, and mRNA Export

Conversion of rough drafts (hnRNA) of transcripts into final form may involve reduction in the primary transcripts from molecules as large as 50,000 nucleotides to abbreviated structures that characteristically range from 500 to 3,000 nucleotides. This is achieved by excision of introns from precursor RNA and ligating the proper ends of the separate coding sequences to yield integrated mature mRNA. Splicing proceeds as follows: cleavage of pre-mRNA at the 5' "donor" site of the exon:intron junction allows formation of a covalent bond between

the 5' end of the intron and a region of the intron 18 to 37 nucleotides from the 3' "acceptor" site of the intron. This generates a lariat-shaped or branched RNA structure (Figure 3-6) [6]. The lariat loop is formed through a single autocatalytic event involving association of pre-mRNA with subunits of several small nuclear ribonucleoprotein species (snRPNs or "snurps") called U (for uridine) RNA that possess conserved "consensus" sequences complementary to those at each end of the intron. In the fevered grammar of molecular biology the complex of the several component pieces of U RNA with nuclear mRNA to form a self-splicing intron is called the spliceosome [7]. As RNA can cut, splice, and reassemble itself in the essential process of extirpating introns, RNA qualifies as a self-splicing enzyme [8].

Introns are not junk Introns are coded for by tRNA and rRNA genes, as well as by mRNA genes, and it is clear that the introns of DNA serve multiple functions. DNA introns code for spacing and controlling elements essential for the assembly of genes for proteins having repeating structures. Separate gene pieces (exons) also code for hydrophobic signal sequences that

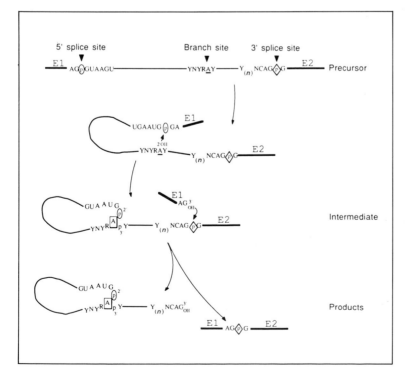

FIGURE 3-6

Mechanism for splicing of nuclear mRNA precursors. The two products of this three-stage reaction are the lariat-shaped introns that are excised and set free from the transcript (bottom left) and the spliced exons, E1 and E2, containing uninterrupted message (bottom right). The fate of the phosphate (p) moieties at the 5' and 3' splice sites is traced by circles and diamonds, respectively. Consensus base sequences are indicated at the splice sites and branch sites by the letters Y, R, and N. (From Sharp PA: Splicing of messenger RNA precursors. Science 235:766, 1987. Copyright 1987 by the AAAS.)

tag a molecule for export. Their transcribed mRNA exons code for useful portions of protein structure. mRNA introns code for turns, folds, or edges of secondary structure that enable peptide members defined by exons to be fitted together. Portions of excised introns possess RNA polymerase activity and are termed ribozymes.

Export of mature mRNA into cytoplasm Trimming and splicing pre-mRNA down to its mature size is accomplished within 20 minutes, and once divested of its introns, mature mRNA exits from the nucleus through "unplugged" pores in the nuclear membrane. Passage through the nuclear pores appears to require the aid of RNA splicing enzymes. Once past this barrier, mRNA is free to commingle with tRNA and ribosomes in the cytoplasm.

The Three-Letter Genetic Code

The first unambiguous evidence that protein sequences were translated from mRNA, and that amino acids were hooked together in useful order obediently by tRNA, stemmed from the demonstration by Nirenberg and Matthai that synthetic polyU coded specifically for phenylalanine. Knowing that there were 20 essential amino acids but only four bases, it had previously been surmised that groups of at least three characters (bases) would be required, groups of two (4^2) being inadequate for 20 amino acids. Completion of the code in 1966 revealed that, of the potential 64 permutations of four bases (4^3), all but three triplet codons specify individual amino acids (Table 3-1) [9]. The code in DNA, as replicated (Table 3-1) in mRNA, is an unpunctuated (commaless) triplet code in which each triplet is called a codon. The meaning (amino acid specification) of each codon is the same in all known organisms, a basis for the argument that life on earth evolved only once. As there are 61 codons for 20 amino acids, many amino acids have more than one codon and some have six. Different codons for a single amino acid are said to be "synonymous," and the redundancy built into the code is derogated as "degenerate," although the degeneracy signifies pleonasty not ambiguity, for codons are subject to a form of primogeniture.

T A B L E 3-1

The genetic code*

		Second position					
		U	C	A	G		
First position (5′ end)	U	UUU ⎤ Phe UUC ⎦ UUA ⎤ Leu UUG ⎦	UCU ⎤ UCC ⎥ Ser UCA ⎥ UCG ⎦	UAU ⎤ Tyr UAC ⎦ UAA Stop UAG Stop	UGU ⎤ Cys UGC ⎦ UGA Stop UGG Trp	U C A G	Third position (3′ end)
	C	CUU ⎤ CUC ⎥ Leu CUA ⎥ CUG ⎦	CCU ⎤ CCC ⎥ Pro CCA ⎥ CCG ⎦	CAU ⎤ His CAC ⎦ CAA ⎤ Gln CAG ⎦	CGU ⎤ CGC ⎥ Arg CGA ⎥ CGG ⎦	U C A G	
	A	AUU ⎤ AUC ⎥ Ile AUA ⎦ AUG Met	ACU ⎤ ACC ⎥ Thr ACA ⎥ ACG ⎦	AAU ⎤ Asn AAC ⎦ AAA ⎤ Lys AAG ⎦	AGU ⎤ Ser AGC ⎦ AGA ⎤ Arg AGG ⎦	U C A G	
	G	GUU ⎤ GUC ⎥ Val GUA ⎥ GUG ⎦	GCU ⎤ GCC ⎥ Ala GCA ⎥ GCG ⎦	GAU ⎤ Asp GAC ⎦ GAA ⎤ Glu GAG ⎦	GGU ⎤ GGC ⎥ Gly GGA ⎥ GGG ⎦	U C A G	

*Bases are given as ribonucleotides; hence U appears in the table instead of T.

Source: From Watson JD et al: Chapt 15, in Molecular Biology of the Gene, vol. 1, 4th ed. Menlo Park, The Benjamin/Cummings Publishing Company, Inc.,1987.

Start and stop codons; frameshifts   The start (initiator) codon AUG specifies methionine: all protein chains begin with this amino acid. Three codons do not specify amino acids but serve as stop signs: these are UAA, UAG, and UGA (Table 3-1). The code provides a precise linear array of ribonucleotides grouped in threes in mRNA, specifying an exact linear sequence of amino acids for each peptide and providing signals that order ribosomes to start and to stop synthesis of the peptide chain. This works so long as the message is dictated and read in register and is not interdicted by suppressor enzymes. If the start signal is shifted in either direction, the reading frame will code for wrong amino acids. Mutations leading to deletions or additions are called frameshifts, and these can cause the message to convey missense or nonsense. Deletion or nonsense of a start signal extinguishes expression or leads to synthesis of an unstable, truncated product, as occurs in some forms of β thalassemia. Deletion or missense of a subterminal stop signal may cause generation of an elongated "read-through" peptide (e.g., hemoglobin Wayne).

Translation

Two kinds of RNA—tRNA and rRNA—do not code for proteins themselves but partici-

pate in decoding the information carried by mRNA. Both are synthesized in the same manner as mRNA and both must be divested of introns to be diffusible and functional.

tRNA: The Adapter Molecule

The mRNA template functions like a track on which ribosomes move and attach to specified amino acids. Free amino acids can become entrained on growing peptide chains only when complexed to specific adapter molecules of tRNA. Molecules of tRNA are small, about 70 to 80 nucleotides long (M_r about 25,000); when viewed flattened-out they have a cloverleaf shape, but x-ray diffraction patterns reveal the tertiary structure of an L-shaped duplex (Figure 3-7) [10].

F I G U R E 3-7

Structure of tRNA. (Left) Cloverleaf diagrams reveal variations in folding patterns and in arrangement of specific bases (black circles) having identity elements for attaching to cognate aminoacyl synthetases. (Right) Tertiary structure of tRNA displays an amino acid attachment site at the 3′ end and an anticodon loop having complementarity for the corresponding mRNA codons. Numbers indicate positions of major recognition elements shown in the cloverleaf. (From Schulman LH and Abelson J: Recent excitement in understanding transfer RNA identity. Science 240:1591,1988. Copyright 1988 by the AAAS.)

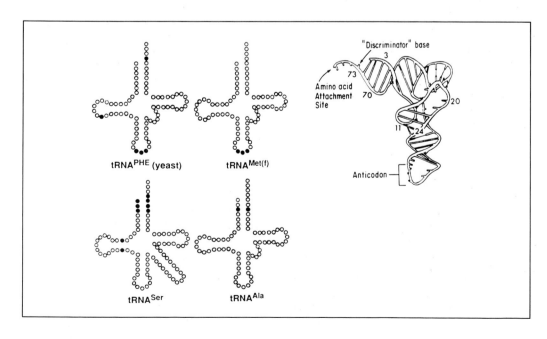

tRNA^{PHE} (yeast)   tRNA$^{Met(f)}$

tRNA^{Ser} tRNA^{Ala}

"Discriminator" base
3
73
Amino acid Attachment Site   70
20
11   24
Anticodon

Each tRNA molecule is specific for a single amino acid. Amino acids in turn are activated to high energy levels by exquisitely specific amino acid synthetases. Aminoacyl synthetases have two binding sites, one that recognizes a particular amino acid, and a second that identifies the codons for the same amino acid on mRNA, assuring high fidelity translation. The chemical linkage between an amino acid and tRNA (AA~tRNA) occurs by formation of a high-energy phosphate bond between the carboxyl group of the amino acid and the third carbon on the ribose ring of the terminal adenosine of tRNA. Thus one end of tRNA captures the correct activated amino acid and the other serves as a navigator which seeks out a docking site on mRNA that is reserved for that particular amino acid. As mRNA moves through or across ribosomes, the successive codons are introduced in an orderly single-file fashion to the conformationally correct AA~tRNA complexes.

Peptide Chain Formation Occurs on Ribosomes

After acquiring their adapters, activated amino acids soon encounter the correct mRNA codon on the surfaces of ribosomes. Ribosomes are very large spheroidal RNA-protein structures that are produced and packaged as subunits in the nucleolus and then are assembled in cytoplasm. All ribosomes are constructed from two subunits, the larger being about twice the size (60S) of the smaller (40S), forming a 70S hamburger-shaped device built from 78 proteins and two major classes of rRNA. Each 70S ribosome unit has two tRNA binding sites: a P (peptidyl) site, where the nascent peptide chain is held to the ribosome by a tRNA molecule, and an A (aminoacyl) site, where aminoacyl tRNAs interact in the process of codon recognition. In the presence of initiation factors (eIFs), translation commences through complementary binding of the methionine (UAC) anticodon aligned at the P site (Figure 3-8) [5]. Once the lead tRNA molecules enter the P cavity, peptide bonds form in faithful compliance with instructions by mRNA codons. Peptide chain elongation then cranks forward by serial, unidirectional, triplet translocation, governed by a complex of enzymes and cofactors.

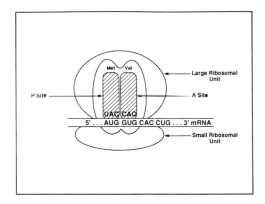

FIGURE 3-8

tRNA binding sites on a ribosome in the act of initiating translation of mRNA for a human β globin chain. The initiator methionine tRNA (UAC) anticodon is aligned at the P site with the AUG start codon. The first codon in the mRNA for human β globin, GUG, is recognized by a valine tRNA through complementary interactions with its anticodon, CAC. (Revised from Nienhuis WE and Maniatis T: Chapt 2, in The Molecular Basis of Blood Diseases, Stamatoyannopoulos G et al, Eds. Philadelphia, WB Saunders Company,1987.)

Polysomes are assembly lines   The segment of an mRNA strand that is in contact with a single ribosome is short, allowing a given mRNA transcript to move over the surfaces of several ribosomes and to serve as a template for several identical lengths of peptide chains simultaneously. A collection of ribosomes bound to a single mRNA chain is called a polyribosome or polysome. The polysomes that make globin chains consist of 5 ± 1 ribosomes. At any given time the lengths of peptide chains attached to successive ribosomes in the polysome vary in proportion to the fraction of the messenger tape each ribosome has already read [11].

The Flow of Information: Redux

The flow of information from gene to polypeptide involves four major sequential steps beginning with the decoding of DNA, as just described. These are reprised, using hemoglobin synthesis as the example [5], in Figure 3-9.

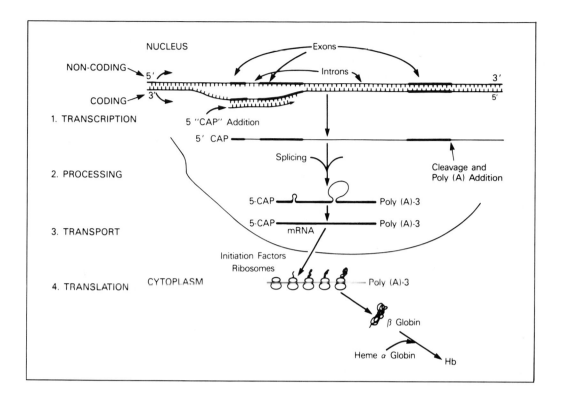

Overview of steps required for gene expression, as exemplified by synthesis of hemoglobin. (From Nienhuis WE and Maniatis T: Chapt 2 in The Molecular Basis of Blood Diseases, Stamatoyannopoulos G et al, Eds. Philadelphia, WB Saunders Company, 1987.)

HEMOGLOBIN BIOSYNTHESIS

Synthesis of hemoglobin (Hb) involves collaboration between two very different biosynthetic pathways. One, synthesis of globin chains, is carried out by cytoplasmic ribosomes. The other, protoheme synthesis, requires extensive participation by mitochondria. Malfunction of either pathway has dire but very different consequences. Errors or failures of globin chain synthesis are responsible for hemoglobinopathies and thalassemias; faulty heme synthesis underlies a colorful array of maladies ranging from porphyrias to sideroblastic anemias.

Hb is a Double Dimer

Normal Hb tetramers are formed by the interlocking of two α-like peptide chains with two β-like chains. During embryonic life two α-like ζ chains unite with two β-like ϵ chains. By combining with α and γ chains these peptides form three kinds of embryonic Hb: Hb Gower I ($\zeta_2\epsilon_2$), Hb Gower II ($\alpha_2\epsilon_2$), and Hb Portland ($\zeta_2\gamma_2$). By the tenth week of gestation, production of ζ and ϵ chains ceases and is superseded by synthesis of γ chains, which combine with α chains to form Hb F, the predominant Hb of fetal life. During the neonatal period γ chain synthesis is repressed and replaced by synthesis of β chains, a transition governed by a pivotal mechanism called the γ to β switch. After the first year of life Hb is a mixture unevenly distributed among red cells composed of 97% Hb A ($\alpha_2\beta_2$), 2 to 3% Hb A$_2$ ($\alpha_2\delta_2$), and less than 1% Hb F ($\alpha_2\gamma_2$).

Chromosomal Organization of Hb Genes

The principal Hb genes reside on different chromosomes. α genes are located on the short arm of chromosome 16, whereas the mixed family of non-α (β-like) genes is broadly distributed distally on the short arm of chromosome 11 beyond band p14. A noteworthy feature of α genes is that the gene loci are duplicated on each chromosome 16 and denoted $\alpha 1$ and $\alpha 2$. The peptides coded for by γ chain genes differ only in a single amino acid (glycine or alanine)—hence the $^G\gamma$ and $^A\gamma$ designation for the two genes; accordingly, γ chain genes are in effect duplicated on chromosome 11. An ontogenic feature of interest is that the human non-α and α globin gene clusters are arrayed on their chromosomes in the same $5' \rightarrow 3'$ order that they are expressed developmentally:

$\epsilon \rightarrow \gamma \rightarrow \delta \rightarrow \beta$ and $\zeta \rightarrow \alpha$, respectively. Interspersed between these functioning genes are four functionless genelike loci that may represent evolutionary relics of harmless gene duplication events; these "pseudogenes" are designated by the prefixed symbol ψ. The organization of α-like and β-like genes on chromosomes 16 and 11 is shown in Figure 3-10 [12].

Globin genes contain three exons and two introns Coding regions of globin genes in people and animals are interrupted by only two intervening sequences, which are purged from initial transcripts by the excision and splicing mechanisms just described. The central exons of the various globin genes appear to code for the major heme-binding structures and the side exons code for stabilizing elements. The fate of the excised introns and the enzymatic potential of the lariat-shaped spliceosome are not well understood. A summary account of the expression of the β globin gene is schematized in Figure 3-11 [13].

Globin Structure

The predominant Hb of adults, Hb A, is formed by the snug fitting together of two identical α chains and two identical β chains. Each α chain possesses 141 amino acids and each β chain has 146 residues, so that the $\alpha_2\beta_2$ ($\alpha^A_2\beta^A_2$) tetramer has a total amino acid con-

FIGURE 3-10

Chromosome location, reading 5' to 3', of human globin genes, and the hemoglobins produced, in each stage of development. Interrupted lines near the top indicate several of the potential globin dimer pairings. (From Schechter AN et al: Genetic, cellular and clinical aspects of the regulation of fetal hemoglobin production, in Hematology—1987. The Education Program of the American Society of Hematology, McArthur JR and Fienstein DI, Eds. Washington, DC, American Society of Hematology,1987.)

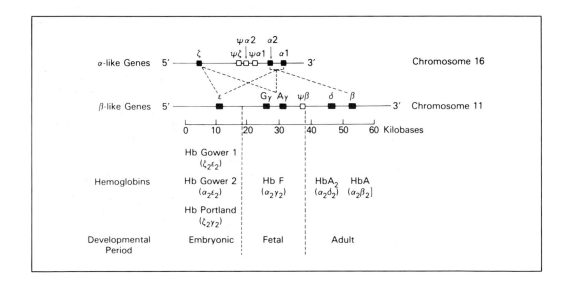

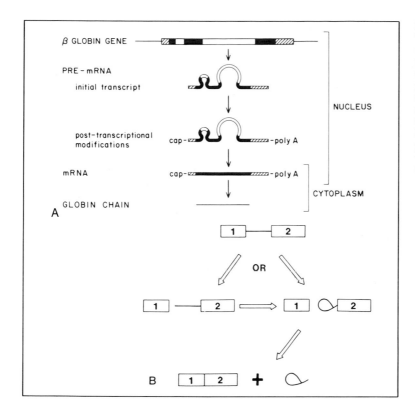

FIGURE 3-11

(A) Schematic representation of β globin gene expression. (B) Proposed fate of introns 1 and 2. (From Ruskin B et al: Excision of an intact intron as a novel lariat structure during pre-mRNA splicing in vitro. Cell 38:317,1984. © Cell Press.)

tent of 574 (M_r: 64,400). X-ray crystallographic studies reveal that each polypeptide possesses seven or eight reflexed α-helical structures that enable the tetramer to fold into a compact ellipsoid about 5 nm in diameter. There is a total of 80 amino acid differences between α and β chains, which confers an unsymmetric three-dimensional shape to the Hb tetramer. The intact tetramer has a twofold axis of symmetry that runs through the water-filled cavity at the center of the molecule. The different regions of the peptide backbone display a nearly symmetric orientation, and therefore if any dimer of globin chains is rotated 180° on the axis it will confront a homologous dimer. Isologous pairings are very weak, and paired protomers barely touch each other; for steric reasons α and β chains pair off into $\alpha\beta$ dimers, the functional subunits of this O_2 transporting protein (Figure 3-12) [14].

Heme Synthesis

The prosthetic (O_2-binding) group of Hb is heme (ferroprotoporphyrin IX), a planar mole-

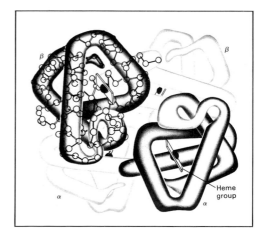

FIGURE 3-12

Compact conformations assumed by the two α and two β chains in a Hb tetramer. The $\alpha\beta$ dimer in front is darkened for sterographic effect, the carbon and nitrogen backbone of the β chain at the upper left is exposed, and the approximate positions of the four planar heme groups are depicted. (From Darnell J et al: Chapt 3, in Molecular Cell Biology. New York, Scientific American Books,1986.)

cule consisting of four pyrrole rings arranged concentrically around a single ferrous ion (Figure 3-13) [15]. Heme synthesis, the most universal of all biosynthetic processes, takes place in eight steps. The initial rate-limiting reaction and the last three steps are catalyzed by mitochondrial enzymes, whereas four intermediate reactions occur in the cytosol. This segregation of the middle steps in heme synthesis from the first and final steps in the mitochondrion ensures strict feedback control. The sequence of the reactions culminating in synthesis of heme, starting with the rate-limiting exergonic reactions leading to formation of δ-aminolevulinic acid (ALA), are summarized in Figure 3-14 [16].

FIGURE 3-13

(A) Structure of heme. (B) Tinker toy view of heme having the same orientation as in A. Atoms are shown as spheres proportional to their size: Fe>>O>N>C>>H. (From Bunn HF and Forget BG: Chapt 2, in Hemoglobin: Molecular, Genetic and Clinical Aspects. Philadelphia, WB Saunders Company,1986.)

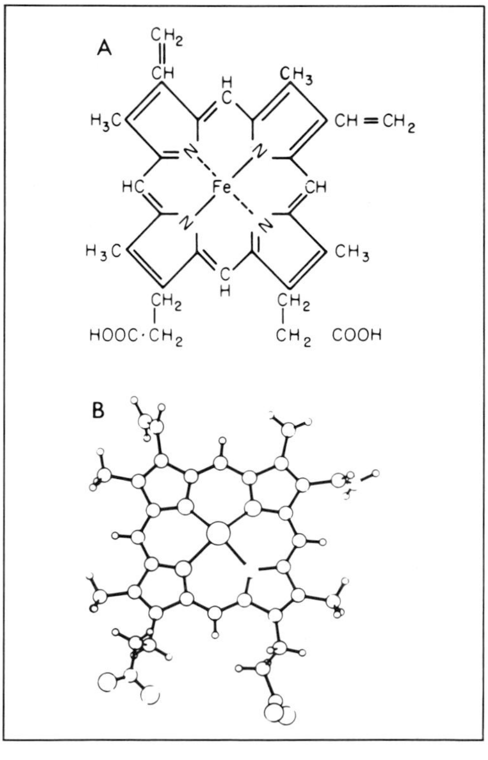

FIGURE 3-14 ▶

The heme biosynthetic pathway. (From Meyer UA and Schmid R: Chapt 50, in Metabolic Basis of Inherited Diseases, 4th ed., Stanbury JE et al, Eds. New York, McGraw-Hill Book Company,1978.)

End-Product Regulation of Hemoglobin Synthesis

Synthesis of heme is self-regulated, but only indirectly through end-product feedback inhibition of both ALA synthesis and incorporation of iron into protoporphyrin IX to form heme. Although free heme participates in regulating its own synthesis in erythroid cells and also stimulates formation of globin, heme synthesis in people (as opposed to rodents) is governed principally by one or more rate-limiting steps that lead to formation of ALA, the first committed precursor in the porphyrin biosynthetic sequence. In addition, subsidiary mechanisms regulate uptake of iron from transferrin and its incorporation by protoporphyrin IX (Chapter 4), assuring that neither excess iron nor a toxic surplus of porphyrin intermediates accumulates. It also appears that accumulations of free α chains and $\alpha\beta$ dimers depress globin chain synthesis, an inhibition evident in iron-starved, heme-depleted erythroid cells. Coordination of heme and globin chain synthesis is so important a matter, and so in keeping with nature's parsimony, that both synthetic processes must be subject to strict feedback controls operating in tandem.

Subunit Assembly: Social Behavior of Hemoglobin Monomers

Efficient biosynthesis of Hb requires balanced production on ribosomes of α and β polypeptide chains. Concurrently heme must be synthesized by mitochondria at a rate sufficient to provide each fresh copy of a globin chain with its prosthetic group. Heme is inserted into its proper niche in globin chains immediately after their emergence. On binding of heme the globin chain folds into its destined 3-D structure, and after encounters of several kinds the functional $\alpha_2\beta_2$ tetramer is formed (Figure 3-15) [17].

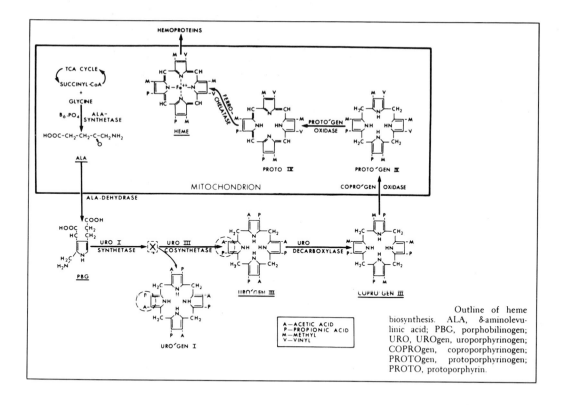

Outline of heme biosynthesis. ALA, δ-aminolevulinic acid; PBG, porphobilinogen; URO, UROgen, uroporphyrinogen; COPROgen, coproporphyrinogen; PROTOgen, protoporphyrinogen; PROTO, protoporphyrin.

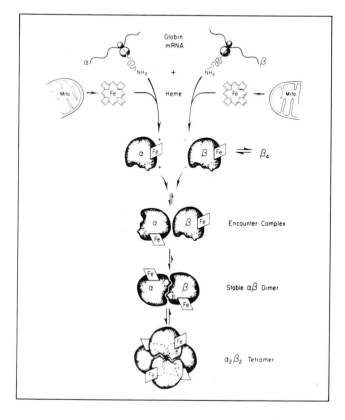

FIGURE 3-15

Assembly of hemoglobin. On binding heme, the completed, unlike globin chains are attracted to each other, form encounter complexes, and then embrace as stable $\alpha\beta$ dimers, precursors of the Hb tetramer. (From Bunn HF: Subunit assembly of hemoglobin: an important determinant of hematologic phenotype. Blood 69:1,1987.)

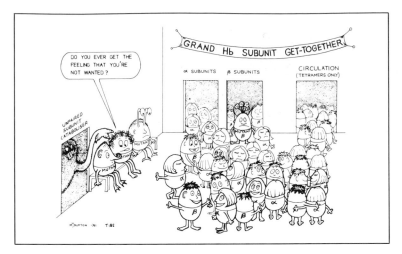

FIGURE 3-16

Social behavior of Hb subunits. (From Schaeffer JR et al: Assembly of normal and abnormal human hemoglobins. Trends Biochem Sci 6:158, 1981.)

Variant subunits may be slow to assemble   In β thalassemia and in heme deficiency states levels of different globin chains may not reach parity, and unpaired α chains may form injurious aggregates subject to proteolysis. As electrostatic attraction excites α and β chains to pair off, mutant chains in patients heterozygous for hemoglobinopathic genes may be slower or faster than normal chains to form dimers and tetramers. Usually, normal α and β chains socialize more rapidly than abnormal chains, and unpaired mutant chains will experience the fate of the unrequited (Figure 3-16) [18].

DECODING THE METHODS OF MOLECULAR GENETICS

The many methods of molecular genetics have simple origins but when used in exotic combinations these have generated a level of arcane complexity that is both wonderful and intimidating. The first insights stemmed directly from the now familiar workings of the deus ex machina of biology, DNA.

Molecular Hybridization: Exploitation of Base Pairing Specificity

Specific base pairing that underlies the flow of genetic information within cells and between generations can be exploited in detecting and isolating genes and in characterizing RNA transcripts and their expressed proteins. As each strand of DNA or RNA will form a double-stranded structure only with DNA or RNA having complementary base sequences, obedient to the base pairing rules discussed earlier, a known DNA or RNA molecule can be used as a hook for fishing out complementary strands from cellular extracts containing mixtures of many sequences. Since reticulocytes are devoid of DNA and rich in mRNAs that code for globin chains, globin mRNAs were the first mammalian messengers to be used as gene probes. Incubation of globin mRNA with RNA-dependent DNA polymerase (reverse transcriptase) in a mixture of nucleotides yields a purified preparation of complementary DNA (cDNA) molecules capable, after RNA templates are removed, of hybridizing only to globin gene DNA or globin mRNA.

As most DNA exists as double-stranded DNA it must be denatured ("melted") into single strands by heating under appropriate conditions and then mixed with a denatured radioactive probe. As the denaturing conditions are relieved, the single strands anneal to form radioactive double-stranded hybrids (of DNA-DNA or DNA-RNA) of those DNA or RNA molecules in the mixture that have sufficient complementarity.

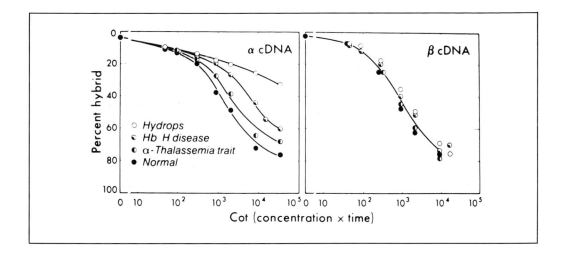

FIGURE 3-17

Molecular hybridization of DNA from individuals with α thalassemia syndromes of various levels of severity, as compared with normal (black circles). The extent of hybridization to α globin cDNA is indicative of four α gene deletions in hydrops fetalis, three in Hb H disease, and two in homozygous α thalassemia trait (white circles). In contrast, hybridization of β chain cDNA (right panel) is normal in all patients. (From Kan YW: The Harvey Lectures, Series 76. New York, Academic Press,1982.)

A common method of detecting complementarity is to attach cDNA to a solid matrix of nitrocellulose paper, which for some reason binds single-stranded DNA tightly. Radioactive RNA or DNA in a test mixture is then added, after which unhybridized strands are washed away. RNA or DNA hybridized to membrane-bound cDNA is resistant to digestion by nucleases; thus any remnants of unhybridized nucleic acid can be trimmed away. By this technique one specific complementary sequence can be removed from complex mixtures containing 10^6 kinds of irrelevant DNA.

Quantitative gene analysis by molecular hybridization The reassociation rate for any DNA sample can be used to quantitate the number of copies of a given gene by ranging the initial concentration of cDNA and the time of reassociation. This strategem was employed by Kan and co-workers to establish that each strand of DNA from chromosome 16 has two α gene loci, and hence diploid DNA could suffer one, two, three, or four deletions (Figure 3-17) [19].

Analysis of Gene Structure

Before plunging deeper into the mysterious waters of molecular biology the reader may wish to refer to a glossary (Table 3-2) [20]. The three general techniques for analyzing gene structure are restriction endonuclease mapping, molecular cloning, and DNA sequencing. The most versatile weapon in the arsenal of recombinant technology is use of unique prokaryotic restriction enzymes known as restriction endonucleases.

Restriction Endonuclease Mapping

Restriction endonucleases are bacterial enzymes that protect bacteria from invasion by restricting foreign DNA. Each of the several hundred known enzymes recognizes specific short oligonucleotides on foreign DNA and cleaves it at specific "restriction sites." Corresponding sequences in the bacterial genome are camouflaged by methylation, but any foreign DNA (such as a globin gene) is promptly recognized by the nuclease and both strands of

TABLE 3-2

Terms used in recombinant technology and molecular cloning

Genomic DNA	All DNA sequences of an organism
cDNA (complementary DNA)	DNA copied from an mRNA molecule
Plasmid	An extrachromosomal small circular DNA molecule capable of reproducing independently in a host cell
Vector	A plasmid or a viral DNA molecule into which either a cDNA sequence or a genomic DNA sequence is inserted
Host cell	A cell (usually a bacterium) in which a vector can be propagated
Genomic clone	A selected host cell with a vector containing a fragment of genomic DNA from a different organism
cDNA clone	A selected host cell with a vector containing a cDNA molecule from another organism
Library	A complete set of genomic clones from an organism, or of cDNA clones from one cell type

Source: From Darnell J et al: Chapt 7, in Molecular Cell Biology. New York, Scientific American Books,1986.

its intrusive DNA helix are cut (Figure 3-18) [21]. Staggered cuts (see the *Eco* RI and *Hin* dIII cleavages in Figure 3-18) create cohesive ends that predispose to form circular DNA by the self-annealing of complementary base pairs under the tutelage of DNA ligase. Combined use of restriction enzymes and DNA ligase has made it possible to graft inserts of any DNA to create hybrid plasmids capable of reproduction and clonal amplification.

Southern blotting   The 3×10^9 base pairs of the genome contain about 1 million recognition sites for the restriction endonuclease *Eco* RI, and digestion of only 10×10^6 cells would yield a messy mixture of at least 1 million fragments of differing lengths. Technology for identifying DNA fragments was devised by a resourceful Scot, E.M. Southern, and thus is known as Southern blotting. After digestion of a DNA population with one or several restriction enzymes, the resulting fragments are separated according to size by electrophoresis on gels and are transferred to a nitrocellulose or nylon membrane. The membrane is then incubated under annealing conditions with a radioactive probe sequence specific for the gene of interest. After hybrid-

ization is complete, x-ray film is exposed to the membrane filter, resulting in an autoradiographic copy. The position and number of radioactive bands on multiple autoradiographs thus generated can be used to deduce the presence and molecular size of DNA fragments containing a specific gene. Figure 3-19 shows an idealized Southern blot of human DNA digested with *Eco* RI and annealed to a mixed $(\alpha + \beta)$ cDNA probe derived by reverse transcription of reticulocyte mRNA [22]. The β gene of the normal individual (specified as NI in Figure 3-19) is split into two fragments of 4.2 and 3.6 M_r because of an intragenic *Eco* RI site. Analysis of DNA from an infant with severe α thalassemia reveals absence of any α globin genes.

Molecular Cloning: Imitation of Life

Molecular cloning enables one to harvest milligram quantities of DNA that contain the sequence of only a single gene or part of a gene. Purification of genes is accomplished by recombining restriction-generated fragments of DNA with an appropriately cleaved vector by enzymatic ligation. Numerous vectors capable

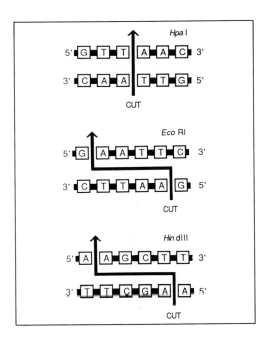

FIGURE 3-18

DNA nucleotide sequences recognized by three commonly used restriction nucleases. As in these examples such sequences are often 6 base pairs long and palindromic. The strand cuts at or near the recognition sequence are often staggered, leaving short, sticky, single-stranded ends. (From Alberts B: Chapt 4, in Molecular Biology of the Cell. New York, Garland Publishing, Inc.,1983.)

of replication in a host bacterium have been exploited, among them bacteriophages, plasmids, or combinations of the two known as cosmids. Amplification is achieved either by multiplication of the transformed bacteria when the vector used is a cosmid or plasmid, or by repetitive cycles of infection and proteolysis if the vector is a bacteriophage.

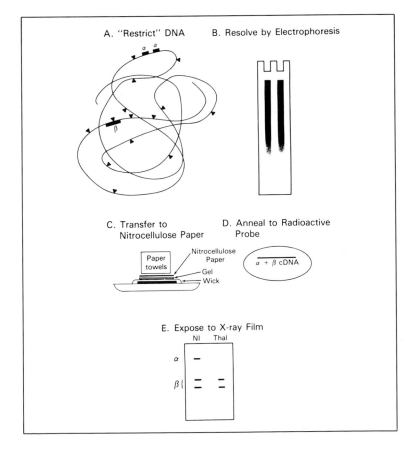

FIGURE 3-19

Southern blotting method of analyzing DNA. This simplified scheme outlines the study of human globin genes in a normal individual (NI) and in a fetus with hydrops fetalis caused by severe α thalassemia (Thal). (From Rowley PT et al: Chapt 1, in Current Hematology and Oncology, vol. 4, Fairbanks VF, Ed. Chicago, Year Book Medical Publishers, Inc.,1986.)

Gene libraries   Gene libraries provide the data-bases for recombinant DNA research; they also are subject to all of the finicky features and hassles of medical libraries, requiring systems for acquisition, cataloging, filing, indexing, searching, and retrieval. Gene libraries can be constructed from genomic cloning or from cDNA cloning. A genomic clone is a cultured host cell containing fragments of genomic DNA after it has been cleaved with restriction enzymes; a cDNA clone is a cultured host cell containing molecules of complementary DNA copied from mRNA.

Bacteriophage λ is widely used in constructing genomic libraries, and, thanks to the fine art of recombinant technology, construction of a 250,000-particle λ library of the entire human genome has become a practical matter. To prepare a genomic library, extracted DNA is broken into fragments by a restriction enzyme such as *Eco* RI which cleaves it in a way that produces short, single-stranded, sticky ends (5'-AA-TT-3', or its reverse) on every fragment [21]. Digestion is not carried to completion but is stopped when the average fragment size is whittled down to about 25 kb plus the two

flanking ends or arms. These fragments are then admixed with a similar number of λ arms having similarly sticky ends as the result of digestion of the bacteriophage by the same (*Eco* RI) enzyme. DNA ligase is used to seal the recombinant molecules, and recombinant DNA is then coated with bacteriophage proteins prepared from infected cells. If DNA fragments are of the correct size, the packaged λ bacteriophages are fully infectious for host cells such as *E. coli*. Entry of the packaged recombinant into *E. coli* or other bacteria susceptible to phage infection is a Trojan horse ruse. The phage-infected bacterial suspension is diluted in a rich medium favoring replication, and as the bacteria divide the plasmids also replicate to produce millions of copies of the original DNA fragment. Plasmids further engineered to contain information necessary for resistance to an antibiotic will flourish in cultures containing antibiotic, whereas bacteria uninfected by the resistant recombinant plasmid vector will die off, facilitating harvest of highly amplified clonal genes. In time a "lawn" is formed of bacterial plaques imprisoned in agar. Plaques containing the desired gene insert can then be identified by

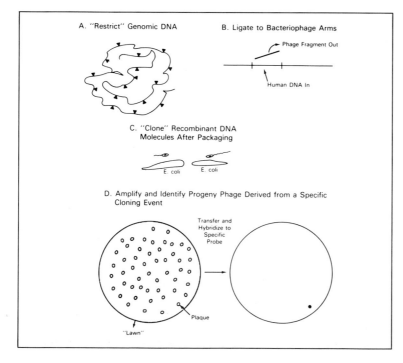

FIGURE 3-20

Outline of methods used in creating a library of DNA fragments in the form of recombinant bacteriophage clones in *Escherichia coli*. (From Rowley PT et al: Chapt 1, in Current Hematology and Oncology, vol. 4, Fairbanks VF, Ed. Chicago, Year Book Medical Publishers, Inc.,1986.)

molecular hybridization and autoradiography by using a sequence-specific radioactive probe (Figure 3-20) [22].

Searching gene libraries   To search a library of cloned genes without a marker or directory is like searching for a book in the National Library of Medicine without a catalog, by strolling through its corridors. A radioactive probe complementary to some portion of the sought gene provides a marker for searching the clone library, employing adaptations of Southern blot methodology. For an unknown gene, a restriction enzyme map of the DNA region containing the gene can be constructed by analysis of overlapping recombinant clones, each of which contains the gene of interest [22]. If no gene-specific nucleic acid probe is available, a vector can be utilized that is capable of directing synthesis (in "expression strains" of bacteria) of the protein product of the pursued gene; an antibody with specificity for the protein product can then be used to probe for the phage plaque containing the corresponding gene. Thus it is feasible to shuttle back and forth between the two languages—that of nucleotides and that of proteins—in perusing libraries and probing genomes.

DNA Sequencing

To sequence DNA by the Maxam-Gilbert method, cloned fragments are labeled at one end (usually 5') with ^{35}S or ^{32}P, and then the samples are exposed to four different chemical procedures designed to break the fragments only at A, G, C plus T, and C residues, respectively. Labeled subfragments created by these reactions all have the isotope label at one end and the cleavage point at the other. After gel electrophoresis and autoradiography, the four sets of labeled subfragments collectively yield one radioactive band for each nucleotide in the original fragment (Figure 3-21) [20]. In an alternative method originated by Sanger, DNA fragments that terminate at a specific base are produced by adding on a base-specific inhibitor during the degradative process. Both methods generate families of fragments differing in length by only a single nucleotide, a difference sufficient for them to be separable

F I G U R E 3-21

DNA sequencing by partial chemical degradation, as devised by Maxam and Gilbert. (Modified from Darnell J et al: Chapt 7, in Molecular Cell Biology. New York, Scientific American Books,1986.)

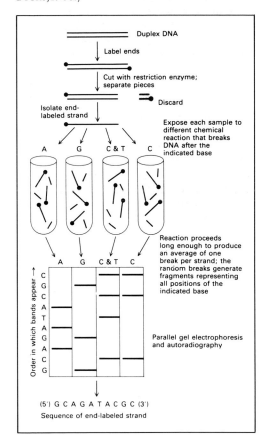

on polyacrylamide gel lanes into autoradiographic sequence ladders (Figure 3-21) from which the base sequence of the end labeled strands can be read.

Polymerase chain reaction   Analysis of specific nucleotide sequences has been facilitated enormously by a recently devised, powerful amplification method known as polymerase chain reaction (PCR). This technique is capable of enriching a specific DNA sequence by a factor of 10^9 within a day or two, permitting analysis of DNA from individual cells. PCR has been an extraordinarily effective tool for high-efficiency cloning of gene sequences, identification of point mutations, and for direct sequencing of mitochondrial and viral DNA. It has opened the way to numerous nonmedical applications, ranging from resurrecting the DNA of extinct species such as the wooly mammoth to forensic use in identifying or exonerating suspects and establishing parenthood. This power to analyze DNA in miniscule samples of hair, blood, or semen left at scenes of violent crimes has proved an enormous boon to forensic medicine.

In the PCR, DNA segments as small as 50 kb or as large as 6,000 kb in length can be amplified exponentially starting from as little as a single gene copy. In this technique, double-stranded DNA is denatured by heat and the separated chains are incubated with two oligonucleotide primers that anneal through complementarity to the opposite ends of the target segment; these primers direct DNA polymerase-dependent synthesis of new complementary strands, doubling the amount of target sequence. As each subsequent amplification step requires a new cycle of heat denaturation, a crucial feature of PCR is exploitation of a heat-stable DNA polymerase derived from *Thermus aquaticus,* a bacterium that thrives in hot springs having temperatures ranging from 70°C to nearly the boiling point. Each cycle is controlled by cyclically varying the temperature to permit denaturation of DNA strands, annealing of the primers, and doubling of DNA [23]. Typically each cycle requires 1 min at 95°C to denature double-stranded DNA, 2 min at 37°C for the primers to anneal their targeted sequence, and 4 min at 70°C for extension of the new DNA strands (Figure 3-22) [24]. By use of automated thermal cyclers, quantities sufficient for nucleotide sequencing can be analyzed for sequence variants by use of allele-specific oligonucleotide probes and for single nucleotide substitutions by means of oligonucleotide ligation assays. This is particularly useful in performing rapid-readout prenatal diagnosis of genetic disorders.

Sequencing the entire genome: The Holy Grail of biology   Recent refinements have made possible colorimetric and isotopic readout systems that permit automated sequencing.

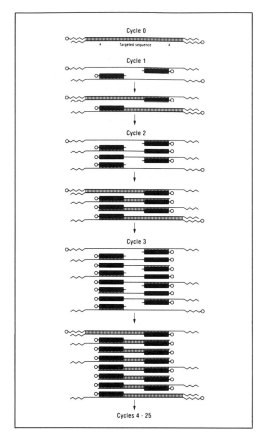

FIGURE 3-22

Polymerase chain reaction. After double-stranded DNA is heated, the separated chains are allowed to bind to primers (black bars) that define the ends of the targeted sequence. The primers in the presence of heat-stable polymerase then initiate synthesis of two replicate chains complementary to the originals. This series of events can be repeated 20 to 30 times, doubling the DNA with each cycle. (From Marx JL: Multiplying genes by leaps and bounds. Science 240:1408,1988. Copyright 1988 by the AAAS.)

Use of alternating pulsed electric fields has also facilitated rapid analysis and separation of much larger fragments, as has the use of yeast artificial chromosomes (YACs). Another order of technical expedition may be attained by improvements in high-speed chromosome sorting.

DNA hybridization techniques can be used to pick out clones from gene libraries that have overlapping sequences, enabling sequence analysis of very large stretches, in what is called overlap hybridization, or "chromosome walking." Complete linking up of fragments from whole chromosomes by chromosome "hopping" is hindered in higher animals by the large numbers of nearly identical repetitive sequences flanking many genes. Nonetheless, the manifest destiny of the increasingly imperialistic world of molecular biology is to map and sequence the entire 100,000-plus genes of the genome. Sequencing the entire dictionary of 3 billion base pairs in the human genome will require imaginative development and coordination of automatic high-speed sequencing and amplification technologies.

Analysis of Gene Expression

Northern Blotting

Analysis of the proximal product of gene expression, RNA, is performed by the northern blotting method—so named through fanciful play on the term Southern blotting. To obtain a northern blot an RNA extract is resolved into molecules of different size in an agarose gel under denaturing conditions; RNA fragments are then immobilized on a membrane filter and subjected to radiographic gene probe analysis. Northern blot analysis is a relatively low-resolution technique used in screening for major alterations in the size and number of RNA transcripts.

S₁ nuclease mapping S_1 nuclease protection mapping provides very precise information by defining the exact position of splice junctions created by removal of introns during RNA processing. Radiolabeled DNA molecules are incubated with an RNA preparation under conditions designed to favor RNA-DNA duplex formation. Annealed molecules are exposed to S_1 nuclease, an enzyme that degrades single-stranded DNA but spares DNA duplexed to RNA. S_1 nuclease protection mapping is particularly serviceable in probing for

errors in splicing, errors that are commonly responsible for variant forms of β thalassemia.

Diagnostic Applications: A Brief Inventory

Recombinant molecular probes can be used for diagnosis and classification of genetic diseases, for antenatal prediction, and for family counselling.

Linkage Methods: RFLPs

Genes located on the same chromosome are transmitted together unless relevant segments of chromosomes are exchanged during the first meiotic division (Chapter 2). The probability that two genes will be transmitted together is an indirect function of the intergene distance and of the number of crossings over. Most linkage studies involve analysis of two common markers (e.g., Rh expression and elliptocytosis) or of a common gene with a rare genetic disease (e.g., ABO expression and adenylate kinase deficiency). The ideal family for linkage studies is an extended pedigree with many matings and swarms of offspring. The application of linkage analysis has been enhanced enormously for less sprawling kindred by assays for restriction fragment length polymorphisms (RFLPs). This method relies on the fact that RFLPs represent naturally occurring neutral variations in DNA lengths that are inherited as codominant traits. In parents who are heterozygous for a restriction site, a given enzyme digest of their DNA will yield specific fragments differing in length. These fragment length polymorphisms serve as classic mendelian markers, as shown in Figure 3-23 [25].

RFLPs have no effect on gene function, but when restriction sites are tightly linked to a mutant gene, they serve as excellent gene markers. As an example, 80% of people of Mediterranean ancestry have a sequence 3' from the β globin gene that is recognizable by *Bam* HI, and 20% do not. In a hypothetical family in which the mother has a thalassemia gene in propinquity to a site for *Hin* dIII on one chromosome (and lacks the site on the homologous chromosome), and the father has a *Bam* HI site on the same chromosome as a thalassemia gene (and lacks that site on the

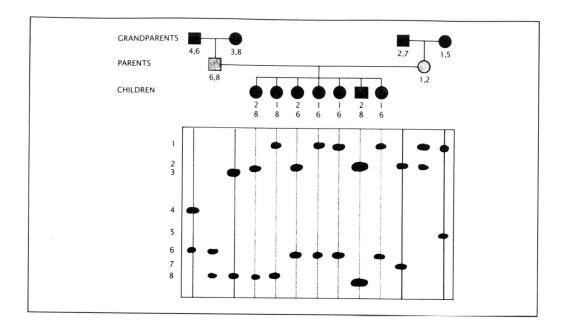

Inheritance of an RFLP can be traced by comparing restriction fragments from blood relatives up and down the family tree. Each individual in this pedigree carries two different alleles of the marker, one from each homologous chromosome. In this example the seven children have inherited either a "size 1 or 2" allelic fragment from the mother and either a "size 6 or 8" allelic fragment from the father, as revealed on Southern blotting. If a particular allele of the RFLP is consistently associated with a genetic disease in an afflicted family, the marker and the gene may be linked. (From White R and Lalouel J-M: Chromosome mapping with DNA markers. Sci Am 258(2):40,1988. Copyright © 1988 by Scientific American, Inc. All rights reserved.)

analysis of the full haplotype for RFLPs yields accurate prenatal diagnosis in almost 100% of cases. In general DNA analysis of parents and grandparents, as well as of siblings, is necessary for adequately tracking the inheritance patterns of mutant genes linked to RFLPs.

Direct Analysis of Globin Genes

If a mutation results in creation or loss of a known restriction enzyme cleavage site, a straightforward Southern blot analysis will distinguish affected individuals. In the sickle cell anemia gene the single nucleotide mutation (substitution) responsible for the $\beta^{6glu\rightarrow val}$ change alters the site for DNA cleavage by the enzymes *Dde* I and *Mst* II. When DNA is cleaved by *Mst* II the nucleotide substitution in the sickle gene renders the region coding for the 5, 6, and 7 residues of β chains resistant to cleavage, resulting in an abnormally large restriction fragment (Figure 3-25) [26].

Synthetic oligonucleotide probe analysis Most point mutations and small deletions do not alter any restriction endonuclease cleavage sites. Synthesis of short oligonucleotide probes have been fashioned to be complementary to known mutant sequences. A 19-nucleotide

homologous chromosome), the offspring may have any of four potential genotypes (Figure 3-24) [22]. DNA for RFLP signatures can be obtained from white blood cells, skin cells, desquamated amniotic fluid cells procured by amniocentesis, or fetal cells isolated from chorionic tissue by cell sorting. DNA of these cells is then subjected to restriction enzyme digestion, Southern blotting, and when necessary PCR amplification. Combined analysis of restriction sites with *Bam* HI plus *Hin* dIII provides a correct prenatal diagnosis in thalassemia families in over 75% of cases;

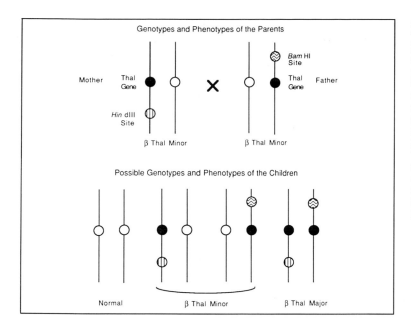

FIGURE 3-24

Restriction endonuclease sites as markers for prenatal diagnosis of β thalassemia major (right), thalassemia minor (center), and normal β globin genes (left). (Modified from Rowley PT et al: Chapt 1, in Current Hematology and Oncology, vol. 4, Fairbanks VF, Ed. Chicago, Year Book Medical Publishers, Inc.,1986.)

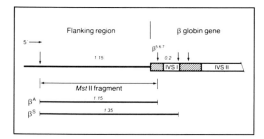

FIGURE 3-25

Direct restriction enzyme method for detection of the sickle mutation. Downward arrows point to *Mst* II sites, including one corresponding to β chain positions 5, 6, and 7. Using a radioactive normal *Mst* II fragment as probe, the expected 1.15 kb fragment is found in normal β^A genes, whereas a 1.35 kb fragment indicates the presence of a sickle (β^s) gene. (From Chang JC and Kan YW: A sensitive new prenatal test for sickle-cell anemia. Reprinted, by permission of the New England Journal of Medicine, 307:30,1982.)

complementary sequence has been designed that hybridizes specifically with the sickle gene locus. Similar synthetic designer probes of 20 to 25 base pair lengths are now available for diagnosing the Hb C gene and the most common of the β thalassemia genes. Systems have been developed for preparing highly sensitive nonradioactive probes that are covalently linked to a fluorescent molecule or enzyme. Fluorescent probes are simpler, safer, and so stable they can be stored in large quantities.

Stones, Bones, and Clones

Creation of the many forms of life has occurred in multitudinous steps. Retracing these steps has depended until recently on relatively crude studies of fossil relics of life after slow mineralization had turned remains of living matter into stone. Unfortunately petrification destroys most organic matter and provides no clues as to the early stages of evolution. Molecular fossils, on the other hand, provide a coherent reading of primordial events, and the number of accumulated mutations in a gene encoding a highly conserved protein (or its DNA or RNA) is a measure of evolutionary distance. Evolutionary (phylogenetic) trees can be established by accepting as an article of faith the principle of parsimony—the reasonable and economic view that contemporary sequences represent the smallest number of base pair changes in the corresponding DNA of ancestral sequences. Relatedness between various globin genes, for example, can be assessed by the number of nucleotide differences between genes, provided the genes counted differ by silent substitutions—mutations that do not alter the amino acid encoded. Strictly speaking, the principle of parsimony can only establish the branching pattern of the phylogenetic tree; to convert evolutionary sequence distances into chronologic differences, it is necessary to accept the notion of a molecular clock.

The molecular clock versus the Darwinians   For decades, heated debate has raged between neutralists, who hold the counterintuitive view that gene mutations are metronomic or stochastic events, and the proponents of Darwinian evolution through selective advantage. The rate of substitution at silent sites in various species is astonishingly constant—about 0.7% per million years for bacteria and 0.9% for the nuclear genes of mammals. Based on the slow ticking of this clock, an evolutionary dendritic (branching) tree of the β gene family has been constructed in which the $\delta:\beta$ divergence is placed at 40 million years (MY) ago, the $\gamma:\epsilon$ divergence at 100 MY ago, and the β, $\delta:\gamma$, ϵ divergence at 200 million years before the present [27]. The metronomic estimates are disputed by Goodman and others who have marshalled strong evidence indicating that the pace of globin gene evolution was adaptive (occurred in surges) and reflective of such evolutionary leaps as the triumphant formation of the first cooperative heterotetramers. Undoubtedly the regularity of the molecular clock also is perturbed by such large-scale genome dynamics known as "molecular drive" and by cross-species transfection.

Eve was black   Molecules like hemoglobin, cytochrome C, or even 16S rRNA evolve too slowly to help construct an evolutionary tree describing the recent emergence of the human race, and there is no firm way to evaluate the fossil (paleontologic) evidence of diggings, for fossil evidence is chancy and cannot exclude the possibilities of altered circumstance and

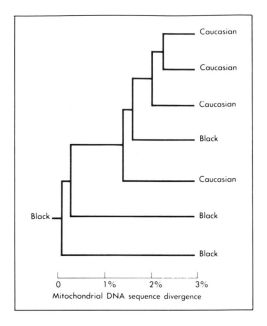

FIGURE 3-26

Human geneologic tree based on mitochondrial DNA sequence divergences, as deduced by the method of maximum parsimony. (Adapted from Cann RL et al: Mitochondrial DNA and human evolution. Nature 325:31,1986. Reprinted from reference 28.)

unrecorded migrations. Instead a "fast clock" molecule such as mitochondrial DNA has been exploited, for mitochondrial DNA (for lack of repair enzymes) mutates 10 times as fast as nuclear DNA. This advantage has made it possible to construct a human geneologic tree (Figure 3-26) [28]. The root of the tree is black African. There are two lines of descent: one leads to blacks only, the other to some blacks and to all other populations. Most modern Africans possess mitochondrial DNA closer to the ancestral kind than do any caucasians, indicating that humanity emerged in Africa and then spread to other continents [29]. The descent of humankind has not been resolved by paleontology but by molecular biology in the context of paleontology. Evolution is now being traced and anticipated in the biology laboratory.

REFERENCES

1. Alberts B et al: Chapt 8, in Molecular Biology of the Cell. New York, Garland Publishing, Inc.,1983.

2. Felsenfeld G: DNA. Sci Am 253(4):58,1985

3. Watson JE et al: Chapt 9, in Molecular Biology of the Gene, vol. 1, 4th ed. Menlo Park, The Benjamin/Cummings Publishing Company, Inc.,1987

4. Darnell J et al: Chapt 4, in Molecular Cell Biology. New York, Scientific American Books,1986

5. Nienhuis WE and Maniatis T: Chapt 2, in The Molecular Basis of Blood Diseases, Stamatoyannopoulos G et al, Eds. Philadelphia, WB Saunders Company,1987

6. Cech TR: RNA as an enzyme. Sci Am 255(5):64,1986

7. Sharp PA: Splicing of messenger RNA precursors. Science 235:766,1987

8. Cech TR: The chemistry of self-splicing RNA and RNA enzymes. Science 236:1532, 1987

9. Watson JE et al: Chapt 15, in Molecular Biology of the Gene, vol. 1, 4th ed. Menlo Park, The Benjamin/Cummings Publishing Company, Inc.,1987

10. Rich A and Kims SH: The three-dimensional structure of transfer RNA. Sci Am 238(1): 52,1978

11. Watson JE et al: Chapt 14, in Molecular Biology of the Gene, vol. 1, 4th ed. Menlo Park, The Benjamin/Cummings Publishing Company, Inc.,1987

12. Schechter AN et al: Genetic, cellular and clinical aspects of the regulation of fetal hemoglobin production, in Hematology— 1987. The Education Program of the American Society of Hematology, McArthur JR and Fienstein DI, Eds. Washington, DC, American Society of Hematology,1987

13. Ruskin B et al: Excision of an intact intron as a novel lariat structure during pre-mRNA splicing in vitro. Cell 38:317,1984

14. Darnell J et al: Chapt 3, in Molecular Cell Biology. New York, Scientific American Books,1986

15. Bunn HF and Forget BG: Chapt 2, in Hemoglobin: Molecular, Genetic and Clinical Aspects. Philadelphia, WB Saunders Company,1986

16. Meyer UA and Schmid R: Chapt 50, in Metabolic Basis of Inherited Diseases, 4th ed., Stanbury JE et al, Eds. New York, McGraw-Hill Book Company,1978

17. Bunn HF: Subunit assembly of hemoglobin: an important determinant of hematologic phenotype. Blood 69:1,1987

18. Shaeffer JR et al: Assembly of normal and abnormal human hemoglobins. Trends Biochem Sci 6:158,1981

19. Kan YW: The Harvey Lectures, Series 76. New York, Academic Press,1982

20. Darnell J et al: Chapt 7, in Molecular Cell Biology. New York, Scientific American Books,1986

21. Alberts B: Chapt 4, in Molecular Biology of the Cell. New York, Garland Publishing, Inc.,1983

22. Rowley PT et al: Chapt 1, in Current Hematology and Oncology, vol. 4, Fairbanks VF, Ed. Chicago, Year Book Medical Publishers, Inc.,1986

23. Saiki RK et al: Primer-directed enzymatic amplification of DNA with a thermostable DNA polymerase. Science 239:487,1988

24. Marx JL: Multiplying genes by leaps and bounds. Science 240:1408,1988

25. White R and Lalouel J-M: Chromosome mapping with DNA markers. Sci Am 258(2):40,1988

26. Chang JC and Kan YW: A sensitive new prenatal test for sickle-cell anemia. N Engl J Med 307:30,1982

27. Bunn HF and Forget BG: Chapt 7, in Hemoglobin: Molecular, Genetic and Clinical Aspects. Philadelphia, WB Saunders Company,1986

28. Watson JD et al: Molecular Biology of the Gene, vol. 2, 4th ed. Menlo Park, The Benjamin/Cummings Publishing Company, Inc.,1987

29. Stringer CB and Andrews P: Genetic and fossil evidence for the origin of modern humans. Science 239:1263,1988

4

Physiology of Red Cells

□

During hypoxia, erythropoietin (EP) is synthesized by renal vascular endothelium in response to insistent signals from the renal O_2 sensor. EP instructs CFU-Es to synthesize and upregulate receptors for EP. The hormone then occupies these receptors and commands erythroid cells on which it is perched to proliferate until equilibrium is restored. This command forces CFU-Es to commit suicidal maturation by blast transformation into the first recognizable erythropoietic cell, the proerythroblast (pronormoblast). Through growth signals transmitted up the stem cell hierarchy, CFU-Es lost through differentiation are replaced by substitutes recruited randomly from the pluripotential pool; each vacancy is then filled through the self-perpetuating offices of the multipotential stem cell, and homeostasis is served.

MATURATION AND DIFFERENTIATION

If all goes well, proerythroblasts undergo a stylized sequence of four consecutive binary reduction-divisions. On the basis of Wright-Giemsa staining the first two generations are classified together as basophilic erythroblasts, followed in order by polychromatophilic erythroblasts, and finally by endstage nucleated red cells, termed orthochromatic erythroblasts (normoblasts). Morphologic identification of the maturational stages following each reduction division is based principally upon cell size, chromatic changes in cytoplasm, and nuclear condensation. During the transition from basophilic erythroblasts to orthochromatic erythroblasts, the blue of cytoplasmic RNA is supplanted by the yellow-pink staining of hemoglobin. These complementary colors are admixed in midmaturation, creating a

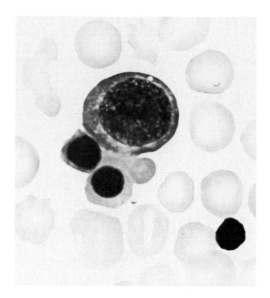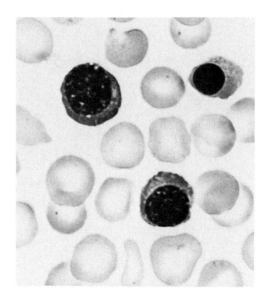

FIGURE 4-1

Morphology of erythroblasts at various stages of maturation in the marrow. (Left) The very large rounded cell with dark (basophilic) cytoplasm is a proerythroblast, precursor of all differentiating erythroblasts. Next to it are late (mature) erythroblasts with condensed nuclei; a disgorged pyknotic nucleus is seen at the lower right. (Right) Progressive stages of erythroid maturation proceeding (left to right) from the large basophilic erythroblast, to a polychromatophilic erythroblast (below), and two orthochromatic erythroblasts about to expel their inactivated nuclei. (Photo by CT Kapff.)

muddy blend, termed polychromatophilia. Black-and-white portraits of erythroblasts at four stages of maturation are shown in Figure 4-1.

During each maturation-division, cell volumes are halved and cell numbers are doubled. Table 4-1 [1] presents a numerical, dimensional, and temporal description of the sum of erythropoietic cells of marrow and of the vastly more numerous denucleated red cells in the circulation. Collectively, these cells comprise the erythron. The most remarkable quan-

titative feature of the erythron is that 100 ml of nucleated erythroid precursors of marrow sustain a red cell population 60 times their number and 20 times their volume. This feat is attributable to the perpetual cell cycling of erythroid progenitors and to the admirable durability of the final and finished product, the red cell. Like Louis Carroll's Red Queen, the erythron must perforce "do all the running it can do, to keep in the same place." Suppression of erythropoiesis inevitably reduces the red cell numbers; shortening of red cell survival (hemolysis) demands enlistment of more erythroid progenitors from the ranks of idle stem cells. The combination of erythrosuppression and heightened hemolysis places cruel demands on the erythron.

The morphologic changes that accompany EP-inspired maturation-division during the 6 or 7 days between matriculation of proerythroblasts and release of mature red cells into circulation are reprised diagrammatically in Figure 4-2 [2].

Advantages of denucleation The penultimate act of orthochromatic erythroblasts is shedding of their pyknotic, inactive nuclei. This occurs either by karyorrhexis (which may leave behind one or more purple-staining nu-

TABLE 4-1

The erythron of a 75-kg adult

Cell type (compartment)	Number of cells	Volume of each cell (fl)	Volume of cell compartment (ml)	Generation time (h)	Transit time (days)
Proerythroblast	10^{10}	900	9	12	0.5
Basophilic erythroblast	4×10^{10}	450	18	20	0.8
Polychromatophilic erythroblast	12×10^{10}	225	27	30	1.3
Orthochromatic erythroblast	24×10^{10}	200	54	——	2.0
Subtotal					
Nucleated red cells	0.4×10^{12}	——	108	——	——
Marrow reticulocyte	20×10^{10}	120	24	——	1.7
Blood reticulocyte	15×10^{10}	110	17	——	1.3
Mature red cell	24×10^{12}	95	2,280	——	120.0
Subtotal					
Nonnucleated red cells	24.4×10^{12}	——	2,300	——	——

Source: From Jandl JH: Chapt 2, in Blood: Textbook of Hematology. Boston, Little, Brown and Company,1987.

clear fragments known as Howell-Jolly bodies), or, more often, by exocytosis (Chapter 1). Denucleation by erythroblasts is a late evolutionary achievement observed only in adult mammals. The cost of this step is addition of a nonproliferative asymmetric division and loss of about 5% of the hard-earned hemoglobin—which winds up as part of the "early-labeling peak" of bilirubin. The benefits are: unloading of 40 pg per cell of dead weight; transformation of a rigid spheroidal cell into a supple biconcave disc capable of reversible deformation in the microcirculation; and prevention of inappropriate resumption of DNA synthesis. Denucleation obviates the cardiac work of moving over 1,000 tons daily of inert nuclei. Erythroid cells are capable of resealing their membranes following nuclear expulsion and

other forms of exocytosis including extrusion of Howell-Jolly bodies. Conversely, growth and maturation of immature red cells, including reticulocytes, are dependent upon their lively capacity for endocytosis.

Receptor-Mediated Endocytosis of Transferrin-Bound Iron

The integrated and controlled process of protoporphyrin production, globin chain synthesis, and assembly of globin subunits in the presence of ferroprotoporphyrin (heme) was described in Chapter 3. The catalytic active site for O_2 binding by hemoglobin (Hb) is the ferrous iron atom (Fe^{2+}) locked covalently into the center of the planar porphyrin ring. Heme is also the prosthetic group of myoglobin,

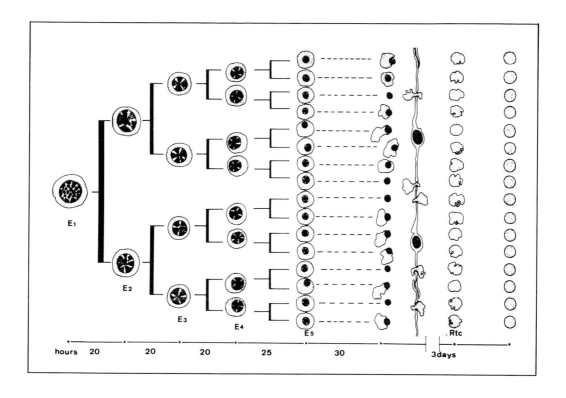

hours   20   20   20   25   30   3days

FIGURE 4-2

Morphologic sequence accompanying amplification by maturation-division of erythroid cells. The notations E1 through E5 successively denote a proerythroblast, early and late erythroblasts, polychromatophilic erythroblasts, and orthochromatic erythroblasts. Denucleation of orthochromatic cells occurs within marrow parenchyma; newly formed reticulocytes then escape the marrow sinuses by downregulating fibronectin receptors (as described in Chapter 1) and bore their way through thinned-out sinus endothelium in the proximity of their junction zones. Rtc = reticulocytes. (From Castoldi GF and Beutler E: Chapt 3, in Atlas of Blood Cells. Function and Pathology, vol. 1, 2nd ed., Zucker-Franklin D et al, Eds. Milan, Edi. Ermes s.r.l.,1988.)

catalase, peroxidase, and cytochromes. The eventual channeling of O_2 to meet tissue energy requirements is made by a redox cascade in which the central vehicles are intracellular iron and its operative heme and nonheme adducts. Iron plays a central role in all oxidative energy metabolism: it is essential to every human cell.

Transferrin and the Transferrin Receptor

The mechanism of seizing iron from foodstuffs and for distributing it to erythroblasts and all other iron-hungry growing or proliferating cells depends entirely on the specific iron transport protein, transferrin. Plasma transferrin is a single-chain bilobed glycoprotein having 678 amino acid residues and an M_r of 79,550. It possesses two identical asparagine-linked biantennary glycans, each containing an iron-binding domain. These similar but non-identical domains bind iron with an effective affinity constant exceeding 10^{30}. Removal of iron from the tight grip of transferrin requires selective binding of iron-transferrin complexes by transferrin receptors on the cell surface [3].

The transferrin receptor is a transmembrane dimeric glycoprotein with two identical subunits, each of which is comprised of 760 amino acids and has an M_r of 85,000. The membrane-spanning dimer is positioned upside-down, with the C terminal end, representing about 70% of the molecule, extending outward from

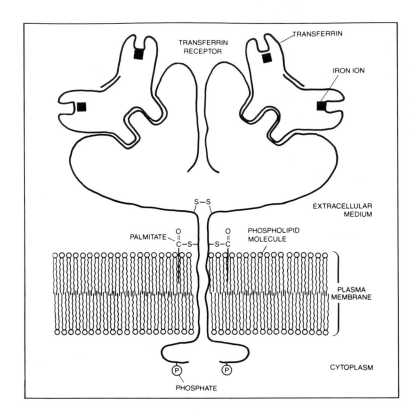

FIGURE 4-3

Transferrin receptor. The bulk of the receptor is outside the lipid bilayer, and each subunit binds 1 molecule of iron-bearing transferrin, the dimer binding 2 molecules holding 4 atoms of Fe^{3+}. The N-terminus domain, the hydrophobic tail of the receptor, keeps the structure anchored to the membrane. (From Dautry-Varsat A and Lodish HF: How receptors bring proteins and particles into cells. Sci Am 250(5):52,1984. Copyright © 1984 by Scientific American, Inc. All rights reserved.)

the cell surface (Figure 4-3) [4]. The human transferrin receptor gene is located at the terminal end of the long arm of chromosome 3 in proximity to the coding domains for transferrin itself [5]. The receptor gene has been cloned and sequenced: it spans a 31-kb genomic segment and is composed of 19 exons interrupted by 18 introns [6]. Identical transferrin receptors have been found in all growing cells, including placental trophoblasts, seminiferous tubules, activated lymphocytes, and all neoplastic cells. The growth of all these cells is arrested by monoclonal antibody (OKT9) to the receptor.

The Transferrin Cycle

Polypeptide receptors on cell membranes can be classified into two general categories. When occupied by ligands, as exemplified by cytokines and the products of oncogenes, class I receptors transmit signals—information relayed via G proteins or other allosteric transducers instructing cells to grow or stop growing, move or stop moving. Class II receptors internalize the ligand, thus providing the cell with nutrients. The paradigm of class II receptors is the fibroblast receptor for low-density lipoprotein (LDL), which escorts cholesterol through the cell membrane. Analogous to the behavior of LDL receptors, transferrin occupancy of the transferrin receptor inaugurates membrane movement leading to selective internalization of the ligand-receptor complex [7].

Clathrin and endosomes form intracellular shuttles Within seconds of the binding of iron-transferrin complexes, occupied receptor molecules move laterally and cluster in selective depressions called coated pits (Figure 4-4) [8]. Coated pits are lacy depressions created by the artful assembly of three fibrillar 180,000 M_r light and 340,000 M_r heavy chains of clathrin, plus a family of supportive proteins [9]. These self-assemble as three-legged members called

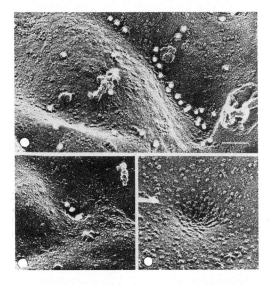

FIGURE 4-4

Scanning EM view of the surface of a freeze-dried reticulocyte exposed to transferrin (Tf) labeled with white-appearing spheres of colloidal gold (AuTf). (Top) Labeled Tf is beginning to cluster into pits. Bar = 100 nm. (Lower left) AuTf clustered into a pit on the cell surface. (Lower right) View of pit on reticulocyte exposed to an excess of unlabeled Tf; binding of labeled Tf was blocked by competition. (Reproduced from the Journal of Cell Biology 1983;97:329 by copyright permission of the Rockefeller University Press.)

triskelions that unite to create geodesic cage-like cones visible in freeze-etched preparations (Figure 4-5) [10]. When occupied by liganded receptors, coated pits pinch off from the inner aspect of the cell membrane to form endosomes 50 to 150 nm across. As they pass deeply into the cytosol, these endosomes are freed of their evanescent coating of clathrin by an ATP-dependent "uncoating enzyme" and then acquire a comma-shaped tubular extension called a CURL (acronym for compartment of uncoupling of receptor and ligand). In the main spheroidal chamber of the endosome the pH is lowered below 5.5 by a Mg^{2+}-dependent ATPase in the endosomal lining that acts as an electrogenic proton pump. This acidification dissociates iron from transferrin. Iron is reduced under these acid conditions and then transported across the vesicle wall by a permeant chelator; this in turn relinquishes iron to mitochondria for heme synthesis, or surrenders any surplus of iron to the iron depot, ferritin. Meanwhile apotransferrin remains complexed to its receptor, segregated along the inner wall of the tapered extension of the CURL, and within a few minutes is returned to the cell surface. There, at pH 7.4, the affinity of apotransferrin for its receptor is so low—about 1% that of iron-loaded transferrin—that the iron-depleted protein is set free and its seat on the resurfaced receptor is quickly

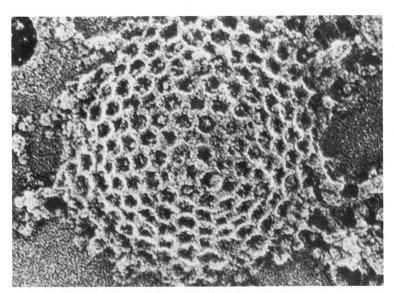

FIGURE 4-5

Freeze-etch view (seen as a dome from the inside of a cell) of a coated pit, exposing the basketlike ultrastructure of the clathrin assembly. (Reproduced from the Journal of Cell Biology 1980;84:560 by copyright permission from the Rockefeller University Press.)

FIGURE 4-6

The transferrin cycle. Note that both the transferrin molecules (black circles) and their receptors are conserved and reutilized, whereas the iron atoms (small white circles) are freed by gentle acid hydrolysis within the uncoated endosome, denoted endosome II, and released to iron proteins such as hemoglobin. Some CURL-type endosomes are routed through the Golgi before conveying the receptor-apotransferrin complex back to the membrane. (From Johnstone RM: Chapt 12, in Red Blood Cell Membranes: Structure, Functions, Clinical Implications. Agre P and Parker JC, Eds. New York, Marcel Dekker, Inc., 1989. Reprinted by courtesy of Marcel Dekker Inc.)

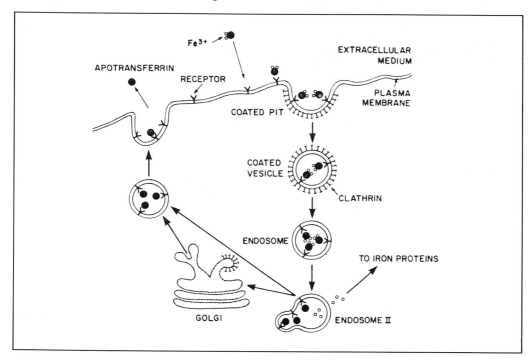

occupied by a new iron-laden transferrin molecule. The transferrin cycle is recapitulated in Figure 4-6 [28]. During cell growth and proliferation the receptor-transferrin complex recycles every 4 to 5 minutes, and each spin of the cycle delivers about 25 atoms of iron per hour per receptor.

Cell cycling is geared to transferrin cycling   The upregulation or synthesis de novo of transferrin receptors is among the first events triggered by proliferative stimuli. All proliferating and all tumor cells express high receptor levels. In activated T cells, induction of IL-2 receptors by IL-2 initiates an autocrine cycle by which T cells proliferate: for this activation to become irreversible, induction of transferrin receptors is necessary and sufficient [11].

RHAPSODY IN RED

The mature red cell is a triumph of evolution. It has disposed of all its biosynthetic equipment (nucleus, ribosomes, mitochondria) and is stripped down to fulfill its roles of delivering O_2 to tissue capillaries and eliminating tissue CO_2 via lung capillaries. Its flexible biconcave wafer shape is perfectly designed to enable mature red cells to survive the trials of hurtling through the circulation and making half a million gruelling roundtrips through the microcirculation, covering a distance of about 300 miles. Normal red cells are 7.8 μm across, 1.7 μm thick, and have a volume of 94 $\pm$ 14 fl and a surface (membrane) area of 135 $\pm$ 16 sq μm. The 35% redundancy in surface area (a perfect sphere of comparable volume would have an area of only 100 sq μm) enables these tough but compliant corpuscles to withstand the hydraulic bending forces of turbulent circulation and to adjust to momentary folding, tumbling, tapering, and twisting configurations without apparent damage. The appearance of a representative population of red cells is shown in Figure 4-7 [2]. The biconcave shape of red cells provides an ideal ratio of surface area to cell volume; this enables these tiny oxyhemoglobin conveyances, 7 to 8 μm across, to traverse cylindrical capillaries having diameters of only 5 μm by assuming an umbrella shape transverse to the direction of flow.

Mechanics of Capillary Blood Flow: Microrheology

When blood cells enter a large cylindrical arteriolar vessel at high velocity, those at the periphery of the stream bounce off the endothelial wall toward the central or axial stream. The densest blood cell elements, the red cells, enter the fast-moving midaxial cur-

rent, the lighter lymphocytes flow more peripherally, and the lightest cells—monocytes, neutrophils, and platelets—tumble slowly along the plasma-rich marginal stream. This rheologic arrangement spares the centralized column of red cells from the friction of scraping along large vessel walls and permits phagocytic and hemostatic cells to patrol the vascular margins outside the tumult and momentum of the axial stream. Red cells are driven to enter the high-speed axial stream of small arteries and arterioles through a collusion of Newtonian forces and the stacking phenomenon known as rouleaux. In the presence of large linear macromolecules such as fibrinogen, red cells stack up like small dishes, held together by weak surface-bridging forces. Entrainment of red cells in rouleaux in vitro is responsible for the erythrocyte sedimentation rate (the ESR—a crude and indirect measure of acute phase reactants such as fibrinogen and macroglobulins). Rouleaux formation in vivo causes red cells to travel through arterioles in trains, minimizing bumping and, by aggregating their weight, facilitating movement into the axial

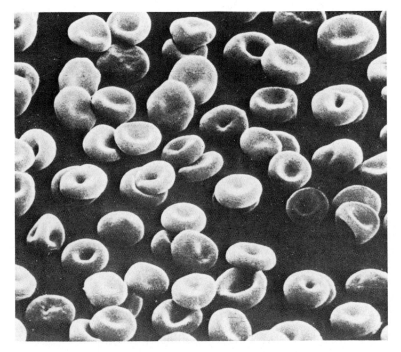

FIGURE 4-7

SEM of normal red cells (erythrocytes). The cells vary modestly in size and shape, with discoidal cells having gentle concavities on opposing faces in the majority. In Wright-Giemsa preparations these cells stain a muted orange-pink and display an area of central pallor occupying over 25% of the topographical area. Cells with thicker-than-average rims simulate bagels, and a minority of normal cells are cup-shaped or triconcave. (From Castoldi GF and Beutler E: Chapt 3, in Atlas of Blood Cells. Function and Pathology, vol. 1, Zucker-Franklin D et al, Eds. Milan, Edi. Ermes s.r.l.,1988.)

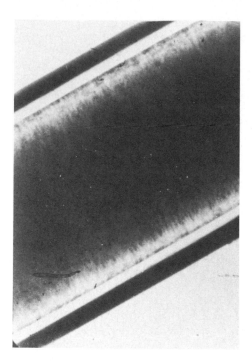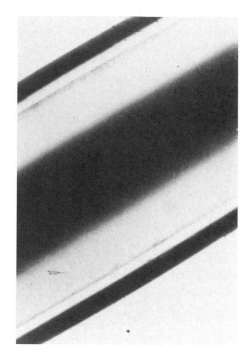

FIGURE 4-8

Whole blood viewed through a transparent fiber cylinder (diameter: 100 μm) at rest (left) and in motion (right). Axial streaming of red cells (right) occurs during nonturbulent flow through arterioles in the presence of fibrinogen or a facsimile thereof. (From Jandl JH: Chapt 1, in Blood: Textbook of Hematology. Boston, Little, Brown and Company,1987; Courtesy of Dr. EW Merrill.)

midstream (Figure 4-8). As the arteriolar diameter lessens, velocity of red cells relative to plasma increases, and the cell concentration is reduced proportionately. In effect the centralized column of red cells is sliding through a sleeve of plasma lubricant. As the cells approach capillary openings they pop sideways into the capillaries and pass through slowly in single file, perpendicular to the axis of flow. The pressure gradient inflates the thin center of the crosswise red cell into the shape of a nose cone, and dragging of the thick rim stabilizes its transverse posture. The parachute shape of

red cells traversing capillaries creates a tight fit with tissue capillaries—ideally suited for exchange of O_2 and CO_2 (Figure 4-9) [12].

Blood Cell Viscosity and Capillary Flow

When red cells enter capillaries having diameters less than their own, the limiting rheologic determinant is the intrinsic viscosity of the cell itself. This is a function of the solubility and concentration of the intracellular hemoglobin and of the viscoelastic properties of the cell membrane.

Intracellular viscosity is determined mainly by the MCHC. A normal MCHC of 33 g/dl contributes 60% of the intrinsic viscosity of red cells; at intracellular concentrations exceeding 36 g/dl red cell viscosity rises sharply, and MCHC levels of 40 g/dl exceed the solubility of hemoglobin, causing the cell to rigidify. Abnormal hemoglobins may be insoluble even at normal intracellular concentrations, forming damaging precipitates that either ensnare the cell in tight passages as exist in the splenic cords, or cause membrane-wrapped hemoglobin inclusions to be torn off. In sickling disor-

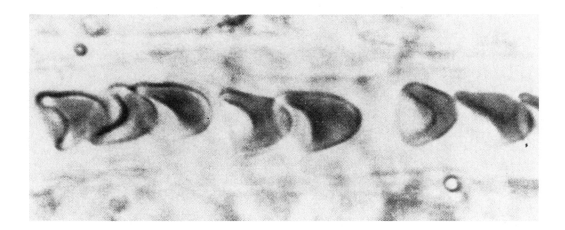

FIGURE 4-9

High-speed microcinematograph shows the umbrella shape of human red cells traversing a capillary. (From Skalak R and Branemark P-I: Deformation of red blood cells in capillaries. Science 164:717,1969. Copyright 1969 by the AAAS.)

ders, polymerization of hemoglobin S may so stiffen red cells that they cannot traverse the microcirculation even under an arterial head of hydraulic pressure.

The viscoelastic properties of red cells, their shape, and their response to and recovery from the shearing forces of the circulation are determined by an integrated system of molecules called the cytoskeleton. Lacking internal organelles or transcellular structures, red cells depend for their intrinsic shape and resistance to deformation upon an interlocking network of skeletal proteins; these are joined into a geodesic framework that provides a scaffolding for the enveloping lipid bilayer in which "integral" membrane proteins are embedded.

The Cytoskeleton

Absent an internal three-dimensional skeleton, red cells depend for their configuration upon a regularly ordered membranous network of crosslinked fibrillar members over which the lipid bilayer is stretched. The cytoskeletal assembly determines cell size and gross configuration, and the bilayer of lipids—an equimolar melange of various phospholipids and of cholesterol—provides a hydrophobic skin. Together, the lipid bilayer and the protein cytoskeleton over which it is wrapped are responsible for an inherent shape having the lowest possible free energy [13].

Polypeptide Composition of Red Cell Membranes

Polypeptides of the red cell membrane are separated conventionally by polyacrylamide gel electrophoresis in sodium dodecyl sulfate (SDS-PAGE) and stained with Coomassie blue. Major membrane proteins are numbered according to their rate of migration toward the cathode. The skeletal proteins, in order of migration, are spectrin, ankyrin, protein band 4.1, and actin. Most nonskeletal membrane proteins fulfill either enzymic, transport, or receptor functions. Two major nonskeletal proteins, band 3 (the anion channel) and the heavily glycosylated glycophorins which comigrate with band 3, span the lipid bilayer and expose functionally different domains on the outer and inner aspects of the membrane. The positioning and nomenclature of the quantitatively major membrane proteins are shown in

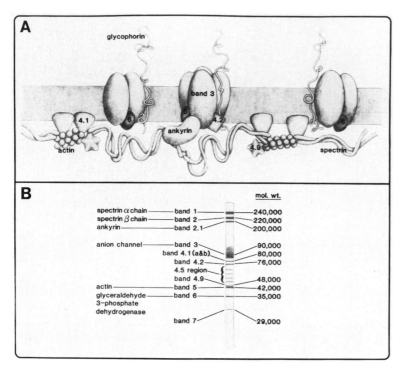

FIGURE 4-10

FIGURE 4-10

Major membrane proteins of red cells. (A) Artist's rendition of the placement of the spectrin-ankyrin-4.1-actin structural lattice lying beneath the lipid bilayer (gray band). The anion channel (band 3) perforce spans the membrane. Glycophorin, like many receptors, is anchored to the bilayer, but extends most of its complex sugar structure outward into the plasma. (B) The size, identification, and band designation of major proteins separated on SDS-PAGE are shown in order of negative charge. (Cathode is at the bottom.) Glycophorin migrates with band 3 in SDS-PAGE systems. (Courtesy Dr. J Palek.)

Figure 4-10. Hundreds of quantitatively minor glycoproteins stud the outer lamina of the bilayer and extend their polar antennae outward into the plasma; this outer shell of glycolipids endows red cells with a high net negative charge (zeta potential) and equips the cell with its surface blood group antigens.

How the Cytoskeleton is Fastened

The red cell skeleton is a protein lattice that laminates the underside of the lipid bilayer. It is formed by linkages between spectrin, actin, protein 4.1, and ankyrin. The most abundant skeletal protein is spectrin, a noodle-shaped fibrous protein composed of two chains, α and β spectrin, that are twisted along each other in antiparallel. At one of their ends, referred to as the "head," spectrin heterodimers possess binding sites that cause them to align as head-to-head tetramers, and occasionally as hexamers and higher-order oligomers (Figure 4-11). Stretched taut, heterodimers and tetramers are 97 nm and 194 nm long, but in their "entropic" state the end-to-end length of relaxed tetramers is much shorter.

The membrane skeleton is a collapsible hexagonal lattice At their distal end, spectrin tetramers are joined into a two-dimensional network by linkage to oligomers of actin, an articulation greatly strengthened by attachment of protein 4.1. This ultrastructural pattern of assembly can be visualized by artificially spreading membrane skeletons derived from Triton-treated red cell "ghosts" and stretching them onto carbon-coated grids (Figure 4-12) [14]. In the intact membrane the flexible spectrin tetramers allow the skeleton to collapse inward like a folded umbrella, held partially open by restraining molecules known as entropy springs [13, 14]. This accommodating skeleton is attached to the membrane by ankyrin, a protein that connects the spectrin β chain to the cytoplasm end of the large transmembrane protein band 3, which shapes the anion channel. The red cell membrane contains over 1,000,000 copies of the 93,000 M_r band 3 homodimer, and the evenly spaced deployment of these numerous transmembrane linchpins assures that the membrane does not slip off its skeletal scaffold. Additional amphi-

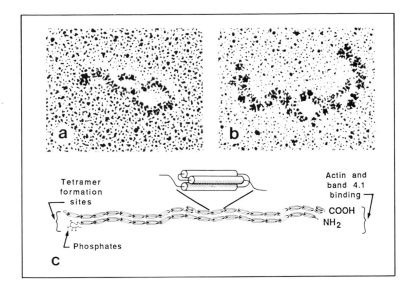

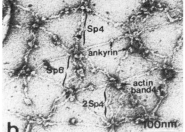

FIGURE 4-11

Anatomy of spectrin.
(a) EM of rotary shad-
owed spectrin hetero-
dimer. (b) Similar EM
of entwined hetero-
dimers in their custom-
ary head-to-head asso-
ciation. (c) Both α and
β spectrin chains are
comprised of 20 and 19
106–amino acid repeat-
ing segments, respec-
tively; each segment is
folded centrally into a
triple-stranded structure
(expanded diagram).
(From Elgsaeter A et al.
Science 234:1217,1986.
Copyright 1986 by the
AAAS.)

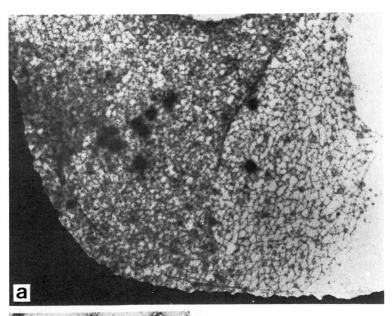

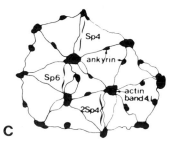

FIGURE 4-12

EM of negatively
stained spread skeletons
of red cells. (a) Low-
power view revealing
mosaic web. (b) At high
magnification the basic
equilateral triangles
formed of spectrin are
seen to generate hexago-
nal modules; junctions
are secured complexes
of short F-actin and
band 4.1. Most spectrin
is in the form of tetra-
mers (Sp_4), but some
hexamers (Sp_6) and double tetramers ($2 Sp_4$) are
evident. Globular com-
plexes of ankyrin are
fastened to ankyrin
binding sites on the
spectrin filaments. (c)
Schematic representa-
tion of (b). (Repro-
duced from the Journal
of Cell Biology
1987;104:527 by copy-
right permission of the
Rockefeller University
Press. Courtesy of Dr. J
Palek.)

pathic anchorage is provided by attachments between protein 4.1 and glycophorins A and C plus direct linkages between spectrin, protein 4.1, and the negatively charged lipids of the inner face of the lipid bilayer [15].

The Lipid Bilayer Is a Two-Dimensional Fluid

Red cells are unique in that all lipid is in the membrane and all membrane is at the surface. Membrane lipids are amphipathic, meaning that each lipid molecule has a nonpolar, hydrophobic end and a polar, hydrophilic end. Consequently, extended bilayers in an aqueous medium self-assemble to form two planes, so that the hydrophobic lipid tails are positioned internally vis-á-vis and the hydrophilic heads face oppositely to form the internal (cytoplasmic) and external (plasma) facades of the bilayer. Lipid bilayers are cooperative structures held together by many reinforcing noncovalent interactions. The lipid bilayer of red cells tends to close on itself so that there are no dangling ends with exposed hydrophobic chains; the lipid bilayer is inherently self-sealing because a hole in the bilayer is energetically unfavorable. Hydrophobic close-packing forces in effect shrink-wrap the lipid bilayer around the cytoskeletal framework.

Membrane Lipid Composition

A noteworthy feature of the red cell lipid bilayer is that the molar ratio of highly hydrophobic lipid, cholesterol, is nearly equal to the sum of the more polar lipids, phospholipids and glycolipids. All red cell membrane cholesterol is in the free (unesterified) form, whereas several classes of phospholipid are represented, of which four predominate (Table 4-2). Lipids are not randomly distributed throughout the membrane, phospholipids being asymmetrically arranged on the apposing leaflets. Choline-containing phospholipids and glycolipids prevail on the outer leaflet, whereas terminal amino-containing phospholipids dominate the inner side, with only a trickle of transmembrane (flip-flop) exchange. In addition the negatively charged phosphatidyl serine is affixed to the inner half by protein 4.1, conferring a significant charge difference between the two membranes.

TABLE 4-2

Lipids of the normal red cell membrane

Total lipids	μmol/10^{11}cells
Cholesterol	36.1
Phospholipids	38.1
Glycolipids	1.0
Free fatty acids	2.6

Phospholipids	% of total phospholipids
Sphingomyelin	26.0
Lecithin	30.5
Phosphatidylserine (and phosphatidylinositol)	13.2
Phosphatidylethanolamine	27.3
Lysolecithin	1.3
Others (polyglycerol phosphatide and phosphatidic acid)	1.7

Source: From Jandl JH: Chapt 2, in Blood: Textbook of Hematology. Boston: Little, Brown and Company,1987.

Cholesterol stiffens the lipid bilayer   Molecular interactions between cholesterol and phospholipids result in a close-packed interpositioning of the two moieties that is crucial to membrane integrity. The single polar hydroxyl group of cholesterol is in submerged contact with the polar head groups of phospholipids while the rigidly planar sterol structure intercalates with fatty acyl chains. This interpolation of cholesterol molecules among phospholipids immobilizes the 10 acyl carbon atoms nearest the membrane surfaces, restraining and stabilizing the subjacent skeletal proteins. Deep within the hydrophobic interior, however, the nonintercalated free ends of the fatty acids of each leaflet are free to wriggle and commingle, creating an "intermediate fluid zone," like jelly in a sandwich. This freedom of motion between the bilayers provides the membrane with flexibility and lateral fluidity. Membrane fluidity is also influenced by the cholesterol:phospholipid (C:P) ratio, the relative proportions of

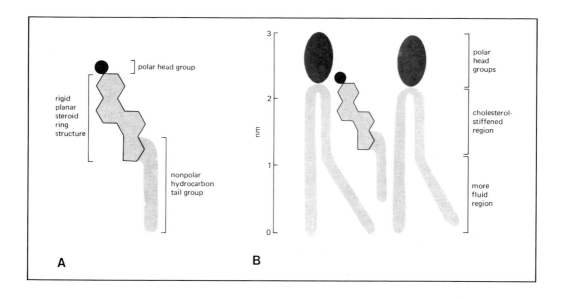

FIGURE 4-13

Schematic drawing depicting the intercalation of cholesterol (A) between phospholipid molecules (B) in a single leaflet of the red cell membrane. Note that the phospholipids appear to be doing the Charleston; the bend in one of their two fatty acids is caused by the presence of a *cis*-double bond about halfway down the hydrophobic tails. (From Alberts B et al: Chapt 6, in Molecular Biology of the Cell. New York, Garland Publishing, Inc.,1983.)

the several phospholipids, and the presence of unsaturated fatty acid side chains (Figure 4-13) [16]. Unsaturated fatty acids (oleic, linoleic, and arachidonic), a low C:P ratio, and lecithin favor fluidity.

The lipid bilayer is 6 nm thick. Acting in union, membrane lipids and the underlying cytoskeleton confer upon intact red cells the resilient viscoelastic properties that enable them to withstand and to adapt to 4 months of abuse in the circulation. The dense thicket of negatively charged heteroglycans and glucosamines sprouting from the membrane outer surface adds to the preservation of this doughty oxyhemoglobin-bearing vehicle by repelling abrasive contact with other cells and other surfaces. These negatively charged sugar groups stem mainly from membrane-embedded glyco-

lipids. The most abundant glycolipids are globosides and hematosides that display branched antennary sugar structures composed of glucose, mannose, galactose, and the hexosamine, N-acetylneuraminic acid, which account for over 80% of the negative charge repulsion of the red cell surface. Fucose-containing glycolipids constitute a minority of these externalized polar groups, but they furnish the cell surface with its most abundant antigenic determinants: the A, B, H, I, and Lewis blood groups. The interlocking and layered molecular structures that comprise the fully assembled red cell membrane are reprised in Figure 4-14.

Red Cell Energetics

During reticulocytehood the high-energy-yielding components of the mitochondrial tricarboxylic acid cycle are lost and the protein-synthetic capability of ribosomes succumbs to RNases. The mature red cell is stripped down metabolically and depends for its livelihood upon the feeble flicker of free energy released by phosphorylated glucose as it is degraded through the fermentative sequence known as the Embden-Meyerhof pathway. The long lifespan of these durable corpuscles is safeguarded by two general metabolic mechanisms of homeostasis: production of

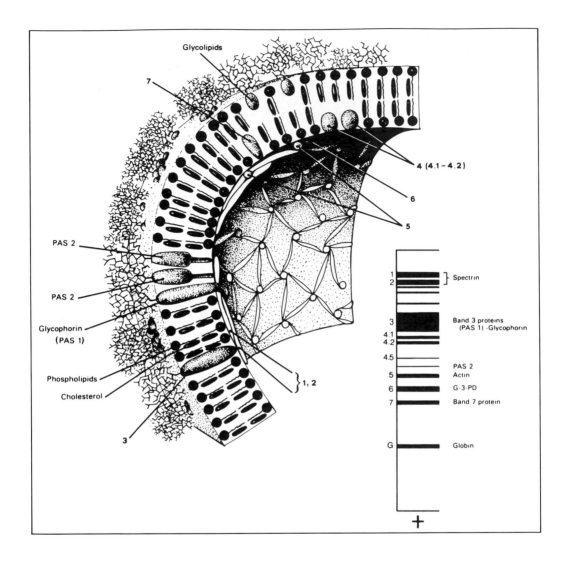

FIGURE 4-14

Simplified model (including SDS-PAGE band no-
menclature) of the intact red cell membrane.
(From Castoldi GF and Beutler E: Chapt 3, in
Atlas of Blood Cells. Function and Pathology,
vol. 1, 2nd ed., Zucker-Franklin D et al, Eds.
Milan, Edi. Ermes s.r.l.,1988.)

ATP, the universal currency of biological energy; and defense against oxidation, nemesis of
the reduced milieu in which cytoplasmic constituents flourish.

ATP Maintains Red Cell Structure and Shape

Energy for operating the sodium and calcium
pumps that regulate cell volume, and phosphorylations required for reversibly modulating cytoskeletal connections responsible for
recovery of cell shape are provided by stepwise
release of free energy of metabolites of phosphorylated glucose made available by the
Embden-Meyerhof pathway (Figure 4-15).

FIGURE 4-15

Metabolism of glucose by red cells. The vertical sequence of reactions (the Embden-Meyerhof pathway) generates 2 molecules (mol) of ATP for each mol invested. The appended cyclic se-

quence—the hexose monophosphate shunt—is regulated by glucose 6-phosphate dehydrogenase (G6PD) and is responsible for maintaining gluta-thione and cellular enzymes in a reduced state.

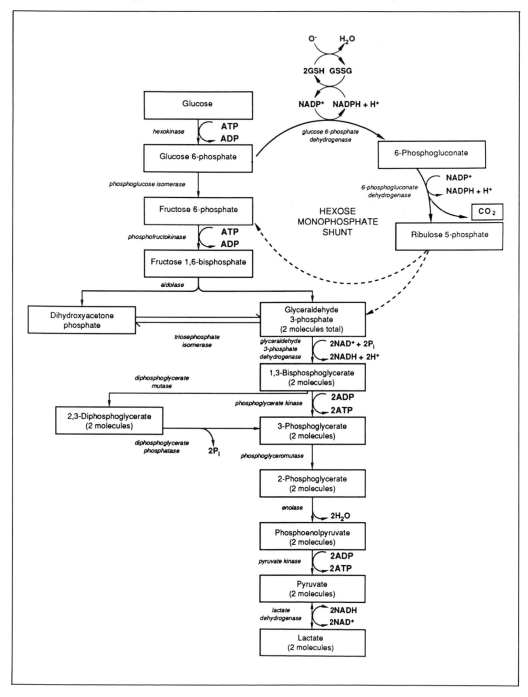

Red cells utilize the fermentative Embden-Meyerhof pathway for generating ATP because this energetic sequence does not require O_2 as substrate. Red cells are able to carry enormous quantities of O_2 safely by strictly limiting inter-action between glycolytic intermediates and this incendiary payload ($E_0' = +0.82V$). Glycolysis proceeding with or without O_2 present is often termed aerobic (or anaerobic) glycolysis, to the confusion of everyone.

HMP Shunt and O_2 Detoxification

Although the function of red cells is to trans-port O_2 without being incinerated by it, limited amounts of O_2 are actually consumed by the hexose monophosphate (HMP) shunt pathway as it regenerates the NADPH needed for reduc-ing oxidized glutathione (GSSG) to its func-tional state (GSH) (Figure 4-15). The HMP shunt is a volatile pathway compared with the imperturbable Embden-Meyerhof sequence; normally, the HMP shunt idles quietly at a rate 3 to 5% of its potential, but when oxidized substrates pile up (e.g., $NADP^+$, GSSG) it can rev up to 30 times baseline activity. This spirited rate of oxidation exerts a drain on glucose 6-phosphate (G6P) levels that is offset by a heightened rate of glucose phos-phorylation. G6P is strategically positioned to divert the flow of phosphohexose either down the ATP-yielding pathway or around the O_2-utilizing HMP shunt pathway. Combustion of O_2 in defense of a redox system such as that governed by G6PD is an edgy arrangement. Intrusion into oxygenated red cells of redox catalysts such as quinones and other permeant oxidants can overwhelm the O_2-utilizing and O_2-detoxifying limits of the HMP shunt. Among the cell components most menaced by excessive oxidations are NADPH ($E_0' = -0.324$), GSH ($E_0' = -0.23$), and hemoglobin ($E_0' = +0.144$). Impairment of the HMP shunt, as occurs most frequently in patients with hereditary deficiency of G6PD, cripples the capacity to detoxify oxidants and predisposes to oxidative hemolysis.

HEMOGLOBIN AND O_2 TRANSPORT

The mission of red cells is to transport the respiratory gasses, O_2 and CO_2. Hemoglobin (Hb) takes up O_2 in the pulmonary capillaries and conveys it to tissue capillaries, where the O_2 is exchanged for CO_2. As O_2 is the primal source of most energy, its regulated delivery to tissues is singularly sensitive to need. A resting person consumes about 250 ml of O_2 and exhales about 200 ml of CO_2 each minute. Dissolved as a gas in plasma water, only about 5 ml of O_2 could be delivered to the tissues each minute. Because of red cell hemoglobin, which can carry 1.34 ml of O_2/g, whole blood can deliver 200 ml of O_2 per liter; in a normal resting adult the necessary 250 ml of O_2 can be transported and unloaded in tissues without lowering the O_2 saturation of blood Hb by more than 20 to 25%. An essential feature of O_2 transport is that Hb must bind O_2 firmly enough to remove it from pulmonary capillar-ies at high O_2 tensions and yet be engineered to unload O_2 at the low PO_2 of tissues; Hb must bind O_2 with an appropriate degree of affinity.

O_2 Binding and Subunit Cooperativity

The O_2 dissociation curve of the monomeric heme protein of muscle, myoglobin, is in the form of a simple rectangular parabola, reflect-ing its very avid binding of O_2 and befitting its role as a thermodynamic driving force in tissue electron transfer reactions [17]. Binding of O_2 by the Hb tetramer is positively cooperative, so that the first O_2 binds weakly to deoxyhemoglobin but profoundly enhances binding of more O_2 by other subunits of the same molecule until saturation is approached. At equilibrium the O_2-binding curve of intact Hb is sigmoidal (Figure 4-16) [18]. The O_2 dissociation curve reveals that arterial blood at a PO_2 of 90 mm Hg releases about 4.5 volumes of O_2/dl as the PO_2 drops to that of mixed venous blood ($PO_2 = 40$ mm). In the process of unloading O_2, the O_2 saturation of normal blood falls from 97% to about 75%—a mod-est decline that affects the PO_2 very little while unloading O_2 generously.

Physics of cooperativity   The intermediate pos-ture and sigmoidal shape of the O_2 dissociation curve is a sensible and highly refined conse-quence of evolved subunit cooperativity. Co-operativity (heme-heme interaction) results from differential movements of the two $\alpha\beta$ dimers at their points of apposition, a rela-

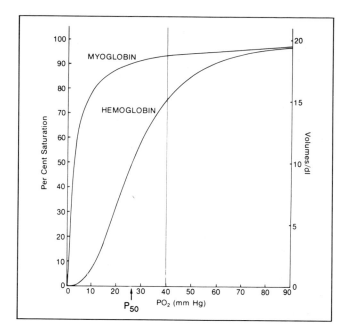

FIGURE 4-16

O_2 binding curves for tissue myoglobin and red cell hemoglobin at 37°C and pH 7.4. The ordinate on the right applies to whole blood containing 15 g Hb/dl. The shorthand expression of the affinity of Hb for O_2 is the term P_{50}, indicating the O_2 pressure that half-saturates Hb. The P_{50} of normal blood (arrow) is 26 ± 1 mm Hg. (Modified from Bunn HF and Forget BG: Chapt 3, in Hemoglobin: Molecular, Genetic and Clinical Aspects. Philadelphia, WB Saunders Company,1986.)

tively stable abutment designated $\alpha_1\beta_1$ and a wobbly contact denoted $\alpha_1\beta_2$. During partial oxygenation the polypeptide chains undergo substantial rotation, bringing the two β chains closer together, and causing the two subunits of the $\alpha_1\beta_2$ interface to slide upon each other, moving from one interfacial notch to another. As the restraints on the subunits lessen, the tetramer shifts from the T (tense) conformation to an R (relaxed) quaternary configuration in which hydrophobic pockets holding the hemes are more openly receptive to further oxygenation. Easier access to these opened pockets increases the O_2 affinity of Hb in the R state by 150 to 300 times that of Hb in the T conformation. The advantage of cooperativity is illustrated by comparing O_2 binding by tissue myoglobin, a monomer, with that of the cooperative tetramer, Hb. To increase the O_2 saturation of myoglobin from 10 to 90%, an 80-fold rise in PO_2 is required; the same increase in O_2 saturation of Hb can be achieved with less than a 5-fold increase in PO_2. Conversely, slight reductions in O_2 saturation of Hb favor rapid unloading of O_2 to tissue myoglobin.

The Bohr effect Within a physiologic range, the P_{50} varies inversely with pH, a phenomenon termed the alkaline Bohr effect. As blood perfuses pulmonary capillaries, CO_2 boils off, raising the pH and shifting the O_2 dissociation curve leftward to the high-affinity state; this promotes uptake of O_2 by the deoxyhemoglobin of red cells. Conversely, as oxygenated red cells enter the high PCO_2 milieu of tissue capillaries, CO_2 is rapidly hydrated by carbonic anhydrase of the red cell membrane to the weak acid, $H^+ + HO_3^-$; the resulting acidification hastens transfer of O_2 from the low-affinity Hb to the O_2-hungry enzymes of tissue cells (Figure 4-17)[18]. The Bohr effect presides over the reciprocal exchange of CO_2 and O_2—the respiratory cycle on which our lives depend.

Allosteric Regulation by 2,3-DPG of O_2 Unloading

Red cells are uniquely rich in a low-energy side-product of glycolysis—2,3-diphosphoglycerate (2,3-DPG) (Figure 4-15). Formed by the unidirectional enzyme, diphosphoglycerate mutase,

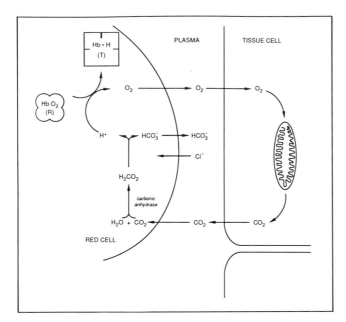

FIGURE 4-17

Unloading of O_2 and uptake of CO_2 and protons by red cells traversing tissues. Formation of carbonic acid (H_2CO_3) from CO_2 and water is catalyzed by carbonic anhydrase. Dissociation of O_2 from Hb and binding of protons are associated with a change of Hb from the R to the T quaternary structure. (From Bunn HF and Forget BG: Chapt 3, in Hemoglobin: Molecular, Genetic and Clinical Aspects. Philadelphia, WB Saunders Company, 1986.)

in an energy-clutch bypass reaction termed the Rapoport-Luebering shunt, 2,3-DPG is concentrated in red cells at levels (4 to 5 mM) approximately equivalent to the molar concentration of Hb and about four times that of ATP. As a trapped anion, 2,3-DPG contributes to both the molality and the slightly acid pH of the red cell interior. Its most important regulatory function is to facilitate unloading of O_2. 2,3-DPG and ATP are called allosteric effectors of Hb because both bind to the protein at a site other than the O_2-liganding catalytic (heme) locus and yet influence the oxygen-binding performance of the entire molecule. As the prime allosteric regulator, 2,3-DPG is responsible for the fact that red cell affinity for O_2 is appropriately intermediate ($P_{50} = 26$), for the O_2 affinity of Hb stripped of 2,3-DPG is intolerably high ($P_{50} = 2$). Each molecule of 2,3-DPG binds to a single tetramer of Hb while it is in the T conformation, but it detaches when the tetramer binds a third O_2 and flips into the R conformation.

2,3-DPG provides temporary relief   In response to hypoxia (high altitude, anemia, cardiopulmonary disorders), the Rapoport-Luebering shunt is swiftly summoned to generate high levels of free 2,3-DPG, inducing a rightward shift in O_2 affinity within several hours. This facilitation of O_2 unloading is an advantage temporarily, particularly at or near sea level, for it enhances O_2 release to tissues at a high PO_2, but the victory may be a Pyrrhic one. By promoting deoxygenation, the energy cost of this allosteric response is charged immediately to the cardiopulmonary system. An energetically more favorable, longterm adaptation to hypoxia is provided by EP-driven expansion of erythropoiesis.

BLOOD FLOW AND O_2 TRANSPORT

Handicaps in O_2 delivery are countered initially by cardiovascular and respiratory adjustments. If the impediment persists beyond a few hours, these homeostatic adjustments are supplemented by alteration in the O_2 affinity of Hb. Definitive correction of imbalances between O_2 supply and demand is achieved by EP-mediated feedback control of red cell production. In chronic anemia the intramedullary erythropoietic mass expands 3-fold within a few weeks and 8- to 10-fold within months. In response to chronic hypoxic stimulation the entire potential marrow cavity becomes occupied by hematopoietic—primarily erythro-

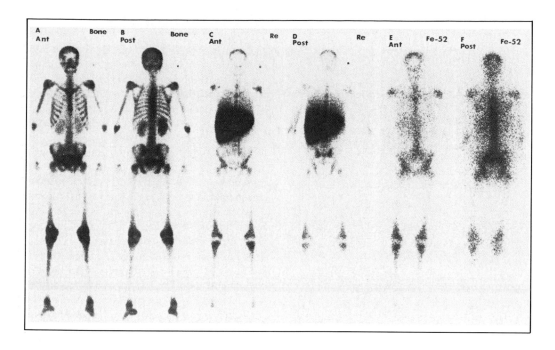

FIGURE 4-18

Geographic extension of erythropoiesis through-out marrow cavity in a patient with chronic hypoxia from sickle cell anemia. Skeletal scintigraphy (A and B) reveals expansion of bony cortex to accommodate proliferating erythroid cells. RES imaging with ^{99m}Tc-sulfur colloid (C and D) confirms expansion of marrow stromal (RES) elements into long bones and calvaria. Imaging with ^{52}Fe (E and F) shows that intramedullary erythropoietic activity codistributes with marrow RES. (From Fordham EW and Amjad A: Radionuclide imaging of bone marrow. Semin Hematol 18:222,1981.)

poietic—tissue (Figure 4-18) [19]. In the feedback mechanism that regulates red cell production, erythropoiesis is governed by sensors that monitor the flow of O_2 to the kidneys and signal renal vascular endothelium to switch on EP production when O_2 delivery is substandard. This mechanism works well when hypoxemia is induced by anemia, but in a setting of O_2 starvation (high altitude, cardiopulmonary disease) heightened EP production will increase hematocrit levels, reducing blood fluidity disproportionately.

Blood Viscosity versus O_2 Flow

In a given vessel perfused at a given pressure, the quantity of O_2 delivered to tissues is the product of the O_2 content (a direct function of hematocrit) and the flow rate of blood (an indirect function of hematocrit). As the consequence of these opposing influences, O_2 transport through tubular vessels as determined in vitro is maximal at hematocrit levels between 40 and 45 vol % (Figure 4-19) [20]. That O_2 flow at high rates of shear is maximal at physiologic levels of hematocrit reaffirms the splendor of natural selection. This ode to evolution and entropy ostensibly stumbles on a point of logic: as hematocrit levels climb above the optimal range portrayed in Figure 4-19, blood flow deteriorates, causing more EP to produce more red cells and more viscosity, leading to a vicious cycle that would generate remorseless, fatal polycythemia. This sequence has been validated by measurement of air pocket PO_2 values in superfluously transfused mice and by studies of regional O_2 transport in dogs transfused to hematocrit levels above 60 to 65 vol %; increases in blood volume, right heart filling pressure, and cardiac output do shift the O_2 delivery curve favorably to the right (at the price of increased cardiac work),

FIGURE 4-19

Oxygen flow (l/viscosity × Hct) at various he-matocrits in vitro. Viscosity was measured with an Ostwald glass viscosimeter at a high fixed rate of shear (uninterrupted heavy line) and with a Brookfield cone-plate viscosimeter at two different shear rates: $115s^{-1}$ corresponds to blood flow in small vessels; $11.5s^{-1}$ character-izes flow in large arteries. (From Erslev AJ: Why the kidney? Nephron 41:213,1985. Re-printed by permission of S. Karger AG, Basel.)

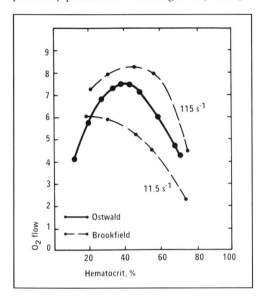

REQUIEM FOR SENESCENT RED CELLS

The actuarial lifespan of red cells is about 120 days. Lifespan is a function of natural aging, whereas pathologic reduction in red cell sur-vival is termed "hemolysis." After prolonged abuse in circulation, red cells begin to show various scars of senescence at about 100 days. Among these are a slowdown of glycolysis, declines in levels of ATP and membrane lipids, and gradual dessication. Aged red cells become rigid and wizened (Figure 4-21) [21]. The most decisive change in red cells that predisposes to their demise appears to be an age-dependent stiffening effect of Hb-spectrin crosslinkages; as in old people this delays recovery from a bent position. How worn-out, effete red cells are finally dispatched remains obscure. Natu-ral IgG antibodies to neoantigens created dur-ing senescence by aggregation of band 3 mole-cules and anti-α-galactosyl autoantibodies are among the suspects. By whatever mechanism, the efficiency with which senescent red cells are culled from blood by macrophages without leaving a trace is impressive.

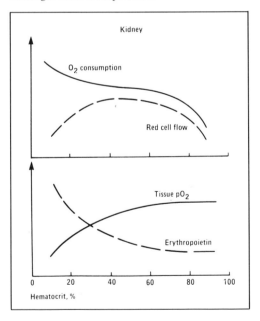

but the downhill slope in PO_2 becomes appar-ent above hematocrit levels of about 65 vol %.

Why the kidneys? Plasma EP levels, mea-sured by radioimmunoassay of unconcentrated plasma, are not elevated in patients with he-matocrits as high as 80 vol %, corresponding to blood viscosities over three times normal. The reason nature has entrusted kidneys with the task of monitoring PO_2 and regulating EP production is that kidneys are the only organ in which O_2 consumption parallels blood flow. As patients become increasingly polycythemic, O_2 consumption and red cell flow to the kidneys decline in tandem, resulting in a level-ing of both renal PO_2 and renal production of EP (Figure 4-20) [20] and avoidance of the vicious viscous cycle.

FIGURE 4-20

Theoretical interplay between hematocrit and O_2 consumption, red cell flow, renal (tissue) PO_2, and erythropoietin production. (From Erslev AJ et al: Why the kidney? Nephron 41:213,1985. Reprinted by permission of S. Karger AG, Basel.)

FIGURE 4-21

Scanning EMs portraying the discocyte-to-echinocyte transformation (A to D) of red cells, accompanying their transfiguration and death. (From Reinhart WH and Chien S: Echinocyte-stomatocyte transformation and shape control of human red blood cells: morphological aspects. Am J Hematol 24:1,1987.)

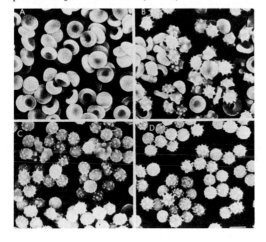

Hemoglobin Catabolism

In keeping with nature's frugality, nearly all of the constituents of the 6 to 7 g of Hb catabolized daily are reused; several backup mechanisms have evolved to prevent the escape of red cell metabolites, the most precious of which is iron.

Haptoglobin and the Renal Threshold

Hb released into plasma is promptly seized with high affinity by haptoglobin (Hp), an 85,000 M_r α_2-glycoprotein synthesized by liver. HpHb complexes are rapidly cleared by hepatic parenchymal cells which degrade the entire complex: during heightened Hb degradation (as in hemolytic anemias) the normal concentration of plasma Hp may fall from 128 ± 25 mg/dl to immeasurably low levels. The HpHb complex is too large (M_r: 150,000) to be filtered through glomeruli, but Hb released after Hp is exhausted is uniquely filtrable. In dilute solution in plasma Hb tetramers dissociate into $\alpha\beta$ dimers:

$$\alpha_2\beta_2 \rightleftharpoons 2\alpha\beta$$

These 32,000 M_r half-molecules are readily filtered through the glomerular basement membrane and are absorbed (resorbed) by the proximal tubular cells. Only when the intraluminal Hb overloads the tubular absorptive capacity (T_m) does Hb appear in the urine. Thus proximal tubular resorption is a second mechanism for conserving Hb catabolites. In these cells, iron is speedily separated from porphyrin and then packaged in ferritin; some ferritin iron is recovered and binds to transferrin in the circulation, but much ferritin is lost through desquamation of iron-laden tubular cells, the presence of which is an indication of hemoglobinemia (Figure 4-22) [22].

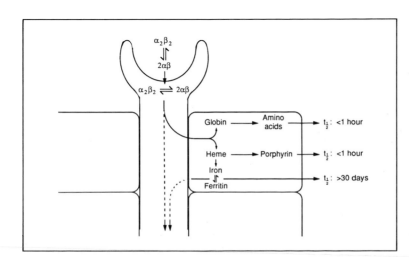

FIGURE 4-22

Renal handling of filtered hemoglobin. (Reproduced from the Journal of Experimental Medicine, 1969;129: 925 by copyright permission of the Rockefeller University Press.)

FIGURE 4-23

Bosom bodies: SEM portrait of a macrophage clutching two effete red cells to its overflowing breast. Phagocytic finales are seldom this picturesque. Ma = macrophage. Er = erythrocyte. Arrows point to advancing edges of the enveloping arms and sleeves of macrophage cytoplasm. (From Tissues and Organs: A Text-Atlas of Scanning Electron Microscopy. By Richard Kessel and Randy Kardon. Copyright © 1979 by W.H. Freeman and Company. Reprinted with permission.)

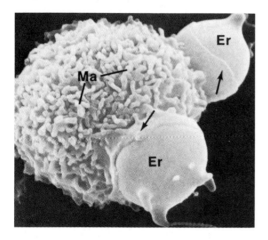

Heme Catabolism

Most senile or otherwise doomed red cells are destroyed by littoral macrophages that line the hepatic and splenic sinuses. Lifeless corpuscles adhere to and are engulfed by macrophages either whole (Figure 4-23) [23] or piecemeal, the globin is oxidatively precipitated, and heme is degraded by a microsomal enzyme system requiring NADPH, molecular O_2, and cytochrome C. The enzyme, heme oxygenase, which is substrate inducible, catalyzes cleavage of the α-methene carbon, causing release of carbon monoxide (CO) and iron; in the presence of NADPH, the linear tetrapyrrole product, biliverdin, is reduced to bilirubin by biliverdin reductase (Figure 4-24) [24, 25]. For each mol of bilirubin and CO formed, 3 mol of O_2 and 3 mol of NADPH are consumed. This reaction represents the only endogenous source of CO in the body, and the rate of CO exhalation (by nonsmoking individuals) is a quantitative measure of the rate of heme degradation.

Bilirubin metabolism If $2\text{-}^{14}\text{C}$-glycine is infused into normal adults the label is incorporated into the porphyrin ring and reappears after heme catabolism as ^{14}C-bilirubin. Most labeled bilirubin is recoverable from feces at 120 ± 20 days, reflecting timely destruction of the cohort of labeled red cells, but about one-quarter of the labeled bilirubin is excreted within several days of the infusion. This "early-labeled peak" is the sum of two components: the earlier, larger portion arises from rapidly cycling heme proteins such as cytochrome P-450; the second part results from catabolism of driblets of Hb released during erythroid division and denucleation and during abortive maturation. The size of this early-labeling fraction is a composite measure of marrow ineffi-

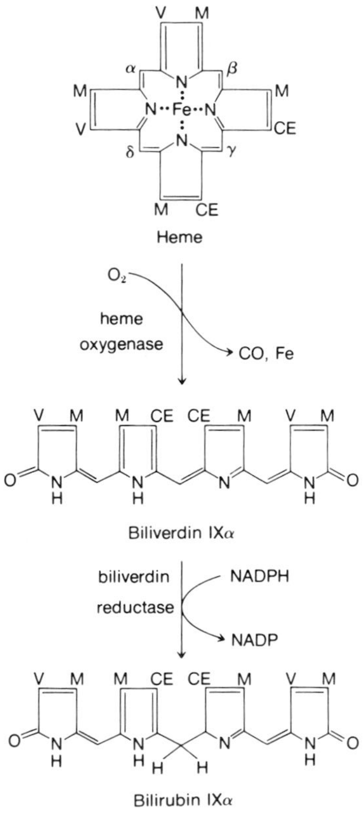

FIGURE 4-24

Formation of bilirubin from heme. CE = β-carboxymethyl, M = methyl, and V = vinyl. (From Awad WM Jr and Wells MS: Chapt 22, in Textbook of Biochemistry with Clinical Correlations, Devlin TM, Ed. New York, John Wiley & Sons, Inc.,1982.)

ciency and may be increased greatly in disorders characterized by growth imbalance during maturation-division; in megaloblastic anemias and thalassemias, in which marrow kinetics are woefully inefficient or "ineffective," the second of the two early peaks may be enlarged prodigiously by intramedullary hemolysis and thereby may become the main source of fecal and serum bilirubin.

Bilirubin entering plasma is solubilized by binding to albumin, which prevents its damaging transit across the blood:brain barrier. Bilirubin on albumin is cleared swiftly by liver hepatocytes, which conjugate the yellow pigment to a water-soluble ("free" or "direct-reacting") diglucuronide that is excreted via the biliary tract through the intestines. Unconjugated (bound or "indirect-reacting") bilirubin accumulates moderately in plasma when the rate of heme degradation is accelerated; hemolytic anemias are characterized by elevations in plasma levels of nonglucuronidated, indirect-reacting bilirubin.

THE ANEMIAS

Anemia is diagnosed most directly on the basis of a reduction in concentrations of red cells, hemoglobin, and hematocrit. Definition of the kind of anemia is usually aided by determination of red cell size and

hemoglobin content and by enumeration of reticulocytes.

Red Cell Size and Hemoglobin Content

Red cell size is best expressed in terms of mean cellular (corpuscular) volume, or MCV; the presence and proportion of subpopulations concealed within the mean can be ascertained and recorded by electronic particle counters. The MCV is calculated by dividing the hematocrit (expressed as l/l) by the red cell count per l:

$$MCV \text{ (fl)} = \frac{\text{hematocrit l/l} \times 1000}{\text{red cell count} \times 10^{12}/l}$$

The mean cellular (corpuscular) hemoglobin content of red cells, or MCH, is computed by dividing the hemoglobin concentration of whole blood by the red cell count per l:

$$MCH \text{ (pg)} = \frac{\text{hemoglobin (g/l)}}{\text{red cell count} \times 10^{12}/l}$$

The mean cellular (corpuscular) hemoglobin concentration, or MCHC, is derived by dividing the hemoglobin concentration—expressed in grams per deciliter of whole blood—by the hematocrit value:

$$MCHC \text{ (g/dl)} = \frac{\text{hemoglobin (g/dl)}}{\text{hematocrit (l/l)}}$$

The normal ranges of values for men and women are given in Table 4-3 [26].

TABLE 4-3

Normal ranges of red cell values in adults

Determination	Men Mean	Men 95% range	Women Mean	Women 95% range
Red cell count, $\times 10^6/\mu l$ (or $\times 10^{12}/l$)	5.1	4.5–5.9	4.6	4.1–5.1
Hemoglobin, g/dl	15.3	14.2–16.9	13.9	12.2–15.0
Hematocrit, l/l × 100	45.9	41.8–49.0	41.4	38.6–45.7
MCV, fl	90	83–99	90	83–99
MCH, pg	30	28–32	30	28–32
MCHC, g/dl	33	32–36	34	32–36
Reticulocytes, %	1.0	0.5–1.8	1.2	0.5–2.2
$\times 10^9/l$	50	25–100	55	25–120

Source: From Jandl JH: Chapt 1, in Blood: Textbook of Hematology. Boston, Little, Brown and Company, 1987.

Reticulocytosis indicates heightened erythro-poiesis The concentration of reticulocytes, recently denucleated young red cells, normally rises in response to anemic hypoxia: absence of reticulocytosis in response to anemia signifies marrow failure; its presence indicates increased red cell destruction (hemolysis). If marrow suppression and hemolysis coexist, the stifled reticulocyte response may mislead.

Classification of Anemias

Almost all anemias can be sorted into either of two primary pathogenetic categories: those caused by impaired release of red cells from marrow and those caused by increased destruction in (or loss from) the bloodstream. An uncomplicated pathogenetic classification of the anemias (excluding blood loss anemia) is presented in Table 4-4.

Signs and Symptoms of Anemia

Most manifestations of any given anemia are common to all anemias. Severity is determined by rate and extent of anemic progression, degree of reduction in blood volume, and adequacy of cardiopulmonary adaptation. Initial compensatory adjustments are cardiovascular and include increases in blood flow and its redistribution to areas most vulnerable to hypoxemia. Centralization of blood flow during the hypovolemia of anemia is responsible for the principal signs of anemia: pallor of tarsal conjunctivae, nail beds, and palmar creases, and absence of blanching of nail beds on palpation [27]. Anemic pallor is not caused by thinness of blood but by reduced perfusion of the skin. The high output circulatory response is attended by thumping palpitation, dizziness, tinnitus, postural faintness, tingling and restlessness of the legs, and other indicators of underperfusion. When hemoglobin levels fall below half-normal, coronary blood flow becomes the limiting factor. Most patients at rest display only modest ventilatory adjustments. Anemic patients are intolerant of exertion, but air hunger at rest is a harbinger of morbid cardiopulmonary decompensation. Among the variable miscellany of anemia concomitants are anorexia, nausea, headache, disturbed mentation, scotomata, and anemic retinopathy (Figure 4-25).

TABLE 4-4

Pathogenetic classification of anemias

Impaired production
  Aplastic and myelodysplastic anemias
  Myelophthisic anemias (infiltrative myelopathies)
  Megaloblastic anemias
  Hypochromic anemias

Increased destruction (hemolytic anemias)
  Primary disorders of red cell membranes
  Secondary disorders of red cell membranes
  Immunohemolytic anemias
  Hemolytic anemias caused by red cell infection
  Heinz body hemolytic anemias
  Hemolytic anemias caused by glycolytic defects
  Hemoglobinopathies
  Anemias of splenomegaly

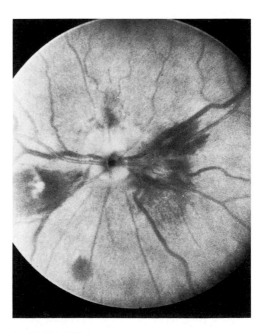

FIGURE 4-25

Anemic retinopathy in a 31-year-old man with anemia (Hb: 5.5 g/dl) of recent onset. The large flame-shaped hemorrhages cleared 1 month after correction of the anemia. (Courtesy Dr. RA Marshall.)

TABLE 4-5

Categorical classification of erythropoietic failures

Category	Functional defect	Marrow morphology	Red cell morphology	Common causes
Aplastic anemias	Disturbed stem cell kinetics	Hypoplastic or dysplastic	Normocytic or macrocytic	Chemicals, radiation, renal insufficiency, marrow infiltration, idiopathic
Megaloblastic anemias	Impaired DNA synthesis	Hyperplastic, megaloblastic	Macrocytic	Cobalamin deficiency, folate deficiency
Hypochromic anemias	Impaired hemoglobin synthesis	Hyperplastic, deficient hemoglobinization	Microcytic, hypochromic	Iron deficiency, anemia of chronic disease, thalassemias, sideroblastic disorders

ANEMIAS CAUSED BY MARROW MALFUNCTION

Production of red cells may be impaired in any of three major ways. Failure of pluripotential stem cells to supply adequate numbers of functional CFU-Es leads to red cell aplasia, and if stem cell failure affects all "myeloid" cell lines (erythroid, myeloid, and megakaryocytic), trilineage aplasia supervenes. The term "aplastic anemia" encompasses not only marrow aplasia (hypoplasia) but also marrow hyperplasia in which the erythroid series is kinetically and clonally defective and unable to generate releasable red cells (myelodysplasia). Included categorically among anemias attributable to stem cell failure are anemias resulting from infiltration of marrow by hostile invaders such as tumor cells; for this form of marrow failure the adjective "myeloinfiltrative" is preferable to the venerable tongue-twister "myelophthisic."

Erythroid precursors that are generated at normal rates by CFU-Es and possess all the RNA apparatus for cytoplasmic growth and hemoglobin accumulation, but cannot garner sufficient DNA to replicate with normal rapidity, suffer and die from unbalanced growth. Marrow fills up with dead and dying cells bearing the morphologic stigmata of failed division. Anemias resulting from replicative impotence are termed "megaloblastic."

In a third major category of faulty erythropoiesis, stem cell kinetics are normal, DNA replication is vigorous, but production and accumulation of hemoglobin falls short; this imbalance in cell growth generates numerous cells small in size and deficient in hemoglobin. These are the hypochromic anemias. A pathophysiologic summary of the categories of erythropoietic failure is given in Table 4-5.

REFERENCES

1. Jandl JH: Chapt 2, in Blood: Textbook of Hematology. Boston, Little, Brown and Company, 1987

2. Castoldi GF and Beutler E: Chapt 3, in Atlas of Blood Cells. Function and Pathology, vol. 1, 2nd ed., Zucker-Franklin D et al, Eds. Milan, Edi. Ermes s.r.l., 1988

3. Jandl JH and Katz JH: The plasma-to-cell cycle of transferrin. J Clin Invest 42:314, 1963

4. Dautry-Varsat A and Lodish HF: How receptors bring proteins and particles into cells. Sci Am 250(5):52, 1984

5. Rabin M et al: Regional localization of the human transferrin receptor gene to 3q26.2→qter. Am J Hum Genet 37:1112, 1985

6. McClelland A et al: The human transferrin receptor gene: genomic organization, and the complete primary structure of the receptor deduced from a cDNA sequence. Cell 39: 267,1984

7. Testa U et al: Differential regulation of transferrin receptor gene expression in human hemopoietic cells: molecular and cellular aspects. J Receptor Res 7(1–4):355,1987

8. Harding C et al: Receptor-mediated endocytosis of transferrin and recycling of the transferrin receptor in rat reticulocytes. J Cell Biol 97:329,1983

9. Moore MS et al: Assembly of clathrin-coated pits onto purified plasma membranes. Science 236:558,1987

10. Stahl P and Schwartz AL: Receptor-mediated endocytosis. J Clin Invest 77:657,1986

11. Neckers LM and Trepel JB: Transferrin receptor expression and the control of cell growth. Cancer Invest 4:461,1986

12. Skalak R and Branemark P-I: Deformation of red blood cells in capillaries. Science 164:717,1969

13. Elgsaeter A et al: The molecular basis of erythrocyte shape. Science 234:1217,1986

14. Liu S-C et al: Visualization of the hexagonal lattice in the erythrocyte membrane skeleton. J Cell Biol 104:527,1987

15. Palek J: Hereditary elliptocytosis, spherocytosis and related disorders: consequences of a deficiency or a mutation of membrane skeletal proteins. Blood Rev 1:147,1987

16. Alberts B: Chapt 6, in Molecular Biology of the Cell. New York, Garland Publishing, Inc.,1983

17. Mayo SL et al: Long-range electron transfer in heme proteins. Science 233:948,1986

18. Bunn HF and Forget GB: Hemoglobin: Molecular, Genetic and Cinical Aspects. Philadelphia, WB Saunders Company,1986

19. Fordham W and Amjad A: Radionuclide imaging of bone marrow. Semin Hematol 18:222,1981

20. Erslev AJ et al: Why the kidney? Nephron 41:213,1985

21. Reinhart WH and Chien S: Echinocyte-stomatocyte transformation and shape control of human red blood cells: morphological aspects. Am J Hematol 24:1,1987

22. Bunn HF and Jandl JH: The renal handling of hemoglobin. II. Catabolism. J Exp Med 129:925,1969

23. Kessel RG and Kardon RH: Chapt 2, in Tissues and Organs. A Text-Atlas of Scanning Electron Microscopy. New York, WH Freeman and Company,1979

24. Awad WM Jr and Wells MS: Chapt 22, in Textbook of Biochemistry with Clinical Correlations, Devlin TM, Ed. New York, John Wiley & Sons, Inc.,1982

25. Yoshida T et al: Human heme oxygenase cDNA and induction of its mRNA by hemin. Eur J Biochem 171:457,1988

26. Jandl JH: Chapt 1, in Blood: Textbook of Hematology. Boston, Little, Brown and Company,1987

27. Strobach RS et al: The value of the physical examination in the diagnosis of anemia. Arch Intern Med 148:831,1988

28. Johnstone RM: Chapt 12, in Red Blood Cell Membranes: Structure, Functions, Clinical Implications. Agre P and Parker JC, Eds. New York, Marcel Dekker, Inc.,1989.

Aplastic and Dysplastic Anemias

□

T he generic term aplastic anemia encompasses disorders caused by attrition of pluripotential stem cells, clonal malfunction of these stem cells, or physical displacement of the stem compartment by malignancy or fibrosis of the marrow.

Some Words on Nomenclature and Etiology

In "classic" aplastic anemia the numbers of stem cells (CFU-GEMMs) are reduced below a critical level necessary for self-renewal; marrow parenchyma becomes depleted of differentiating blood cells and the marrow cavity fills with fat. This morbid and relentless atrophy leading to pancytopenia and death is known by the unqualified term "aplastic anemia." Many patients with pancytopenia have a similar course of stalking progression, but the marrow paradoxically is hypercellular. In this more complicated process pluripotential stem cell function has been commandeered by a clonal population originating from a single cytogenetically flawed but kinetically advantaged ancestor. Stem cell numbers are normal, but the differentiating offspring are morphologically and functionally deranged in multiple ways and fail to thrive. These heterogeneous "aplastic" disorders associated with marrow hyperplasia are known collectively as the myelodysplastic (or dysmyelopoietic) syndromes and are often precursive to acute myelogenous leukemia—hence the prevenient but popular appellation of "preleukemia." A third major sort of marrow failure results from brute eviction of marrow parenchyma, most often by malignant infiltration. This hostile takeover of marrow space also causes pancytopenia, but characteristically small numbers of differentiating marrow precursors escape through the disrupted marrow: blood barrier, creating eye-catching "leukoerythroblastic" changes in the blood. Often classified nostalgically as myelophthisis, dis-

TABLE 5-1

Etiologic classification of aplastic and dysplastic anemias

I. Aplastic anemias
    A. Primary (idiopathic)
    B. Secondary to chemical or physical agents
        1. Agents causing dose-dependent marrow injury
            a. Ionizing radiation
            b. Agents used in chemotherapy
            c. Benzene
            d. Arsenic
            e. Alcohol
        2. Agents causing idiosyncratic marrow injury
            a. Chloramphenicol
            b. Phenylbutazone and congeners
            c. Carbonic anhydrase inhibitors
            d. Gold
            e. Miscellaneous
    C. Infection
    D. Metabolic derangements
    E. Hereditary
    F. Anemia of chronic renal disease
    G. Pure red cell aplasia
        1. Acquired
        2. Congenital
II. Myelodysplastic syndromes
III. Infiltrative myelopathies

eases caused by marrow replacement are more aptly designated infiltrative myelopathies. The aplastic and dysplastic anemias are classified according to etiology in Table 5-1.

APLASTIC ANEMIA

Pathophysiology

Hematopoietic stem cells have two duties: to self-renew and to generate differentiated offspring. If the numbers of pluripotential stem cells are reduced below critical levels, estimated at about 10% of normal [1], primacy is given to self-renewal. If the stem cell compartment cannot be restocked, production of differentiating progenitors lapses, and blood counts decline at rates reflecting their intrinsic lifespans. Most aplastic anemias result from incomplete stem cell failure and hematopoietic marrow recedes unevenly, leaving behind foci or "hot pockets" of struggling survivors (Figure 5-1). The collective mass of red marrow is diminished but geographically scattered so that random sampling of marrow may reveal fatty tissue or dry taps on some specimens and atypical cellular marrow on others. In puzzling patients, diagnosis of aplastic anemia can be confirmed by ferrokinetic studies, which reveal a high saturation of transferrin with iron and slowed clearance of radiolabeled iron from plasma. A more vivid appreciation of the extent and employment of fatty replacement in marrow can be gained through magnetic resonance (MR) imaging (Figure 5-2) [2].

Most stem cells in these desperate colonies of survivors are placed under intense pressure by EP; remnant marrow cells are rushed into dysplastic maturation and the blood often contains macrocytic red cells, elevated levels of fetal hemoglobin, and cells abnormally sensitive to acidified serum and complement. In a minority of aplastic anemia patients a clonal transformation occurs in the damaged marrow, and the syndrome of paroxysmal nocturnal hemoglobinuria (PNH) may evolve as a form of clonal escape; about 20% of patients with PNH have a prior record of several years of aplastic anemia. That the diminution in hematopoietic activity in uncomplicated aplastic anemia represents a stem cell disability rather than a disturbance in the hematopoietic microenvironment is affirmed by the fact that about 70% of patients are cured by allogeneic marrow transplantation [3] whereas stromal cells are nontransplantable [4].

Incidence and Prognosis

In the United States and Western Europe the annual age-specific new case incidence of aplastic anemia is about 5 per million, with a steep rise in people over 65. About 25% of patients suffer a fulminant course, with an average survival of 4 months and 50% of patients die within 1 year of onset. The remainder survive with or without transfusion support for 1 to 10 years, but in about 10% of

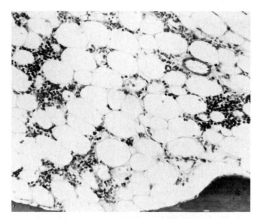

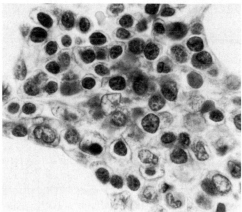

FIGURE 5-1

Marrow biopsy from a patient with aplastic anemia. (Above) At low power most areas are seen
to be occupied by adipocytes, throwing into relief vascular structures and stromal scaffolding,
but scattered small islands of struggling hematopoietic cells are visible in the sea of fat. (Below)
High-power view of a compact "hot pocket" of
proliferating marrow cells in which erythroid
elements predominate. Wright-Giemsa. (Photos
by CT Kapff and DS Weinberg.)

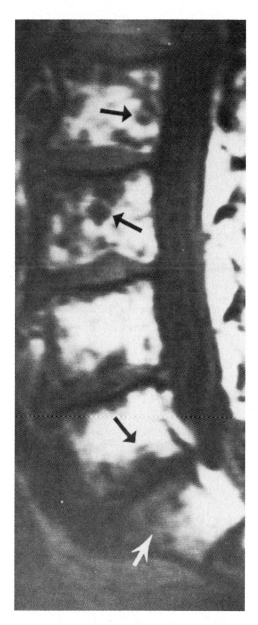

FIGURE 5-2

Saggital MR image of the lumbar spine in a 50-
year-old patient with idiopathic aplastic anemia.
Most marrow space appears white because of
high signal intensity (SI), indicating fat. Scattered focal areas of low SI (black arrows) correspond to islands of hematopoiesis; intermediate
SI signifies fibrosis (white arrow). (From Kaplan
PA et al: Bone marrow patterns in aplastic anemia: observations with 1.5-T MR imaging. Radiology 164:441,1987.)

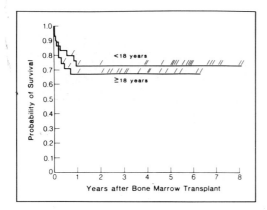

FIGURE 5-3

Projected longterm survival in severe aplastic anemia of 30 children (<18 years) and 28 adults (≥18 years) who received allogeneic marrow transplants from sibling donors. (From McGlave PB et al: Therapy of severe aplastic anemia in young adults and children with alloge neic bone marow transplantation. Blood 70:1325,1987.)

established aplasias the process gradually abates. The statistics for this uncommon disease are grim. In patients with negative prognostic indicators (a "corrected" reticulocyte count of less than 1% and neutrophil and platelet counts less than 500 and 20,000 cells/ μl, respectively), the 1-year survival rate is only 20% [1]; hence successful marrow transplantation offers the only hope for survival (Figure 5-3) [3].

Idiopathic Aplastic Anemia

In most Western populations about 50% of cases of aplastic anemia are idiopathic, but in Asia, where aplastic anemia is far more prevalent, 90% of cases have no known cause, and paradoxically the young age groups are at higher risk than the old, suggesting contagion. The expression idiopathic is an admission of ignorance, for absence of proof is not proof of absence. In all instances patients presenting with aplastic anemia should be interrogated and examined thoroughly for evidence of causative factors.

Aplastic Anemias Secondary to Agents Causing Dose-Dependent Damage to Marrow

Ionizing Radiation

Radiation that removes electrons from atoms is called ionizing radiation. Included among ionizing radiations are electromagnetic emanations such as x-rays and γ-rays, and energetic particles such as α particles (helium nuclei) and β particles (electrons). Neutrons, being uncharged particles, do not ionize directly but by elastic collisions with protons induce secondary ionizations. Marrow cell (and other biologic) damage by ionizing radiation depends on the quantity of radiant energy absorbed by target tissues. The principal units employed to express doses absorbed by tissues are the rad (1 rad = 100 ergs/g tissue) and the gray or Gy (1 Gy = 1 joule/kg tissue, or 100 rads). To compare different kinds of radiation, units called the rem and the sievert have been introduced. One rem is the amount of any radiation that has a biologic effect equivalent to that inflicted by 1 rad of γ-rays. One sievert is the amount of radiation equivalent in biologic effect to 1 Gy of γ-rays. Defined loosely, 1 sievert equals 100 rems and 1 Gy equals 100 rads.

Highly penetrant radiations (neutrons, x-rays, and γ-rays) are hazardous to cells even at a distance, whereas the depth of penetration of α particles is limited to a few μm and that of β particles is intermediate. X-rays and γ-rays have a low rate of energy transfer, whereas particulate radiations impart intense linear energy transfer along densely ionized tracks. Internalized α or β particles create secondary charged particles, ions, and free radicals capable of reacting as "nucleophiles" with DNA; these lead to an assortment of stable and unstable aberrations that in sufficient number can prove lethal to the cell (Figure 5-4) [5].

Determinants of susceptibility to absorbed radiation
The susceptibility of cells to irradiation—either as internalized particulate radiation or as whole body penetrating radiation—is several orders of magnitude greater in actively cycling cells than in cells reposing in the G_0 phase of cell cycle. Among cell popula-

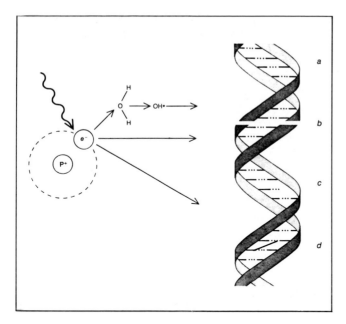

FIGURE 5-4

Damage to DNA by ionizing radiation can be direct or indirect. At the left an electron is dislodged when a hydrogen atom absorbs a photon of radiation (wiggly arrow). This may give rise indirectly to a free radical OH· (top horizontal arrow) or to electrons that react directly with DNA (lower arrow). Three of the many kinds of damage caused by ionization of DNA are denoted by the letters on the right of the double helix. (a) = normal DNA. (b) = a double-stranded break. (c) = deletion of a base. (d) = covalent crosslinking of the DNA duplex. (From Upton AC: The biological effects of low-level ionizing radiation. Sci Am 246(2):41,1982. Copyright © 1982 by Scientific American, Inc. All rights reserved.)

tions, vulnerability is proportional to the fraction of cells in S phase, and thus the most radiosensitive tissues are the germinal cells of testes, hematopoietic cells, and gut mucosal cells. A single brief overexposure to ionizing radiation may cause extensive damage to marrow and gut, leading to death by acute neutropenia, thrombocytopenia, and bleeding from intestinal ulcerations. Should the patient survive the first 2 to 3 weeks, recovery usually follows because most multipotential and pluripotential cells are normally in the radioresistant G_0 phase of cell cycle. These stem cell survivors swing into active cycle and eventually repopulate the marrow. If, on the other hand, exposure to ionizing radiation is chronic or repetitive, reserve stem cells are aroused to action, rendering them vulnerable to irradiation. As exposure continues, the rate of stem cell dysplasia and death increases until aplastic anemia supervenes.

Benzene

It is incumbent upon the physician caring for a patient with aplastic anemia to search for historical evidence of overexposure to benzene, for benzene is the best documented of the dose-dependent chemical causes of toxicologic myelosuppression. At low levels (<0.1 ppm) benzene is a ubiquitous component of the ecology, but its unique prowess as a solvent and degreaser has led to widespread epidemics of industrial overexposure, resulting in marrow suppression, aplastic anemia, and, less often, acute myelogenous leukemia. Once widely used in manufacturing of rubber and leather goods, as a universal degreasing agent, in dry cleaning, in printing, and as an antiknock component of gasoline (white gas), benzene has been supplanted in most instances by toluene, Stoddard solvent, and other nonmyelotoxic solvents. Overexposure in modern times occurs mainly in small workshops or as a peril of cellar or cottage crafts, for most industries at risk are advisedly attentive to the health hazards posed by benzene vapor. One persisting source of overexposure is an ironic consequence of guidelines regulating the use of lead additives to gasoline; to restore antiknock properties, nonleaded gasolines now contain benzene as an additive in concentrations in the United States of about 2% and in levels as high as 10% elsewhere. A threshold level below which benzene does not jeopardize marrow function is not clearly established. Most individuals who developed aplastic anemia or acute myelogenous leukemia from benzene overexposure in the past were chronically exposed to levels in excess of 200 ppm. It is uncertain whether intermittent exposure to levels below 100 ppm is hazardous. The current federal benzene standard applicable to the workplace is 1 ppm.

Unlike idiopathic aplastic anemia, marrow aplasia from overexposure to benzene often is reversible after the cessation of overexposure. Patients who fail to show evidence of recovery within 2 months of abstention are candidates for marrow transplantation.

Alcohol (Ethanol)

The most prevalent and popular dose-dependent hematosuppressive is alcohol. Alcohol in doses in excess of 100 g/day has a direct depressive effect upon marrow sufficient to cause moderate anemia, occasionally accompanied by thrombocytopenic purpura. A generic indication of the cytotoxic effect of alcohol or other toxins on marrow cells is the appearance of large clear vacuoles in proerythroblasts (Figure 5-5). Alcohol-induced hematosuppression and proerythroblast vacuolation, plus the dimorphic anemia with ringed sideroblasts sometimes found in the more dedicated

dipsomaniacs, are self-limited, usually moderate anomalies that vanish within 2 weeks of abstention.

Agents Causing Idiosyncratic Marrow Injury

About 90% of secondary aplastic anemias (excluding chemotherapy-induced aplasia) occur as an unpredictable side effect of medication. At least 400 chemicals and drugs have been indicted as causing unexpected, idiosyncratic marrow failure, usually on circumstantial grounds. The most notorious example is chloramphenicol, which in the period 1950 through 1984 was responsible for nearly 20% of all cases of aplastic anemia in the United States. Taken in large doses chloramphenicol causes mild reversible marrow hypoplasia, associated with vacuolation of erythroid and myeloid cells, a low reticulocyte count, and elevation of unutilized transferrin-bound iron in plasma. Toxicity ceases promptly on drug withdrawal in this dose-related process. A frightening discovery first made in the 1950s was that in some individuals chloramphenicol in any dose—even in the trivial amounts absorbed from eyedrops or surface embrocations—causes a profound, intractable aplastic anemia, usually lethal within 1 year. The genetic basis for this tragic

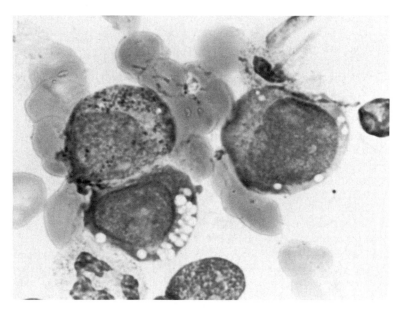

FIGURE 5-5

Vacuolation of proerythroblasts in the marrow of a patient with acute and chronic alcoholism. (Photo by CT Kapff.)

idiosyncratic reaction has never been unveiled, and no means is available for identifying in advance the 1 person in 20,000 who is lethally hypersusceptible. Use of chloramphenicol has declined in recent years, and the leading current causes of idiosyncratic aplastic responses to drugs (according to an international survey of 22.3 million people) are the pervasive analgesics indomethacin, diclofenac, and the butazones (phenylbutazone and oxyphenbutazone) [6]. Idiosyncratic aplasia, like the idiopathic kind, is obstinately unresponsive to conventional nostrums and yields only to transplantation of HLA-matched marrow.

Autoimmune Aplastic Anemia

Suspicion that some forms of aplastic anemia are mediated by immunologic rejection akin to graft-versus-host disease (GVHD) has come from the following observations: aplastic anemia often accompanies thymoma or severe immunodeficiency disease such as X-linked lymphoproliferative syndrome; aplasia frequently develops in immunodeficient children following transfusion of blood containing viable histocompatible lymphocytes; and in coculture studies of normal and aplastic marrow, expurgation of suppressor T cells sometimes enhances formation of BFU-E colonies. These indications, however indirect, have led to extensive trials of infusions of antithymocyte globulin (ATG) and antilymphocyte globulin (ALG) [7,8]. Hematologic improvement occurs in 40 to 60% of patients treated with ALG. In contrast to results with marrow transplantation, most responses to antilymphocyte infusions are incomplete, patients manifesting residual macrocytosis, neutropenia, and thrombocytopenia. Nevertheless longterm survival is greatly improved in those aplastic anemia patients who do not qualify for marrow transplantation for lack of suitable donors and other auspicious factors including suitable age. The successes with ATG and ALG are of enormous heuristic value and have inspired efforts to employ more natural means of modulating suppressor T cell function by using combinations of regulatory cytokines such as γ-interferon. Proof that idiopathic aplastic anemia is commonly caused by cell-mediated immunosuppression is still wanting, and it appears that aplastic anemia (unlike pure red cell aplasia of childhood) rarely is the result of autoantibodies. Erroneous concepts can pave the way to accurate observations and fortunate therapies, however, and immune modulation may well prove to be the key to dependable salvation. At this writing, between 50 and 80% of patients with idiopathic or idiosyncratic aplastic anemia can be salvaged by employing marrow transplantation or ATG infusions [1].

Infections

Most infections are myelosuppressive. Acute self-limited infections characteristically curtail hematopoiesis partially for 10 days to 2 weeks, causing minor, seldom troublesome reductions in blood counts. Chronic infection or inflammation causes a sustained anemia (anemia of chronic disorders) that may diminish the patient's vitality but is no threat to life. In patients with short red cell survival and chronic hemolytic anemia, on the other hand, acute and chronic myelosuppression can be ruinous, for the compensatory erythropoietic response is silenced; in patients with severe hemolytic anemia any infection can become life-threatening within several days, precipitating so-called aplastic crisis. The principal cause of calamitous aplastic crisis in patients with hemolytic disease is infection with the B19 strain of human parvovirus (HPV).

Parvovirus Infection: The Nemesis of Hemolytic Anemia Patients

The B19 strain of parvovirus is host-specific for people and usually is called human parvovirus (HPV). HPV, a tiny single-stranded DNA virus, is responsible for a highly communicable grippelike contagion consisting of fever, headache, myalgia, and respiratory symptoms. This nondescript prodrome is followed within a week by an exanthem and (in adults) by polyarthropathy—a syndrome know in pediatric circles as fifth disease or erythema infectiosum. HPV has a specific tropism for erythroid cells, as revealed by immunofluorescence, in situ hybridization, and Southern blot analysis of DNA replicative forms. Proerythroblasts are most vulnerable to infection by HPV, but the virions also cause arrest in CFU-E and

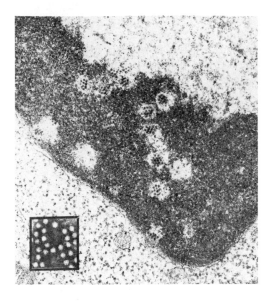

FIGURE 5-6

Electron micrographs of B19 parvoviruses in infected erythroblast and in serum (inset) during transient aplastic crisis. Parvoviruses are small (23 nm across), single-stranded DNA particles that are fastidiously erythrotropic; as shown in the micrograph the icosahedral particles of HPV form crystalline arrays and inhabit lacunae within the marginated chromatin of erythroid precursors. HPV particles are selectively tropic for CFU-Es and dividing erythroid cells as they enter S phase. (From Young N: Hematologic and hematopoietic consequences of B19 parvovirus infection. Semin Hematol 25:159,1988.)

BFU-E colony growth [9]. Single-stranded viruses in a double-stranded world, parvoviruses employ a singular strategy for replication. Parvoviruses are endowed with palindromes of 125 to 150 nucleotides at each end of the DNA strand; these mirror-image sequences form T-shaped duplex hairpin structures, and replication proceeds through enzymatic cleavage of the duplex intermediates. The infectious strands (negative with respect to RNA) give rise to two negative and two positive DNA strands. In patients with hereditary spherocytosis, sickle cell anemia, thalassemia, pyruvate kinase deficiency, and other kinds of severe hemolytic anemia, HPV organisms invade the nuclei of erythroid progenitor cells (Figure 5-6) [10], causing virtual disappearance of reticulocytes from blood and of erythroblasts from marrow. Until infection abates, patients with hemolytic disease may depend for their lives on transfusional support. Recovery from this erythropathic infection is heralded by the appearance in marrow of giant proerythroblasts that display large eosinophilic inclusion bodies, split nucleoli, and variable numbers of pseudopods and vacuoles (Figure 5-7) [11]. HPV infection is responsible for 86% of aplastic crises in children with sickle cell anemia.

Viral Hepatitis

Most fatal cases of virus-associated chronic aplastic anemia occur within 1 to 3 months of

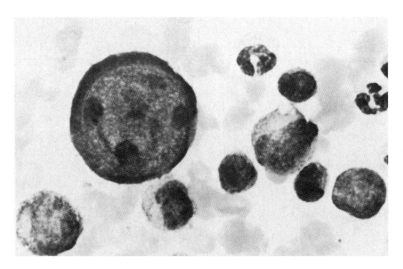

FIGURE 5-7

Giant proerythroblast exhibiting large eosinophilic nuclear inclusions in Wright-stained marrow. Note normal assortment of myeloid cells and absence of erythroblasts. (From Van Horn DK et al: Human parvovirus-associated red cell aplasia in the absence of underlying hemolytic anemia. Am J Pediatr Hematol Oncol 8:235,1986.)

onset of viral hepatitis, usually commencing during convalescence. Although hepatitis B virus (HBV) is often tropic for hematopoietic cells, HBV infections are usually associated with mild hematosuppression, rarely causing aplastic anemia. Over 80% of cases of posthepatitis aplastic anemia are attributable to infection by non-A, non-B virus: so-called hepatitis C. The risk of chronic aplasia after hepatitis, all kinds combined, is estimated at 0.1 to 0.2%; conversely, among patients with established aplastic anemia, about 5% have an antecedent history of clinically overt hepatitis. The likelihood and severity of aplastic anemia after viral hepatitis are unrelated to the severity of liver damage. Posthepatitis aplastic anemia carries an exceptionally grim prognosis, and the diagnosis mandates vigorous efforts to locate an HLA-compatible transplant donor. That transplantation of HLA matched normal marrow rapidly restores hematopoiesis [12] affirms that hepatitis does not despoil the hematopoietic microenvironment.

Hereditary (Constitutional) Aplastic Anemias

Approximately 30% of aplastic anemias that appear in childhood are hereditary, and in two-thirds of these patients aplasia is preceded by heterogeneous combinations of congenital anomalies, signifying the diagnosis of Fanconi's anemia.

Fanconi's Anemia: A Syndrome of Defective DNA Repair

In Fanconi's anemia relentlessly progressive aplastic anemia emerges during childhood or adolescence amidst a setting of multiple congenital anomalies, the most common of which are: patchy brown pigmentation of the skin, dwarfism, microcephaly, renal anomalies, and an assortment of skeletal aberrations, the most singular of which is absence or underdevelopment of the thumbs (Figure 5-8) [13]. The mode of inheritance is recessive, with phenotypic diversity, and a gene frequency of about 1 in 600. Children with characteristic malformations or who have siblings with Fanconi's anemia can be diagnosed by chromosome stud-

FIGURE 5-8

Hands of a 9-year-old child with Fanconi's anemia show symmetrical hypoplasia of the thumbs, which resemble short fingers. (From Hoffbrand AV and Pettit JE: Chapt 6, in Clinical Hematology Illustrated. An Integrated Text and Color Atlas. London, Gower Medical Publishing Ltd., 1987.)

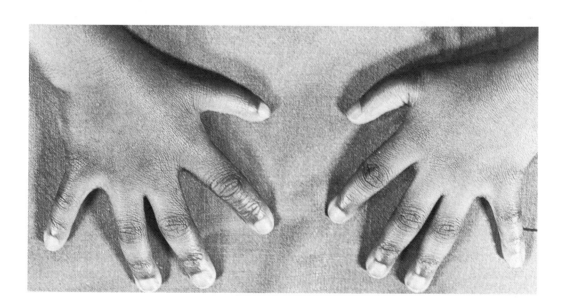

ies; indeed cytogenetic tests are available for prenatal, postnatal, and carrier detection of the chromosome instability characteristic of Fanconi's anemia. The molecular basis of the defect in DNA repair that marks this disease is unknown, but exposure of dividing blood or marrow cells to clastogenic stress by alkylators or ionizing radiation in culture generates weird and elaborate chromatid exchange figures, attesting to extensive breakage and faulty rejoining (Figure 5-9) [14].

Fanconi's anemia is a premalignant disorder

Pancytopenia evolves inexorably during childhood, red marrow recedes centripetally, and pressure by EP forces release of "stress reticulocytes," macrocytes, and red cells containing hemoglobin F and bearing the fetal i antigen. Even on androgen therapy half-survival is less than 10 years from onset, and most victims succumb within 5 years after commencement of pancytopenia. In over 10% of cases the aplastic process terminates as a variant of AML, and (as in other disorders of DNA repair) Fanconi patients are prone to develop malignancies other than leukemia. Marrow transplantation from HLA-identical siblings can cure the marrow failure but does not protect the recipient against other neoplasms to which these patients are predisposed.

Congenital Dyserythropoietic Anemias (CDAs)

CDAs comprise a group of rare familial disorders in which anemia and ineffective erythropoiesis are associated with binuclearity or multinuclearity of marrow erythroblasts. CDAs are characterized by anemia, florid erythroid hyperplasia of the marrow without reticulocytosis, and mild icterus. In each of the three major types of CDA that have been defined on morphologic grounds the genetic abnormality is restricted to committed erythroid stem cells. A common mechanism accounting for the trapping of many abnormal erythroblasts in the marrow, where they are doomed to disintegrate, is that the cells are immobilized by their sheer bulk. In the mildest of these disorders (type I CDA) some erythroblasts are binucleate or multilobulated, their nuclei tethered together by thin Feulgen-positive bridges. In type II CDA, multinuclearity of marrow erythroblasts is associated with the finding that denucleated circulating red cells lyse in acidified serum, giving rise to the conflated acronym HEMPAS (hereditary erythroblast multinuclearity with a positive acid serum test). In the rare type III variant, about 30% of erythropoietic cells are massively enlarged and contain up to 12 nuclei;

FIGURE 5-9

Metaphase spreads of lymphocytes from a patient with Fanconi's anemia. Multiple complex chromatid exchange figures and endo-reduplications create antic kaleidoscopic designs characteristic of this deadly ailment. (From Auerbach AD et al: Prenatal and postnatal diagnosis and carrier detection of Fanconi anemia by a cytogenetic method. Reproduced by permission of Pediatrics Vol 67 page 128 copyright 1981.)

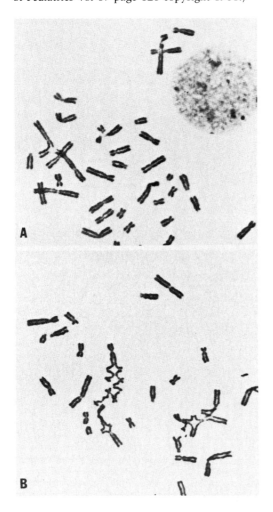

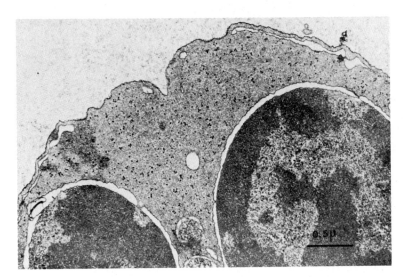

FIGURE 5-10

TEM of a binucleated late erythroblast from a patient with type II CDA. Note two cisternae just beneath the cell membrane. (From Punt K et al: Chapt 4, in Dyserythropoiesis, Lewis SM and Verwilghen RL, Eds. New York, Academic Press, 1977.)

clearly such "gigantoblasts" (as described in hematologic argot) are too big to travel. The pathogenesis of most CDAs is uncertain, but studies of type II CDA—the most common of these erythropoietic curiosities—indicate that late erythroblasts acquire a double membrane enclosing a cisterna lying 40 to 60 nm beneath the cell membrane (Figure 5-10) [15]. This thickened shell of reduplicated membrane may incarcerate the dividing nuclei, locking them in various multiples within a single membraneous chamber. Fortunately the constraints to division are incomplete and highly variable. The main features characterizing the three well-defined types of CDA are listed in Table 5-2 [16].

TABLE 5-2

Types of congenital dyserythropoietic anemias

Feature	Type I	Type II	Type III
Red cell size	Macrocytic	Normocytic	Macrocytic
Anemia	Mild to moderate	Mild to severe	Mild
Marrow erythroblasts	Megaloblastoid; 1–3% binucleated; 1–2% chromatin bridges	10–50% bi- and multinucleated	Gigantoblasts
Genetics	Recessive	Recessive	Dominant
Sugar water test	Negative	Negative	Negative
Acid serum test	Negative	Positive	Negative
Reaction with:			
Anti-i	Slight	Strong	Slight
Anti-I	Positive	Strong	Slight

Source: From Alter BP: Chapt 7, in Hematology of Infancy and Childhood, 3rd ed., Nathan DG and Oski FA, Eds. Philadelphia, WB Saunders Company, 1987.

Pure Red Cell Aplasia

Marrow aplasia confined to erythroid progenitors is known in hematologic patois as pure red cell aplasia (PRCA). PRCA may occur as a hereditary disease (Diamond-Blackfan anemia) which presents within the first 18 months of life as a chronic severe anemia of obscure genetic provenance, sometimes arising in a Fanconilike setting of multiple congenital anomalies. This "constitutional" anemia can be cured by transplantation of marrow from an HLA-identical sibling [17], a happy fact that refutes postulations of humoral inhibitors or flaws in the hematopoietic environment. More common are the acquired forms of PRCA, acute and chronic.

Acute PRCA

Most cases of acute PRCA are caused by HPV infection or occur as idiosyncratic responses to drugs. Common among provocative pharmaceuticals are sulfonamides, anticonvulsants, isoniazide, phenylbutazone, and carbonic anhydrase inhibitors. In nearly all instances full recovery has occurred shortly after cessation of drug therapy.

Chronic Acquired PRCA

Chronic acquired PRCA usually occurs in middle or later life and in at least half of cases erythroid growth is halted by IgG antibodies directed against erythroblasts, erythroblast nuclei, or erythropoietin, and erythropoiesis occasionally recovers following plasmapheresis or repeated infusions of intravenous gamma globulin. In many instances erythroid colony suppression is mediated by suppressor T cells, and recovery from T cell–mediated inhibition has been achieved by administration of ALG or cyclosporine. In a subset of patients with T cell chronic lymphatic leukemia, erythrosuppression is caused by a cytotoxic clone of leukemic T cells bearing the morphology and cell surface phenotype of immature natural killer (NK) cells. Collectively these several observations indicate that in many or most instances PRCA is caused either by growth suppressor factors elaborated by clones of T cells or by autoantibodies reacting specifically with CFU-Es or other erythroid precursors [18]. Frequent association of PRCA with an assortment of unrelated antibodies, with lupus erythematosus, and with benign thymomas suggests that PRCA is a syndrome culled from the melange of ill-defined autoimmune disorders. Even the "purity" of this syndrome is sullied by the fact that nearly one-third of patients eventually develop pancytopenia. This uncertainty of definition should not deter therapeutic use of the full panoply of immunosuppressive therapies (corticosteroids, antilymphocyte globulin or antithymocyte globulin, cyclophosphamide, azathioprine, or—if all else fails—marrow transplantation), for the disease can be deadly and immunosuppression usually helps.

Anemia of Chronic Renal Failure

Hypoplastic anemia is a constant accompaniment of chronic renal failure and is proportional in its severity to the degree of failure as measured by urea or creatinine retention. As there are at present over 10,000 patients in the United States with endstage renal disease awaiting renal transplantation, renal failure ranks first among causes of severe hypoplastic anemia. Anemia of renal failure is an endocrine deficiency state entirely correctable by regular infusions of recombinant human erythropoietin.

Anemia of Renal Failure: A Correctable Hormone Deficiency

With renal failure two functions are lost: renal excretory function and renal endocrine function. During excretory failure circulating red cells are damaged by accumulation of toxic metabolites and imbalances in acid-base and salt-water regulation. These derangements cause modest disturbances in red cell glycolysis, red cell lifespan is mildly or moderately shortened, and roughly 50% of red cells display a pathognomonic but benign "burr cell" deformity (Figure 5-11). Prevalence of burr cells correlates poorly with the rise in BUN and not at all with red cell survival.

As renal function worsens, normocytic anemia without neutropenia or thrombocytopenia progresses until a steady state is achieved at hemoglobin levels of 5 to 7 g/dl. Blood transfusions are necessary in patients with cardiovas-

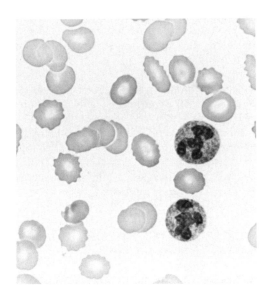

FIGURE 5-11

Burr cell deformity of uremia. Uremic burr cells differ from other echinocytes in possessing about 1 dozen rounded crenulations, most of which are spaced evenly around their margins. Note preservation of central pallor in most burr cells, a characteristic increase in the number of elliptocytes, and moderate hypersegmentation of neutrophils. (Photo by CT Kapff.)

cular problems; systematic transfusions provide an additional and unanticipated benefit in somehow enhancing the survival of subsequent renal transplants—possibly by inducing immunologic toleration.

Recombinant erythropoietin   Rational therapy of the anemia of renal disease is replacement of erythropoietin, normally synthesized by renal vascular endothelium (Chapter 1), by infusing recombinant human erythropoietin (rEP or rHuEpo), a 34,000 M_r glycoprotein mass-produced in mammalian cell expression systems [19]. In hemodialyzed patients with endstage renal disease the hematologic response to rHuEpo infusions given three times weekly is dose-dependent and unassociated with immunologic retaliation (Figure 5-12) [20]. Maintenance of hematocrits between 35 and 40 requires infusions of roughly 100 units/kg three times weekly. Recombinant erythropoietin is nontoxic and nonimmunogenic, and patients receiving replacement therapy enjoy increased vitality, improved disposition and appetite, warmer body temperature, sounder sleep, and reawakened sexual interest and performance. Victory as always claims its price: in renal failure, EP-driven resumption of

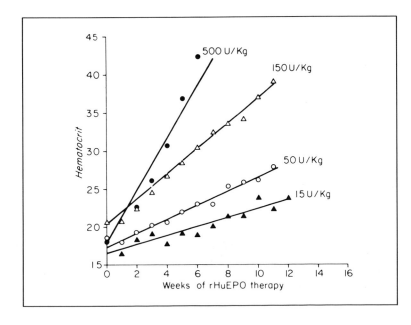

FIGURE 5-12

Dose-dependent rises in hematocrits of anemic hemodialysis patients with endstage renal disease during thrice-weekly infusions of recombinant erythropoietin. Each symbol represents four or five patients. (From Eschbach JW et al: Correction of the anemia of end-stage renal disease with recombinant human erythropoietin. Results of a combined phase I and II clinical trial. Reprinted, by permission of the New England Journal of Medicine, 316:73, 1987.)

erythropoiesis often accelerates or induces hypertension, increased blood viscosity provokes "dialyzer clotting," and serum creatinine levels rise somewhat as plasma volume is diminished [21]. Correction of anemia solves only some of the problems besetting renoprival patients, but replacement therapy with recombinant EP represents an inspiring triumph of genetic engineering; application to other refractory anemias is receiving sedulous attention.

MYELODYSPLASTIC SYNDROMES AND PRELEUKEMIA

Myelodysplastic syndromes are a heterogeneous group of clonal disorders of hematopoiesis exhibiting in common hypercellular but dysfunctional marrow, refractoriness to known hematopoietic factors, and a propensity to progress to acute myelogenous leukemia (AML). In all likelihood the neoplastic clone does not make its debut as overt leukemia, for G6PD isozyme analyses indicate that marrow is populated by cells of clonal (single stem cell) origin before the evolution of clonal karyotypic abnormalities and prior to overgrowth by leukemic cells. For this reason myelodysplastic anemias are lumped together as preleukemia by individuals who emphasize their clonal nature and commonality with AML [22], and are separated as independent entities by committees more concerned with guidelines for classification and fortified in their stance by the fact that most (over 60%) myelodysplastic processes never do transform into overt leukemia [23].

Natural History of the Preleukemic Syndrome

Myelodysplastic syndromes are stealthy, chameleon processes, unpredictable in pace, that particularly affect the elderly or persons of any age who have been treated with alkylating agents or radiotherapy or both. In the natural course, a series of mutagenic events launches a neoplastic clone that competes successfully with normal hematopoietic cells and ultimately dominates them. Over a period of months, years, or decades, the robotic progeny blindly overrun the more civilized ranks of normal marrow cells, and excessive numbers of

unprogrammed blasts start to accumulate. The future course of patients at this point is determined by the kinetic vigor of the clone. If sufficiently dysplastic, malignant cells either fail to flourish or vacillate, resulting in either a stalemate (chronic myelodysplastic or preleukemic syndrome) or marrow hypoplasia. If the cells gain in vitality and become indifferent to regulatory cytokines, myeloblasts accumulate and the process may eventually transform into frank AML in any of its seven guises. For a detailed exposition of myelodysplastic disorders, see Chapter 13.

INFILTRATIVE MYELOPATHIES (MYELOPHTHISIC ANEMIAS)

Infiltration of marrow by nonhematopoietic cells disrupts the marrow:blood barrier and causes untimely release of immature cells into the bloodstream, creating a morphologic pattern known as leukoerythroblastic anemia. When marrow occupation by nonresident cells is extensive, blood-forming elements are evicted, some to take refuge in the spleen, and

FIGURE 5-13

Leukoerythroblastic changes in blood of a patient with myelofibrosis. The anomalous finding in blood of nucleated red cells, young myeloid cells, and teardrop forms is diagnostic of marrow infiltration. (Photo by CT Kapff.)

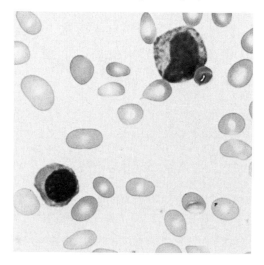

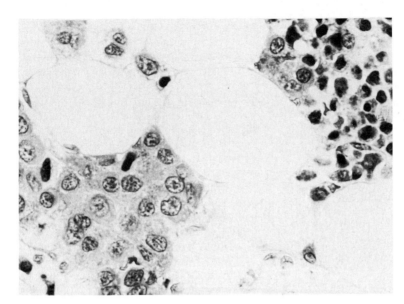

FIGURE 5-14

Marrow biopsy in a patient with leukoerythroblastic blood changes and a "dry tap" reveals islands and clusters of large anaplastic cells having numerous mitotic figures. Normal mixed hematopoietic elements are crowded aside (upper right). (Photo by CT Kapff.)

pancytopenia sets in. The end result is a syndrome of: marrow replacement, often to the extent that efforts to aspirate marrow cells are rewarded only by "dry taps"; premature appearance in blood of nucleated red cells, immature myeloid cells, and giant platelets; and anemia, usually marked by teardrop deformities (Figure 5-13). The term "infiltrative myelopathy" is recommended as being more explicit and less melodramatic than the venerable word "myelophthisis."

The most prevalent causes of infiltrative myelopathy are metastatic carcinoma (Figure 5-14), lymphoreticular malignancies, and miliary or disseminated tuberculosis. Diagnosis and rational therapy depend upon marrow biopsy.

REFERENCES

1. Gewirtz AM and Hoffman R: Current considerations of the etiology of aplastic anemia. CRC Crit Rev Oncol Hematol 4:1,1985

2. Kaplan PA et al: Bone marrow patterns in aplastic anemia: observations with 1.5-T MR imaging. Radiology 164:441,1987

3. McGlave PB et al: Therapy of severe aplastic anemia in young adults and children with allogeneic bone marow transplantation. Blood 70:1325,1987

4. Laver J et al: Host origin of the human hematopoietic microenvironment following allogeneic bone marrow transplantation. Blood 70:1966,1988

5. Upton AC: The biological effects of low-level ionizing radiation. Sci Am 246(2):41,1982

6. The International Agranulocytosis and Aplastic Anemia Study: Risks of agranulocytosis and aplastic anemia. A first report of their relation to drug use with special reference to analgesics. JAMA 256:1749,1986

7. Speck B et al: A comparison between ALG and bone marrow transplantation in treatment of severe aplastic anemia. Thymus 10:147,1987

8. Doney K et al: Treatment of aplastic anemia with antithymocyte globulin, high-dose corticosteroids, and androgens. Exp Hematol 15:239,1987

9. Potter CG et al: Variation of erythroid and myeloid precursors in the marrow and peripheral blood of volunteer subjects infected with human parvovirus (B19). J Clin Invest 79:1486,1987

10. Young N: Hematologic and hematopoietic consequences of B19 parvovirus infection. Semin Hematol 25:159,1988

11. Van Horn DK et al: Human parvovirus-associated red cell aplasia in the absence of underlying hemolytic anemia. Am J Pediatr Hematol Oncol 8:235,1986

12. Witherspoon RP et al: Marrow transplantation in hepatitis-associated aplastic anemia. Am J Hematol 17:269,1984

13. Hoffbrand AV and Pettit JE: Chapt 6, in Clinical Hematology Illustrated. An Integrated Text and Color Atlas. London, Gower Medical Publishing Ltd., 1987

14. Auerbach AD et al: Prenatal and postnatal diagnosis and carrier detection of Fanconi anemia by a cytogenetic method. Pediatrics 67:128,1981

15. Punt K et al: Chapt 4, in Dyserythropoiesis, Lewis SM and Verwilghen RL, Eds. New York, Academic Press, 1977

16. Alter BP: Chapt 7, in Hematology of Infancy and Childhood, 3rd ed., Nathan DG and Oski FA, Eds. Philadelphia, WB Saunders Company, 1987

17. Lenarsky C et al: Bone marrow transplantation for constitutional pure red cell aplasia. Blood 71:226,1988

18. Ammus SS and Yunis AA: Acquired pure red cell aplasia. Am J Hematol 24:311,1987

19. Powell JS et al: Human erythropoietin gene: High level expression in stably transfected mammalian cells and chromosome localization. Proc Natl Acad Sci USA 83:6465,1986

20. Eschbach JW et al: Correction of the anemia of end-stage renal disease with recombinant human erythropoietin. Results of a combined phase I and II clinical trial. N Engl J Med 316:73,1987

21. Eschbach JW and Adamson JW: Recombinant human erythropoietin: implications for nephrology, Am J Kidney Dis 11:203,1988

22. Bagby GC Jr: The concept of preleukemia: clinical and laboratory studies. CRC Crit Rev Oncol Hematol 4:203,1986

23. Bennett JM et al: Proposals for the classification of the myelodysplastic syndromes. Br J Hematol 51:189,1982

6

Megaloblastic
Anemias

□

Megaloblastic anemias are a morphologically similar group of pancytopenic disorders caused by selective reduction in the rate of DNA synthesis relative to the rate of RNA synthesis. As transcription, translation, stem cell kinetics, and protein synthesis proceed normally, retardation of DNA but not RNA replication leads to unbalanced cell growth, with reluctant generation of slowly dividing daughter cells having abundant cytoplasm but deranged nuclei. The brisk production of cytoplasmic RNA and protein in cells whose thymine-starved nuclei synthesize DNA too slowly for timely division protracts cell cycling. Cells commanded by cytokines to divide fail to do so or do so fitfully or too slowly. As a result marrow space fills with kinetically lethargic, overstuffed cells, creating a spurious appearance of hyperplasia. The nuclear:cytoplasmic imbalance ("dyssynchrony") becomes more flagrant with each strained division; eventually the frustrated cells either die in the marrow, a process called "ineffective hematopoiesis," or they omit a terminal division and enter the bloodstream as large, misshapen endstage cells having a shortened lifespan.

All dividing cells in the body are similarly affected by impaired DNA synthesis, but the changes are most evident in nonstop proliferative tissues such as marrow and intestinal mucosa, and the cellular stigmata are most vivid in the orderly ranks of erythropoietic and myelopoietic cells. Familiarity with the distinctive and picturesque morphology of megaloblastic anemias is imperative because the vast majority of these anemias are caused by deficiency of either cobalamin (vitamin B_{12}) or folate and can be cured by appropriate replacement therapy.

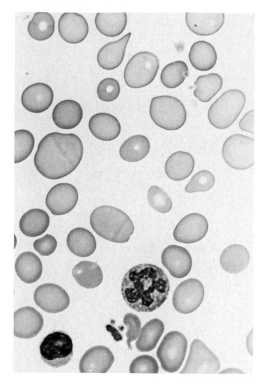

FIGURE 6-1

Morphologic dyad pathognomonic of megaloblastic anemias: hypersegmentation of neutrophils and oval macrocytes (macroovalocytes). The neutrophil is large and its nucleus contains eight or nine segments, indicating that one to two terminal nuclear divisions were omitted. Most red cells are large (compare with the lymphocyte nucleus—the microyardstick of morphology): many are two to four times normal in size, and some have a characteristic ovoid (egg) shape. Among the common accompaniments of megaloblastic anemia shown here are teardrop forms. (Photo by CT Kapff.)

Hypersegmentation and Macroovalocytes: Logos of the Megaloblastic Disorders

Blood cells in megaloblastic anemias bear two distinctive deformities (Figure 6-1). Hypersegmentation of neutrophils is the first, most unequivocal cachet of megaloblastic disease; hypersegmentation is the consequence of one or more omitted terminal divisions, giving rise to large cells containing surplus lobulated nuclear material. The second sign of megaloblastic arrest is the pathognomonic presence of red cells that are both large and egg-shaped; their large size and ovoid shape are also the result of an omitted division, creating a fused product that was intended to be two cells of slightly different diameter. Macroovalocytes are about twice normal in volume, but blood films and cell diameter profiles in megaloblastic anemias reveal extreme variation in size and shape, with macrocytes commingled with small fragmented, teardrop, and spheroidal forms. Thus the average MCV in severe anemia usually falls in the range of 115 to 140 fl.

Progression of anemia is often so gradual that red cell counts may fall below 1 million cells/μl before symptoms appear—a tribute to adaptive responses to chronic hypoxia. Moderate rather than severe leukopenia is the rule, but platelets may decline to counts below 10,000/μl, albeit thrombocytopenia is the least regular accompaniment of anemia.

The Marrow in Megaloblastic Anemias

Marrow morphology reveals the pathogenesis of megaloblastic anemia in caricature. The unique cytologic features of megaloblastic arrest are most flagrantly displayed by intermediate and late erythroblasts, for nuclear deformities are cumulative with each labored division, and nuclear:cytoplasmic asynchrony becomes most apparent in the normally regimental erythroid series. Nevertheless, nuclear chromatin in both erythroid and myeloid series acquires an unevenly speckled pattern, much like that of sliced salami (Figure 6-2). In the less orderly myeloid cells, the most emphatic aberrations are found in giant metamyelocytes and band forms. Unbalanced growth also affects megakaryocytes: these normally polyploid cells may show redundant hypersegmentation and some multinuclearity, and megakaryocyte fragments and giant platelets may slip into the bloodstream.

Pathogenetic Basis of Megaloblastic Anemias

Cytologic deformities arising from deficiency of cobalamin and of folate look alike because the two vitamins act in series to generate thymidylic acid (dTMP) necessary for DNA synthesis. The molecular lesion underlying megaloblastic anemias is impaired conversion of deoxyuridylate monophosphate (dUMP) to

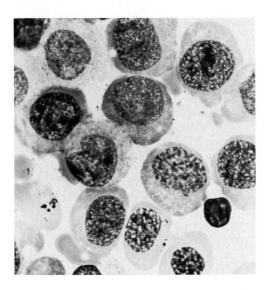

FIGURE 6-2

Marrow aspirate from a patient with megaloblastic anemia, showing abundant large erythroblasts of differing ages. At center stage is a large but relatively normal-looking proerythroblast. Proceeding downward, one can see abundant accumulation of cytoplasm, which is clear and filled with hemoglobin, but nuclear chromatin fails to condense. The motley chromatin clumping is most conspicuous in maturing erythroblasts and creates a pattern reminiscent of sliced salami. Beside the proerythroblast are (bottom to top) a giant band form and giant metamyelocytes, bearing the same nuclear aberrations. Note the nuclear fragments—Howell-Jolly bodies—in the orthochromatic erythroblast and the macrocyte at the bottom center and lower left. (Photo by CT Kapff.)

dTMP. The converting enzyme, known in short form as methyltransferase, is dependent on cobalamin-mediated transfer of a 1-carbon group from the inert folate metabolite, N^5-methyltetrahydrofolate (N^5-methyl FH_4), to homocysteine; this transfer, mediated by the coenzyme methylcobalamin, generates methionine from homocysteine and demethylates FH_4. Demethylation of metabolically "trapped" N^5-methyl FH_4 makes FH_4 available for conversion to the folate coenzyme, $N^{5,10}$-methylene FH_4. dTMP is then synthesized by the enzyme thymidylate kinase, which negotiates the transfer of a 1-carbon fragment from $N^{5,10}$-methylene FH_4 to dUMP (Figure 6-3) [1].

Uracil Misincorporation into DNA Creates Errors in Strand Copying

As $N^{5,10}$-methylene FH_4 is the coenzyme of thymidylate synthetase, the relevant limiting role of cobalamin is as a cofactor to this folate coenzyme. In the absence of FH_4 and its adducts, thymidylate synthesis is slowed or blocked, leading to a pathologic increase in the dUTP/dTTP ratio. Consequently, dUMP is phosphorylated at a rate that swamps dUTP pyrophosphatase, and dUTP accumulates in the cell. Some uridine is then misincorporated into nascent strands of DNA in place of thymidine because DNA polymerase is unable to distinguish between the two nucleotides. Normally

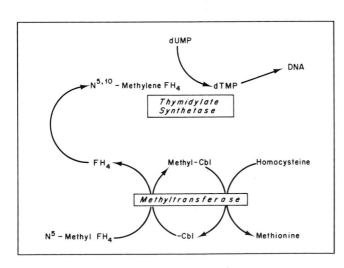

FIGURE 6-3

Consecutive and linked participation of cobalamin (Cbl) and folate (FH_4) in the synthesis of thymidylic acid (dTMP), which is then incorporated via dTTP into DNA. In the absence of either vitamin, DNA synthesis is halted or prolonged in S phase, and dUMP accumulates. (From Beck W: Chapt 34, in Hematology, 3rd ed., Williams WJ et al, Eds. New York, McGraw-Hill Book Company,1983.)

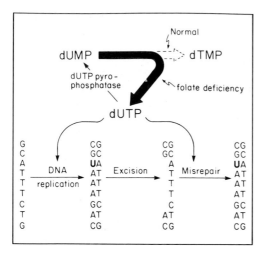

FIGURE 6-4

Explanation for DNA strand breakage responsible for megaloblastic arrest in folate deficiency. The same mechanism operates if folate metabolism is crippled by cobalamin deficiency. From failure to methylate deoxyuridine monophosphate (dUMP) to deoxythymidine monophosphate (dTMP), dUMP is shunted into dUTP and uracil (U) is misincorporated into DNA in place of thymine (T). Repeated efforts by editorial enzymes to excise the false base are futile, and some uracil persists. This leads to the breakage and fraying of DNA strands responsible for megaloblastic morphology and arrested maturation-division. (From Babior BM and Stossel TP: Chapt 6, in Hematology. A Pathophysiological Approach. New York, Churchill Livingstone,1984.)

an editorial enzyme, uracil-DNA-glycosylase, detects misincorporated uracils and excises them by hydrolyzing the N-glycosyl bond linking the false base to the deoxyribose phosphate backbone [2]. In megaloblastic anemias, there is insufficient dTTP on hand for efficient correction by this DNA repair enzyme, and several protracted cycles of excision and resynthesis may be required to incorporate the traces of thymine available into defective daughter strands (Figure 6-4) [3].

The overwhelming majority of megaloblastic anemias result from deficiency of cobalamin (vitamin B_{12}) or folate, but comparable megaloblastic arrest may result from suppression of DNA synthesis by drugs, from inborn errors

TABLE 6-1

Pathogenetic classification of megaloblastic anemias

I. Cobalamin (vitamin B_{12}) deficiency
   A. Dietary deficiency
   B. Deficiency of gastric intrinsic factor (IF)
      1. Pernicious anemia
      2. Gastrectomy
   C. Intestinal malabsorption
      1. Ileal resection or ileitis
      2. Familial selective cobalamin malabsorption
      3. Competitive parasites or infections
         a. Fish tapeworm
         b. Bacterial overgrowth in malformed small bowel
   D. Increased requirement

II. Folate deficiency
   A. Dietary deficiency
   B. Impaired absorption
      1. Sprue
      2. Extensive small bowel disease or resection
      3. Intestinal short circuits
      4. Anticonvulsants, oral contraceptives
   C. Increased requirement
      1. Pregnancy
      2. Hemolytic anemia
      3. Myeloproliferative and other hyperproliferative disorders

III. Drug-induced suppression of DNA synthesis
   A. Folate antagonists
   B. Metabolic inhibitors
      1. Of purine synthesis
      2. Of pyrimidine synthesis
      3. Of thymidylate synthesis
      4. Other inhibitors
   C. Alkylating agents
   D. Nitrous oxide

IV. Inborn errors
   A. Hereditary orotic aciduria
   B. Defective folate metabolism
   C. Lesch-Nyhan syndrome
   D. Defective transport of cobalamin

V. Erythroleukemia

Source: From Jandl JH: Chapt 5, in Blood: Textbook of Hematology. Boston, Little, Brown and Company, 1987.

affecting cobalamin or folate metabolism, and from the erythropoietic malignancy erythroleukemia (Table 6-1) [4].

COBALAMIN (VITAMIN B$_{12}$) DEFICIENCY

The corrinoid compound long familiar as vitamin B$_{12}$ is now known by the semisystematic name, cobalamin. Cobalamin consists of three basic components: the hemelike corrin ring, having cobalt at its planar center; a nucleotide bonded to cobalt below the plane; and one of four kinds of ligands known as β-groups that are attached to cobalt above the plane (Figure 6-5). Cyanocobalamin (CNCbl) and hydroxocobalamin (OHCbl) have no coenzyme role but are rapidly converted to active adducts by tissue enzymes and are convenient forms for use in parenteral therapy. The coenzyme methylcobalamin is essential to the folate-cobalamin connection upon which DNA synthesis depends (Figure 6-3), and deficiency of methylcobalamin is responsible for megaloblastic anemia and intestinal and epithelial atrophy. The coenzyme adenosylcobalamin (AdoCbl) is required for rearrangement of methylmalonyl CoA to succinyl CoA, the latter serving as the basic fuel of the high-energy-yielding Krebs (tricarboxylic acid) cycle. Some (but not all) evidence suggests that failure of the AdoCbl-dependent methylmalonyl CoA mutase reaction indirectly leads to incorporation of odd-chain fatty acids into lipids such as myelin sheaths, possibly explaining the myelopathy found in deficiency of cobalamin but not of folate.

Assimilation of Cobalamin

Cobalamin is assimilated via a unique sequence of three high-affinity transport proteins which relay the vitamin from gut to tissue cells, protecting it en route from digestion, excretion, or bacterial competition.

Intrinsic factor

Cobalamin entering the stomach encounters binding proteins of several kinds. So-called R binders (R is for rapid on electrophoresis) are a family of ubiquitous cobalamin-avid proteins of unknown physiologic function. Biologically, R binding is a false, fleeting reaction that terminates when the complex reaches the digestive enzymes of the duodenum. Cobalamin does not complex to the binder of destiny—Castle's gastric intrinsic factor (IF)—at the low pH of the stomach, but high-affinity binding by IF occurs promptly when gastric juice enters the alkaline circumstance of the duodenum. IF is a 44,000 M_r glycoprotein secreted (along with HCl) by gastric parietal cells. IF binds cobalamin covetously on a mole-for-mole basis (association constant: 1.5×10^{10}), following which IF dimerization encapsulates the cobalamin ligands within an intestinal transport vehicle that is shielded from proteolysis.

IF-Cbl complexes bind to ileal receptors IF-Cbl complexes are granted safe conduct through

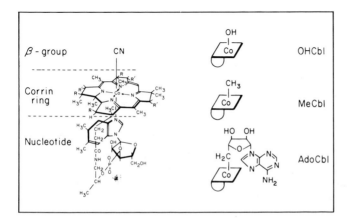

FIGURE 6-5

The cobalamins. The chemical structure of cyanocobalamin (CNCbl) is portrayed on the left. Note that the nucleotide of cobalamins contains the unique base, 5,6-dimethylbenzimidazole. On the right are abbreviated representations of the structures of hydroxocobalamin, methylcobalamin, and adenosylcobalamin. (From Babior BM and Stossel TP: Chapt 6, in Hematology. A Pathophysiological Approach. New York, Churchill Livingstone, 1984.)

the small intestine until they reach the terminal ileum, where they bind avidly to specific receptors on the brush border surfaces of ileal mucosal cells (Figure 6-6) [5].

TC II is the cobalamin transport protein   R proteins, including transcobalamin I and III, are present in all body fluids, but their physiologic role has not been elucidated. The internal conveyor of cobalamin is the 30,000 M_r transport protein, transcobalamin II (TC II), a product of hepatocytes, macrophages, and ileal enterocytes. TC II plucks cobalamin from the ileal cells and distributes the vitamin throughout the body by a selective receptor-mediated transport process. Uptake of cobalamin from blood is accomplished mainly by endothelial cell internalization of the TC II-Cbl complex through a system of coated pits and vesicles [6]. Endothelium is the active and limiting intermediary in transferring TC II-bound cobalamin to tissue cells, either for storage (liver cells) or metabolism (dividing cells). Congenital lack of TC II (but not of TC I or TC III) leads to severe, potentially fatal megaloblastic anemia commencing in the first

weeks after birth. If diagnosed, these patients can be maintained in good health by massive (2 mg) daily doses of hydroxocobalamin given parenterally or orally [7].

Cobalamin levels of serum   Measured by radioisotope dilution assay, the normal range for serum cobalamin is 150 to 650 pg/ml. Clinical evidence of deficiency generally begins to appear when the level drops below 100 pg/ml, but levels between 100 and 200 pg/ml should be looked upon with suspicion.

Cobalamin deficiency only rarely results from a poor diet and then is largely limited to dedicated vegetarians who also abstain from eggs and milk (ovolactovegetarians, or vegans). Cobalamins are synthesized by numerous microorganisms and pervade soil, sewage, and the surroundings of human habitation. In most populations the daily diet contains 5 to 30 μg of the vitamin, of which 1 to 2 μg are absorbed and retained daily. Protection against temporary dietary deprivation is considerable, for the hepatic reserves in normally nourished adults are bountiful, averaging over 1,000 μg of the vitamin—a 3- to 4-year supply. In temperate zones, cobalamin deficiency is almost always caused by deranged absorption.

FIGURE 6-6

Hypothetical portrayal of uptake of IF-Cbl complexes by receptors on ileal mucosal cells. The receptor at the mucosal surface is formed by pairs or tetrads of heterodimers consisting of small hydrophilic α subunits and large transmembrane β subunits. Binding is calcium-dependent and induces a conformational change in the oligomeric receptor that somehow opens an avenue to the circulation. (Adapted from Grasbeck R and Kouvoren I: The intrinsic factor and its receptor—are all membrane transport systems related? Trends Biochem Sci 8:203,1983.)

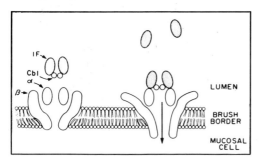

Pernicious Anemia

The most prevalent cause of cobalamin deficiency is failure of gastric parietal cells to manufacture IF. The syndrome of parietal cell atrophy and achlorhydria (achylia gastrica) combined with cobalamin deficiency and megaloblastic arrest still bears the alarming name of pernicious anemia (PA), although the disorder has been treatable for over 60 years. Adult-onset PA is relatively common among individuals of Northern European origin, particularly Scandinavians, and usually occurs after the age of 50.

PA may be an autoimmune disease   Over 90% of PA patients have cytotoxic IgG antibodies to parietal cells in their sera, and polyclonal IgG or IgA antibodies to IF are detectable in the serum, saliva, and gastric juice of over three-fourths of cases. Some antibodies to IF block its binding to cobalamin and others impede absorption of cobalamin by the ileum. In the presence of both kinds of antibody, IF is

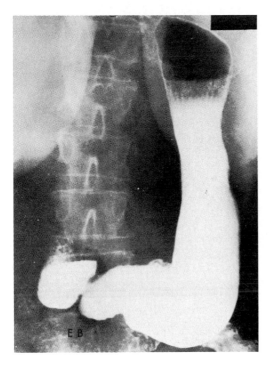

FIGURE 6-7

Barium meal radiograph of the stomach in PA. The stomach has a long, lax, slumping shape free of rugal markings, and the fundus is bald. (From Laws JW and Pitman RG: The radiological features of pernicious anaemia. Br J Radiol 33:229,1960.)

functionally double teamed. It is not known whether these intriguing immunologic markers are cause or effect.

The PA Syndrome

PA is a unique syndrome that when fully expressed consists of: megaloblastic anemia, gastric parietal cell atrophy followed by generalized epithelial atrophy, and subacute combined degeneration of the spinal cord and brain. The megaloblastic arrest is morphologically identical to that of folate deficiency, as indicated earlier. Progression of anemia need not parallel progression of epithelial atrophy or the neuropathy.

Epithelial atrophy Cobalamin deficiency leads to attrition and nuclear dysplasia in all exfoliating cell populations, causing visible atrophy, depapillation, and a thinning of epithelium at the sides and tip of the tongue.

Thinning of tongue epithelium allows the red color of blood to show through, often creating a beefy red appearance. Dogma notwithstanding, burning glossitis in PA patients suggests secondary deficiencies of other B vitamins. Atrophy of tongue, lips, skin, and enteric and vaginal mucosa is secondary to cobalamin deficiency. Atrophy of gastric mucosa, on the other hand, is the initial lesion responsible for PA, and all of the major abnormalities of PA are mimicked within a few years after total gastrectomy.

Atrophy of gastric mucosa involves the proximal two-thirds of the stomach, which becomes flattened to parchment thinness. Roentgenologic examination reveals a flattening and laxity of the fold pattern; the fundal dome is small with an absence of rugae (Figure 6-7) [8]. On gastroscopy the mucosa appears gray and translucent, mucosal thickness is about one-third of normal, and biopsy reveals sparse glands lined mainly by mucus-secreting cells and surrounded by infiltrates of lymphocytes and plasma cells (Figure 6-8) [8].

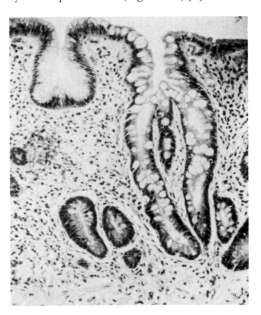

FIGURE 6-8

Appearance of gastric biopsy in PA. Atrophy of surface epithelium is associated with intestinal metaplasia and appearance of numerous mucus-filled goblet cells—a hallmark of "achylia gastrica." (From Chanarin I: The Megaloblastic Anemias, 2nd ed. Oxford, Blackwell Scientific Publications,1979.)

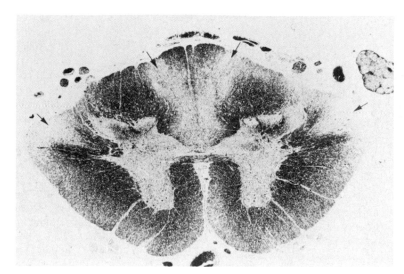

F I G U R E 6-9

Degeneration of the pos-
terior and lateral col-
umns of the spinal cord
in PA. Arrows point to
areas of demyelination
and loss of nerve fibers.
(From Kass L: Perni-
cious Anemia. Philadel-
phia, WB Saunders
Company, 1976.)

Neurologic abnormalities in PA   Hematologic
and epithelial lesions accompany all megaloblastic disorders, but only cobalamin deficiency causes a characteristic neuropathy best
known as subacute combined degeneration
(SCD). Severity and progression of the
neuropathy do not correlate with progression
of anemia, and in patients receiving plentiful
dietary or supplemental folate the diagnosis
may be masked, for folate corrects the
megaloblastic effects of cobalamin deficiency
but does not prevent and may even hasten the
crippling myelopathy. The symptoms and signs
are caused by patchy demyelination and eventual axonal degeneration of the dorsal and
lateral columns of the spinal cord (Figure 6-9)
[9].

The neurologic symptoms of PA (and other
cobalamin deficiency states) begin with symmetrical weakness and paresthesias of hands
and feet associated with loss of vibratory sense
in the lower extremities. Soon afterward the
gait grows unsteady and then ataxic, and the
Romberg test becomes positive, attesting to
severe dorsal column malfunction. As the disease progresses to involve the lateral columns,
the legs grow increasingly weak and spastic
and flexion deformities occur. During this
grievous deterioration patients are prey to
hosts of infirmities, including painful paresthe-

sias, optic neuropathies, and assorted cognitive
disturbances ranging from confusion to dementia [10].

Treatment of PA is a lifetime commitment
Diagnosis of PA is based on demonstration of
low levels of cobalamin in the serum of patients having two or more correlative findings
characteristic of the disease: achlorhydria or
achylia, absence of IF by radioimmunoassay,
increased methylmalonate in the urine, or the
presence of serum antibodies to IF. In case of
doubt and in patients pretreated with cobalamin, diagnosis can be verified by the Schilling
test. In this test an enormous "flushing" dose
of nonradioactive vitamin is given to saturate
TC I and TC II; a small dose of radioactive
cobalamin is then given by mouth, and the
extent of oral absorption is determined by the
renal excretion of labeled vitamin. In PA,
cobalamin is poorly absorbed. That cobalamin
malabsorption is due to IF deficiency is established by repeating the test with the modification that IF is given by mouth along with
labeled cobalamin. Cobalamin malabsorption
of gastric origin (PA or gastrectomy) is corrected by this "stage 2" Schilling test; malabsorption caused by ileal disease or intestinal
parasitization by competitive microorganisms
is not. The Schilling test has been modified in

several additional ways to make it more versatile in differentiating causes of cobalamin deficiency [11].

Parenteral cobalamin circumvents intestinal malabsorption and induces a characteristic hematologic response, as seen in Figure 6-10 [12], in which the pattern of daily reticulocyte counts assumes a Gibraltarlike configuration. PA patients should receive 100 to 1,000 μg of cyanocobalamin daily intramuscularly for at least several days, after which the patient requires monthly injections for life. The hematologic response should be complete; on the other hand the neuropathy usually improves only partially. Neurologic problems of recent onset may clear completely, but those that have been established for 3 months or longer are beyond remedy.

Intestinal Malabsorption of Cobalamin

Ileal Malfunction

As receptors for IF-Cbl complexes are concentrated in the terminal ileum, a PA-like syndrome develops in patients with ileal resection, regional enteritis (Crohn's disease), or lymphoma of the ileum. Patients deprived of ileal function require lifelong cobalamin therapy.

Competitive Parasites and Microorganisms

A celebrated cause of parasitic competition for foodstuffs occurs in patients parasitized by sufficient numbers of the fish tapeworm *Diphyllobothrium latum*. Worms lodged in large numbers high in the jejunum are in position to usurp cobalamin (which they require for their own growth). Expulsion of the worms and a course of parenteral cyanocobalamin are both recommended.

An analogous mechanism by which dietary cobalamin can be preempted occurs in patients with intestinal fistulas, blind loops, or multiple diverticulas. These gut malformations may become stagnating cesspools containing swarms of vitamin-starved microorganisms that rob the host of cobalamin and displace serum cobalamin with biologically inactive analogs of bacterial origin. The most severe and graphic form of the "blind loop syndrome" is seen in patients with multiple diverticulosis involving the mesenteric aspect of the jejunum. Bacteria flourish in these corrupted saccules and, being upstream of the ileal receptors, have first opportunity to consume cobalamin (Figure 6-11). Diagnosis, if in doubt, can be confirmed by performing the "stage 3" Schilling test and showing cobalamin malabsorption to be remedied by oral antibiot-

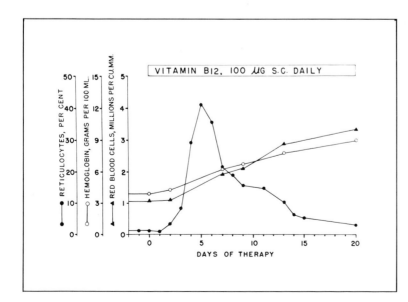

FIGURE 6-10

Hematologic response to parenteral vitamin B_{12} (cyanocobalamin) in a severely anemic patient with PA. Reticulocyte levels start to rise on the third day of therapy, reaching a peak on the fifth or sixth day. (From Jandl JH: in Cecil-Loeb Textbook of Medicine, 13th ed., Beeson PB and McDermott W, Eds. Philadelphia, WB Saunders Company, 1971.)

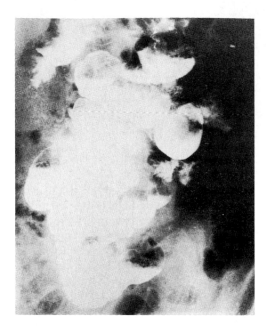

FIGURE 6-11

Barium meal radiograph showing multiple jejunal diverticula in a patient with cobalamin-responsive megaloblastic anemia. (From Chanarin I: The Megaloblastic Anemias, 2nd ed. Oxford, Blackwell Scientific Publications, 1979.)

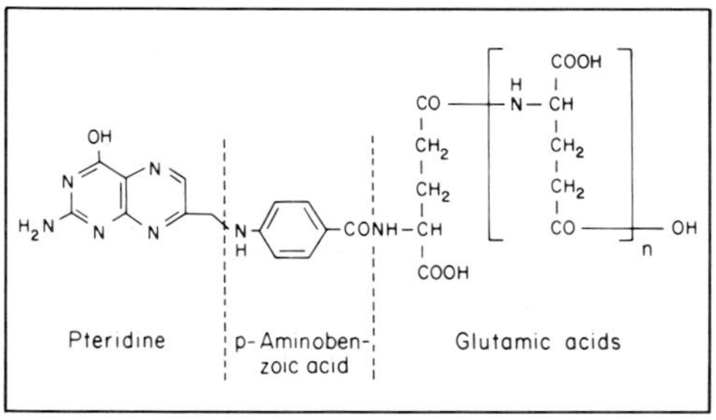

FIGURE 6-12

Folic acid (pteroylglutamic acid) occurs in nature as a polyglutamate having variable numbers of γ-glutamyl carboxy linkages in series (indicated by bracketed repeat structure on the right). For clarity some hydrogens have been omitted. (From Babior BM and Stossel TP: Chapt 6, in Hematology. A Pathophysiological Approach. New York, Churchill Livingstone, 1984.)

ics. Broad-spectrum antibiotics often produce a reticulocyte response, but the effect is not lasting. Parenteral cobalamin therapy is necessary for a full hematologic response; when possible, surgery should be performed to restore intestinal hydraulics and hygiene, enabling resumption of cobalamin absorption.

FOLATE DEFICIENCY

Folate is the trivial name for pteroylmonoglutamate, parent for a large family of compounds occurring in nature conjugated to polyglutamate chains. Synthesized by higher plants, folate in leafy green vegetables is the primary natural source of this hematopoietic vitamin. Folate consists of three parts: the pteridine ring; a p-aminobenzoic acid residue, and an L-glutamate residue. Almost all natural folate occurs in the form of polyglutamates in which from five to six glutamic acid residues are attached in series to PGA by peptidase-resistant γ-carboxyl peptide bonds (Figure 6-12).

Folate (F) itself is metabolically inert, and requires two 2-step reductions, first to FH_2, then to FH_4, under the auspices of a single NADPH-linked enzyme, dihydrofolate reductase. Dihydrofolate reductase is extremely sensitive to inhibition by folate analogs such as methotrexate, accounting for the efficacy of methotrexate when used as an antimetabolite (antifol) in cancer chemotherapy. Methylated derivatives of the biologically active FH_4 play important and versatile roles in transferring 1-carbon fragments to various acceptors. The main reaction that equips folate with 1-carbon fragments is the transfer of a methylene ($-CH_2-$) group to the business end of the pteridine ring, creating a methylene bridge and generating the folate coenzyme of thymidylate synthetase: $N^{5,10}$-methylene FH_4. As noted earlier, transfer of the 1-carbon fragment to dUMP is essential to DNA synthesis (Figure 6-3), and, in the absence of sufficient folate, a thymineless state develops, leading to the uracil misincorporation, strand breakage, and arrested S phase characteristic of megaloblastic anemias.

Assimilation of Folate

For intestinal absorption, natural folate conjugated to polyglutamate requires intervention by special hydrolytic enzymes called "conjugases." Conjugases (deconjugases) located in the brush border throughout the small intestinal mucosa are γ-glutamyl-carboxy-peptidases, which split off the polyglutamate chains and enable absorption of folate as the inert methylated form (N^5-methyl FH_4). Methylated folate (the sole form measured by microbial assay of serum) is transported into growing cells including erythroblasts via specific receptors [13]; the methyl group is relinquished to homocysteine, yielding FH_4 and methionine, as part of the methyltransferase cycle (Figure 6-3). Demethylated FH_4 is then reconjugated within tissue cells by means of an ATP-dependent synthetase designed for converting FH_4 to the polyglutamyl storage form. The balance between tissue conjugases and the folylpolyglutamate synthetase activities is instrumental in regulating the rate of DNA synthesis.

Dietary Deficiency

A normal balanced diet contains about 1,000 μg of folate. The minimum daily requirement for folate (or its polyglutamated equivalent) is about 100 to 200 μg daily, and an average well-nourished adult possesses about 5,000 μg in body stores. Hence the margin of safety is small compared with cobalamin, and within a few months of deprivation megaloblastic changes may commence. Deficiency of folate is endemic among the poor, elderly, reclusive, and alcoholic. Nutritional folate deficiency usually occurs in a setting of generalized malnutrition, and folate deficiency patients, unlike PA patients, look malnourished. Severe ulcerative gastrointestinal lesions may afflict the patient from end to end, causing stomatitis, cheilosis, dysphagia, meteorism, and watery diarrhea, and biopsy and radiologic changes mimic those of sprue (Figure 6-13) [14]. Subacute combined degeneration of the cord does not occur, but peripheral neuropathies and burning paresthesias of the feet are common. Patients are generally too apathetic or

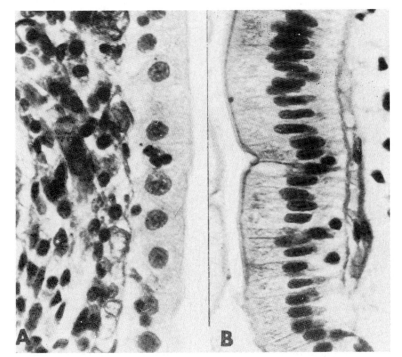

FIGURE 6-13

Peroral intestinal biopsies of the duodeno-jejunal junction in a folate-deficient alcoholic patient before and after folate therapy. Before treatment (A), villous epithelial cells are sparse, squat, and have large rounded nuclei. After folate therapy (B), cells are much taller, more numerous, and become compressed by their multitude. (Reproduced, with permission, from: Hermos JA et al: Mucosa of the small intestine in folate-deficient alcoholics. Ann Intern Med 76:957,1972.)

too alcoholic to help themselves, and diagnosis is commonly made at receiving hospitals. Diagnosis is confirmed by serum folate levels below 3 ng/ml and red cell folate concentrations less than 100 ng/ml [15]. Administration of oral folate (5 mg daily) produces a prompt hematologic response, and intestinal lesions and malfunctions disappear within a few weeks. Durable restoration is likely only in those willing and able to eat well and reform their life-styles.

Impaired Absorption

Folate is well absorbed throughout normal intestine, and loss of intestinal surface or function must be extensive to disturb absorption.

Tropical Sprue

Tropical sprue is endemic to the tropics but also affects visitors from temperate areas, implying an infectious origin—an ancient deduction still awaiting proof. It starts as an abrupt diarrhea followed by persistent anorexia and evidence of malabsorption. Response of the entire debilitating syndrome of obstinate diarrhea, weight loss, and eventually megaloblastic anemia to folate is so prompt and invariable as to constitute an affirmative diagnostic test.

Nontropical Sprue: Gluten-Sensitive Enteropathy, Alias Adult Celiac Disease

Nontropical sprue in adults is a rekindling of childhood celiac disease: both are a generalized malabsorptive enteropathy provoked by ingestion of either of the wheat proteins: gluten or gliadin. Gluten-sensitive enteropathy is initiated by an immunologic reaction that damages intestinal mucosa cells, causing flattening of villi, baring of crypts, and denudation of brush borders (Figure 6-14) [16]. About 80% of patients with nontropical sprue begin to improve absorptive function within a few weeks of instituting a gluten-free diet. The megaloblastic anemia responds rapidly to oral or parenteral folate, and folate supplements should be continued for life.

Increased Folate Requirements

Folate requirements are heightened by any added burden of cellular growth, physiologic or pathologic.

Megaloblastic Anemia of Pregnancy

During the third trimester of gestation the fetus begins to compete successfully for all of the ingredients required for DNA synthesis, the most marginal of which is folate. During late

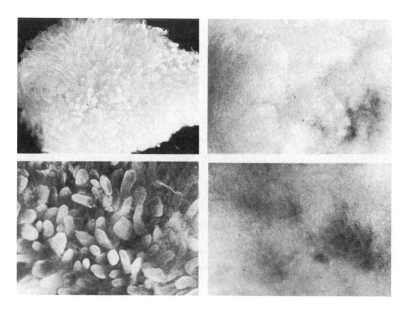

FIGURE 6-14

Adult celiac disease. Panels on the left show normal villi and (at higher power, lower left) finger and leaf patterns. Panels on right show flattened mosaic pavement (upper right) and exposed crypt openings (lower right). (From Hoffbrand AV and Pettit JE: Chapt 3, in Clinical Hematology Illustrated. An Integrated Text and Color Atlas. London, Gower Medical Publishing Ltd., 1987.)

pregnancy and for several weeks postpartum, folate requirements increase by 5- to 10-fold. Folate-responsive megaloblastic anemia (long misnamed "pernicious anemia of pregnancy") occurs in about 3% of pregnant women, and at term 60 to 90% of parturient women have subnormal serum levels of folate. Routine supplementation of the diet during pregnancy with 1 to 5 mg of folate daily will avert this common, occasionally severe, complication of pregnancy with little likelihood (in this age group) of masking unsuspected PA.

Heightened Hematopoiesis and Hyperproliferative Disorders

In severe hemolytic anemias, erythropoiesis may accelerate 10-fold, enough to double the total body rate of DNA synthesis and to create "relative nutritional deficiency." All patients with severe sustained hemolytic anemia should be given folate supplements of 5 mg daily. In myeloproliferative disorders and other forms of widespread malignancy that parasitize folate stores, morphologic evidence of folate deficiency may be obscured or confused by the underlying process, but most patients benefit from folate supplements.

Drug-Induced Suppression of DNA Synthesis

In chemotherapy of leukemias and solid tumors DNA synthesis is interfered with by intent. Megaloblastic anemia is usually a mild concomitant of agents that inhibit purine and pyrimidine synthesis, but drugs that block dihydrofolate reductase (methotrexate), thymidylate synthetase (5-fluorouracil), ribonucleotide reductase (hydroxyurea), or DNA polymerase (cytosine arabinoside) can cause severe megaloblastic arrest and their use must be carefully monitored, for anemia is unresponsive to folate or cobalamin.

Methotrexate and folinic acid (Leukovorin) rescue Methotrexate, a widely used chemotherapeutic agent, is a specific inhibitor and avid binder of dihydrofolate reductase ($K_i = 7 \times 10^{-10}$M). It blocks de novo purine synthesis by FH_2 [17], indirectly halting dTMP synthesis in all proliferating tissues. Megaloblastic arrest, generalized sloughing of the

gastrointestinal mucosa, and even death can occur from overdosage. Fortunately cytotoxic effects of methotrexate can be overcome by circumventing the block with parenteral N^5-formyltetrahydrofolate (folinic acid, alias Leukovorin). Availability of this antidote permits use of high-dose methotrexate, but it is imperative that folinic acid be given immediately after the methotrexate. A strategem applicable to leukemias or other malignancies of body cavities such as spinal fluid is to give methotrexate intrathecally followed by an intravenous chaser of folinic acid.

Nitrous oxide N_2O, a strong oxidant, causes oxidation of cob(I)alamin (vitamin B_{12}s) to the inert cob(III)alamin (vitamin B_{12}a), preventing regeneration of the folate cofactor to thymidylate synthetase. This agent produces an acute and profound form of cobalamin deficiency, complete with megaloblastosis, elevation of serum (methylated) folate, and reduction in methionine levels. N_2O-induced megaloblastic anemia is a common happening among patients admitted to intensive care or surgical and dental services. It can be prevented by parenteral administration of folinic acid just before and 12 h following anesthesia [18].

Inborn Errors Leading to Megaloblastic Anemia

Even collectively, inborn errors leading to megaloblastic anemia are too rare for the compass of this book. For reference, these include hereditary orotic aciduria, faulty production of transcobalamin II, inborn errors of folate absorption and metabolism, and the macabre, autistic X-linked disorder of purine metabolism known as the Lesch-Nyhan syndrome.

Unexplained Megaloblastic Disorders

Megaloblastic morphology is a prominent and unexplained feature of about 20% of patients with disorders of heme synthesis that respond partially to pharmacologic doses of pyridoxine—the pyridoxine-responsive anemias (Chapter 7). Some of these patients also respond partially to folate. A more common and deadly disorder that can be a morphologic facsimile of megaloblastic anemia was originally described by Di Guglielmo.

Erythroleukemia

Erythroleukemia (Di Guglielmo's syndrome), the M6 variant of AML, is discussed here briefly because the leukemic erythroblasts appear megaloblastic, particularly early in the course. Marrow becomes occupied by dysplastic erythroid cells, most of which are megaloblastic, some being truly bizarre, displaying occasional giant multinucleated forms. The protean hematologic findings in erythroleukemia are subject to swift transitions, and usually within several months of presentation the marrow is overrun by swarming myeloblasts.

REFERENCES

1. Beck W: Chapt 34, in Hematology, 3rd ed., Williams WJ et al, Eds. New York, McGraw-Hill Book Company,1983

2. Koistinen P et al: Hematopoietic and gastric uracil-DNA glycosylase activity in megaloblastic anemia and in atrophic gastritis with special reference to pernicious anemia. Carcinogenesis 8:327,1987

3. Babior BM and Stossel TP: Chapt 6, in Hematology. A Pathophysiological Approach. New York, Churchill Livingstone, 1984

4. Jandl JH: Chapt 4, in Blood: Textbook of Hematology. Boston, Little, Brown and Company,1987

5. Grasbeck R and Kouvonen I: The intrinsic factor and its receptor—are all membrane transport systems related? Trends Biochem Sci 8:203,1983

6. Soda R et al: Receptor distribution and the endothelial uptake of transcobalamin II in liver cell suspensions. Blood 65:795,1985

7. Zeitlin HC et al: Homozygous transcobalamin II deficiency maintained on oral hydroxocobalamin. Blood 66:1022,1985

8. Chanarin I: The Megaloblastic Anemias, 2nd ed. Oxford, Blackwell Scientific Publications,1979

9. Kass L: Pernicious Anemia. Philadelphia, WB Saunders Company,1976

10. Shields RW Jr and Harris JW: Subacute combined degeneration of the spinal cord and brain, in Current Therapy in Neurologic Disease–2, Johnson RT, Ed. Philadelphia, BC Decker Inc.,1987

11. Carethers M: Diagnosing vitamin B_{12} deficiency, a common geriatric disorder. Geriatrics 43(3):89,1988

12. Jandl JH: in Cecil-Loeb Textbook of Medicine, 13th ed., Beeson PB and McDermott W, Eds. Philadelphia, WB Saunders Company, 1971

13. Antony AC et al: Effect of perturbation of specific folate receptors during in vitro erythropoiesis. J Clin Invest 80:1618,1987

14. Hermos JA et al: Mucosa of the small intestine in folate-deficient alcoholics. Ann Intern Med 76:957,1972

15. Herbert V: Making sense of laboratory tests of folate status: folate requirements to sustain normality. Am J Hematol 26:199, 1987

16. Hoffbrand AV and Pettit JE: Chapt 3, in Clinical Hematology Illustrated. An Integrated Text and Color Atlas. London, Gower Medical Publishing Ltd.,1987

17. Baram J et al: Effect of methotrexate on intracellular folate pools in purified myeloid precursor cells from normal human bone marrow. J Clin Invest 79:692,1987

18. Amos RJ et al: Prevention of nitrous oxide-induced megaloblastic changes in bone marrow using folinic acid. Br J Anaesthesiol 56:103,1984

7

Hypochromic Anemias and Disorders of Iron Metabolism

□

Iron is not only essential to life; it is essential for the function of every cell. The second most abundant metal in the earth's crust, iron is admitted to the body and to the body's cells through a series of transport vehicles and guarded checkpoints that serve to protect against the high toxicity of free ferric ions. Once taken in, however, iron atoms are trapped, for no physiologic mechanism exists for iron excretion. This narrow conservatism is responsible for the comparably high incidence of both iron deficiency and iron overloading [1]. Iron homeostasis is dependent upon two specialized iron-sequestering proteins: transferrin and ferritin. Ferritin is responsible for safeguarding iron entry to the body and for keeping any iron surplus in an accessible storage form. Transferrin is in charge of transporting and recycling iron between plasma and the transferrin receptors of cells (Chapter 4). The biosynthetic rates for both the transferrin receptor and ferritin are regulated coordinately by iron.

THE IRON CYCLE

In adults about 90% of iron movement results from recycling of iron released from dead red cells, transported by transferrin, and reutilized by marrow erythroblasts. Each day about 20 mg of iron are recycled for erythropoiesis, several mg are reutilized to replenish heme and nonheme iron of cycling tissue cells, and less than 1 mg is absorbed by gut mucosa to offset losses incurred by fecal and urinary excretion and in sweat and desquamated skin. Recycling of iron from effete red cells is essential to the economy of iron [2].

Iron Absorption

Iron is retained jealously in the body by iron-liganding mechanisms. Most iron that people are born with is still present at their death. A small amount normally is lost from the gastrointestinal tract every day, largely as leaked blood and sloughed epithelium. Losses are replenished by absorption of iron from food; dietary iron is supplied largely as heme but also as inorganic iron derived from nonheme iron-containing enzymes and from animal storage iron. Heme is absorbed as such by special heme receptors located throughout the intestinal tract, but absorption of inorganic iron salts is affected by blocking (phytate and phosphate) and enhancing (ascorbate) substances within the diet. Inorganic iron in the ferric form is solubilized and shifted to the ferrous state in the presence of gastric acid, facilitating absorption. The first encounter between soluble iron salts and gut epithelium takes place in the duodenum and upper jejunum, and most absorption occurs there; below this point pancreatic bicarbonate raises the pH sharply, converting iron to insoluble and unabsorbable aggregates of ferric polyhydroxides.

In the intestinal mucosal cell, heme iron is released from the porphyrin ring by heme oxygenase, and the free iron joins Fe^{2+} atoms taken up as such to enter a common pool. Iron entering the mucosal cell is somehow ferried into the extravascular spaces of the lamina propria where it is complexed to transferrin and rapidly appears in circulation. Iron atoms absorbed in amounts exceeding immediate needs are sequestered by the specific iron storage protein, ferritin (Figure 7-1) [3]. If in the short (3- to 4-day) lifespan of the mucosal cell ferritin iron is not surrendered, unused ferritin iron is sloughed into the intestinal lumen during normal exfoliation of the cell. Ferritin plays a pivotal role in the absorption as well as the storage of iron.

Ferritin

Ferritin is a large (440,000 M_r) iron storage protein composed of 24 apoferritin subunits arranged to form a hollow geodesic sphere 13 nm in diameter. The central core, 6 nm across, is capable of holding about 4,500 atoms of ferric iron, although the molecule is normally only two-thirds iron-saturated. mRNA for apoferri-

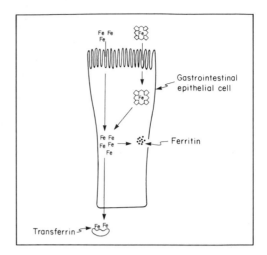

FIGURE 7-1

Absorption of iron by the intestinal epithelial cell. The mechanisms by which internalized iron is transported across the cell and relinquished to transferrin is unknown, for transferrin does not enter the cell. Unused iron is packaged in ferritin. (From Babior BM and Stossel TP: Chapt 4, in Hematology. A Pathophysiologic Approach. New York, Churchill Livingstone, 1984.)

tin is found in every somatic cell of the body. Apoferritin molecules are released from polyribosomes only after incorporation of iron. In the absence of free iron, apoferritin remains bound to polyribosomes, blocking unnecessary formation of additional apoferritin. Hence, ferritin biosynthesis is regulated without a corresponding change in total ferritin mRNA by redistribution of mRNA between polysome and nonpolysome pools [4]. Synthesis of apoferritin is stimulated by iron atoms and inhibited by negative feedback. The alacrity with which apoferritin can be assembled posttranslationally in the presence of iron atoms—as during absorption and tissue distribution of iron unbound to transferrin—reflects nature's care to keep this potentially toxic mineral insulated.

Ferritin structure   Human ferritin is composed of subunits of two types: H and L. H-rich isoferritins (found in heart and red cells) and L-rich molecules (predominant in liver, spleen, and placenta) are products of large families of genes that have been mapped to several chromosomes. Each subunit is folded into cylindrical molecules; when assembled into the 24-subunit shell, the quaternary structure possesses six channels for to-and-fro passage of iron, and displays a 4-fold axis of symmetry that passes through the shell (Figure 7-2) [2, 5].

During isoelectric focusing, ferritin molecules from various tissues form distinctive bands reflecting differences in the balance of H and L chains. Ferritin extracted from macrophages has been shown to differ from that in erythroblasts, a fact that contradicts the postulated mechanism whereby erythroid cells gain iron from "nurse" cells by suckling macrophage ferritin.

Hemosiderin Iron in ferritin is in a paracrystalline form composed of mixed hydrates and phosphates. Ferritin molecules become close-packed within lysosomes into larger amorphous aggregates called hemosiderin, which coalesce as golden granules that are visible by light microscopy and are stained vividly by prussian blue.

The entire iron cycle is reprised in Figure 7-3 [6].

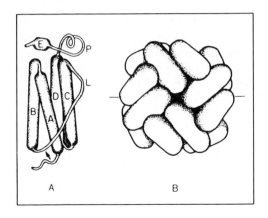

FIGURE 7-2

Ferritin structure. (A) 3-D conformation of an apoferritin subunit. Letters A to E and P indicate helical segments and L is a connecting loop. (B) Quaternary structure of the apoferritin shell as viewed down a 4-fold axis of symmetry. Iron enters and exits through hourglass-shaped channels surrounded at their narrowest part by four E helices—one from each subunit. Iron within the shell forms crystalline micelles. (Adapted from Clegg GA et al: Prog Biophys Molec Biol 36:56,1980 and from Seligman PA et al: Chapt 7, in The Molecular Basis of Blood Diseases, Stamatoyannopoulos G et al, Eds. Philadelphia, WB Saunders Company,1987.)

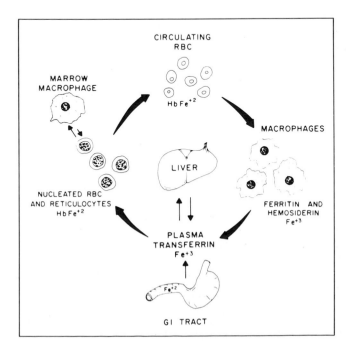

FIGURE 7-3

Schematic recapitulation of the iron cycle. Most body iron is used for erythropoiesis and is trapped within circulating red cells. Hemoglobin of expired red cells is degraded in macrophages of liver, spleen, and marrow; and hemoglobin iron is returned to the erythron by transferrin. Transferrin regulates the flow of iron by interacting with its receptor (Chapter 4). Ferritin synthesis for storage of surplus iron is governed by negative feedback. The iron cycle is so efficient and conservative that only about 1 mg of iron must be assimilated via the intestine daily to assure homeostasis. (From Erslev AJ and Gabuzda TG: Pathophysiology of Blood, 3rd ed. Philadelphia, WB Saunders,1985.)

Tissue Distribution of Iron

Although iron plays a pivotal role in oxidative energy metabolism in all cells, it is unevenly allocated to various iron pools according to the metabolic needs and proliferative behavior of the several cell systems (Table 7-1) [7]. The status of the various iron pools can be evaluated by indirect (noninvasive) methods, most of which are available as routine laboratory procedures, or by indirect methods that are either painfully invasive or painfully expensive and limited to hematology referral centers.

Indirect Methods

Tests employed routinely in evaluating the iron status of patients include the following: serum iron level, serum transferrin level measured as iron-binding capacity, transferrin saturation, and serum ferritin level—four measurements that together constitute an "iron profile." Measurement of free erythrocyte protoporphyrin is of more limited use, being most informative in distinguishing iron-lack disorders from iron-

loading diseases such as the thalassemias and pyridoxine-responsive anemias. Quantitating the amount of iron excreted into the urine after injecting an iron-chelating agent such as deferoxamine (Desferal) is restricted for use in estimating crudely the extent of known or suspected iron overload. Values obtained by these several indicators are given in Table 7-2, which compares normal ranges with representative findings in iron deficiency, iron overload, and chronic inflammatory disease [7].

Direct Methods

Quantitation of iron in specimens secured by marrow or liver biopsy is the most direct of direct methods of assessing iron status. Reticuloendothelial stores of iron can be assessed with practical accuracy by grading hemosiderin content on an arbitrary scale of 0 to 6+ using prussian blue–stained core biopsies or acceptable aspirates. By this scale normal marrow is graded 1+ to 3+, iron deficiency marrow registers 0, and in inflammatory,

TABLE 7-1

Tissue distribution and functions of iron

Protein	Tissue/cells	Iron, mg*	Total body iron (%)	Function of iron compound
Hemoglobin	Red blood cells	2,500	66	O$_2$ transport by blood
Myoglobin (and other nonenzyme muscle proteins	Muscle	500	13	O$_2$ transport in muscle
Heme enzymes (e.g., cytochromes, oxidoreductases)	All cells	50	1	O$_2$ transport, utilization, and consumption in all cells
Nonheme iron-dependent enzymes and proteins	All cells	200	5	O$_2$ transport, iron reserve in all cells
Ferritin and hemosiderin	Liver, spleen, and marrow	500	13	Iron storage
Transferrin	Plasma and extravascular fluids	14	<1 (0.4)	Iron transport
Total	——	3,800	98	——

*Quantities of iron specified are the averaged values for normal men and women.

Source: From Jandl JH: Chapt 6, in Blood: Textbook of Hematology. Boston, Little, Brown and Company, 1987.

TABLE 7-2

Noninvasive indicators of iron stores

Measurement	Clinical state			
	Normal	Iron deficiency	Iron overload	Chronic inflammatory disease
Serum iron (μg/dl)	120 ($\pm$30)	<40	120–280	20–50
Total iron-binding capacity (μg/dl)	330 ($\pm$30)	300–480	<300	<260
Transferrin saturation (%)	35 ($\pm$10)	<16	40–100	10–25
Ferritin (μg/l)	100 ($\pm$60)	<10	>250	>150
Protoporphyrin (FEP) (μg/dl red cells)	30 (15 to 80)	100–1,000	<100	100–800
Urinary excretion of chelated iron (mg/day)	0.8 ($\pm$0.2)	<0.3	>2.2	0.8–1.2

Source: From Jandl JH: Chapt 6, in Blood: Textbook of Hematology. Boston, Little, Brown and Company, 1987.

thalassemic, or sideroblastic anemias marrow hemosiderin is usually grossly increased (5+ to 6+). The correspondence between marrow nonheme iron measured chemically or by neutron activation and that estimated by histologic (prussian blue) grading is sufficiently good to discriminate cleanly between extreme aberrations in iron stores (Figure 7-4) [8]. Chemical measurement of iron in liver biopsy specimens is justified only for the diagnosis of iron overload in patients at risk of developing hemochromatosis.

Specialized methods for quantitating iron stores Direct noninvasive magnetic measurements of hepatic iron stores can be made with a specially designed superconducting quantum-interference device (SQUID), which senses quantitatively the magnetic property of paramagnetism possessed by storage iron [9]. Magnetic-susceptibility measurements provide a phantom biopsy that quantitates ferritin and hemosiderin (as distinct from diamagnetic heme iron) and is the method of choice for

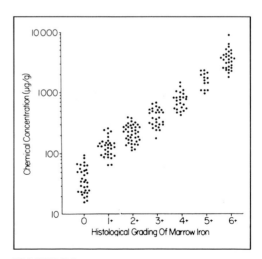

FIGURE 7-4

Range of correspondence between chemical concentrations of iron in marrow specimens versus histologic grading based upon staining with potassium ferrocyanide. (Reproduced from the Journal of Clinical Investigation, 1963,42:1076 by copyright permission of the American Society for Clinical Investigation.)

evaluating the progression and regression on therapy of the iron overload disorders, hemochromatosis and transfusion-dependent refractory anemias. At present, unfortunately, SQUID has only a single referral tentacle. Dual-energy computed tomography (DE-CT) has the advantage of high-resolution focus; although it measures both heme and nonheme iron, it has the potential for quantitating the iron content of individual organs at risk, such as pancreas.

Physiologic Variables in Iron Metabolism

In certain stages of life, iron balance can be precarious. The first of these is in infancy when the rate of growth may outstrip both the inherited and newly acquired stores of iron. Adolescence, an edgy stage to begin with, is another period of rapid growth and iron jeopardy. In women the demands of growth are compounded by the desiderata of menstruation and pregnancy. Obligatory iron losses in males are at most 1 mg daily, an amount easily matched by absorption of dietary iron. In menstruating women iron needs (averaged out over the entire cycle) are increased by 0.5 mg daily, and during late pregnancy as much as 5

to 6 mg are added to the daily iron requirements needed to satisfy fetal impositions [10]. The inequality between men and women with regard to iron requirements is shown in Figure 7-5 [11]. The impact of this nutritional inequity on four standard parameters of iron homeostasis is demonstrated in Figure 7-6 [12].

Hypochromic Anemias

In hypochromic anemias stem cell kinetics and DNA synthesis are normal but cytoplasmic synthesis of the gene product, hemoglobin, is reduced. Under pressure by EP the proliferative marrow continues to produce erythroid progeny but with each division the failure in hemoglobin synthesis creates an increasingly damaging nuclear:cytoplasmic imbalance which is the antithesis of that in megaloblastic anemias. When the cumulative amount of hemoglobin in late erythroblasts falls short of the required 20 pg/cell, an extra division is triggered. The end result is either a nonviable shell of a cell or a barely viable one that is both pale and small. The two principal causes of hypochromic anemias are defective synthesis of heme and impaired synthesis of globin chains. A pathogenetic classification of hypochromic anemias is presented in Table 7-3.

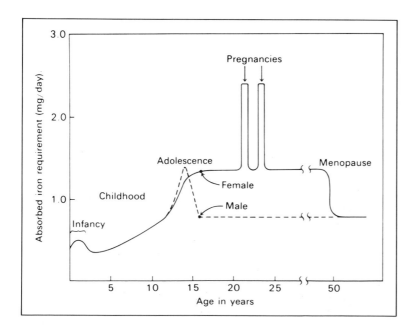

FIGURE 7-5

Daily iron requirements in females (continuous line) and males (interrupted line) of various ages. (From Wintrobe MM et al: Clinical Hematology, 8th ed. Philadelphia, Lea & Febiger, 1981.)

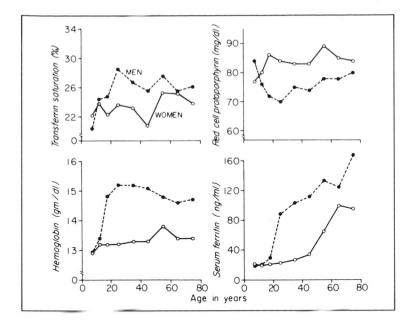

FIGURE 7-6

Median values in a survey population of 1,564 individuals for transferrin saturation, red cell protoporphyrin, hemoglobin, and serum ferritin levels. Serum ferritin levels were the most dramatically skewed: over 20% of adult females (aged 18 to 45 years) had subnormal levels of ferritin, as compared with less than 2% of age-matched males. (From Cook JD et al: Evaluation of the iron status of a population. Blood 48:449,1976.)

TABLE 7-3

Pathogenetic classification of hypochromic anemias

I. Disorders of iron metabolism
   A. Iron deficiency anemia
      1. Decreased iron intake
      2. Blood loss
      3. Impaired iron transport
   B. Anemia of chronic disease
      1. Chronic inflammatory diseases
      2. Malignant diseases

II. Disorders of heme synthesis: the sideroblastic anemias
   A. Hereditary sideroblastic anemia
   B. Idiopathic sideroblastic anemia
   C. Secondary sideroblastic anemias
      1. Drug-induced
      2. Alcohol-induced
      3. Lead poisoning

III. Disorders of globin synthesis: the thalassemias
   A. β Thalassemia
   B. α Thalassemia
   C. Other thalassemias

Source: From Jandl JH: Chapt 6, in Blood: Textbook of Hematology. Boston, Little, Brown and Company, 1987.

IRON DEFICIENCY ANEMIA

Iron deficiency and protein-calorie malnutrition are believed to be the two most common medical ailments. As iron deficiency is prevalent, treatable, and often is the first evidence of gastrointestinal bleeding, early diagnosis is imperative. Iron deficiency sufficiently severe to slow down erythropoiesis is almost always preceded by a latent phase during which macrophages are depleted of storage iron and plasma ferritin levels decline to the lower limits of normal. As deficiency progresses plasma iron levels fall, in response to which transferrin concentrations rise and free erythrocyte protoporphyrin accumulates for lack of its ferrous ligand. Only after this prodrome do hypochromic microcytic cells appear in the blood (Figure 7-7) [13].

Causes of Iron Deficiency Anemia

In adult males and postmenopausal females the occurrence of iron deficiency anemia in the absence of overt hemorrhage is tantamount to a diagnosis of occult gastrointestinal bleeding. Excessive menstrual loss, the leading cause of iron deficiency in young women, is usually self-evident. In tropical areas hookworm infection

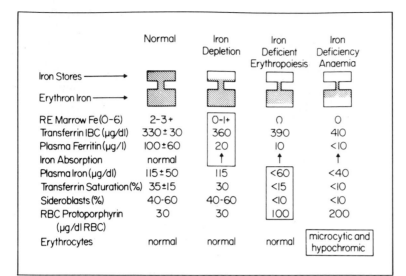

	Normal	Iron Depletion	Iron Deficient Erythropoiesis	Iron Deficiency Anaemia
Iron Stores ⟶				
Erythron Iron ⟶				
RE Marrow Fe(0–6)	2–3+	0–1+	0	0
Transferrin IBC (µg/dl)	330±30	360	390	410
Plasma Ferritin (µg/l)	100±60	20	10	<10
Iron Absorption	normal	↑	↑	↑
Plasma Iron (µg/dl)	115±50	115	<60	<40
Transferrin Saturation (%)	35±15	30	<15	<10
Sideroblasts (%)	40–60	40–60	<10	<10
RBC Protoporphyrin (µg/dl RBC)	30	30	100	200
Erythrocytes	normal	normal	normal	microcytic and hypochromic

FIGURE 7-7

Sequential changes in the development of iron deficiency anemia. (From Bothwell TH et al: Chapt 2, in Iron Metabolism in Man. Oxford, Blackwell Scientific Publications, 1979.)

is the preeminent cause of blood loss and iron deficiency anemia. About 500 million people harbor hookworms, and the quantity of blood lost daily is proportional to the number of these intestinal leeches. Each hookworm, its head burrowed into the small intestinal wall and its anal end dangling into the gut lumen, pumps peristaltic plumes of blood into the alimentary tract at a rate of over 100 suctions per minute. In heavy infections total blood loss may reach 100 ml daily.

Any hemorrhagic lesion of the alimentary tract may be responsible for blood loss and iron deficiency, and one of the most important routine responsibilities of the physician is performance of stool screening tests for occult blood—a mandatory practice often necessitating the posting of unusual packets through the mails.

Malabsorption of iron is comparatively uncommon in the general public but is sufficiently frequent in patients who have had gastric resection to warrant prophylactic iron supplementation. Intestinal malabsorption of iron can be a puzzling problem in patients with diffuse enteritis, particularly in the cryptic form of adult celiac disease.

Blood and Marrow Morphology

The appearance of flat, pale, small hypochromic red cells in the blood is the morphologic prelude to iron deficiency anemia. As anemia ensues, hypochromia and microcytosis generally develop in tandem, and values for MCV, MCH, and MCHC are all reduced proportionally. Red cell pallor can become so striking the cells resemble wafers, and when hemoglobin concentrations decline below 5 or 6 g/dl the population of pale discoidal cells is admixed with an assortment of poikilocytes, creating a chaotic morphology reminiscent of thalassemia. Contrary to the assertions of many iron mavens, iron deficiency anemia usually can be differentiated on morphologic grounds from the trait form of thalassemia, the only other hematologic abnormality associated with MCV levels below 70 fl (Figure 7-8). The differentiation of iron deficiency anemia and β thalassemia minor can be resolved unequivocally by the finding of siderocytes and punctate basophilic stippling, which is found in thalassemia but not in iron deficiency. A customary but not unique feature of iron deficiency anemia is an associated increase in platelet counts to levels about twice normal.

Iron lack and iron misappropriation (thalassemia) require antithetical therapies, and even the most illustrious morphologists must turn to supportive biochemical measurement before making this crucial differentiation. Several discriminate algorithms have been proposed, the most productive formularies including serum ferritin levels and electronic red cell counts. None is perfect, however, for patients with β thalassemia trait have iron deficiency and a

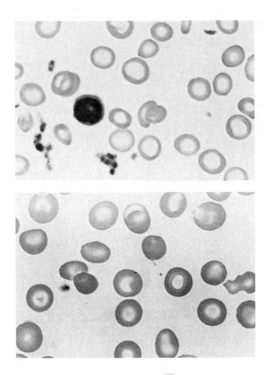

FIGURE 7-8

Hypochromic red cells of iron deficiency anemia (above) compared with those of β thalassemia minor (below). In iron deficiency anemia the red cells appear patently pale, many possessing a mere peripheral rim of hemoglobin. Nearly all cells have an enlarged central area of pallor, with only faint targeting. Despite moderately severe anemia, poikilocytes are not numerous. In thalassemia minor, despite little or no anemia, the cells are even more microcytic (use the lymphocyte nucleus as a yardstick), but the cells do not look pale, and target forms are more numerous. (Photos by CT Kapff.)

low serum ferritin from blood loss with the same frequency as normal individuals. The finding of an elevated proportion of hemoglobin A_2 (Hb $\alpha_2\delta_2$) is characteristic of β thalassemia, whereas A_2 is low or normal in iron deficiency, but normal A_2 levels are found in α-thalassemic disorders. Morphologic diagnosis should be fortified with a full iron profile (Table 7-2), combined when appropriate with family studies.

Marrow morphology does not distinguish iron deficiency from thalassemia, for in both disorders erythroblasts are small and possess only scant shaggy cytoplasm, mottled with small puddles of hemoglobin. Defective, late-stage erythroblasts with condensed nuclei nearly naked of cytoplasm create a spurious look of hyperplasia, but many or most erythroblasts die within the marrow. The finding of prussian blue–staining hemosiderin deposits in marrow excludes iron deficiency; absence of hemosiderin does not prove that anemia was caused by iron deficiency, but it affirms the possibility.

Manifestations of Iron Deficiency

Iron deficiency anemia is insidious, allowing time for mobilizing remarkably effective adaptations comparable to those in pernicious anemia. Patients usually do not seek medical attention until hemoglobin levels fall below 7 to 8 g/dl, when impaired work performance and cardiovascular intolerance of sustained exertion become troublesome [14].

Behavioral Effects

Iron-deficient children show mental and behavioral impairment that can be improved gradually by iron repletion. Iron-deficient infants display depressed spontaneous activity, impaired cognitive functions, and numerous noncognitive disturbances such as short attention span, withdrawal, and a characteristic silent solemnity [15]. An outré behavioral oddity found in about half of iron deficiency patients of all ages is compulsive chewing or gnawing, known as pica. In adults the compulsive eating of starch, clay, symbolic nonfood items, and noisy or brittle foods (pretzels, potato chips, and peanuts) may arouse misplaced merriment among otherwise friendly observers, who may not recognize that devouring several kilograms of ice daily (pagophagia) is diagnostic, not merely eccentric, behavior. In infants pica can exact a vicious toll, for iron-deficient infants may be driven to gnaw on surfaces coated with lead paint, a wicked irony leading to ingestion of a toxin (lead) that further impairs hemoglobin synthesis and mental development.

Epithelial Manifestations

Atrophy of epithelium affects at least 30% of patients with chronic iron deficiency. The resul-

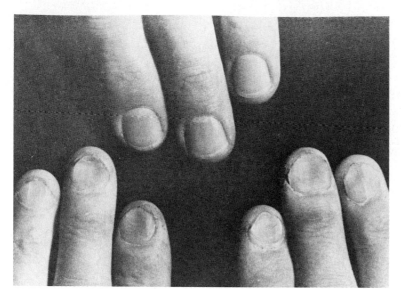

FIGURE 7-9

Spoon-shaped nails
(koilonychia) of a pa-
tient with chronic iron
deficiency (below) are
compared with normal
nails. (Reproduced,
with permission, from:
Rosenbaum F. and Leon-
ard JW: Nutritional
iron deficiency anemia
in an adult male. Re-
port of a case. Ann In-
tern Med 60:683,1964.)

tant thinning and fragility of epithelial structures sometimes results in a pathognomonic
triad of koilonychia, papillary atrophy of the
tongue, and esophageal webbing.

Koilonychia In chronic iron deficiency, finger-
nails become brittle and weak and split easily
at the ends. With loss of natural resilience the
nails become flattened in the course of normal
gripping and pressing, and eventually the outer
aspects become concave rather than convex
(Figure 7-9) [16]. Koilonychia is diagnostic of
iron deficiency. It recedes within about 4
months of iron replenishment.

Tongue, mouth, and esophagus Early in iron
deficiency, atrophy of the filiform papillae on
the anterior portion of the tongue becomes
evident, but with time the fungiform papillae
also flatten out and eventually the tongue
becomes smooth, glistening, and transparent,
often in association with painful chapping and
cracking of the corners of the mouth.

A singular feature of chronic iron lack is the
development of one or more transverse esophageal webs just below the cricoid and above
the aortic arch. These fragile epithelial shelves
may cause gradually worsening dysphagia and
even become imperforate (Figure 7-10) [17].
Esophageal webs do not resolve with iron
therapy, and relief from dysphagia requires

bougienage. If neglected, esophageal webs
sometimes progress to carcinoma in situ and
later to esophageal cancer.

Management of Iron Deficiency

A diagnosis of iron deficiency demands two
things of the physician. First, every means must
be employed to discover a source of bleeding; in
patients with intermittent or denied bleeding,
this may require painstaking perseverance. Second, the iron deficit must be corrected in full.
Oral ferrous sulfate tablets providing 120 to
180 mg of elemental iron daily are as promptly
effective and safer than parenteral preparations
in correcting the deficit; therapy should continue at least 4 months after restoration of the
red cell count to assure replenishment of depleted iron stores. The response to iron is rarely
dramatic, newly formed reticulocytes being outnumbered by the myriads of small red cells.
Reticulocyte counts ordinarily reach a maximum 7 to 10 days after therapy is started, with
peak levels seldom exceeding 10%; the red cell
count returns to normal within about 8 weeks
regardless of the starting level of hemoglobin.
Epithelial recovery takes longer and may be
incomplete; atrophic gastritis, if present as part
of the epithelial wasting, usually does not respond to replacement therapy.

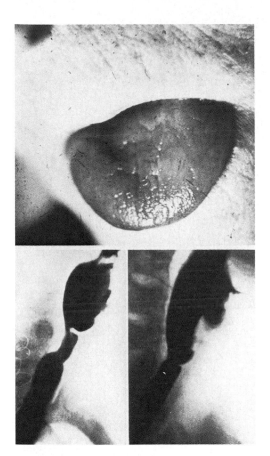

FIGURE 7-10

Epithelial abnormalities characteristic of chronic iron deficiency anemia. (Above) Smooth, depapillated tongue and shrivelled chapped lips of a patient with chronic iron deficiency. (Below, left) Barium swallow showing characteristic web filling defect in the anterior wall of the pharynx just below the cricoid. Below the web is a narrowed segment of the upper esophagus ending in a second constriction. (Below, right) Persistence of the upper web in the same patient despite 1 year of iron therapy. (Barium swallow views from Hutton CF: Plummer Vinson syndrome. Br J Radiol 29:81,1956.)

ANEMIA OF CHRONIC DISORDERS

The vague term "anemia of chronic disorders" (ACD) alludes to the nonthreatening anemias that commonly accompany chronic inflammatory or neoplastic diseases. In ACD, hypoferremia is associated with a reduced transferrin level, low transferrin saturation, elevated serum ferritin, and a surplus of storage iron. Anemia appears within a few weeks of chronic infection or neoplasia, but hematocrit levels seldom decline below about 32%. In most patients the red cells are mildly hypochromic or hypochromia is evident in blood smears even when the MCHC falls within normal limits. Differentiation from iron deficiency is resolved by two findings: serum levels of ferritin are elevated, not depressed, and marrow storage iron is increased, not absent.

In ACD macrophages compete with erythroblasts for iron   Activated, proliferating macrophages upregulate receptors that are specific for apotransferrin, thereby preventing a large fraction of iron-binding protein from participating in the recycling of iron to the erythron.

Lactoferrin   During inflammation iron-free lactoferrin (apolactoferrin) is secreted by neutrophils in gram quantities. Lactoferrin is a transferrinlike glycoprotein (M_r: 76,000) that is released by the secondary granules of neutrophils and becomes bound to apolactoferrin receptors on macrophages, further augmenting the appetite of the burgeoning macrophage population for iron. Macrophage-bound apolactoferrin is an iron trap: iron bound to the lactoferrin-receptor complex is internalized by receptor-mediated endocytosis and accumulates in macrophages as ferritin. Excessive trapping of iron and transferrin by aroused macrophages explains the defective iron cycling of ACD, but the underlying erythrosuppressive response to inflammation is mainly traceable to the discharge into plasma of growth-inhibitory cytokines including interleukin 1, tumor necrosis factor, gamma interferon, and transforming growth factor. As anemia is moderate and self-limited, blood transfusion is rarely necessary.

SIDEROBLASTIC ANEMIAS

Sideroblastic anemias are a heterogeneous group of hypochromic disorders caused by defective iron utilization within erythropoietic cells. Consequently during erythroblast maturation unused iron accumulates as ferritin, which in turn collects in toxic quantities between the mitochondrial cristae. During the late stages of maturation mitochondria laden with iron slag gather tightly around the pyknotic nucleus to create the telltale morphologic totem of sideroblastic anemias, the ringed sideroblast.

Ringed Sideroblasts: The Hallmark of Sideroblastic Anemias

The morphologic triad of sideroblastic anemias is: hypochromic red cells, with erythroid dimorphism; hyperferremia; and unique perinuclear rings or arcs of prussian blue–positive granules in orthochromatic erythroblasts (Figure 7-11) [18]. Ringed sideroblasts occur in small numbers in several erythropoietic disorders, but when nuclei in over 10% of orthochromatic erythroblasts are ringed by a necklace of prussian blue–staining granules the diagnosis of sideroblastic anemia is made. For authentication, three criteria must be met: (1) the iron granules must be abnormally large, (2) they must exceed five or six in number, and (3) they must form an arc extending around at least 30% of the nucleus.

Pathogenesis of Sideroblastic Anemia

In sideroblastic anemias iron uptake from transferrin is unimpaired, but there is a block in iron utilization that causes a pileup in mitochondria that can be lethal; heavily iron-laden cells expire within the marrow, creating a spurious appearance of erythroid hyperplasia. A multiplicity of metabolic defects has been reported in the various sideroblastic anemias. Most frequent has been the finding of diminished activity of the first and rate-limiting enzyme in heme synthesis, mitochondrial δ-aminolevulinic acid (ALA) synthetase (Chapter 3). In several reports activity of ferrochelatase, the distal enzyme in the heme biosynthetic pathway, has been subnormal,

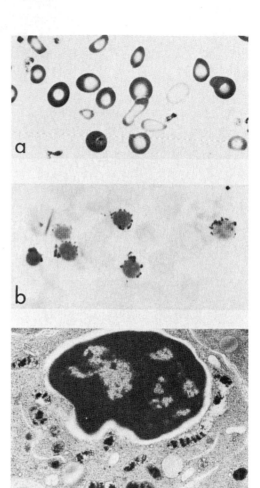

FIGURE 7-11

Morphologic findings diagnostic of sideroblastic anemia. (a) Most red cells are mildly hypochromic and microcytic, but a subpopulation of cells is extremely pale (red cell "dimorphism"). (b) Marrow erythroblasts stained with prussian blue and counterstained with safranin display perinuclear collars of large iron granules (ringed sideroblasts). (c) EM view of the perinuclear mitochondria reveals dense deposits of iron lodged between the mitochondrial cristae, creating a ladder effect. (From Bottomley SS: Sideroblastic anaemia. Clin Haematol 11:389,1982.)

TABLE 7-4

Classification of sideroblastic anemias

Hereditary
   X-linked
   Heredity undetermined
Acquired
   Idiopathic
   Secondary
      Drug-induced (antituberculosis drugs,
      chloramphenicol chemotherapeutic
      agents)
      Alcohol-induced
      Chronic lead poisoning

and in others a defect of coproporphyrinogen oxidase was implicated. In most subsets of sideroblastic anemias there is no clear molecular explanation for the failure to utilize iron and for the uncontrolled self-destructive cellular gulosity for iron. A crude descriptive classification of these unusual but not rare anemias is presented in Table 7-4.

Hereditary Sideroblastic Anemias

In most family studies, hereditary sideroblastic anemia has shown an X-linked recessive pattern, and hemizygotes have been afflicted with lifelong hypochromic and dimorphic (or polymorphic) anemia, often severe, accompanied by severe iron overloading, which progresses in survivors to clinical hemochromatosis. In about half of kindreds anemia has responded partially to very high doses of pyridoxine, generating the expression "pyridoxine-responsive anemia." Response to pyridoxine is not through alleviation of pyridoxine deficiency; for sustained remission, pharmacologic doses of pyridoxine must be given for life and even in response the microcytosis and hypochromia are not corrected. In at least some X-linked cases, benefit from large doses of pyridoxine can be explained by the presence of genetic variants of ALA-synthetase that either have an increased K_m for pyridoxal 5'-phosphate (the obligate coenzyme for ALA synthesis) or are unstable and abnormally sensitive to mitochondrial protease.

Idiopathic Sideroblastic Anemia

Idiopathic sideroblastic anemia (ISA), a disease acquired by older people, is the most common sideroblastic disorder, accounting for about 1% of all patients referred for hematologic consultation. Like the hereditary forms, ISA stems from a pronounced reduction in ALA-synthetase activity, but paradoxically this iron-loading disorder is associated with high levels of free erythrocyte protoporphyrin, proving that ferrochelatase activity and possibly other terminal steps in heme synthesis are also compromised. The response rate to pharmacologic doses of pyridoxine is far lower (about 5%) than in hereditary sideroblastic anemias. Many ISA patients have macrocytic red cells, megaloblastic morphology, and respond sufficiently well to folate to warrant continued folate supplementation. About half of patients with ISA have recurrent clonal chromosomal abnormalities, and 10 to 15% of these cases eventually evolve into acute myelogenous leukemia. ISA never undergoes spontaneous remission, and it is probable that all patients with this disorder should be classified among the myelodysplastic refractory anemias (Chapter 13).

Drug-Induced Sideroblastic Anemias Are Reversible

Some acquired sideroblastic anemias are reversible processes caused by exposure or overexposure to medications or myelotoxic chemicals. INH is the most common cause of drug-induced sideroblastic anemias, particularly when used in combination with other antituberculosis drugs.

Severe alcoholics are punished in many ways for their intemperate thirst, suffering as they do from multiple nutritional deficiencies and disturbed liver function. Folate deficiency with megaloblastic anemia is commonplace, but the transition to a sideroblastic marrow with hyperferremia generally signifies superimposed pyridoxine deficiency. Alcohol interferes with conversion of pyridoxine to the coenzyme, pyridoxal 5'-phosphate. Alcohol also activates a hemin-controlled repression of globin synthesis, which may contribute to the reversible block in iron utilization [19].

Chronic Lead Poisoning

Chronic lead poisoning (plumbism, saturnism) warrants special consideration for it is both dangerous and preventable. It is most prevalent among infants and children, who often face the triple jeopardy of iron deficiency, pica, and access to lead-painted surfaces, and among occupationally exposed adults. In both young and old, lead poisoning causes chronic hypochromic anemia, but in children the leading iron indicators may misguide because of coexistence of iron deficiency [20].

Effects of lead on heme synthesis   Lead absorbed by ingestion or inhalation is rapidly transferred to red cell and erythroblast membrane lipids; being lipophilic, lead penetrates readily to reach the organelles, resulting in multiple derangements. In marrow, lead concentrates in the phospholipid inner matrix of mitochondria, where it impedes delivery of iron to the internal acceptor site in which protoporphyrin and ferrochelatase are situated and waiting. The effect of lead is to starve ferrochelatase of iron. This causes both an

FIGURE 7-12

Coarse basophilic stippling and hypochromia in the anemia of chronic lead poisoning. Stippling is especially prominent in the orthochromatic erythroblast (upper left). Wright-Giemsa stain. (From Jandl JH: Chapt 6, in Blood: Textbook of Hematology. Boston, Little, Brown, and Company,1987.)

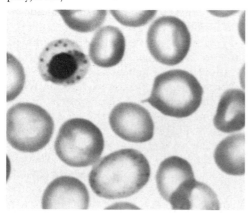

accumulation of iron in the mitochondria and a marked pileup of free erythrocyte protoporphyrin in the cytoplasm.

Anemia is a late feature of chronic lead poisoning, unless exposure is extreme—as among carpenters ordered to "delead" a lead-painted surface by sanding. Hemoglobin levels decline when blood lead levels rise above about 50 μg/dl. In most patients reticulocyte levels are elevated, reflecting hemolysis caused by lead-induced damage to the lipid bilayer. Coarse basophilic stippling, a notorious feature of lead poisoning, results from toxic inhibition of pyrimidine 5'-nucleotidase, an enzyme that normally cleaves ribonucleotide residues shortly after nuclear extrusion. Coarse basophilic stippling is limited to the youngest red cells, however, and thus only a small percentage of cells are heavily stippled in lead poisoning (Figure 7-12) [7].

All patients with symptomatic or hematologic evidence of lead poisoning require chelation therapy, preferably combining dimercaprol (BAL) and calcium EDTA.

CHRONIC IRON OVERLOAD

When iron utilization is crippled, as in refractory sideroblastic states and thalassemia, and when management of intractable anemia of any sort necessitates periodic blood transfusions, the iron burden imposed eventually overwhelms the iron storage capacity of the macrophage system, for there is no mechanism for excreting surplus iron. When the total surplus of storage iron exceeds about 10 g, iron becomes deposited harmfully in the parenchymal cells of liver and other organs. The purest form of iron overloading is not caused by faulty iron utilization or transfusional siderosis but occurs as an inherited nonhematologic disorder, hereditary hemochromatosis—the exemplar of disorders associated with iron overloading.

Hereditary Hemochromatosis

Hereditary hemochromatosis (hemochromatosis) results from an inborn error of intestinal iron absorption, in which dietary iron is inappropriately hyperabsorbed throughout life regardless of need. The autosomal recessive gene

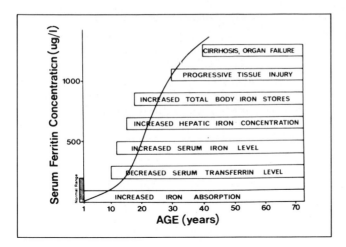

FIGURE 7-13

Biochemical and pathologic progression of iron overload in hemochromatosis. (From Halliday JW and Powell LW: Iron overload. Semin Hematol 19:42,1982.)

for hemochromatosis is linked tightly to the HLA (human leukocyte antigen) portion of the major histocompatibility (MHC) locus on the short arm of chromosome 6; full expression occurs only in homozygotes. In large surveys using a transferrin saturation exceeding 62% as the diagnostic criterion, the frequency of homozygosity is 0.0045, corresponding to a gene frequency of 0.067 (1 person in 16) [21]. Expression of this common and cryptic genetic anomaly is subject to the quantity of iron in the diet, and presumably even a single gene for hemochromatosis poses an added problem for patients with chronic iron overloading diseases such as thalassemia and other anemias marked by ineffective erythropoiesis ("erythropoietic hemochromatosis").

Pathogenesis: The Iron Curtain Is Raised

The amount of iron absorbed from the diet in homozygous hemochromatosis exceeds normal by only 1 to 2 mg daily, but the problem is that even iron-replete intestinal mucosa cells allow continued entry of iron, acting as though there were a raised or defective barrier and no feedback mechanism for regulating iron uptake. Thus iron absorption continues senselessly, and by adulthood men (who have no menstrual outlet for iron) can accumulate 15 to 20 g of excess iron, most of it stored in the liver. Early in the evolution of hemochromatosis, transferrin saturation rises well above 50%

and transferrin concentration falls. As iron is errantly admitted by intestinal mucosa cells to the portal circulation while transferrin is nearly saturated, atoms of unbound iron may undergo many passages through the liver before they can occupy open sites on transferrin. Consequently, in hemochromatosis 30% of plasma iron perfusing liver and other organs may be in hydrated ionic complexes. Like other transition metals, ionized iron has the ability to accept and donate single electrons, making it a dangerous catalyst of free radical reactions. Specifically, Fe^{2+}/Fe^{3+} in the presence of O_2 and NADPH generates reduced radicals of oxygen, the most indiscriminate and instantly cytotoxic of which is OH· [22]. As most freshly absorbed iron is unbound to transferrin, it is not surprising that hepatocytes bear the brunt of iron catalyzed oxidations. All hemochromatosis patients have extreme hepatic siderosis, and in nearly 95% liver biopsy reveals fibrosis. Iron deposition with accompanying damage by free radical O_2 metabolites in other tissues is responsible for the familiar clinical features of the disease: pigmentation of the skin, "bronze" diabetes, chondrocalcinosis, complex neuropathies, cardiomyopathy, and hepatoma. Of these, iron-mediated cardiomyopathy with intractable congestive failure is the principal cause of death, followed by hepatoma, which develops in 20 to 30% of patients. The age-dependent chemical and clinical progression of hemochromatosis is portrayed in Figure 7-13 [23]. A notable difference between hemochromatosis and transfusional iron overloading is that in hemochromatosis the macrophages of marrow and spleen are usually spared; marrow hemosiderin tends to be low or absent in patients whose liver parenchymal cells are glutted with iron deposits.

Management   With recent awareness of the prevalence of hemochromatosis and application of early screening procedures that include measurement of serum ferritin and HLA typing of suspect families, prognosis has improved dramatically in the last 10 to 15 years. Vigorous venisection, involving weekly or twice-weekly 500-ml phlebotomies, is necessary to remove the iron overload with appropriate expedition (i.e., within 12 to 18 months) (Figure 7-14) [24]. Patients depleted of iron within 18 months by programmed venisections enjoy a normal life expectancy [25]. In untreated patients 5-year survival rates after diagnosis are below 30%. Early diagnosis and an appropriate follow-up regimen of less frequent phlebotomies (usually 2 to 6 per year) are essential to successful therapy, for undertreated patients face risks of cardiomyopathy and liver cancer that are 200 to 300 times that of the general age-matched population.

Other Causes of Iron Overload

Iron overload is a potential problem in patients with alcoholic cirrhosis or porphyria cutanea tarda, and tissue damage can occur rarely as the result of unreasonably protracted iron medication. Iron overload was once endemic in the black population of South Africa (so-called "African siderosis"). The steady decline in traditional amateur brewing in iron drums and its replacement by commercial breweries appears to be extinguishing this regional variety of iron overload, while further enriching the coffers of the white population.

Transfusional Iron Overloading and Chelation Therapy

Children with severe hereditary hemolytic anemias and patients of all ages with severe aplastic or refractory dysplastic anemias depend for their lives on transfusional support. For full benefit the transfusion rate should be adjusted to maintain hemoglobin levels about 11.5 g/dl. This may require transfusing 100 to 400 ml/kg body weight annually, thereby loading the body with up to 10 g of unexcretable iron each year. The consequences are the same as for full-blown homozygous hemochromatosis, and about 40% of patients dependent

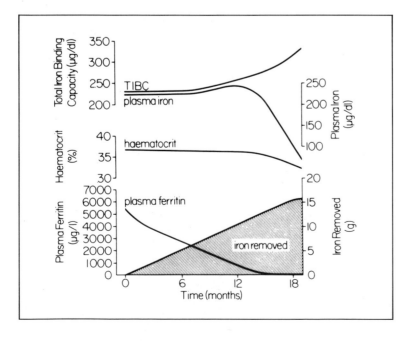

FIGURE 7-14

Serial changes in transferrin, plasma iron, hematocrit (haematocrit), and plasma ferritin levels in response to systematic venesection therapy and removal of over 15 g of red cell iron. Note that plasma iron and hematocrit concentrations hold up until ferritin levels fall to normal. (From Bothwell TH et al: Chapt 6, in Iron Metabolism in Man. Oxford, Blackwell Scientific Publications,1979.)

since birth on transfusional support die early of acute or chronic heart failure. The only effective means of fending off this dismal denouement is the daily or continuous subcutaneous administration of an iron-chelating agent, of which deferoxamine (desferrioxamine, Desferal) is most widely used.

THE THALASSEMIAS

Thalassemias are hereditary hypochromic anemias caused by absent or defective synthesis of one or more of the polypeptide chains of globin. In most thalassemias synthesis of either α or β chains of Hb A ($\alpha_2\beta_2$) is impaired. Normally α-like and β-like globin chains are synthesized coordinately. If not, unbalanced synthesis harms the erythron in two ways. First, failure of α and β globin chains to match up reduces total hemoglobinization of erythroblasts to concentrations (less than 20 pg/cell) inadequate for their survival; therefore, most erythroblasts die in the marrow, a process called "intramedullary hemolysis" or "ineffective erythropoiesis." The minority of cells that complete maturation and are released into circulation are too pale, small, and deformed to transport O_2 satisfactorily. Second, unbalanced synthesis of α or β chains leads to intracellular accumulations of unmatched chains, which aggregate as inclusion bodies. If sufficiently large, these inclusions ensnare or injure the cells within the marrow, adding to the intramedullary carnage. Those that escape into circulation carry aggregates of denatured globin, and many of these cells are unable to slip through the trapping defiles and strictures of the splenic cords.

Collectively thalassemias are among the commonest hereditary disorders. α thalassemias are the most prevalent and widely distributed of the genetic hemoglobin disorders, and in some Asian and black populations the α thalassemia gene frequency exceeds that of the normal genotype. The high frequencies of the benign trait form of α thalassemia (α^+ thalassemia) in malarial areas appear to be the most refined result of natural selection known, for sickle cell trait and G6PD deficiency, the other main evolutionary adaptations to falciparum malaria, exact a heavy toll among homozygotes

and hemizygotes, and a protective advantage of β thalassemia remains to be established [26]. In the endless warfare between people and Plasmodia, the evolution of α-thalassemic balanced polymorphism (best defined as inheriting something bad that protects against something worse) has been the most cost-effective and highly conserved adaptive genetic defense.

Most α Thalassemias Result From Large Deletions in the α Globin Gene Complex

The α globin complex resides on the short arm of chromosome 16 (Figure 3-10) and contains two expressed α globin genes (α1 and α2), plus an embryonic ζ gene and two pseudogenes. The extensive sequence homology surrounding the two α structural genes reflects the process of concerted evolution, accomplished by unequal crossing over between duplicated gene regions. Each α globin gene is embedded within a 4-kb region of duplication within which are shorter homology units. The extensive homology surrounding α genes, which is not seen in the β globin complex on chromosome 11 (Figure 3-10), accounts for the proclivity of this region to sustain deletional events, eight genotypic kinds having been described. The most common deletions are those that generate chromosomes bearing a single gene. Misalignment and crossing over create a single fused gene from which 3.7 kb of DNA are missing; the single gene complex is the product of a $-\alpha^{3.7}$ "rightward deletion." About 30% of American blacks are heterozygous for this deletion ($-\alpha^{3.7}\alpha/\alpha\alpha$) and 2% are homozygous ($-\alpha^{3.7}\alpha/-\alpha^{3.7}\alpha$). Less often, misalignment and crossing over cause a "leftward deletion" of 4.2 kb of DNA. The $-\alpha^{3.7}$ deletion removes the entire α1 gene (or produces a hybrid α1–α2 gene), and the $-\alpha^{4.2}$ deletion eliminates the α2 gene (Figure 7-15) [27]. As the majority of α globin is encoded by the α2 gene, loss or mutation affecting the α2 locus, which is common in Asians, creates a more serious imbalance in the α/β synthetic ratio and a higher percentage of Hb Bart's (γ_4) than loss or mutation of the α1 locus [28].

Nondeletion forms of α thalassemia   Not all α thalassemias are the result of large deletions in the α globin complex. An assortment of uncom-

FIGURE 7-15

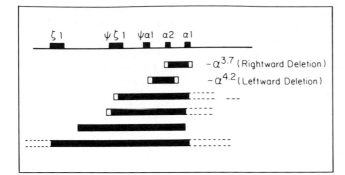

Samples of deletions within the α globin gene complex. Black regions indicate gene regions known to be deleted. White boxes depict the possible extremes of known deletions, and interrupted lines current uncertainties as to the boundaries of extensive deletions. (From Orkin SH: Chapt 4, in The Molecular Basis of Blood Diseases, Stamatoyannopoulos G et al, Eds. Philadelphia, WB Saunders Company,1987.)

mon molecular lesions has been described in which expression of the α globin gene has been depressed. These include: mutations in the termination codon, as in the case of the elongated variant, Hb Constant Spring; a splicing defect caused by a small base pair deletion of the first intron; point mutation of the polyadenylation site or of the $\alpha 1$ initiation codon; and formation of extremely unstable α globin structural variants. In some patients with myeloproliferative disorders, profound α thalassemia occurs as an acquired accompaniment of erythroid dysplasia.

The α-Thalassemic Syndromes: Gene Number, Gene Order, and cis Versus trans

The four basic α-thalassemic syndromes correspond to deletions or mutations of one, two, three, or all four of the α globin genes expressed in erythropoietic cells. The various α thalassemias arise from all the permutations of α gene number, α gene position, and cis or trans pairing of deletional and nondeletional defects (Table 7-5).

α thalassemia minor   Deletion of a single α gene has no hematologic consequence, and even genetic absence of two α globin genes has a very minor lowering effect on hemoglobin levels and is notable chiefly for causing moderate hypochromia and microcytosis. In Asians both deletions are in cis and affect the same chromosome, but in individuals of black African descent a single α locus is deleted from each of the two pairs of chromosomes. Accordingly all clinically evident thalassemia syndromes are possible within Asian populations, whereas among blacks, in whom the α-thal-2

gene predominates (Table 7-5) and α-thal-1 is rare, Hb H disease is uncommon and hydrops fetalis with Hb Bart's is virtually nonexistent; in blacks the double deletions occur in trans, a gene deployment that precludes severe thalassemia. A factor in addition to gene number and position that affects the expression of α thalassemia minor is the "leftwardness" of the deletion. Individuals (primarily Asians) homozygous for the leftward $-\alpha^{4.2}$ deletion have higher levels of Hb Bart's than persons (primarily black) who are homozygous for the rightward $-\alpha^{3.7}$ deletion [28].

α thalassemia of either double-deletion phenotype causes only a modest accumulation of unmatched β chains, with limited damage to red cells and mildly ineffective erythropoiesis. Damage is held in check by an ATP-dependent proteolytic custodial enzyme unique to immature red cells.

Hemoglobin H Disease

Deletion or mutation of three of the four α globin genes is usually caused by double heterozygosity for the α-thal-1 and α-thal-2 genes, resulting in a $--/-\alpha$ genotype. The resulting syndrome, most prevalent in Asians, is characterized by chronic hemolytic anemia caused by the injurious pileup within red cells of unpaired β chains, which arrange themselves as unstable tetramers (β_4). β_4 tetramers of Hb H have a very high O_2 affinity and lack the Bohr effect and cooperativity, and hence are useless in O_2 transport. The Hb H molecule is so arranged that eight (rather than two) highly reactive sulfhydryl groups are exposed, rendering the protein vulnerable to oxidative denaturation. The precipitates of Hb H are not

TABLE 7-5

The α-thalassemia syndromes

Syndrome	Genotype*	Hematologic abnormalities	Hemoglobin variants	
			At birth	Later
Normal	αα/αα	None	None	None
Silent carrier state (α-thal-2)	−α/αα	None	Hb Bart's (0–2%)	None
α-thal-minor				
α-thal-1 (heterozygous)	−−/αα	Mild anemia plus	Hb Bart's (2–10%)	None
α-thal-2 (homozygous)	−α/−α	thalassemic morphology		
Hb H disease	−−/−α −−/XX −−/αCS	Chronic hemolytic anemia	Hb Bart's (10–40%)	Hb H (5–30%) Hb Bart's (trace)
Hydrops fetalis	−−/−−	Fatal anemia in utero	Hb Bart's >80% (also Hb H and Hb Portland)	———

*X = nondeletional gene of α locus; CS = gene for Hb Constant Spring.

Source: From Jandl JH: Chapter 6, in Blood: Textbook of Hematology. Boston, Little, Brown and Company, 1987.

FIGURE 7-16

Red cells from an unsplenectomized patient with Hb H disease, after blood had been stained supravitally with BCB dye and then air dried. Hb H precipitates account for the fine speckling; the coarse, black clumps represent the aggregated RNA of reticulocytes. (Photo by CT Kapff.)

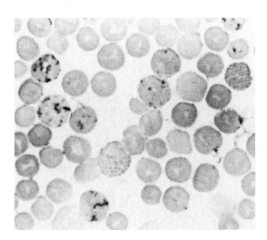

visible on routine Wright-Giemsa staining but can be seen as fine, evenly dispersed granular inclusions after red cell suspensions have been exposed to a few drops of a redox dye such as brilliant cresyl blue (BCB) (Figure 7-16).

Hb H disease is characterized by mild to moderate hemolytic anemia, with hypochromic microcytic red cells, and elevated reticulocyte levels. The spleen is usually enlarged by "work hyperplasia" as well as red cell engorgement; in patients with severe anemia and exceptional splenomegaly, splenectomy is often beneficial.

β Thalassemias

The β globin gene cluster contains five expressed genes and one pseudogene and spans 60 kb of DNA on the short arm of chromosome 11 (Figure 3-10). Unlike most α thalassemias, which are caused by gross gene deletions, the common forms of β thalassemia are due to single base substitutions or small insertions or deletions within the β globin gene that result in errors of transcription, RNA processing, or translation. Over 40 point mutations have been described, but pinpointing the heterogeneous mechanisms underlying malfunction of β globin genes has required the most resourceful technology, combining gene amplification by DNA polymerase chain reactions with dot blot hybridization using designed oligonucleotide probes [29]. Less frequently β thalassemia is caused by large or even massive deletions that remove part or all of the β globin gene cluster.

Although numerous kinds of hereditable mutations may underlie impairment of β globin synthesis, inheritance is straightforward: as each chromosome 11 possesses but a single β globin locus, individuals are either heterozygous (β-thal minor) or homozygous (β-thal major) for the β-thal gene. The most common form of β thalassemia spares the δ globin locus and therefore is marked by an increased proportion of Hb A_2. In the homozygous state the high A_2 kind of β thalassemia can be separated into two major subtypes: in one, β^+-thal, β chains are produced in subnormal amounts; in the other, $\beta°$-thal, no β chains are produced. In addition homozygosity for crossover $\beta\delta$ fusion variants such as the Lepore hemoglobins may cause severe β thalassemia. The relative amounts of the hemoglobin fractions produced in the β-thal major syndromes are shown in Table 7-6.

β Thalassemia Major

All four genetic variants of β thalassemia are capable of causing severe, lifelong, transfusion-dependent anemia and attendant iron overloading. The clinical and hematologic courses of the four variants can be described collectively although some differences exist in laboratory findings.

Anemia   Anemia in β thalassemia major is severe, with hemoglobin levels ranging from 2 to 7 g/dl. Red cells are very small (MCV: 50 to 60 fl), pale, and wildly varied in size, shape, and coloring: in no other anemia is there more grotesque and kaleidoscopic polymorphism (Figure 7-17).

Anemia is caused by two problems compounded. Foremost, the erythropoietin-driven marrow is unable to produce erythroblasts that are adequately stocked with hemoglobin, and 80 to 90% of the cells expire wretchedly in the crowded chambers of the marrow sinuses, depositing heaps of hemosiderin as they die. Second, those few erythropoietic cells that synthesize viable quantities of hemoglobin are forced to go through an added division to do so. The pitiful products entering the circulation are pale, small, and deformed and are laden with bulky precipitates of denatured α chains. Damage to cell membranes by α chain debris contributes to intramedullary hemolysis, and in circulation the inclusions cause red cells to be snared in the spleen, superimposing extramedullary hemolysis. Transit from the crypts of splenic cords to the broad boulevards of the spleen sinuses is an exquisite test of size and suppleness. Red cells loaded with α chain baggage are arrested at the slitlike passageways, resulting either in trapping of the cell or in a tugging affair in which the cell may escape the trap but acquire a tail as a memento (the

TABLE 7-6

Hemoglobin fractions in variants of β-thal major

Genotype	Hb A (%)	Hb A_2 (%)	Hb F (%)	Others
β^0/β^0	0	1–6	>94	Free α chains
β^+/β^+	5–50	2–8	40–80	Free α chains
β^0/β^+	2–10	1–3	>85	Free α chains
$\delta\beta^{Lepore}/\delta\beta^{Lepore}$	0	0	80	Hb Lepore (20%)

Source: From Jandl JH: Chapt 6, in Blood: Textbook of Hematology. Boston, Little, Brown and Company, 1987.

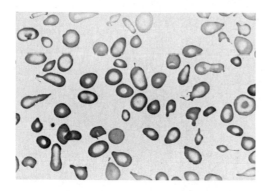

FIGURE 7-17

Blood smear from a patient with β thalassemia major. Anisocytosis is so extreme that no two cells look exactly alike. Amidst the menagerie of bizarre forms and fragments, three characteristic aberrations stand out: teardrop or tapered forms, target cells, and broad, colorless wafers. (Photo by CT Kapff.)

teardrop form). After splenectomy, cells loaded with inclusions are allowed to circulate, and tailed (teardrop) forms disappear.

As production of hemoglobin F is phased out in the first year of life, the first signs of anemic hypoxia and general failure to thrive become evident. Hepatosplenomegaly causes abdominal distension and feeding problems. As the child grows older a disfiguring physiognomy characteristic of thalassemia and other severe congenital hemolytic anemias results as the most visible aspect of generalized adaptive expansion of the marrow space (Figure 7-18). Pathologic expansion of erythropoietic tissue in a vain effort to compensate for the inefficiency of erythropoiesis leads to widening of the long bones and separation of the diploe of the skull, with dissolution of the outer tables, creating a radiologic imaging resembling "hair on end" (Figure 7-19) [30]. Openings or ero-

FIGURE 7-18

"Thalassemic facies" of a child with β thalassemia major. Marked overgrowth of the expanded maxillary cavity leads to extreme bucktooth deformity, severe malocclusion, and mongoloid broadening of the cheeks. (Courtesy DHA Pearson.)

FIGURE 7-19

"Hair on end" or "sunray" appearance of the skull in thalassemia is caused by trabecular striations radiating outward, accompanied by demineralization of the outer table. Similar changes occur in similarly severe congenital hemolytic anemias of other origins. (From Hoffbrand AV and Pettit JE: Chapt 5, in Clinical Hematology Illustrated. An Integrated Text and Color Atlas. London, Gower Medical Publishing Ltd.,1987.)

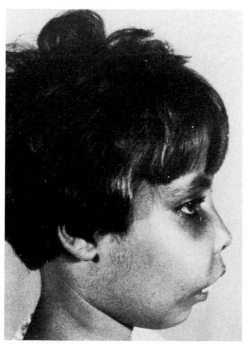

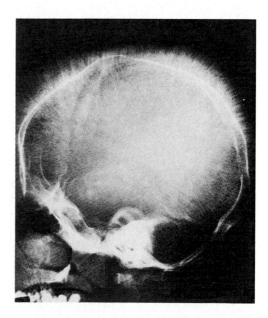

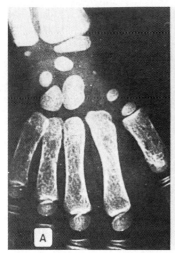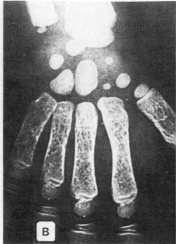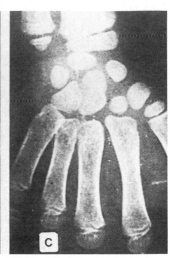

FIGURE 7-20

Trabecular radiologic pattern of the metacarpals of a patient with β thalassemia major 12 months (A) and 1 month (B) before transfusion. The filigreed trabecular pattern and reduced bone mass was transformed to normal 12 months after initiation of transfusional support (C). (From Sbyrakis S et al: A simple index for initiating transfusion treatment in thalassaemia intermedia. Br J Haematol 67:479,1987.)

sions through the bony cortex may lead to irruption of erythropoietic tissue into neighboring areas; these escaped but benign growths are most commonly seen by x-ray as large, smoothly lobulated masses located in the posterior mediastinum.

Management β thalassemia major patients who depend for their survival on aggressive transfusion therapy are doomed to die of transfusional myocardial hemosiderosis unless this is vigorously combatted by daily chelation therapy. Transfusional support, often supplemented by splenectomy, can restore hemoglobin levels to an acceptable range and resolves the erythropoietic housing problem (Figure 7-20) [31]. In severely affected patients who cannot tolerate the mixed hazards of transfusional siderosis and chelation, the desperate alternative is transplantation of HLA-compatible marrow [32].

β Thalassemia Minor

The heterozygous states for β^+-thal or β°-thal are characterized by little if any anemia, with hemoglobin levels rarely falling below 10 g/dl, and by striking, uniform microcytosis. The incongruous association of a nearly normal blood hemoglobin with marked microcytosis helps differentiate this trait from iron deficiency (Figure 7-8).

Large Deletions in the β Globin Gene Cluster and HPFH

Large deletions that remove 50 to over 100 kb of the β-like gene cluster on chromosome 11, but spare the $^G\gamma$ and $^A\gamma$ genes for fetal hemoglobin, in effect abrogate F-to-A switching. Similar disruption is caused less often by various point mutations or small deletions that indirectly stimulate synthesis of Hb F. Mutations that increase Hb F production may be categorized into those in which Hb F is distributed nonuniformly (heterocellularly) among cells displaying hypochromic microcytic morphology, and those in which Hb F is pancellular and the cells are nearly normal in appearance. The former are thalassemic mutations; the latter are called "hereditary persistence of fetal hemoglobin" (HPFH).

In some HPFH mutants the deletion excises the entire β and δ loci plus intergene DNA extending upstream and downstream. The defi-

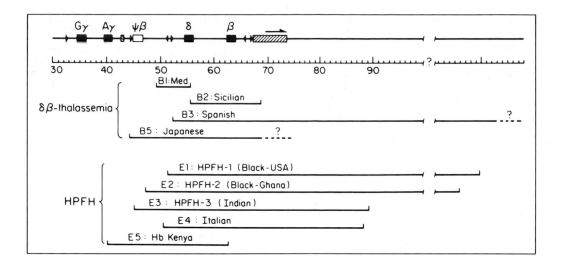

FIGURE 7-21

Location and size of deletions in various $\delta\beta$ thalassemia and HPFH mutants. (From Stamatoyannopoulos G and Nienhuis AW: Chapt 3, in The Molecular Basis of Blood Diseases, Stamatoyannopoulos G et al, Eds. Philadelphia, WB Saunders Company,1987.)

cit in β-like gene expression is compensated for by stimulation of the HPFH gene. In homozygotes 100% of hemoglobin is Hb F, and because of the higher O_2 affinity of intracellular fetal hemoglobin these persons may be mildly polycythemic. Depending on the extent of the deletion, synthesis of both $^G\gamma$ and $^A\gamma$ may be highly active, or only $^G\gamma$ may be expressed. (In the "Greek" form of HPFH, unlike the deletional forms found largely in black populations, the singular production of the $^A\gamma$ form of fetal hemoglobin is unaccompanied by any known gene deletion.) In patients heterozygous for $^G\gamma^A\gamma$ HPFH, Hb F levels range from 15 to 35%.

In patients with the rare thalassemic disorder $\delta\beta$-thal, both δ and β loci are deleted and hemoglobin A_2 levels are low or absent. Homozygotes have thalassemia intermedia with 100% hemoglobin F; in heterozygotes, anemia is mild, hypochromic, and microcytic, and hemoglobin F (range of concentration: 5 to 20%) is distributed nonuniformly. The sizes

of the heterogeneous deletions responsible for the enlivened production of hemoglobin F in $\delta\beta$ thalassemia and HPFH are represented in Figure 7-21 [33].

REFERENCES

1. Cook JD et al: Estimates of iron sufficiency in the US population. Blood 68:726,1986

2. Seligman PA et al: Chapt 7, in The Molecular Basis of Blood Diseases, Stamatoyannopoulos G et al, Eds. Philadelphia, WB Saunders Company,1987

3. Babior BM and Stossel TP: Chapt 4, in Hematology. A Pathophysiologic Approach. New York, Churchill Livingstone,1984

4. Rogers J and Munro H: Translation of ferritin light and heavy subunit mRNAs is regulated by intracellular chelatable iron levels in rat hepatoma cells. Proc Natl Acad Sci USA 84:2277,1987

5. Clegg GA et al: Ferritin: molecular structure and iron-storage mechanisms. Prog Biophys Molec Biol 36:53,1980

6. Erslev AJ and Gabuzda TG: Pathophysiology of Blood, 3rd ed. Philadelphia, WB Saunders, 1985

7. Jandl JH: Chapt 6, in Blood: Textbook of Hematology. Boston, Little, Brown and Company,1987

8. Bothwell TH et al: Chapt 4, in Iron Metabolism in Man. Oxford, Blackwell Scientific Publications,1979

9. Brittenham GM et al: Magnetic-susceptibility measurement of human iron stores. N Engl J Med 307:1671,1982

10. Bothwell TH and Charlton RW: A general approach to the problems of iron deficiency and iron overload in the population at large. Semin Hematol 19:54,1982

11. Wintrobe MM et al: Chapt 23, in Clinical Hematology, 8th ed. Philadelphia, Lea & Febiger,1981

12. Cook JD et al: Evaluation of the iron status of a population. Blood 48:449,1976

13. Bothwell TH et al: Chapt 2, in Iron Metabolism in Man. Oxford, Blackwell Scientific Publications,1979

14. Cook JD and Lynch SR: The liabilities of iron deficiency. Blood 68:803,1986

15. Lozoff B and Brittenham GM: Behavioral aspects of iron deficiency. Prog Hematol 14:23,1986

16. Rosenbaum E and Leonard JW: Nutritional iron deficiency anemia in an adult male. Report of a case. Ann Intern Med 60:683,1964

17. Hutton CF: Plummer Vinson syndrome. Br J Radiol 29:81,1956

18. Bottomley SS: Sideroblastic anaemia. Clin Haematol 11:389,1982

19. Bottomly SS: Chapt 10, in Iron in Biochemistry and Medicine, II. Jacobs A and Worwood M, Eds. London, Academic Press, Inc. (London) Ltd.,1980

20. Clark M et al: Interaction of iron deficiency and lead and the hematologic findings in children with severe lead poisoning. Pediatrics 81:247,1988

21. Edwards CQ et al: Prevalence of hemochromatosis among 11,065 presumably healthy blood donors. N Engl J Med 318:1355,1988

22. Halliwell B: Oxidants and human disease: some new concepts. FASEB J 1:358,1987

23. Halliday JW and Powell LW: Iron overload. Semin Hematol 19:42,1982

24. Bothwell TH et al: Chapt 6, in Iron Metabolism in Man. Oxford, Blackwell Scientific Publications,1979

25. Niederau C et al: Survival and causes of death in cirrhotic and in noncirrhotic patients with primary hemochromatosis. N Engl J Med 313:1256,1985

26. Hill AVS et al: α-Thalassemia and the malaria hypothesis. Acta Haematol 78:173,1987

27. Orkin SH: Chapt 4, in The Molecular Basis of Blood Diseases, Stamatoyannopoulos G et al, Eds. Philadelphia, WB Saunders Company,1987

28. Bowden DK et al: Different hematologic phenotypes are associated with the leftward $(-\alpha^{4.2})$ and rightward $(-\alpha^{3.7})$ α^+-thalassemia deletions. J Clin Invest 79:39,1987

29. Cai S-P et al: A simple approach to prenatal diagnosis of β-thalassemia in a geographic area where multiple mutations occur. Blood 71:1357,1988

30. Hoffbrand AV and Pettit JE: Chapt 3, in Clinical Hematology Illustrated. An Integrated Text and Color Atlas. London, Gower Medical Publishing Ltd., 1987

31. Sbyrakis S et al: A simple index for initiating transfusion treatment in thalassaemia intermedia. Br J Haematol 67:479,1987

32. Brochstein JA et al: Bone marrow transplantation in two multiply transfused patients with thalassaemia major. Br J Haematol 63:445,1986

33. Stamatoyannopoulos G and Nienhuis AW: Chapt 3, in The Molecular Basis of Blood Diseases, Stamatoyannopoulos G et al, Eds. Philadelphia, WB Saunders Company,1987

8

Hemolytic Anemias

☐

Normal red cells circulating in a normal environment have an actuarial lifespan (mean longevity) of about 120 days. In clinical usage the term "hemolysis" encompasses all mechanisms that cause red cells to expire prematurely. In some cases untimely demise results from accelerated senescence, but in the vast majority of hemolytic diseases hemolysis is caused by active destruction. Rarely red cells are dissolved while in circulation ("intravascular hemolysis"), but in most hemolytic processes destruction is initiated by trapping of cells in the sinuses of the spleen or liver, a process ineptly termed "extravascular hemolysis." Hemolytic disorders are marked by evidence of increased hemoglobin catabolism (Chapter 4) combined with persistent reticulocytosis and other indicators of increased erythropoiesis. Most anemias have a hemolytic component, but for practical purposes it is desirable to segregate disorders in which hemolysis occurs during circulation from disorders (such as thalassemia) that are dominated by intramedullary hemolysis.

Pathologic destruction of red cells may be initiated by abnormalities or infirmities intrinsic to the red cell or by hostile processes arising extrinsic to the red cell. Most hemolytic anemias stemming from intrinsic defects are hereditary, and virtually all forms of damage and destruction originating extrinsic to the red cell are acquired.

PRIMARY DEFECTS OF THE RED CELL MEMBRANE

Hereditary Spherocytosis

Hereditary spherocytosis (HS) is the most prevalent hereditary hemolytic anemia among people of Northern European descent. HS usually is transmitted by a single autosomal dominant gene and the lifelong hemolysis is of moderate severity, but in a minority of families transmission occurs via recessive inheritance, and homozygotes may have transfusion-dependent hemolytic anemia. The cardinal features of HS are: congenital hemolytic anemia with spherocytosis, variable elevations of indirect-reacting (nonglucuronide) bilirubin, splenomegaly, and invariable benefit from splenectomy.

HS Results from an Intrinsic Skeletal Defect

The molecular defects that cause HS have not been elucidated fully, but there is ample evidence that the cells are born with a slight native spheroidicity resulting from a deficit in surface area. The shortage of surface area relative to cell volume (S/V ratio) creates a slightly obese, rigidified structure having an elevated MCHC and lacking the suppleness necessary for traversal through the tight exits of the splenic cords; like fat people, fat red cells, however small, bend with difficulty. The shape change and inelasticity of HS cells are so slight that their circulation is unimpaired except through the demanding defiles of the spleen. Thus presence of the spleen is necessary for expression of this hereditary disorder, and extirpation of the spleen corrects hemolysis without correcting the intrinsic cellular defect (Figure 8-1).

HS can be caused by any of several closely related abnormalities that affect spectrin or interactions between spectrin and protein 4.1 or ankyrin; these defects, although similar, are heterogeneous.

Aberrations of spectrin and its associates   The hexagonal protein lattice that laminates the inner surface of the membrane and governs the shape and flexibility of red cells is formed by three articulated proteins: spectrin, protein 4.1, and actin, which are attached to the integral membrane linchpin, protein band 3, by ankyrin (see Chapter 4, Figures 4-10 and 4-11). Most forms of HS are associated with a spectrin deficit, the magnitude of which correlates with the severity of hemolysis and sphericity [1]. To distinguish HS variants in shorthand, a system of nomenclature has been proposed in which superscripts $^+$ and ^{0} indicate partial and complete deficiency, respectively. In the patients with deficient spectrin in whom the αI domain has been genetically shortened

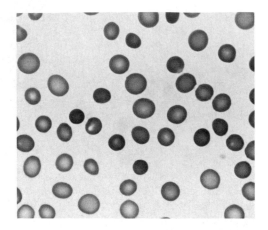

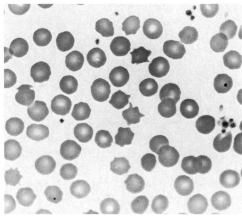

FIGURE 8-1

HS red cells before and after splenectomy. (Above) Before splenectomy many red cells are darkly condensed, smooth spherocytes, and the remainder are spheroidal, having diminished areas of central pallor. (Compare red cell sizes with that of the small lymphocyte nucleus.) (Below) After splenectomy red cells display more central pallor, but 10 to 20% of them resemble acanthocytes (spiculed cells). Note the black Howell-Jolly bodies, markers of the asplenic state, in several of the red cells. (Photo by CT Kapff.)

from 80,000 M_r to 74,000 M_r, the concise notation is abbreviated to Spα$^{I/74}$.

In the uncommon but deadly recessive variant of spectrin deficiency (HS [Sp$^+$]), spectrin levels range from 30 to 74% of normal, are inversely related to osmotic fragility (an accurate measure of surface/volume ratio) and are predictive of the efficacy of splenectomy. Pa-

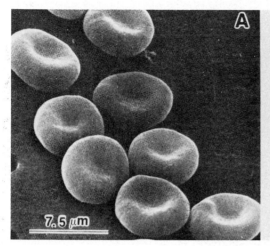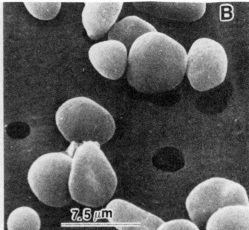

FIGURE 8-2

Scanning EMs of red cells on 3-μm-pore filters. (A) Normal-appearing red cells of patient's heterozygous mother. (B) Small (MCV: 74 fl), dense (MCHC: 39 g/dl), spherical cells of a patient homozygous for a defective α spectrin gene. (From Agre P et al: Deficient red-cell spectrin in severe, recessively inherited spherocytosis. Reprinted, by permission of the New England Journal of Medicine, 306:1155,1982.)

tients with spectrin levels above 70% achieve normal blood counts, just as do patients with "typical" dominant HS. Patients with spectrin levels between 40 and 70% have extreme microspherocytosis (Figure 8-2) [2] and respond imperfectly to splenectomy, displaying instead persisting compensated hemolysis. In homozygous recessive spectrin-deficient HS transmission has been linked to inheritance of a structural variant of the spectrin αII domain [3]; this implies a thalassemialike defect of the gene locus for α spectrin, which is located (along with that for protein 4.1) on chromosome 1.

In typical HS, representing almost 90% of all HS cases, the disease is the expression of a single dominant gene. Hemolysis is moderate or mild, but sufficient to cause splenomegaly, compensatory erythroid hyperplasia, and all the biochemical trappings of hemolytic disease. Reticulocyte levels range from 3 to 20%, haptoglobin is low or absent, and the MCHC usually exceeds the upper limit of normal (36 g/dl). Spectrin content of typical HS red cells is

about 80% of normal [3], making it uncertain that this deficiency is a primary expression of the disease. Furthermore the common form of HS has been associated with deletions and translocations involving the short arm of chromosome 8. In some kindred with moderately severe dominant HS, half of the β spectrin chains have a mutation localized to the βIV domain that inhibits vertical binding of spectrin to protein 4.1. In addition to causing uniform spherocytosis, this HS (Sp-4.1) mutation induces acanthocytosis involving 10% of the cells. Abnormalities or deficient synthesis of other skeletal proteins such as ankyrin [4] may unstabilize the cytoskeleton, thereby reducing spectrin inclusion in the assembly or leading to increased spectrin degradation. The various genetic flaws leading to HS cause loss of small but precious amounts of membrane surface.

Splenic conditioning and spherocytosis Shortage of surface area relative to cell volume, with loss of normal deformability, slows down the passage of HS red cells from the cordal to the sinus passages of the spleen. Each transit removes more surface and increases the likelihood of reentry of the ever-smaller, ever-denser "conditioned" cells into the narrow confines of the cordal compartment. About 2% of red cells entering the "red pulp" of the spleen pass into the vascular cords, which are partially collapsed discontinuous chambers interposed between the capacious sinuses through which most red cells pass unmolested. To escape the cords and

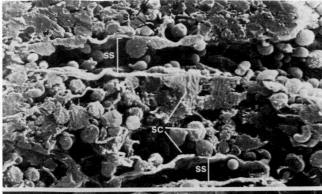

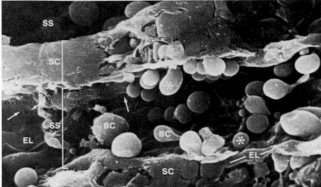

FIGURE 8-3

SEMs of cryofractured longitudinal
sections of splenic red pulp, exposing cakelike alternating compartments of the splenic sinuses (SS)
and splenic cords (SC) as seen at
low power (above) and higher
power (below). For blood cells (BC)
to migrate from cords to sinuses (below) they must squeeze through 2-
to 3-μm openings (arrows) between
the shingles of endothelial cells (EL)
lining the sinuses. Red cells lacking
the litheness required to negotiate
transmural passage are delayed (asterisks) or detained in the teeming
confines of the cords—exposed to
the tender mercies of macrophages,
the gendarmarie of cordal structures. Detention and packing within
splenic cords results in "erythrostasis" and stagnation. (From Tissues and Organs: A Text-Atlas of
Scanning Electron Microscopy. By
Richard Kessel and Randy Kardon.
Copyright © 1979 by WH Freeman
and Company. Reprinted by permission.)

return to the venous sinuses red cells must
squeeze through the intervening slitlike openings. HS cells are small but obese, and their
restricted membrane redundancy impedes this
tight passage, which is an exquisite test of cell
suppleness (Figure 8-3) [5]. Stasis in the cords
subjects metabolically hapless red cells to deficiency of glucose, low pH, O_2 free radicals
discharged by the cramped macrophages, and
piecemeal loss of the lipid bilayer [6]. Adding to
their peril, HS cells leak sodium inward at an
excessive rate, increasing the ATPase-driven
drain on ATP stores. On each excursion
through the cordal compartment more surface
membrane is sacrificed. Eventually—within an
estimated 30 to 40 cordal transits—the small,
unbending spherocyte dies in the crowded
crypts of the spleen.

Direct evidence that the spleen is both the
conditioner and graveyard of HS cells has been
obtained by comparing the osmotic fragility of
red cells secured simultaneously from the
bloodstream, the splenic vein, and the splenic
red pulp (Figure 8-4) [7]. These observations,
in which osmotic "fragility" is used to measure
the surface/volume ratio, indicate that HS cells

detained and conditioned in the spleen become
increasingly spherical, a transformation that
can be mimicked by incubating HS cells at
37°C in vitro.

Diagnosis and Management

Diagnosis of HS should be suspected in any
patient with chronic hemolytic anemia whose
blood smear exhibits numerous spherocytes.
Suspicion is enhanced by a family history of
anemia (particularly if "cured" by splenectomy), pigment gallstones, or unexplained jaundice. Diagnosis is validated by examining red
cells of family members and of the patient,
using the "incubation fragility" and "autohemolysis" tests.

Incubation fragility and autohemolysis tests
The hallmark of HS is spherocytosis. Spherocytes (having a diminished surface-to-volume
ratio) will burst in slightly hypo-osmolal
("hypotonic") solutions of NaCl. In mild or
typical HS the subpopulation of conditioned
cells may be quite minor; to elicit their inherent
defect, the cells are subjected to erythrostasis in

vitro. Normal red cells withstand sterile incubation comparatively well, as judged by the modest symmetric and sigmoidal leftward shift in osmotic fragility curves. In HS, the curve is slightly asymmetric before sterile incubation (Figure 8-4) and becomes markedly skewed to the left following incubation.

If HS cells are allowed to settle out, pack, and exhaust their supply of glucose and ATP, the cells both lose membrane lipid and shrink as their cation pumps fail; eventually (usually at about 30 h) the minimal S/A ratio—the "critical hemolytic volume"—is reached, and the cells lyse through the classic process of colloid osmotic hemolysis. In the 48-h autohemolysis test, HS cells hemolyze spontaneously unless fortified by addition of glucose, whereas normal red cells withstand the deprivation well. The 48-h autohemolysis test is a supportive but imperfect diagnostic test that is less specific than the incubation fragility test.

Splenectomy corrects anemia but not spherocytosis   In HS patients with moderate or severe hemolytic anemia splenectomy is imperative, for chronic hemolysis retards growth and vitality, transfusions create undesirable risks, and the patient faces the collective hazards of gallstones, cholecystitis, and the perennial peril of aplastic crisis. In mild cases splenectomy should be deferred to later childhood to avoid the risk of overwhelming sepsis that is an uncommon but catastrophic complication of the asplenic state. As fatal sepsis is caused by pneumococcal septicemia in over 60% of cases, polyvalent pneumococcal vaccine should be given all children prior to surgery, followed by prophylactic penicillin postoperatively. Benefit from splenectomy is lasting except in rare instances in which small accessory spleens were overlooked during surgery or splenic fragments escaped into the peritoneal cavity. Hemolytic relapse in such cases is usually mild and can be diagnosed by radionuclide scanning and corrected by removal of born-again splenic tissue.

Hereditary Elliptocytosis

Hereditary elliptocytosis (HE) constitutes a heterogeneous group of disorders of red cell skeletal components that confer in common an elliptical, sausage, or canoe shape to affected cells (Figure 8-5) [8]. HE is usually transmitted

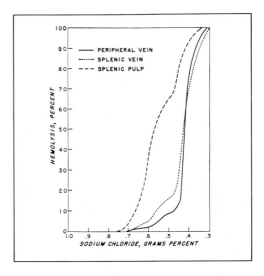

FIGURE 8-4

Influence of the spleen on the osmotic fragility (OF) of HS cells. Most HS cells are only slightly spheroidal, as judged by their OF, but a subpopulation of spheroidal cells are lysed at NaCl concentrations exceeding 0.50 g/dl, creating a bulge on the otherwise erect summation curve (uninterrupted line). Blood from the splenic vein contains about twice as many spheroidal cells (dotted line), and most cells eluted from incised splenic red pulp are very osmotically fragile, indicating sphericity. (From Jandl JH and Cooper RA: Chapt 58, in The Metabolic Basis of Inherited Disease, 4th ed., Stanbury JB et al, Eds. New York, McGraw-Hill Book Company, 1978.)

FIGURE 8-5

Scanning EM of a conventional HE cell, revealing the shape of a dugout canoe, with parallel sides and hemoglobin concentrated at the opposite poles. The form is elliptical, not oval, the venerable term "hereditary ovalocytosis" being a misnomer. (From Bessis M: Chapt 11, in Corpuscles. Atlas of Red Cell Shape. Berlin, Springer-Verlag, 1974.)

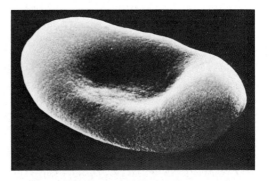

by a single (dominant) autosomal gene, but the molecular defect, the gene locus, and intensity of gene expression vary extensively among kindreds. Collectively, the incidence at birth of HE, all variants combined, is 400 per million. One of the common elliptocyte genes is linked closely to the Rh locus on the short arm of chromosome 1 (1p33), another for the protein 4.1 gene is at the terminus of the same region (1p32 → pter), and a third (1q24) is located on the long arm of chromosome 1 (near the Duffy blood group locus) amidst the region containing the α spectrin gene. Nine clinical variants of HE have been delineated, but these have been combined into three major categories on the grounds of clinical severity and red cell morphology: the typical (common) HE, and two uncommon variants—spherocytic elliptocytosis and stomatocytic elliptocytosis.

In the common form of HE, representing 85% of the total, affected individuals have little or no hemolytic anemia, hemolysis if present is usually compensated, and between 30 and 90% of red cells are elliptic or boat-shaped (Figure 8-6).

Pathophysiology of HE

HE cells do not acquire their elongated shape until they enter the circulation, indicating lateral skeletal instability and defective shape recovery when the cell is exposed to shear stress. The most common molecular defect underlying this instability is a defect in spectrin dimer (SpD) self-association. Normally 95% of spectrin extracted from red cells is in the tetrameric (SpT) conformation, but in most of the common HE variants up to one-third of the spectrin exists as free dimers. On a structural level the defects responsible for impaired SpD-SpD self-association are detected by limited tryptic digestion of spectrin, which cleaves the α and β chains into their subunit domains: αI through αV and βI through βIV. To date, three major variants of the αI domain of spectrin have been defined in HE in which this 80,000 M_r peptide has been variously truncated: Sp $\alpha^{I/74}$, Sp $\alpha^{I/46}$, and Sp $\alpha^{I/65}$. Truncation of the C-terminal end of the spectrin β chain (βI domain) ablates both the self-association and phosphorylation sites of that chain, resulting in a moderately severe form of HE.

Most patients deficient in protein 4.1 are simple heterozygotes lacking about 50% of the

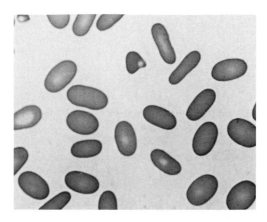

FIGURE 8-6

Red cell morphology in common HE associated with moderate hemolytic anemia. The marker cell is ellipsoidal with an axial ratio of over 2:1. Presence of cell fragments and microelliptocytes signifies ongoing hemolysis. (Photo by CT Kapff.)

protein and presenting with mild HE. The mutant gene has a DNA rearrangement upstream from the initiation codon for translation; the mRNA from the mutant locus is aberrantly spliced, leading to deficiency of protein 4.1. Protein 4.1 helps secure the skeleton to the membrane bilayer through its linkage to the integral protein, glycophorin. Patients homozygous for protein 4.1 deficiency suffer a severe transfusion-dependent hemolytic anemia, marked by pronounced spherocytic elliptocytosis and red cell budding.

Hereditary Pyropoikilocytosis (HPP)

HPP, a rare congenital hemolytic disorder once described as a distinct entity, is closely related to HE and shares with it the same molecular defects of spectrin, differing mainly in that over half the total spectrin is in the free dimer form and many mutant spectrin chains are shed from the cell. HPP red cells and their spectrin proteins are very sensitive to heating at 46°C. Many if not most cases of HPP are homozygous or doubly heterozygous for the same defects (e.g., Sp $\alpha^{I/74}$ and Sp $\alpha^{I/46}$) found in heterozygous form in HE, and homozygous common HE is indistinguishable morphologically from HPP (Figure 8-7). The severity of poikilocytosis is unmatched in any other hemolytic disease. Unlike HE, HPP cells are

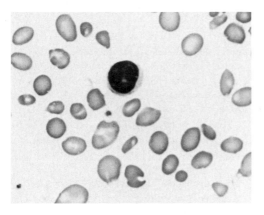

FIGURE 8-7

Mutilated red cell morphology in HPP. Virtually all cells are misshapen, with fragmented, spherical, and elliptical forms predominating. For sizing, compare red cells with lymphocyte nucleus (9 μm across). (Photo by CT Kapff.)

deficient in membrane and extremely microcytic, with MCV values ranging from 55 to 75 fl. The various complications of severe congenital hemolytic anemia become apparent early: growth impairment, deformities caused by expansion of erythroid marrow, and pig-

ment gallstones. The close association between HPP and HE is emphasized by the fact that, in some affected newborns, HPP transforms during the first year into common HE—a progression that precludes unequivocal diagnosis of HPP in early infancy.

Skeletal shape change versus skeletal fragmentation The "spectrin diseases" and analogous skeletal disorders vary from mild, when mutant spectrins lead only to skeletal destabilization, to severe, when instability is so severe that fragments are lost. In HE, mutations impairing spectrin chain self-assembly or interfering with "horizontal" connections with other skeletal members weaken the cytoskeleton and red cells become elongated by circulatory shear stress. In HPP the mutant spectrin chains actually bud off in marrow and in circulation, causing severe membrane instability, loss of both surface area and volume, and formation of micropoikilocytes. The less drastic "vertical" defect of HS cells results in vesicular oozing off of lipid bilayer, with formation of membrane-poor spherocytes [9]. These hypothetical generalizations are summarized in caricature in Figure 8-8 [4].

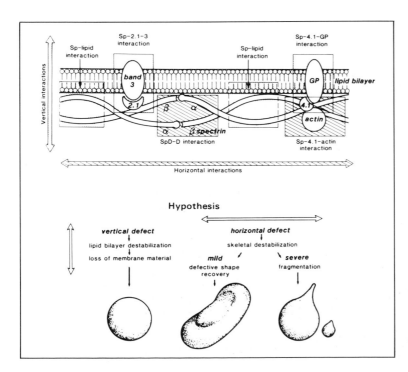

FIGURE 8-8

Pathogenesis of membrane lesions in HS, HE, and HPP. (From Palek J: Hereditary elliptocytosis, spherocytosis and related disorders: consequences of a deficiency or a mutation of membrane skeletal proteins. Blood Rev 1:147,1987.)

Management

Most individuals with HE are symptomless and require no therapeutic intervention. In severe HE, homozygous HE, and certified HPP, splenectomy is indicated. After splenectomy, anemia is either cured or alleviated, despite persistence or even exaggeration of the morphologic deformities.

Acanthocytosis and Spur Cell Anemia

Acanthocytes are dense contracted cells having numerous thorny spicules (Figure 8-9) [10]. They are prevalent in the blood of two very different disorders: abetalipoproteinemia and spur cell anemia. Abetalipoproteinemia is a rare derangement of apolipoprotein B synthesis and assembly by jejunal mucosa: this leads to severe reductions in all major plasma lipids and reverses the normal 1.2:1.0 lecithin:sphingomyelin ratio and increases the cholesterol:phospholipid (C:P) ratio of red cells entering the circulation. These lipid imbalances severely deform and slightly stiffen red cells, but membrane viscosity is not sufficient to impede capillary transit in vivo and there is little if any hemolysis. This is not the case with the look-alike acanthocytes associated with chronic hepatocellular disease.

Spur Cell Anemia

Some patients with severe chronic hepatocellular disease—usually alcoholic cirrhosis—acquire a rampant, usually fatal hemolytic anemia associated with splenomegaly and acanthocytosis. The acanthocytes resemble those of abetalipoproteinemia but the cells tend to be more spheroidal and the spicules are often sharper and shorter, hence the name spur cell anemia.

Pathophysiology   In 5 to 10% of patients with advanced alcoholic cirrhosis an abnormal high-density lipoprotein accumulates that is extremely rich in free (unesterified) cholesterol. In normal red cells the C:P molar ratio is about 1.0, but in spur cell anemia free cholesterol is loaded onto the cell membrane by exchange equilibrium, increasing the C:P ratio and proportionately expanding the surface area of the lipid bilayer. Mild increases in cholesterol and surface area (+10 to 20%) cause red cells to spread out and acquire a targetlike appearance as an artifact of drying; this deformity does not disturb rheologic properties of red cells and is seen as a reversible event in patients with biliary tract obstruction (Figure 8-10) [11]. In cirrhotic patients cholesterol overloading is extreme, with increases in the C:P ratio of 40 to 70%; the

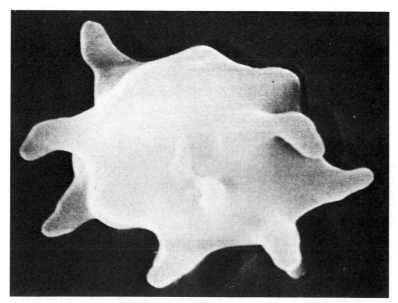

FIGURE 8-9

SEM view of an acanthocyte. The shape is that of a lumpy spheroid adorned with 8 or 10 tassels. (From Jandl JH: Chapt 7, in Blood: Textbook of Hematology. Boston, Little, Brown and Company, 1987.)

resulting redundancy of lipid bilayer exceeds the physical limits of the cytoskeletal framework, causing the surface to buckle, wrinkle, and eventually extend cholesterol-rich protrusions (Figure 8-11). Cholesterol is a stiff lipid, and the spiculated cholesterol-burdened cells are rudely remodeled during their trying passage through the spleen. The spicules are broken off, the cell is reduced to a prickly spherocyte, and eventually the spur cells, wounded by conditioning, are trapped and destroyed in the spleen. Spur cell anemia is a relentless hemolytic process, and the only recourse is splenectomy in those patients in whom the risks of abdominal surgery are deemed acceptable.

Paroxysmal Nocturnal Hemoglobinuria

Paroxysmal nocturnal hemoglobinuria (PNH) is an acquired clonal disorder of blood cell membranes, usually arising from a somatic mutation in the multipotential stem cell compartment occurring in the course of marrow hypoplasia. The PNH syndrome encompasses chronic intravascular hemolysis, pancytopenia, and recurrent thrombotic episodes. This uncommon but celebrated hemolytic syndrome is sometimes initiated by drug-induced marrow aplasia and occasionally terminates as acute myelogenous leukemia.

Pathophysiology: PNH Cells Have an Anchorage Problem

The salient cellular defect in PNH—an aberration that has inflamed the curiosity of legions of investigators—is their increased susceptibility to hemolytic complement. Blood cells of PNH are chimeric, comprising a mixture of cells normally insensitive to activated complement and an expanding clonal population of marrow and blood cells that are moderately to extremely sensitive to complement. The relative proportions of sensitive and insensitive cells varies from patient to patient, with good correlation between the proportion of mutant cells and severity of hemolysis. Intravascular hemolysis is mild when the proportion of sensitive cells is below 20%, it is episodic or sleep-related when 20 to 50% of red cells are hypersensitive, and higher proportions lead to perpetual hemoglobinuria and hemoglobine-

FIGURE 8-10

Target cells (codocytes) as viewed by SEM. In suspension these harmless cells are broader and flatter than normal and thus have diminished osmotic fragility: these are the parameters of a cell with an increased surface:volume ratio. During drying, hemoglobin aggregates; in these broad cells, islands of aggregate are left behind, usually centroidally, to create the gestalt of targeting. (From Bessis M: Chapt 9, in Corpuscles. Atlas of Red Cell Shape. Berlin: Springer-Verlag, 1974.)

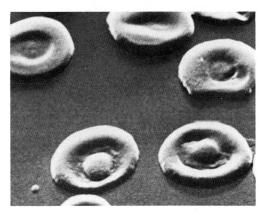

FIGURE 8-11

Red cell morphology in spur cell anemia. Nonspiculated cells are broad and show wavy contours. Most cells in this malign disorder are dark, wizened, and spheroidal; spicules are numerous, unevenly distributed, and often sharp. (Photo by CT Kapff.)

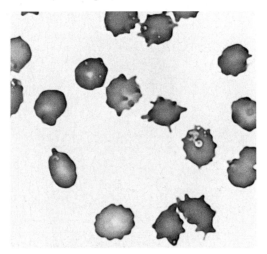

mia. Increased sensitivity to complement can be shown in vitro by activation through either the classic or alternative pathways, by lowering the pH or increasing Mg^{2+} levels, or by addition of cobra venom. Several proteins are missing from the membranes of red cells and other blood cells in PNH, only some of them predisposing to hemolysis. All of these deficiencies have been traced to a defective anchoring of proteins to membrane glycophospholipids containing phosphatidylinositol.

Complement-mediated lysis normally is inefficient when complement and target cells are from the same species: this "species restriction" is attributable to a protein that binds and inhibits C8, a penultimate actor in the terminal pore-forming complement cascade responsible for perforating and hemolyzing target cells. PNH cells are lacking in C8 binding protein (C8bp), making them vulnerable to the autologous membrane attack complex (C5–C9) of complement. PNH cells are also deficient in decay-accelerating factor (DAF), a 70,000 M_r membrane glycoprotein that inhibits C3 convertase formation, resulting in unrestrained amplification of midstage activation of the complement cascade. Absence of both defenses adequately explains the extreme sensitivity of PNH red cells to the low-level quotidian activation of complement.

Lack of C8bp may also explain the enhanced stimulation of platelets and thrombotic complications that assail PNH patients [12]. In addition, however, the clonal population of PNH cells is deficient in acetylcholinesterase, a harmless anomaly, and affected neutrophils exhibit low levels of leukocyte alkaline phosphatase, without untoward effect. The basis for this galaxy of anomalies, explanatory and meaningless alike, is that all of these proteins are anchored within cell membranes to glycophospholipid-containing phosphatidylinositol (PI). The underlying defect in PNH cells of all kinds—red cells, granulocytes, platelets, and

FIGURE 8-12

Association of hemoglobinemia with sleep regardless of time of day in a patient with PNH. Note hemoglobinemia was deferred to daytime when the patient was kept awake 27 h. Association of hemolysis with sleep is attributed to physiologic lowering of pH. (From Ham TH: Studies on destruction of red blood cells. I. Chronic hemolytic anemia with paroxysmal nocturnal hemoglobinuria: investigation of the mechanism of hemolysis, with observations on 5 cases. Arch Intern Med 64:1271,1939. Copyright 1939, American Medical Association.)

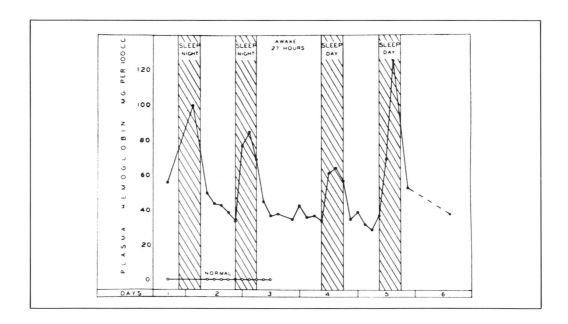

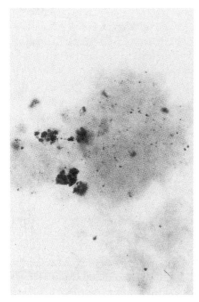
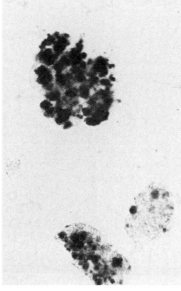

FIGURE 8-13

Renal tubular cells laden with hemosiderin and ferritin in urine of a patient with PNH. Prussian blue–positive material is seen at low power in urinary sediment (left) and (at higher power) in individual renal tubular cells (right). (From Hoffbrand AV and Pettit JE: Chapt 4, in Clinical Hematology Illustrated. An Integrated Text and Color Atlas. London, Gower Medical Publishing Ltd.,1987.)

certain subsets of lymphocytes—is defective tethering of these (and possibly other) proteins to membrane PI [13].

Description and Management

Red cells of PNH are unique in that their defect is intrinsic but acquired, and the cells usually appear normal microscopically. This is the only severe hemolytic disorder in which spherocytes are absent. Diagnosis is most simply established by use of the sucrose hemolysis test, but a more definitive (and painstaking) method is the Ham acid-serum test. Clinical evolution is very gradual, and recognition of the disease is often delayed by the confusing prelude of erythroid hypoplasia. A classic circadian pattern of nocturnal (or sleep-associated) hemoglobinuria occurs in only one-quarter of patients, but the finding of red urine on awakening and the association of hemoglobinemia with sleep are incriminating (Figure 8-12) [14]. In severe PNH, haptoglobin and hemopexin are chronically depleted, and the only "renal threshold" is provided by renal tubular degradation of filtered hemoglobin. If plasma levels of hemoglobin exceed about 30 mg/dl in haptoglobin-depleted patients, hemoglobin is spilled into the urine. This may be visibly evident only episodically, but hemosiderinuria is perpetual due to excessive sloughing of iron-laden cells from the proximal tubules (Figure 8-13) [15]. Patients with longstanding hemoglobinuria suffer renal functional impairment, and some PNH patients eventually die of slowly progressive uremia and interstitial nephritis.

Among other complications are iron deficiency resulting from loss of hemoglobin iron (up to 20 mg daily) into urine, and pyogenic infections, which are responsible for about 10% of fatalities. PNH patients are predisposed to intravascular thrombosis, presumably due to the platelet activation by complement noted earlier. Fatal thromboses generally involve the portal circulation, the hepatic vein, or the venous circulation of the brain.

Intravascular hemolysis is commonly severe enough to require a maintenance transfusion. In some patients transfusion requirements can be minimized by alternate-day prednisone, and androgens should be given a trial. Actual or impending thrombotic occlusions may benefit from the combination of anticoagulation, fibrinolytic agents, and prednisone therapy, although results are uneven. Patients with severe, established PNH should be considered for marrow transplantation, particularly if HLA-identical sibling donors are available to help out victims of this deadly but nonfamilial disease.

SECONDARY DEFECTS OF THE RED CELL MEMBRANE

During the 2 to 3 miles of daily commuting to the regional vasculature, red cells are cushioned from abrasion and collision by slipping into the axial stream and forming trains of rouleaux. Turbulence in the arterial vasculature leads to head-on collisions, and roughening, rigidification, or impedance in the microcirculation may scrape off pieces of membrane or fracture the cytoskeleton. Hemolytic anemias caused by turbulence, abrasion, and cleavage are known collectively as "red cell fragmentation syndromes."

Macroangiopathic Hemolytic Anemias

The most uncomplicated and stark example of fragmentation hemolysis occurs in long-distance runners who stomp forcefully and repetitiously on hard surfaces ("runner's hemolysis" or "march hemoglobinuria"). Transient hemoglobinemia and hemoglobinuria are common in marathon runners and devotees of karate, conga drumming, and other percussive activities because of violence done to red cells in vessels perfusing the points of impact. Macroangiopathic hemolytic anemia may be chronic and severe in patients equipped with an aortic valve prosthesis. Mild hemolytic anemia sometimes occurs in individuals with severe calcific aortic stenosis, but only if the pressure gradient across the valve exceeds about 50 mm Hg. Red cell fragmentation, with appearance in the blood of schistocytes—a mixture of cleaved cell fragments and helmetlike or bib-shaped cells—can become a serious problem during resumption of physical activity following insertion of an aortic prosthesis. Mechanical hemolysis of life-threatening magnitude may result from a tear in the moorings of prostheses of either aortic or mitral valves, for the pounding by regurgitant jets with each heartbeat is sufficient to rupture red cell membranes. Direct hemodynamic hammering explains the severe hemolysis commonly observed in early-model prostheses, but shearing forces at the roughened blood-plastic interfaces account for most of the fragmentation observed with more refined devices; indeed, absent regurgitation, hemolysis has been observed to cease once the artificial surface is covered over by endothelium. In addition to replacing faulty regurgitant valves, supplemental iron should be given to restore that lost through urinary excretion of hemosiderin and hemoglobin.

Microangiopathic Hemolytic Anemias

Collectively, microangiopathic hemolytic anemias are among the most common of hemolytic disorders. Microangiopathy—disruption or denudation of the nonthrombogenic endothelium of the microvasculature—exposes perfusing blood cells to the sticky procoagulants of the subendothelium, triggering local or disseminated intravascular deposition of fibrin. Disseminated intravascular coagulation (DIC), with plating of the vasculature with fibrin deposits, release of anticoagulant "split" products of fibrin, and consumption of platelets and certain coagulation factors, is a feared and often final complication of many common disorders, plus several rare ones. The imminent prospect of DIC menaces patients with infection, obstetric disorders, hypertension, disseminated carcinoma, and an assortment of immunologic vascular diseases (Chapter 24).

Pathophysiology

The hallmarks of microangiopathic hemolytic anemias caused by DIC are appearance of fibrin degradation (split) products in high titer, hemolytic anemia, and red cell fragmentation deformities (Figure 8-14). During intravascular coagulation red cells hurtling through vessels coated and crisscrossed by fibrin strands may adhere to and become draped over transverse fibrils; some cells slip their noose, others are garroted (Figure 8-15) [16]. When hung clothesline-fashion over a fibrin strand, red cells usually slump one way or the other before they are cleaved along the axis of suspension: the two unequal products of cleavage are half-spheroids (helmet forms) and kite-shaped fragments, both of which may survive several days in the circulation.

Microangiopathic hemolytic anemia generally occurs as a complication of an obvious and dangerous disease, such as gram-negative septicemia, malignant hypertension, and disseminated hematogenous carcinoma. A syndrome of microangiopathic hemolytic anemia, intravas-

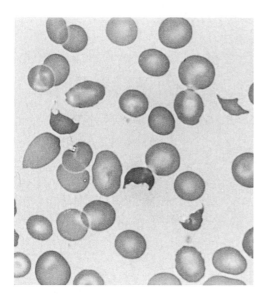

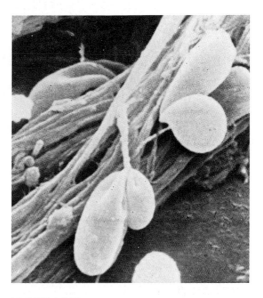

FIGURE 8-14

Red cell deformities in a patient with sepsis, shock, and DIC. The helmet-shaped and fragmentation deformities are emblematic of microangiopathic hemolytic anemia. (Photo by CT Kapff.)

FIGURE 8-15

Scanning EM of red cells suspended by filaments of fibrin during intravascular coagulation. (By permission, from Bull BS and Kuhn IN: The production of schistocytes by fibrin strands [a scanning electron microscope study]. Blood 35:104,1970.)

cular thromboses, renal impairment, and pulmonary edema is especially common in mucin-producing adenocarcinomas of stomach, colon, lung, or breast treated with mitomycin C or bleomycin [17]. A more stealthy but equally deadly microangiopathic syndrome afflicts women with severe preeclampsia. A minor amount of defibrination accompanies normal delivery, but in patients with preeclampsia or eclampsia, lingering defibrination may ignite suddenly into an acute DIC that threatens the survival of both mother and unborn child and too often goes undiagnosed. When the patient presents with hemolysis, elevated liver enzymes, and low platelets (the "HELLP syndrome"), immediate exchange transfusion and induced delivery are imperative [18].

The first clues to onset of diffuse thrombotic microangiopathy and fragmentation hemolysis are a rapid unexplained fall in hematocrit, reduction in haptoglobin levels, hemoglobinuria, purpura, and adult respiratory distress syndrome. Several variants or facsimiles of microangiopathic hemolytic anemia warrant separate consideration because of singular differences in pathogenesis and clinical expression. Among these are thrombotic thrombocytopenic purpura and hemolytic uremic syndrome.

Thrombotic thrombocytopenic purpura (TTP)
TTP or Moschcowitz syndrome, is an arcane, fickle, and complex disorder of young adults. The cardinal features of this uncommon, remittent, but often fatal disorder are severe microangiopathic hemolytic anemia, thrombocytopenic purpura, fluctuating central nervous system crises, fever, and renal failure. This frightening syndrome commences with petechiae, bleeding, and bizarre, fleeting cerebral malfunctions. It appears to be initiated by immunologically mediated damage to endothelium, with release of endothelial secretory products that clump platelets and generate emboli composed of platelet-fibrin aggregates. The resulting intravascular platelet consump-

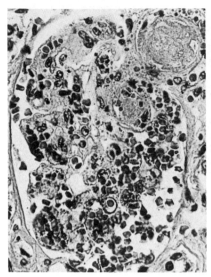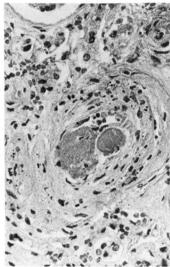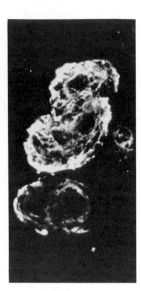

FIGURE 8-16

Renal vascular thrombosis and necrosis in HUS. (Left) Necrosis and thrombosis of an afferent arteriole and thickening of the glomerular endothelium, with extravasation of red cells into Bowman's space. (Middle) Thrombosed small renal artery with necrosis and red cell fragments in the vessel wall. (Right) Direct immunofluorescent staining revealing circumferential deposits of IgM in the arteriolar walls. These vessels also stained (not shown) for C1q and C3. (From Brown RS and Marion A: An 83-year-old woman with anemia, oliguric renal failure, and past lymphoma. Case records of the Massachusetts General Hospital, case 16-1988. Reprinted, by permission of the New England Journal of Medicine, 318:1047,1988.)

tion is responsible for bleeding, and soft platelet-fibrin emboli plug vessels in the brain, kidney, and marrow. In a patient with unexplained thrombocytopenic purpura, the added findings of numerous spherocytes, schistocytes, and erythroblasts in the blood virtually clinches the diagnosis. DIC is not essential to the pathogenesis of this syndrome, and from ignorance of causation, no fail-safe therapy has been devised. Best and most immediate, but seldom permanent, results are obtained by a program of plasma exchange.

Hemolytic uremic syndrome   Hemolytic uremic syndrome (HUS) is a TTP-like immunologic

disorder of vascular endothelium that is largely localized to renal arteries and glomeruli. Vascular damage is provoked by a variety of microorganisms and antigens. In the "classic" HUS afflicting infants in summertime epidemics, infection by strains of *Escherichia coli* that produce a fecal cytotoxin (verotoxin) causes bloody diarrhea followed in the convalescent phase by accretion of platelets mixed with fibrin in renal glomeruli; the glomerular process is evanescent and full recovery is the rule. In children and adults, HUS also occurs as a postinfective process, but the antibody-inciting organisms are streptococci, staphylococci, and various enteric pathogens. Antibody-directed, cell-mediated damage to vascular endothelium causes injurious deposition of immune complexes, fibrin, platelets, and neutrophils in the arteries and arterioles, as well as in glomeruli. Fibrin deposition in the subendothelium with microthrombi in glomerular capillaries and arterioles lead to focal or confluent cortical necrosis, with hypertension and a poor prognosis (Figure 8-16) [19].

Giant hemangioma   Microangiopathic hemolytic anemia, thrombocytopenia, and focal DIC often complicate massive proliferative hemangiomas (Kasabach-Merritt syndrome). Red cell fragmentation, platelet consumption, and activation of procoagulants take place within the angioma. If the vascular tumor is superficial it should be resected; localized intratumoral consumption of platelets and coagulation factors in deep unresectable hemangiomas can be halted by infusions of cryoprecipitate and the protease inhibitor, epsilon-aminocaproic acid (EACA).

IMMUNOHEMOLYTIC ANEMIAS

In immunohemolytic anemias, red cell destruction may be caused by alloantibodies (isoantibodies) or autoantibodies. Alloantibodies, which cause hemolysis only as a result of transfusion or transfer across the placenta, are conventional antibodies specific for "foreign" antigens on incompatible cells. Autoantibodies are generally nonspecific and often represent a case of mistaken identity, an immunologic error provoked either by alteration of self-antigens by extrinsic agents or by genetic or acquired derangements of immunologic recognition. Autoimmune hemolytic anemias (AHA) have been associated with impaired T cell suppressor activity, immune deficiency syndromes, thymic disorders, various lymphoproliferative disorders, hapten-inspired or hapten-dependent (drug-induced) antibodies, and global autoimmune disorders such as systemic lupus erythematosus. However inspirational these associations may be, there is remarkably little mechanistic understanding of why self-toleration breaks down in AHA or why the ubiquitous red cell is so often selected as the target. At present the term autoimmune hemolytic anemias should be used for convenience and with suspicion.

Pathophysiology of Immune Hemolysis

Immune hemolysis is initiated by attachment of antibodies to the red cell surface. Subsequent events are determined by the class of antibody and the density and distribution of surface antigens. If the antibody is of the IgM class, of which anti-A antibodies are exemplary, destruction is caused by agglutination or by activation of serum complement. If anti-

body is of the IgG class, of which Rh antibodies are the prototype, destruction is mediated by binding of the Fc portion of cell-bound IgG molecules by macrophages residing in sinuses of the spleen and liver. The function of macrophages is facilitated enormously by their residence in sinus endothelial structures, a cellular collaboration popularly recognized by the vague but useful term, RES ("reticuloendothelial system").

Hemolysis by IgM Antibodies

IgM antibodies (M_r: 850,000) are composed of five identical subunits, each consisting of two μ (heavy) chains and two κ or λ (light) chains, that are assembled in a starfish configuration. The large, flexible IgM pentamers can easily bridge the 20- to 30-nm gap separating circulating red cells and hence are capable of agglutinating red cells by forming a lattice, causing the cells to lodge in the systemic circulation or be trapped by the RES. Because IgM antibodies dissociate from antigen rapidly at body temperature, agglutination is minimal except in chilled regions of the circulation, but as these large pentamers skip about from cell to cell in the warm regions they are capable individually of activating the complement cascade. The 155,000 M_r (7S) IgG molecules of the IgG1 and IgG3 subclasses can also activate the first component (C1) of the complement pathway (Figure 8-17)[20], but two or more closely positioned 7S molecules are required (Figure 8-18) [20].

Complement-mediated hemolysis Complement can be activated beginning at C1 by antibody-coated targets or antibody-antigen complexes (the classical pathway) or beginning at C3 by certain polysaccharides and lipopolysaccharides such as zymosan and endotoxin (the alternative pathway). In antibody-mediated hemolysis of red cells, the first of the 11 components of the classical pathway, C1q, functions as the complement recognition unit for the Fc portion of antibodies attached to the cell membrane. C1q, a bouquet-shaped, collagenlike molecule travelling as a complex with the proenzymes C1r and C1s, senses immobilized Fc fragments and in making contact acti-

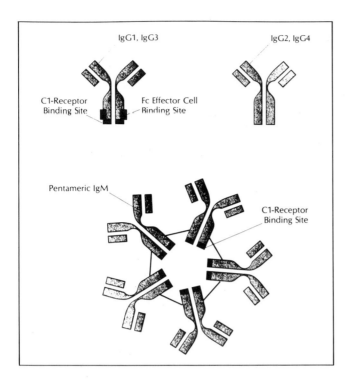

FIGURE 8-17

Immunoglobulin classes and subclasses determine the kind of effector mechanism brought into play in immune hemolysis. IgG1 and IgG3 subclass antibodies possess Fc binding sites that promote phagocytosis and terminal binding sites that initiate complement activation. IgG2 binds only weakly, and IgG4 molecules lack this capability. Pentameric IgM antibodies possess multiple binding sites for C1 and are highly efficient in initiating complement-mediated lysis. (From Rosse WF: Autoimmune hemolytic anemia. Hosp Pract 20(8):105, 1985.)

FIGURE 8-18

(A) Rh antigens (and most antigens involved in AHA) are spaced too far apart to be bridged by the initial recognition protein (CIq) of the complement pathway. The IgG anti-Rh antibody binds to antigen at its Fab end with high affinity, causing the Fc portion to extend outward where it is available to the Fc receptors on macrophage surfaces. (B) In contrast, a single IgM antibody to an ABO antigen fixes C1 promptly, for it has multiple C1 binding sites and the antigens are deployed in closely packed patches. (From Rosse WF: Autoimmune hemolytic anemia. Hosp Pract 20(8):105, 1985.)

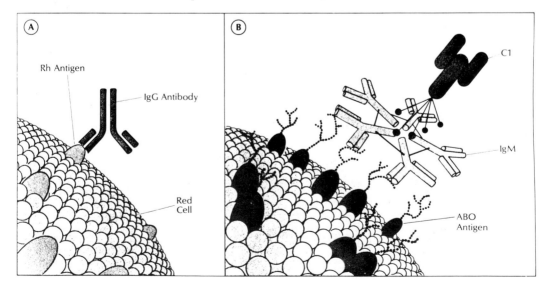

vates C4 and C2 through limited proteolysis (Figure 8-19) [21]. C4,2 convertase complex generates C3 in a crucial amplification step that liberates split products of C3, including a major fragment, C3b, that adheres to neighboring areas of the membrane. C3b launches the explosive terminal C5–C9 membrane attack complex of the cascade, eventuating in the insertion of C5b6789 complexes into the lipid bilayer and creation thereby of discrete membrane pores 10 nm across—twice the diameter of hemoglobin (Figure 8-20) [22]. If complement activation proceeds unhindered to completion the perforated red cell exsanguinates.

Complement is governed by a system of checks and balances The cytolytic potential of the complement cascade is tightly controlled by a system of antagonists that operate at different stages of activation: activated C1 is stymied by C1 esterase inhibitor; C4,2 convertase is degraded by DAF; C3b is cleaved to an inactive form (iC3b) by factors H and I plus the C3b receptor (CR1); and C8 is balked by C8bp. Coating of red cells with functionless C3d, a

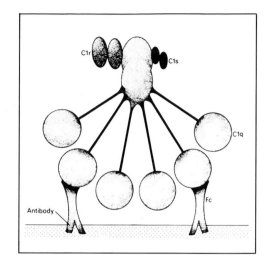

FIGURE 8-19

Each of the six spherical subunits of C1q possesses a binding site for the Fc portion of antibody molecules (an IgG doublet is illustrated). Once contact is made, C1r and then C1s are proteolytically activated; C1s, an esterase, generates the C4,2 complex, the convertase for C3. (From Petz LD and Garraty G: Chapt 3, in Acquired Immune Hemolytic Anemias. New York, Churchill Livingstone,1980.)

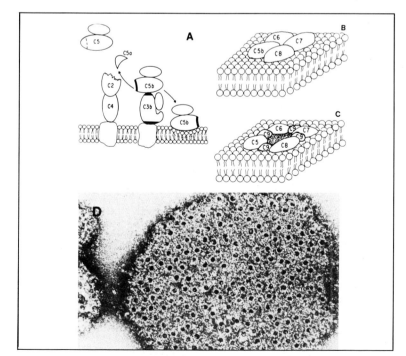

FIGURE 8-20

Terminal steps of hemolysis by complement. (A) Activation of C5 by classic pathway components. (B) Embedding of C5–C8 complexes into the outer lamina of the bilayer. (C) Formation of lytic pore by insertion of C9. (D) Honeycombed ruins of a red cell punctured by multiple membrane attack complexes, as seen by EM after negative staining. (From Rosse WF: Interaction of complement with the red-cell membrane. Semin Hematol 16:128, 1979.)

split product of C3b, blocks antigenic determinants and protects the cells against further encounters with antibody and complement. This firm C3d coating—not the potent but fleeting IgM antibodies—accounts for agglutination by anticomplement Coombs sera of red cells from patients with cold-active IgM antibodies.

Hemolysis by IgG Antibodies

Destruction of red cells by IgG antibodies is an orderly process in which the caprices of complement are circumvented, red cells being cleared from circulation by macrophages of the RES. Clearance is by first-order kinetics and occurs preferentially in the sinuses of the spleen, secondarily in the hepatic sinuses, and to a small extent if at all in the marrow.

Fc receptor–mediated immune hemolysis The surfaces of macrophages ensconced in the spleen and liver sinuses are studded with receptors (about 10^6 per cell) having high affinity for the Fc portions of IgG1, IgG3, and (to a lesser extent) IgG2 antibodies. Fc gamma receptors (FcγRs) bind avidly to a region of IgG molecules near the carboxy terminal (tail) ends, which

project like prongs when the forked hypervariable (head) ends of antibodies are attached to red cell surface antigens (Figures 8-17 and 8-18). As IgG-coated red cells glide past lurking macrophages the Fc projections lock on to the macrophage receptors, causing the apposed cell membranes to adhere in patches, and then, by a "Velcro" effect, to fuse together (Figure 8-21) [23]. Macrophage binding of IgG-coated red cells can be inhibited and even reversed by high concentrations of free IgG, particularly if aggregated so as to immobilize the Fc regions. During their initial intimate attachment to macrophages, antibody-coated red cells rapidly become spherical (osmotically fragile) and their membranes submit to softening and exploration by busy probing fingers that emerge like serpents from the macrophage surface; if at this moment the macrophage releases its quarry, the red cell escapes to the circulation as an umbilicated spherocyte. Macrophages are capable of grasping numerous IgG-coated red cells at one time, forming rosettes in which ensnared red cells are the petals. Even the gluttonous macrophage has its physical limits, being constrained by the surface area necessary for enveloping its prey. In most immunohemolytic ane-

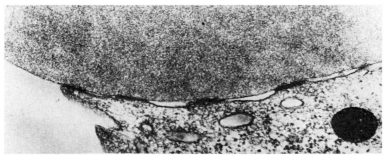
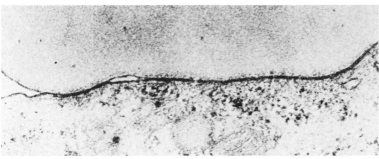

FIGURE 8-21

EM views of early steps in the binding of an antibody-coated red cell to a macrophage. (Above) The intact red cell (above) is bound at evenly spaced points of fusion, representing Fc receptor–IgG linkages. (Below) Apparent trilaminar merging of the external leaflets of the two cells. (From Jandl JH: Chapt 9, in Blood: Textbook of Hematology. Boston, Little, Brown and Company, 1987.)

mias, the number of antibody-coated red cells greatly exceeds the capacity of the burgeoning macrophage population to bind and ingest. Consequently, a steady state is reached, during which many red cells are altered beyond repair or are actually phagocytized, but even more are regurgitated temporarily into the bloodstream as spherocytes.

During immune hemolysis in vivo most antibody-sensitized red cells are destroyed piecemeal on the surfaces of heavily engaged macrophages, which simultaneously imprison or nibble off portions of trapped cells within an arborizing network of thin branching processes. Antibody-coated cells that encounter an unengaged macrophage one-on-one are swallowed whole without nice preliminaries; afterward the hemoglobin is oxidatively precipitated and degraded within the phagosome, hemoglobin iron is relinquished to transferrin, and dismantled components of the phagosome diffuse back to the macrophage surface for reconstitution of membrane structure. The callous efficiency with which a macrophage can devour a single antibody-garnished red cell is portrayed in Figure 8-22 [24]. Fc receptors of mononuclear cells are primarily responsible for the orderly clearance of IgG-coated red cells from circulation, but the attachment process may be strengthened and hastened by synergistic participation of receptors for C3b and C3d. In immunohemolytic disorders caused by warm-active IgG autoantibodies, red cells display C3 as well as IgG coating in roughly half of cases.

The Coombs Test

Diagnosis of immunohemolytic processes requires demonstration that immunoglobulins or complement components (or both) are attached to the patient's red cells. This is achieved by an immunologic trick in which heterologous (animal) antibodies to human immunoglobulins are employed to bridge together cells coated with antibodies or other proteins having too small a reach to agglutinate cells directly, as do cell-spanning IgM antibodies; this "antiglobulin" strategem is known as the Coombs test. In the direct Coombs test (direct antiglobulin test, or DAT), the patient's red cells are washed free of plasma and then exposed to antibodies pre-

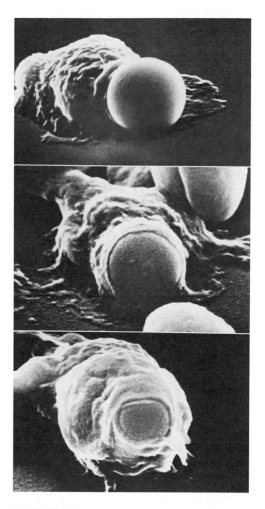

FIGURE 8-22

SEMs arranged to depict the process of erythrophagocytosis. (Top) By Fc receptor–mediated attachments the macrophage cups its prey, drawing in surface membrane. (Middle) A thin veil of cytoplasm creeps over the doomed cell, and (bottom) envelopment advances toward completion. An undisturbed macrophage is capable of gulping down an intact antibody-coated red cell within 1 to 2 minutes. (From Bessis M: Chapt 16, in Corpuscles. Atlas of Red Cell Shape. Berlin, Springer-Verlag, 1974.)

pared by immunizing animals against human serum or preferably against purified human immunoglobulins, Fc fragments, or complement components C3 and C4. The resultant antisera are pasteurized, and irrelevant anti-

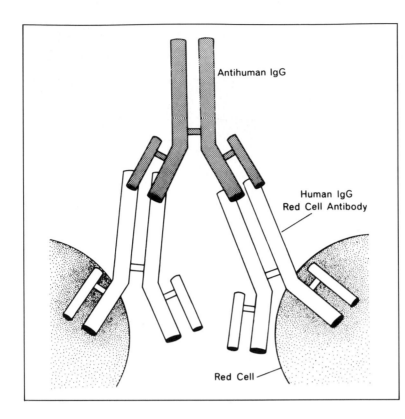

Antihuman IgG

Human IgG
Red Cell Antibody

Red Cell

FIGURE 8-23

The Coombs
(antiglobulin) test.
Neighboring red cells
coated with nonagglu-
tinating IgG are aggluti-
nated by heterologous
antibody to human IgG.
The cells are cross-
linked by antihuman
IgG bridges between the
protruding Fc portions
of heavy chains. Anti-
bodies monospecific for
the Fc fragments of
heavy chains can be
used to distinguish the
class and subclass of
bound antibody. (From
Petz LD and Garraty G:
Acquired Immune
Hemolytic Anemias.
New York, Churchill
Livingstone, Inc.,
1980.)

bodies are absorbed out by incubation with large volumes of washed normal human red cells; alternatively monoclonal antibodies may be employed. Either strategem yields a monospecific reagent that causes a lattice-structured agglutination of antibody-coated red cells (Figure 8-23) [25]. Agglutination can be hastened by mild centrifugal packing ("spin Coombs test") or expeditiously enhanced by combined use of PVP-augmentation and use of an autoanalyzer: the PVP-augmented Coombs test can detect attachment of as few as 8 to 10 IgG molecules per red cell—a 50-fold improvement over routine manual Coombs tests.

Indirect Coombs test   The indirect Coombs test detects antibodies in plasma unattached to red cells. In immunohemolytic anemias this is an operational backup test indicative of dissociation of surplus or weakly avid antibodies. Antibody in plasma in absence of antibody attached to red cells indicates that the antibody is an alloantibody, not an autoantibody.

Autoantibodies, alloantibodies, and typing of Coombs-positive cells   The autoantibodies in plasma or eluates from red cells of patients with immunohemolytic anemias usually react with all normal red cells, creating difficulties in using the Coombs test for crossmatching potential donor blood. Usually transfused normal red cells that are compatible at the ABO and Rh loci fare no worse than the patient's cells, despite acquiring a coating of autoantibody. The most important consideration in selecting donor blood is the detection of alloantibodies in a setting where the patient's autoantibody reacts with all donor cells. Several procedures are available for identifying serum alloantibodies reactive with minor blood group determinants of donor cells and for determining the phenotype of the patient's Coombs-positive red cells. The most direct method for distinguishing alloantibodies from free antibody is the differential absorption technique. Apart from an inexcusable ABO mismatch, most hemolytic transfusion reactions are caused by alloantibodies to

TABLE 8-1

Use of differential absorption of anti-Jk^a serum to determine blood type in a patient with a positive Coombs test

Red cells used to absorb anti-Jk^a typing serum	Dilutions of absorbed anti-Jk^a tested against Jk (a+b+) red cells						
	1	2	4	8	16	32	Score
Jk(a+b+)	2+	1+	1+	1/2+	0	0	16
Jk(a+b−)	1+	1+	0	0	0	0	8
Jk(a−b+)	3+	3+	2+	2+	1+	0	32
Patient's	2+	1+	0	0	0	0	10*

*These results indicate that the patient is Jk(a+).

Source: From Petz LD and Garratty G: Chapt 5, in Acquired Immune Hemolytic Anemias. New York, Churchill Livingstone, 1980.

Rh, Kell, Kidd, and Duffy (Fy^a) blood group antigens. If in-saline Rh typing antibodies are available, the screening panel for differential absorption need only contain test cells negative for Kell, Kidd, and Fy^a determinants. The antigen makeup of the patient's Coombs-positive red cells also can be determined by differential absorption. For example, if the patient's red cells contain the antigen Jk^a of the Kidd blood group system, the cells will absorb antibody from anti-Jk^a typing serum, lowering the titer; heterozygous cells (Jk[a+b+]) will absorb less antibody than homozygous cells (Jk[a+b−]) and Jk[a−b+] cells will absorb none (Table 8-1) [25].

Description of Autoimmune Hemolytic Anemias (AHA)

Classification of AHAs can be based on the nature of causative antibodies and on whether autoimmunity is idiopathic or secondary to disease or medication. The most practical distinction is between cold-active (usually IgM) antibodies and warm-active (usually IgG) antibodies that are most damaging at body temperature (Table 8-2) [23].

TABLE 8-2

Autoimmune hemolytic anemias

Cold-active antibodies
  Primary (idiopathic) cold agglutinin disease
  Secondary cold agglutinin disease
    Infections
      Mycoplasma pneumonia
      Infectious mononucleosis
      Other
    Paroxysmal cold hemoglobinuria
    Lymphoproliferative disorders
Warm-active antibodies
  Primary (idiopathic) immunohemolytic anemia
  Secondary immunohemolytic anemias
    Lymphoproliferative disorders
    Nonlymphatic neoplasms
    Connective tissue disorders
    Infections
    Drug-induced immunohemolytic anemias
      Hapten type
      α-Methyldopa type

Source: From Jandl JH: Chapt 9, in Blood: Textbook of Hematology. Boston, Little, Brown and Company, 1987.

AHA Caused by Cold-Active Antibodies

About 95% of cold-active IgM autoantibodies are specific for the I antigen. Nearly all adults are I-positive and yet normal plasma contains low concentrations of cold-active anti-I. Auto-agglutination and autohemolysis are forfended by a thermal barrier. Pathologic anti-I causing cold agglutinin disease with or without hemolytic anemia most often occurs during convalescence from infection by *Mycoplasma pneumoniae;* immunologic specificity is identical to normal anti-I, but antibody occurs in higher concentrations and has a broader thermal range. Unlike polyclonal elevations in response to infection, cold agglutinins responsible for primary cold agglutinin disease or associated with aberrant B cell clones in lymphoproliferative disorders are monoclonal IgMκ, and specificity may be directed against I, i, P, Pr, or rarely ABO or Rh antigens. High titers of cold agglutinins activate complement but hemolysis is highly variable, for the complement sequence is interrupted when red cells coated with C3 in the cool acrocyanotic regions of the peripheral circulation return to the warm central regions. As the warmed IgM rapidly dissociates, C3b is inactivated, and degradation products of C3b bind to glycophorin A with increased efficiency, terminating the cascade. Avoidance of cold exposure is fundamental to management of this malady; this can be accomplished by use of homely deterrents such as long underwear and ear-muffs, temporary donning of an "environmental suit" (cost: $650), or oft-welcome advice to seek a balmier climate (cost: rapidly increasing). Cold agglutinin disease caused by malignant clonal populations of B cells in lymphoproliferative diseases requires chemotherapeutic control.

AHA Caused by Warm-Active Antibodies

AHAs associated with warm-active antibodies are idiopathic in roughly 55% of patients; they are drug-induced in about 20%, associated with lymphoproliferative disorders in 15%, and secondary to miscellaneous other immune or infectious disorders in 10%.

Description   Fulminant onset is typical of idiopathic, drug-induced, or postinfection forms of AHA, whereas immunohemolysis secondary to lymphoreticular malignancies or SLE is more gradual and often indolent. In nearly 90% of AHA patients, red cells are coated with IgG (accompanied by variable amounts of inactivated C3 in about half of cases), and in two-thirds of cases the antibody subclass is IgG1. Usually hemolysis occurs when 100 to 200 or more molecules of IgG attach to the red cell surface, but as few as 10 to 20 molecules of IgG3 suffice to initiate cell clearance. When the process is explosive or massive, both liver and spleen participate in Fc receptor–mediated cell removal, and some heme pigments (hemoglobin, methemoglobin, and methemalbumin) may appear in the plasma. Splenomegaly almost always develops within a few days or weeks of onset, and a precarious balance may be achieved within 2 to 3 weeks between the hemolytic efficiency of the hyperplastic spleen and the amplified erythropoietic activity of the hyperplastic marrow. In a typical patient with severe AHA, blood hemoglobin falls to about 5 to 7 g/dl, reticulocyte levels rise hectically to between 20 and 40%, and the blood smear shows two major populations of red cells: small, dark-staining microspherocytes, and large, pale, polychromatophilic cells (Figure 8-24). In many patients with idiopathic AHA this unpredictable disease self-terminates within several weeks, but more often it has a waning-and-relapsing or chronic pattern spanning several years.

Management   After stabilizing the severely anemic patient with transfusions, the physician's mandate is to search for an underlying cause; the most lamentable oversight is failure to recognize that hemolysis is caused by a drug or infection, elimination of which would cure the disease. The "upfront" therapy for controlling the rate of hemolysis is prednisone (or its congeners), which causes prompt, durable remissions in over 30% of patients and therapy-dependent amelioration in another 40%. Corticosteroid actions are multifactorial and carry numerous adverse side effects; their efficacy in AHA is explained by a dose-dependent downregulation of Fcγ receptor activity. The finding that FcγR activity is rate limiting in AHA has led to the use of high-dose intravenous IgG infusions for blockading these recep-

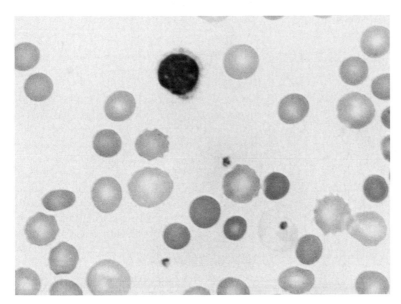

FIGURE 8-24

Red cell morphology in severe immunohemolytic anemia induced by warm-active IgG autoantibodies. Spherocytes and microspherocytes, the small, dark red cells lacking central pallor, are admixed with large round or oblong macroreticulocytes. Spherocytosis of this prominence is only seen in Coombs-positive hemolytic anemias and in severe HS. (Photo by CT Kapff.)

tors. Commercial preparations contain aggregated IgG; this preempts receptor sites for IgG antibody-coated red cells, sharply braking red cell clearance. A more direct suppression of Fc receptor activity can be achieved by infusing monoclonal antibody to the receptors, but this approach has been frustrated by the induction of anti-idiotypic antibodies to the anti-Fc molecules. In those patients requiring longterm maintenance courses of high-dose IgG, backup modes of therapy include splenectomy and cytotoxic drugs. Cytotoxic agents are a last resort in patients refractory to other therapies, but novel strategies have been devised to make these toxic agents more selective: one method is to package toxic warheads in antibody-coated platelets or pellets—a poison-bait or Trojan horse ruse.

Splenectomy is the therapy of choice in patients refractory to, or excessively dependent upon, prednisone. Splenectomy is usually beneficial in patients with splenomegaly who are shown beforehand to sequester selectively ^{51}Cr-labeled autologous red cells, as determined by directional scintillation counters or radioisotope imaging.

Drug-induced AHA About 20% of immunohemolytic disorders are initiated by pharmaceutical agents, and a search for such agents is mandatory, for the key to management is simple abstinence. The mechanism of induction of antibodies reactive with red cells can be classified broadly into two categories: the "hapten type" and the unknown. Hapten-type mechanisms can be subdivided into those in which antibody is directed against a drug–red cell complex (the penicillin model) and those in which the initiating process is binding of drug to a protein, forming immune complexes that deposit passively on the innocent red cells (the stibophen model). Penicillin (and streptomycin) bind covalently to red cells if given in very large quantities intravenously; the drugged cells are recognized as foreign by the immune system and hapten-specific IgG antibodies cause splenic trapping and hemolysis. This process ceases abruptly after penicillin is stopped and the Coombs test becomes negative within 2 to 3 months. Hemolysis by the immune complex mechanism accounts for the majority of sporadic forms of drug-induced immune hemolysis. Antibodies to drug-protein complexes are usually complement-activating IgM, and the hemolytic reaction may be violent and associated with hemoglobinemia, hemoglobinuria, and hypovolemic shock.

The antihypertensive agent methyldopa (α-methyldopa or Aldomet) is the commonest known cause of drug-induced immunohemolytic anemia. Over 10% of patients on methyldopa therapy for 6 to 12 months acquire a positive Coombs test, usually involving IgG1. The polyclonal antibodies react with antigens of the Rh locus, usually at low titer and with weak affinity. In a small portion of Coombs-positive individuals the direct and indirect Coombs tests are both strongly positive and hemolysis ensues through Fc receptor–mediated mechanisms. The "methyldopa model" is beguiling because the immunohemolytic process exactly mimics idiopathic AHA but the drug does not participate in the immune process it has provoked. (Unlike antibody provoked by penicillin or stibophen, antibody eluted from affected red cells does not require presence of the drug to bind to normal red cells in vitro.) Nevertheless hemolysis gradually abates after withdrawal of the medication, and the Coombs test reverts to negative within 1 to 2 years. There is no satisfactory explanation for the loss of toleration in some but not other methyldopa-treated persons. The drug does impair T cell suppressor function, which (in spacious language) may lead to misreading of self-antigens and decontrolled synthesis of antibody by B cells. That the causative role of methyldopa in this common subset of AHA was discovered by epidemiologic means and is not demonstrable by serologic tests in vitro raises concern that other idiopathic cases of AHA may also be induced by drugs or other extrinsic antigens.

HEMOLYTIC ANEMIAS CAUSED BY INFECTION OF RED CELLS

In global terms, infection of red cells by protozoa or bacteria is the most widespread cause of hemolytic anemia. Malaria alone has a current prevalence of about 300 million cases and the annual mortality exceeds 1 million.

Malaria

Malaria is a protozoan infection transmitted by female *Anopheles* mosquitoes, which serve as the reservoir and vector for the infective sporozoites from any of four species of the genus *Plasmodium*: *P. vivax*, *P. ovale*, *P. malariae*, and *P. falciparum*.

Pathophysiology

Sporozoites enter the bloodstream via the saliva of female anopheles during blood meals. Inoculated sporozoites are cleared rapidly by slipping beneath littoral cells of the hepatic sinuses and somehow securing sanctuary in the nourishing cell sap of hepatocytes. In this liver or exoerythrocytic phase, merozoites flourish, transform to schizonts, and through frenzied multiplication known as schizogony generate enough merozoite offspring within 1 to several weeks (up to 50,000 per sporozoite) to rupture the distended hepatocytes. Millions of minute merozoites then flood the circulation and adhere to red cells by means of unique receptors.

Receptors, knobs, and immunity   *P. vivax* binds selectively to Duffy determinants (Fy^aFy^b) on red cells, and natural resistance to vivax infections has developed as a genetic adaptation among blacks of West African ancestry, among whom the frequency of Duffy-negative phenotype is extraordinarily high (90%). *P. falciparum* merozoites are equipped with a receptor complex that recognizes and attaches to glycophorin on red cell surfaces; the apical end of the small (1 to 2 μm across) merozoite burrows into the red cell wall, creating a depression that serves as the point of parasite entry (Figure 8-25) [26]. As the parasite invades the cell within its own bubble or vacuole, the spectrin-actin framework of the cytoskeleton parts and then draws together again like a purse, sealing in its hungry guest.

During the erythrocytic phase of malaria, receptor-mediated endocytosis (of one to five merozoites per red cell) is complete within 30 seconds of first contact. Safe within the savory interior of its host cell, parasites quickly assume ring shapes (ring stage), and these ring forms transform to trophozoites which grow by feeding on hemoglobin (excreting lumps of brownish hematin as they do so) to become large amoeboid structures. As they feed on their host, trophozoites commandeer red cell metabolites, manufacture their own G6PD and transferrin receptors, and synthesize hundreds of parasite proteins; some of these proteins are exported into the circulation, and others assemble into membrane complexes (including a histidine-rich protein) that form sticky knobs

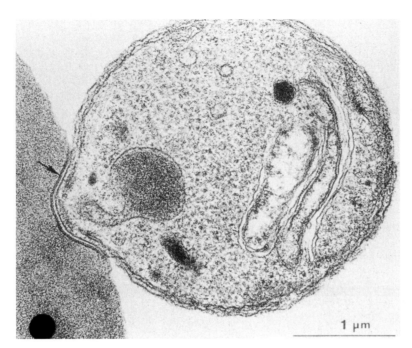

FIGURE 8-25

EM of *P. falciparum* merozoite creating a depression in the red cell membrane, which becomes thickened at the site of invagination. (From Aikawa M and Miller LH: Malaria and the Red Cell. Ciba Foundation Symposium 94. Copyright 1983. Reprinted by permission of John Wiley & Sons, Ltd.)

FIGURE 8-26

Knobs on the surface of a red cell infected with *P. falciparum* form focal junctions (arrows) with the surface of an endothelial (En) cell, as revealed by EM. (Inset) High-power micrograph shows multiple microfilaments securing the red cell knobs to the endothelium. (From Aikawa M and Miller LH: Malaria and the Red Cell. Ciba Foundation Symposium 94. Copyright 1983. Reprinted by permission of John Wiley & Sons, Ltd.)

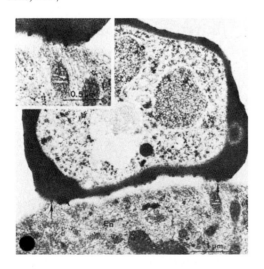

on the red cell surface. Parasite-derived proteins on the protruding knobs cause cells to adhere to vascular endothelium and to other red cells expressing knobs (Figure 8-26) [26]. In *P. falciparum* and *P. malariae* infections, as trophozoites mature to the "preschizontic" phase the hapless, half-devoured host cells become very knobby, and IgG antibodies to parasite proteins congregate on the exposed proteins. This immune response finishes off the red cells before they burst and serves as a means of controlling infection by remanding IgG-coated parasitized cells to the vascular prisons of the spleen. The subsequent course is determined by the antithetical rates of parasitization and splenic sequestration.

The malaria cycle Before the full force of the immune system is aroused, trophozoite nuclei undergo segmentation and divisions to form multinucleated schizonts, cytoplasm condenses around each daughter nucleus, outfitting a new generation of merozoites. When the shelled-out red cell disintegrates, its cargo of 12 to 24 merozoites is unleashed and free to infect virginal red cells, initiating a new, amplified cycle of red cell infection and hemolysis.

As these cycles are repeated the surges of multiplication gradually become synchronized into 2- to 3-day intervals, dependent on the erythrocytic life cycle of the plasmodium species. Through some arcane process a small number of merozoites are chosen to transmute into large sexual forms called gametocytes that will resume proliferative activity only if ingested by another anopheline mosquito as she engorges on the patient's blood. From the mosquito standpoint the cycle is consummated in the stomach of the female mosquito; in this covert cavern the male microgamete, after sprouting and then losing his threadlike flagellae, mates with the female macrogamete. The issue of this union, a wormlike oökinete, encysts in the lining of the egg cavity, and as the abdomen is inflated by osmotic force (from degradation of hemoglobin), the egg-derived sporozoites are popped free and migrate to the salivary gland, primed for inoculation into another victim. The life cycle of this author of pestilence is reprised in Figure 8-27.

Description

Clinical and hematologic manifestations vary with the species of *Plasmodium*. Conventional

symptoms are fever, chills, headache, muscle pain, and prostration, reflecting an explosive cytokine-directed outburst with IL-1 in the vanguard. The individual characteristics of the several human malarias are listed in Table 8-3 [27]. The hallmark of this disease is the malarial paroxysm of chills (rigor) and fever (the "hot stage") lasting several hours and followed during defervescence by profuse sweating and exhaustion; except for their rhythmicity, malarial paroxysms simulate severe transfusion reactions.

Hematologic Findings

Early in the course of malaria the foremost cause of hemolysis is rupture of parasitized cells. The severity of hemolysis is proportional to the number of red cells infected and thus is greatest in falciparum malaria; hemolysis by *P. vivax* is delimited by the preferential attachment of merozoites to reticulocytes. At first hemolysis is confined to parasitized cells, but within a week of clinical onset hemolysis worsens as increasing numbers of nonparasitized red cells are destroyed by immunologic mechanisms and by the increasing efficiency of the enlarging spleen in trapping damaged red cells. Preformed immune complexes composed of parasite protein and glycophorin attach to red

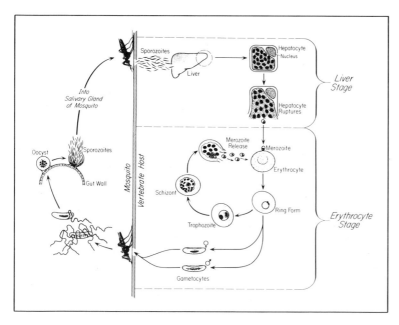

FIGURE 8-27

The eternal triangle responsible for perpetuating malaria. (Courtesy Dr. M. Jungary.)

TABLE 8-3

Characteristics of infection with four species of human plasmodia

Feature	Species			
	Plasmodium vivax	*Plasmodium ovale*	*Plasmodium malariae*	*Plasmodium falciparum*
Incubation period (days)	13 (12–17) or up to 6–12 months	17 (16–18) or longer	28 (18–40) or longer	12 (9–14)
Approximate number of merozoites per tissue schizont	Over 10,000	15,000	2,000	40,000
Erythrocytic cycle (h)	48	40–50	72	48
Parasitemia (per μl)				
Average	20,000	9,000	6,000	20,000–500,000
Maximum	50,000	30,000	20,000	2,000,000
Primary attack severity	Mild to severe	Mild	Mild	Severe in nonimmunes
Febrile paroxysm (h)	8–12	8–12	8–10	16–36 or longer
Relapses	+ +	+ +	+ + +	–
Period of recurrence	Long	Long	Very long	Short
Duration of infection (yr)	1.5–3	Probably same as *P. vivax*	3–50	1–2

Source: From Bruce-Chwatt LJ: Essential Malariology. London, William Heinemann Medical Books, Ltd., 1980.

cell membranes, whether or not the cell harbors parasites; as the result variable amounts of IgG and C3 are detectable by the Coombs test.

Morphologic findings   Diagnosis of malaria depends on identification of *Plasmodia* in red cells, using Wright-Giemsa stained blood smears. *Vivax*-parasitized red cells are distinctive for they are enlarged and pale and may be diffusely freckled with bright red dots (Schüffner's dots); trophozoites extend delicate blue hoop-shaped rings, and all stages of schizogeny as well as sexual forms may coexist in the same blood film. In *P. falciparum* malaria late trophozoites and schizonts are rare, but blood smears abound in small delicate ring forms, measuring about one-sixth the red cell diameter, and often occurring several per red cell, sometimes as marginal (accolé) forms.

Resistance to Malaria

The most robust defense against plasmodial infections is cell-mediated and humoral immunity. The T cell network reacts violently to parasite antigens and through persuasion by interleukins, B cells generate IgM and IgG antibodies in abundance; these opsonize and steer parasitized cells into the xenophobic sinuses of the spleen. Killing of the trapped parasites is performed by macrophages, which (following receptor-mediated binding) secrete cytocidal agents including tumor necrosis factor and free radical oxygen. Malaria is an immunosuppressive infection, however, and efforts of the host to eradicate plasmodia usually lead to a standoff unless chemotherapeutic help is provided. Control of blood-stage forms of malaria is made difficult by the constant shifting of antigenic determinants that accompanies parasite differentiation. Untreated patients in whom host and parasite have achieved uneasy equilibrium gradually develop marked (often massive) splenomegaly, with extensive red cell pooling in splenic sinuses plus plasma expansion caused by pronounced increases in IgM concentrations: the combination of massive splenomegaly, hemolysis, and dilutional anemia is known as the tropical splenomegaly syndrome.

Genetic mechanisms of resistance   The historical distribution of common hemoglobin variants, thalassemia, and G6PD deficiency mirrors that of endemic malaria [28]. In areas where *P. falciparum* has been holoendemic, malaria appears to have acted as a selective force favoring evolution of high-frequency genes that confer resistance. Genetic resistance is advantageous primarily in early life before immunologic defenses are in place. Red cells from individuals heterozygous for sickle cell anemia or with hereditary persistence of fetal hemoglobin possess comparatively indigestible hemoglobin and are partially protected by their variant proteins. In theory G6PD deficiency cells are marvelously adapted to survive falciparum malaria, for their high levels of oxidized glutathione should be toxic to growing trophozoites; the resourceful parasites produce their own superior brand of G6PD, however, and the extreme prevalence of G6PD deficiency in populations historically exposed to *P. falciparum* remains unexplained. The putative genetic advantage conferred by inheritance of genes for thalassemia, hemoglobins C and E, and Melanesian elliptocytosis also awaits clarification.

Management: Chemotherapy and Malaria Vaccines

Appropriate chemotherapy can suppress or cure most forms of malaria, but emergence of drug-resistant strains of *P. falciparum* has enabled this ancient pestilence to evade eradication. Chemotherapeutic regimens must be tailored to suit the stage of infection and the species and strain of plasmodium involved. The long quest for immunoprophylactic and immunotherapeutic means for controlling malarial infections has been tripped up by the facility with which plasmodia, like trypanosomes, are able to change their antigenic identity to evade even the resourceful T cell network. Plasmodia possess variable surface antigens that can be shifted in "casettes," enabling the cells to change immunologic clothes selected from a large wardrobe. This quick-change mechanism is made possible by cutting surface antigens loose from membrane phosphatidylinositol through the action of phospholipase C. To be successful vaccines will need to be directed against stable or immunodominant surface epitopes specific for all three stages of the parasite: sporozoites, asexual erythrocyte parasites, and sexual forms. Facsimiles of several immunodominant repeating peptides have been synthesized and are being tested as vaccines: malaria vaccination may be available for worldwide use within a few years.

Babesiosis

Babesiosis (piroplasmosis) is a hemolytic disorder similar to falciparum malaria that occurs in island and coastal areas of northeastern United States, in the lake and forest regions of northcentral states, and in California, France, Ireland, and Scotland. Most infections are caused by *B. microti*, which is transmitted from feral deer mice to people (particularly persons over 50 years of age) by hard ticks of the genus *Ixodes*. *Ixodes* are 3-host ticks and at each stage of development (larva, nymph, and adult), bites by female ticks inoculate sporozoites into the victim's bloodstream. Sporozoites penetrate red cell membranes directly via a complement (C3b) receptor-mediated mechanism, and the interiorized trophozoites rapidly assume ring shapes similar to those of *P. falciparum* (Figure 8-28). Babesias divide by budding rather than schizogony; each parasite generates a maximum of four merozoites, some of which form tetrads or "maltese cross forms."

Description

The peak incidence of babesiosis is in early August and symptoms first appear 1 to 4 weeks after the tick bite. The disease ranges from an evanescent, subclinical malaise to severe hemolytic anemia with hectic fever,

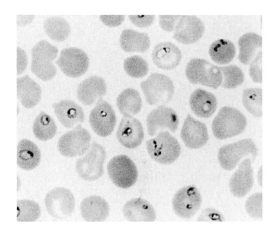

FIGURE 8-28

Numerous *B. microti* ring forms and two tetrads in red cells of a patient with severe babesiosis. Ring forms are as numerous as in *P. falciparum* malaria and often form similar joined structures having clear centers. Note the lack of heme pigment and absence of schizonts or gametocytes. (Photo by CT Kapff.)

chills, and prostration. In splenectomized individuals babesiosis can cause catastrophic intravascular hemolysis, with hemoglobinemia, hypovolemic shock, and renal shutdown. As with malaria, *B. microti* can be transmitted from symptomless carriers via transfusion of blood or blood components. Babesiosis can be cured or aborted by the antibiotic clindamycin.

Bartonellosis (Carrión's Disease)

Bartonellosis is an acute hemolytic infection of abrupt onset and high mortality that is caused by a small pleomorphic gram-negative organism, *Bartonella bacilliformis*. It is transmitted by the bite of female sandflies of the genus *Phlebotomus*, and the distribution of this crepuscular vector is responsible for delimiting bartonellosis to those who dwell in (or venture into) the Andean slopes of Peru, Colombia, or Ecuador at altitudes between 700 and 2,500 m.

Description

Within 3 weeks after being bitten by an infected sandfly the victim is stricken by fever,

chills, and hemolytic anemia of alarming severity in which the red count may plunge below 1,000,000 cells/μl within a few days. During the initial onslaught Bartonella organisms may be found swarming on the surfaces of over 90% of red cells, adhering at first in appliqué fashion, and then forming cone-shaped depressions, trenches, and deep invaginations. Propelled and spun about by long polar flagella, the bacilli twist and bore their way into the doomed red cells through forced endocytosis (Figure 8-29) [29]. During severe bacteremia a dozen or more organisms may cling to, deform, and enter each red cell. On smears stained with Wright-Giemsa the organisms are

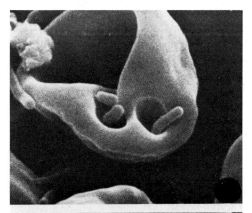
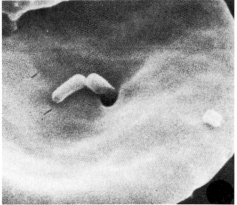

FIGURE 8-29

Scanning EMs showing bartonella bacilli burrowing into and penetrating the membranes of red cells during hemolytic septicemia. (From Benson LE et al: Entry of Bartonella bacilliformis into erythrocytes. Infect Immun 54:347,1986.)

red-purple and remarkably pleomorphic, varying from stubby coccoid forms to thin bacilli up to 4 μm long.

Acute bartonellosis is extremely dangerous if not treated promptly with antibiotics (chloramphenicol or tetracycline), causing death in about 40% of neglected patients. Among survivors, a second eruptive, verrugal stage appears, consisting of multitudes of unsightly cutaneous hemangiomas, which cause the patient to appear studded with cranberries. The sessile nodules are richly vascular and contain bacteria on and within vascular endothelium. Clearing of the verrugal phase can be hastened by antibiotic therapy.

METABOLIC DISORDERS OF RED CELLS

Red cells depend for their survival on transporting O_2 without being burned by it and on preserving their dimensions and viscoelastic properties during 4 months of service as O_2 transport vehicles. Protection against oxidation is provided by the hexose monophosphate shunt (pentose phosphate pathway), and structural repair and maintenance depend on generation of ATP by the Embden-Myerhof pathway (Chapter 4). Failure to detoxify free radical metabolites of reduced O_2 leads to oxidative hemolysis and precipitation of hemoglobin (Heinz body hemolytic anemias), and defective synthesis of ATP from metabolic deprivation or genetic inadequacy causes failure of essential membrane functions. In either case, red cell life span is shortened, with the oldest cells dying first—usually in the proving grounds of the RES.

Pathophysiology of Oxidative Hemolysis

Red cells are designed metabolically to carry enormous quantities of O_2 safely by strictly delimiting interaction between their incendiary payload of O_2 ($E_0' = +0.82V$) and the various vulnerable proteins, enzymes, and cofactors essential to cell function. Mature red cells draw upon nonoxidative glycolysis (fermentation) for energy, avoiding risky dependence upon oxidoreductive mitochondrial mechanisms, and they are armed in depth by antioxidative enzymes. Among these systems for detoxifying O_2 activated by reacting with reduced substrates are catalase, superoxide dismutase, glutathione (GSH) reductase, and GSH peroxidase. Collectively these enzyme systems are capable (within limits) of scavenging superoxides and peroxides, preventing accumulation of harmful free radicals such as hydroxyl ions (OH·) and singlet O_2 (O*).

Thiol Oxidation and G6PD

The first lines of defense against oxidation are NADPH ($E_0' = -0.32$) and GSH ($E_0' = -0.23$), which together safeguard SH-containing enzymes and membrane thiols. Maintenance of GSH at normal levels (2–3 mM) is the assignment of NADPH, which is generated and regenerated by the HMP shunt (Figure 4-15). Hence glutathione stability depends ultimately on the activity of G6PD in returning $NADP^+$ to its functional, reduced form. This antioxidative system is highly responsive, and HMP shunt activity is quite capable of revving up to 30 times normal in response to oxidative stress. If exceptionally high levels of free radical metabolites of reduced O_2 are generated in the cell, or if the shunt is crippled by deficiency of a key enzyme such as G6PD, stepwise oxidations occur. If oxidation persistently overwhelms the shunt, as occurs during cycling interactions between O_2 and redox drugs that reduce O_2 to free radical metabolites, GSSG accumulates and the two reactive thiols of hemoglobin are converted to mixed disulfides and then to sulfates. This irreversible denaturation of globin causes ferrihemes to dissociate, poorly soluble greenish hemochromes (sulfhemoglobins) accumulate, and finally large aggregates of precipitated hemoglobin form as end products of the oxidative assault. The aggregates are called Heinz bodies.

Pathologic effects of Heinz bodies   The presence of one or a few free-floating Heinz bodies within a red cell is relatively harmless in vitro, but in vivo the inclusions become bonded to the inner aspect of the membrane skeleton, altering the resilience, rheology, and other physical properties of the cell. Membrane-bound Heinz bodies at first pout from the cell and then are shed by exocytosis as membrane-bound particles, creating bite-out deformities as mementos of the event (Figure 8-30) [30].

Exocytosis of hemoglobin precipitates in the general circulation is the random consequence

FIGURE 8-30

Red cell deformities caused by Heinz bodies in a patient with oxidative hemolysis induced by an aniline derivative. Inset (at center) demonstrates by phase microscopy the stepwise expulsion of individual Heinz bodies. Upper and lower panels are Wright-Giemsa—stained smears displaying telltale bite-out deformities that remain after dislodgment of the inclusions (From Andre R et al: Deux observations d'anemie hemolytique aigue apres prise de phenyl-semi-carbazide. Remarques sur la poikilocytose et revue de la litterature. Nouv Rev Fr Hematol 5:431,1965.)

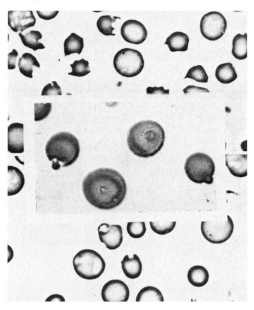

of hydraulic battering and shear, but in traversing the spleen, red cells burdened with Heinz body aggregates are arrested as they attempt to squirm through the shingled fenestrations connecting cords to sinuses (Figure 8-31) [31]. Heinz body–filled cells trapped attempting to escape through the screenlike basement membrane and endothelial slats of the splenic red pulp face one of two fates: either the cell remains tethered by its tail and the membrane skeleton breaks up, or the leash is snapped and the cell resumes circulating. The membrane bilayer mends itself by lateral rearrangements, but one or more bite-out deformities remain with the cell as scars of its trek through the splenic filter.

Drugs that cause Heinz body hemolytic anemias   Oxidized forms of aromatic redox compounds possess the risky potential of transferring electrons one at a time from donors such as NADPH and GSH to molecular oxygen. This cyclic interaction generates free radical forms of both the drug and of O_2. Most drugs that cause oxidative hemolysis are actual or potential quinones: among these are antimalarials, sulfonamides, sulfones, and many analgesics, antipyretics, and antibiotics. In sufficient quantity quinones and other free-radical forming drugs are capable of inducing Heinz body hemolytic anemia in any individual. The most common circumstance predisposing to oxidative hemolysis is administration of sulfon-

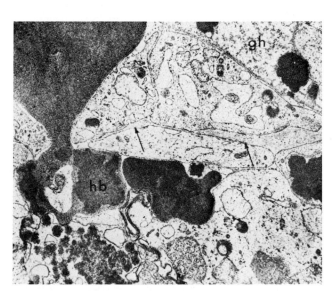

FIGURE 8-31

EM showing that the bulk of a red cell previously exposed to an oxidant drug had slithered through a gap in the basement membrane (arrows) separating a cord (below) from a sinus (above), but further progress was prevented by the bag of Heinz bodies (hb) in its "tail." (From Rifkind RA: Heinz body anemia: an ultrastructural study. II. Red cell sequestration and destruction. Blood 26:433,1965.)

amides or nitrofurans to patients with renal failure. Several genetic aberrations underlie increased susceptibility to oxidant drugs: the most important and prevalent of these is G6PD deficiency.

G6PD Deficiency

G6PD deficiency is the most prevalent inborn metabolic disorder of red cells, affecting over 100,000,000 people. G6PD is the first and rate-limiting enzyme of the HMP shunt and governs the speed with which blood cells consume or detoxify O_2. G6PD is encoded by genes located on the X chromosome: accordingly, G6PD deficiency is fully expressed in hemizygous males and homozygous females, and enzyme activity is partially diminished in heterozygous females, depending on the balance of lyonization. Genetic mosaicism is demonstrable in red cells from heterozygous women, but some degree of nongenetic mosaicism affects red cells of both sexes because enzyme activity declines arithmetically with cell age.

Normally G6PD is a dimer of two peptides (M_rs: 55,000) that possess a high affinity for NADP$^+$; enzyme binding to its cofactor is strongly inhibited by NADPH and by ATP through competition for G6P.

Variants of G6PD

G6PD variants have been classified on the basis of three major criteria: clinical significance, enzyme activity, and electrophoretic mobility. The normal enzyme, designated G6PD B, is the product of the Gd^B gene and is the most prevalent isozyme, all population groups considered. G6PD A, product of the Gd^A gene, is an electrophoretically faster variant having normal catalytic activity; G6PD A$^-$ comigrates with G6PD A but has subnormal catalytic activity, as signified by the minus sign. All other variants are designated by geographic names. As over 300 variants of G6PD have been described, a simplified grouping into five classes has been promulgated, in which clinical severity is the dominant consideration (Table 8-4) [32]. Class 1 variants are extremely unstable and are associated with congenital nonspherocytic hemolytic anemia (CNSHA). Class 2 and Class 3 variants, representing 90% of G6PD deficiency states, are not associated with

TABLE 8-4

G6PD variants

			Electrophoretic mobility of representative variants*		
Class	Clinical features	Enzyme activity	Fast	Normal	Slow
1	Congenital nonspherocytic hemolytic anemia	Severely deficient	Charleston (8)	Boston (20)	Chicago (17)
2	Hemolytic attacks on exposure to oxidants or (in some) *Vicia fava*	Severely deficient	Markam (10)	Mediterranean, Corinth (12)	Panay (19)
3	Hemolytic attacks on exposure to oxidants, acidosis, or certain infections	Mildly or moderately deficient	A$^-$, Canton, Debrousse (18)	Mahidol (6)	Athens (18)
4	None	Normal	A (A$^+$) (6)	B (B$^+$) (1)	Baltimore-Austin (7)
5	None	Increased	Hektoen	———	———

*Numbers in parentheses indicate number of authentic variants in each electrophoretic category.

Source: From Jandl JH: Chapt 11, in Blood: Textbook of Hematology. Boston, Little, Brown and Company, 1987.

chronic hemolysis but do impose hypersusceptibility to oxidant drugs. The Mediterranean variant (G6PD^{Med}) is the most widespread Class 2 deficiency state, and its prevalence among Greeks, Sardinians, and Sephardic Jews and their descendants ranges from 3% to 50%. The most prevalent of the Class 3 variants, A$^-$, affects 12% of American black males, 19% of African black males, and 15% of men in Thailand and Vietnam. Class 2 and Class 3 G6PD deficiency states have a tropical and subtropical distribution mirroring that of endemic malaria.

Hemolysis of G6PD-Deficient Red Cells

Clinical expression of G6PD deficiency can be sorted into three distinct syndromes. CNSHA occurs in the rare Class 1 variants, in which G6PD is too unstable to measure: for lack of a sound NADPH-reducing system, spectrin and other skeletal components of the membrane undergo oxidative crosslinking and aggregation, and the cells become too rigid to negotiate the sinuses of liver and spleen. Moderately severe lifelong hemolytic anemia is the rule, often commencing with hemolytic disease of the newborn.

In the common forms of G6PD deficiency (G6PD A$^-$ and G6PD^{Med}) the enzyme deficit ordinarily is harmless unless HMP shunt activity is stressed by exposure to oxidant drugs. Most oxidant medications (such as antimalarials and sulfonamides) are not direct oxidants but are activated only during metabolic degradation within oxygenated red cells to semiquinones, which through "redox cycling" leads to catalytic reduction of O_2 to O_2^- and to the dreaded OH· radical. The sequential results following administration of a prototype indirect oxidant, the 8-aminoquinoline antimalarial primaquine, is portrayed in Figure 8-32 [33]. In patients receiving drugs of the primaquine sort on a daily basis, a resistant or equilibrium phase usually is achieved in which hemolysis is well compensated; resistance results from selective elimination of older red cells, in which G6PD levels are lowest, and replacement by younger cells have fresher enzymes. Resistance is relative, for progressively younger age brackets of cells are hemolyzed if drug dosage is progressively increased.

Hemolysis in Class 2 and 3 variants of G6PD can also be triggered by acute or subacute infections (particularly viral hepatitis and pneumococcal pneumonia) and by diabetic ketoacidosis. The mechanisms underlying the vulnerability of G6PD-deficient red cells to these metabolic importunities are unknown but are presumed to reflect factors

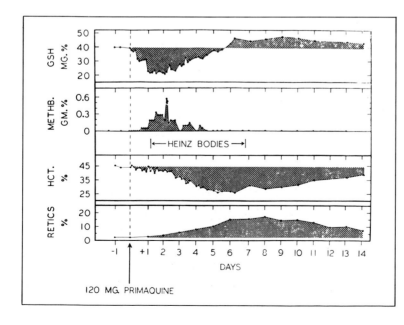

FIGURE 8-32

Sequential oxidative response to a single large dose of primaquine in a black male having the A$^-$ variant of G6PD. As primaquine is converted to a quinone, GSH is oxidized, methemoglobin appears as a transient step in the eventual degradation of hemoglobin to Heinz bodies, and a bout of hemolysis ensues as the result of membrane damage. (From Brewer GJ et al: The hemolytic effect of primaquine. XV. Role of methemoglobin. J Lab Clin Med 59:905,1962.)

such as hyperthermia and acidosis that worsen enzyme instability. Some evidence indicates that the profound hemolytic effect of infection in G6PD-deficient patients is caused by release of oxidants from granulocytes goaded by complement-activating immune complexes. Red cells possess C3b receptors that serve the useful purpose of mopping up C3b; G6PD-deficient cells engaged in this mop-up pay dearly for their Good Samaritanism.

Favism   The third syndrome to which certain G6PD-deficient individuals may be predisposed is intravascular hemolysis triggered by exposure to the common broad bean, *Vicia fava*. Favism does not occur in persons with the A$^-$ variant of G6PD but is prevalent among Greek, Italian, and other Mediterranean populations where the incidence of G6PD^{Med} ranges up to 35%. As broad beans are a popular staple among those of Mediterranean ancestry, culture and genetics have conspired to make favism an ethnic affliction. Fava beans contain uniquely high concentrations of pyrimidine aglycones that activate amounts of O_2 in the presence of GSH sufficient to overwhelm the feeble reductive apparatus of G6PD-deficient red cells. The O_2 free radicals generated cause oxidative crosslinking of skeletal proteins to hemoglobin, forming large polypeptide aggregates and engendering membrane damage, spherocytosis, and bite-out deformities indistinguishable from those caused by oxidant medication (Figure 8-33). G6PD deficiency is necessary but not sufficient to engender a hemolytic reaction to fava beans. Only certain variants of G6PD predispose to favism and even in patients with G6PD^{Med}, hemolytic reactions are inconstant, subject to some undefined, possibly immunologic caprice.

Diagnosis and Screening

Oxidative hemolysis can usually be suspected from historical circumstance and the finding on blood smears of bite-out deformities; Heinz bodies may or may not be detectable using supravital staining with crystal or methyl violet. Of many screening tests employed, the ascorbate-cyanide test is most useful as a generic test encompassing all metabolic defects leading to oxidative instability: in addition to the preponderant problem, G6PD deficiency, this test gives positive results in glutathione

Red cell deformities during acute favism. (Photo by CT Kapff.)

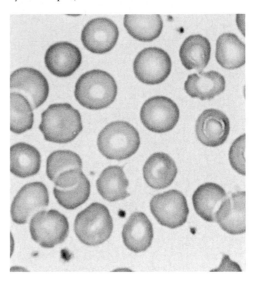

deficiency, unstable hemoglobin disease, and pyruvate kinase deficiency.

Unstable hemoglobin disease   Congenital Heinz body hemolytic anemia (CHBHA) is an uncommon hemolytic disorder inherited by autosomal codominant genes and caused by structural aberrations of hemoglobin (usually in the region of the heme pocket or the $\alpha_1\beta_1$ interface) that predispose to oxidation. The structural alteration in hemoglobin Zürich renders hemoglobin doubly sensitive to oxidative precipitation: substitution of arginine for the distal histidine at βE7 pries open the heme pocket, making the heme iron freely accessible to oxidant drugs such as sulfonamides. Exposed ferrihemes readily dissociate from their niche, globin thiols are laid bare, and the unstabilized globin dissociates into dimers and flocculates into denatured inclusion bodies. The inclusions formed during drug exposure are similar to Heinz bodies and have the same deleterious effects upon cell survival, causing chronic hemolysis, bite-out deformities, and increased excretion of dipyrrole pigments. Unlike Heinz body hemolytic anemias, inclusions of genetically unstable hemoglobin are unusually large and irregular and are particularly numerous in reticulocytes. The extreme vulnerability of unstable hemoglobins to thermal denaturation at 50°C and to precipitation in buffered isopropanol provides the basis for simple screening tests.

PYRUVATE KINASE DEFICIENCY

Although far less prevalent than G6PD deficiency, pyruvate kinase (PK) deficiency ranks as the most common enzymatic disorder associated with severe chronic nonspherocytic hemolytic anemia (CNSHA). PK deficiency is transmitted by autosomal recessive genes and most cases arise from double heterozygosity for different mutant genes. Mutant forms of dysfunctional PK have differing kinetic properties, accounting for the clinical heterogeneity between affected families.

Pathophysiology

PK is a key glycolytic enzyme that catalyzes the following reaction:

$$\text{Phosphoenolpyruvate} + \text{ADP} \xrightarrow[\text{Mg}^{2+} + \text{K}^+]{\text{PK}} \text{pyruvate} + \text{ATP}$$

The enzyme is a tetramer formed by two pairs of electrophoretically separable subunits that exhibit conformational changes characteristic of allosterism, in accordance with the

$$R \rightleftharpoons T$$

model of Monod. The substrate phosphoenolpyruvate (PEP) and the allosteric effector fructose-1,6-diphosphate (FDP) cooperate in shifting equilibrium toward the highly catalytic R form, favoring hyperbolic reaction kinetics. In most patients doubly heterozygous for PK deficiency, the hybrid mutants responsible for hemolytic disease possess low residual activity, weak affinity for PEP, and insensitivity to FDP (Figure 8-34) [34]. This ineffectual enzyme is unable to convert the high-energy intermediate, PEP, to pyruvate, preventing mature red cells from regenerating adequate ATP, the universal biologic source of free energy. This is no problem for immature erythroid cells, for these are equipped with mitochondria—those omnivorous organelles that flourish on fatty acids,

FIGURE 8-34

Comparison of PK kinetic activity in a normal subject (interrupted line) versus that of a PK-deficient subject doubly heterozygous for PK variants (continuous line). The patient's mutant PK reached half-maximum activity only at substrate (PEP) concentrations that are unattainable in mature red cells, rendering the enzyme functionally useless. (Redrawn from Valentine WN et al: Chapt 73, in The Metabolic Basis of Inherited Disease, 5th ed., Stanbury JB et al, Eds. New York, McGraw-Hill Book Company, 1983.)

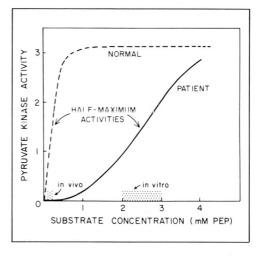

amino acids, and dicarboxylic acids—and oxidative phosphorylation by mitochondria is 18 times as efficient in generating ATP as is glycolysis. When mitochondria are phased out during reticulocyte maturation, red cells severely deficient in PK activity are destined to expire within a few days. Cells less deficient in PK may last many weeks or months, accounting for the paradoxical finding that mildly anemic patients have lower ATP levels than severe cases. Glycolytic intermediates proximal to the defect accumulate; 2,3-DPG is markedly elevated, causing a rightward shift in the P_{50} (Chapter 4) that partially ameliorates tissue hypoxia in severely anemic patients. Levels of 2,3-DPG exceeding twice normal (8 to 10 mM) are virtually diagnostic of PK deficiency.

Red cell survival is curtailed because all ATP-dependent systems fail. Cation pumps flag, K^+ is lost along with obligate water, causing cellular desiccation, and membrane spicules and other deformities emerge. Damage is compounded during each trip to the spleen, where metabolic deprivation exhausts the marginal energy reserves of these disadvantaged cells. As splenic hyperplasia ensues in response to the hemolytic "workload," the large, sticky reticulocytes become selectively sequestered. This is particularly unfortunate in the most severely anemic patients in whom reticulocytes may be the principal carriers of O_2.

Description

Clinical expression of PK deficiency ranges from severe congenital hemolytic anemia with jaundice to a fully compensated subclinical hemolytic trait. Generally anemia is moderate or severe, with steady-state levels of hemoglobin ranging from 6 to 12 g/dl, but the course may be punctuated by aplastic crises precipitated by infection with human parvovirus or other myelopathic organisms. Red cell morphology is relatively bland, but in severe cases (particularly after splenectomy), spiculed, crenated, and contracted forms may abound (Figure 8-35). Before splenectomy, reticulo-

cyte levels range from 5 to 20%, but afterward reticulocytes—no longer impounded in the spleen—undergo a pronounced and paradoxical rise despite improvement in the hemoglobin level. The peculiar spiculed forms (shown in Figure 8-35) become associated with conventional morphologic markers of the postsplenectomy state: Howell-Jolly bodies, Pappenheimer bodies, siderocytes, target cells, and acanthocytes.

Patients who are transfusion-dependent require splenectomy to forestall transfusional iron overload. Splenectomy is not curative but it eliminates or minimizes transfusion requirements and improves growth and development. The worse the anemia, the greater the benefit from splenectomy; most patients who survive childhood maintain acceptable levels of hemoglobin (compensated hemolysis) with recourse to transfusion only during aplastic crises.

REFERENCES

1. Agre P et al: Partial deficiency of erythrocyte spectrin in hereditary spherocytosis. Nature 314:380,1985

2. Agre P et al: Deficient red-cell spectrin in severe, recessively inherited spherocytosis. N Engl J Med 306:1155,1982

3. Waugh RE and Agre P: Reductions of erythrocyte membrane viscoelastic coefficients reflect spectrin deficiencies in hereditary spherocytosis. J Clin Invest 81:133,1988

4. Palek J: Hereditary elliptocytosis, spherocytosis and related disorders: consequences of a deficiency or a mutation of membrane skeletal proteins. Blood Rev 1:147,1987

5. Kessel RG and Kardon RH: Tissues and Organs: A Text-Atlas of Scanning Electron Microscopy. San Francisco, WH Freeman and Company,1979

6. Zail S: Clinical disorders of the red cell membrane skeleton. CRC Crit Rev Oncol Hematol 5:397,1986

7. Jandl JH and Cooper RA: Chapt 58, in The Metabolic Basis of Inherited Disease, 4th ed., Stanbury JB et al, Eds. New York, McGraw-Hill Book Company,1978

8. Bessis M: Chapt 11, in Corpuscles. Atlas of Red Cell Shape. Berlin: Springer-Verlag,1974

FIGURE 8-35

Red cell morphology in severe PK deficiency after splenectomy. (Photo by CT Kapff.)

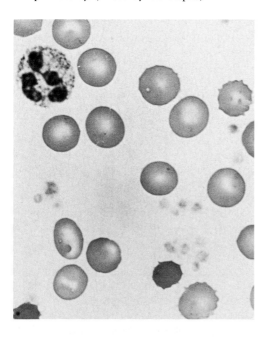

9. Allen DW and Kaplan ME: Chapt 2, in Current Hematology and Oncology, vol. 6. Fairbank VF, Ed. Chicago, Year Book Medical Publishers, Inc.,1988

10. Jandl JH: Chapt 7, in Blood: Textbook of Hematology. Boston, Little, Brown and Company,1987

11. Bessis M: Chapt 9, in Corpuscles. Atlas of Red Cell Shape. Berlin: Springer-Verlag, 1974

12. Blaas P et al: Paroxysmal nocturnal hemoglobinuria. Enhanced stimulation of platelets by the terminal complement components is related to the lack of C8bp in the membrane. J Immunol 140:3045,1988

13. Burroughs SF et al: The population of paroxysmal nocturnal hemoglobinuria neutrophils deficient in decay-accelerating factor is also deficient in alkaline phosphatase. Blood 71: 1086,1988

14. Ham TH: Studies on destruction of red blood cells. I. Chronic hemolytic anemia with paroxysmal nocturnal hemoglobinuria: investigation of the mechanism of hemolysis, with observations on 5 cases. Arch Intern Med 64:1271,1939

15. Hoffbrand AV and Pettit JE: Chapt 4, in Clinical Hematology Illustrated. An Integrated Text and Color Atlas. London, Gower Medical Publishing Ltd.,1987

16. Bull BS and Kuhn IN: The production of schistocytes by fibrin strands (a scanning electron microscope study). Blood 35:104, 1970.

17. Murgo AJ: Thrombotic microangiopathy in the cancer patient including those induced by chemotherapeutic agents. Semin Hematol 24:161,1987

18. Weinstein L: Preeclampsia/eclampsia with hemolysis, elevated liver enzymes, and thrombocytopenia. Obstet Gynecol 66:657,1985

19. Brown RS and Marion A: An 83-year-old woman with anemia, oliguric renal failure, and past lymphoma. Case records of the Massachusetts General Hospital, case 16-1988. N Engl J Med 318:1047,1988

20. Rosse WF: Autoimmune hemolytic anemia. Hosp Pract 20(8):105,1985

21. Petz LD and Garraty G: Chapt 3, in Acquired Immune Hemolytic Anemias. New York, Churchill Livingstone,1980

22. Rosse WF: Interaction of complement with the red-cell membrane. Semin Hematol 16: 128,1979

23. Jandl JH: Chapt 9, in Blood: Textbook of Hematology. Boston, Little, Brown and Company,1987

24. Bessis M: Chapt 16, in Corpuscles. Atlas of Red Cell Shape. Berlin, Springer-Verlag,1974

25. Petz LD and Garraty G: Chapt 5, in Acquired Immune Hemolytic Anemias. New York, Churchill Livingstone,1980

26. Aikawa M and Miller LH: Structural alteration of the erythrocyte membrane during malarial parasite invasion and intra-erythrocyte development, in Malaria and the Red Cell. Ciba Foundation Symposium 94. London, John Wiley & Sons, Ltd.,1983

27. Bruce-Chwatt LJ: Essential Malariology. London, William Heinemann Medical Books, Ltd.,1980

28. Weatherall DJ: Common genetic disorders of the red cell and the 'malaria hypothesis.' Ann Trop Med Parasitol 81:539,1987

29. Benson LE et al: Entry of Bartonella bacilliformis into erythrocytes. Infect Immun 54:347,1986

30. Andre R et al: Deux observations d'anemie hemolytique aigue apres prise de phenyl-semi-carbazide. Remarques sur la poikilocytose et revue de la litterature. Nouv Rev Fr Hematol 5:431,1965

31. Rifkind RA: Heinz body anemia: an ultrastructural study. II. Red cell sequestration and destruction. Blood 26:433,1965

32. Jandl JH: Chapt 11, in Blood: Textbook of Hematology. Boston, Little, Brown and Company,1987

33. Brewer GJ et al: The hemolytic effect of primaquine. XV. Role of methemoglobin. J Lab Clin Med 59:905,1962

34. Valentine WN et al: Chapt 73, in The Metabolic Basis of Inherited Disease, 5th ed., Stanbury JB et al, Eds. New York, McGraw-Hill Book Company,1983

C H A P T E R

9

Abnormal Hemoglobins and Hemoglobinopathies

☐

More than 400 hemoglobin (Hb) variants of known structure have been characterized. Those with high gene frequencies and clinical impact were recognized first and assigned alphabetical initials signifying order of discovery (Hbs A, C, D, and E) or hematologic features (Hbs F, S, and M). As investigators realized that the alphabet would soon be exhausted, they named hemoglobins according to the patients' origin or hospital or on blithe impulse: playful names range from the chauvinistic (Hb Brigham and Hb Beth Israel) to the operatic (Hb Aïda). Although these colorful cognomens have stuck, more formal designations were devised which cite in order the variant chain, the sequential and helical number of the deviant amino acid, and the amino acid substitution. Hb S is designated $\beta6(A3)Glu{\rightarrow}Val$ or merely $\beta6\ Glu{\rightarrow}Val$: this shorthand notation signifies that glutamic acid has been replaced by valine at the sixth amino acid from the N-terminus (the third amino acid in the A helix) of the β chain.

Common Hb Variants and Their Detection

Most Hb variants can be identified provisionally if the results of electrophoresis in cellulose acetate and in citrate agar are combined with electrophoretic patterns of globin chains after denaturation in 6 M urea. Virtually all variants can be separated cleanly by the higher resolution achieved with isoelectric focusing on thin slabs of polyacrylamide gel. Definitive identification of mutant Hbs can be made by use of monoclonal antibodies, and radioimmune and immunoabsorbant assays have been automated for routine clinical use. The most common clinically important Hb variants are classified in Table 9-1 [1].

TABLE 9-1

Clinically important hemoglobin variants

I. The sickle syndromes
  A. Sickle cell trait
  B. Sickle cell disease
    1. SS
    2. SC
    3. SD$_{Los Angeles}$
    4. SO$_{Arab}$
    5. S/β-Thalassemia

II. The unstable hemoglobins → congenital Heinz body anemia (~ 90 variants)

III. Hemoglobins with abnormal oxygen affinity
  A. High affinity → familial erythrocytosis (~40 variants)
  B. Low affinity → familial cyanosis (Hbs Kansas, Beth Israel, St. Mandé)

IV. The M hemoglobins → familial cyanosis (6 variants)

V. Structural variants that result in a thalassemic phenotype
  A. β-Thalassemia phenotype
    1. Lepore hemoglobins ($\delta\beta$ fusion)
    2. Abnormal mRNA processing: Hbs E, Knossos
    3. Extreme instability: Hb Indianapolis
  B. α-Thalassemia phenotype
    1. Chain termination mutants: Hb Constant Spring
    2. Extreme instability: Hb Quong Sze

Source: From Bunn HF and Forget BG: Chapt 10, in Hemoglobin: Molecular, Genetic and Clinical Aspects. Philadelphia, WB Saunders Company,1986.

Genetic Mechanisms

Hb variants are inherited as autosomal codominants and 95% of these represent single amino acid substitutions in a globin chain, reflecting a single base change in the corresponding triplet codon of globin gene DNA. As was depicted in Figure 3-10, β chain genes are simple alleles located on the β chain coding region of the short arm of chromosome 11. Hence patterns of inheritance are most clearly demonstrated by β chain variants, for a single β chain gene is inherited from each parent. In accordance with classic mendelian genetics, if both parents are heterozygous for the β chain variant, Hb S, the offspring have a 50% chance of being heterozygous (sickle cell trait, or Hb AS), 25% will be normal (Hb AA), and 25% will have sickle cell disease (Hb SS). β-thal genes are also allelic to β chain structural genes, and children of parents, each of whom is heterozygous for Hb S or β-thal, have a 25% chance of being doubly heterozygous for Hb S and β-thal (Figure 9-1) [2].

In contrast to the β gene, the α genes, which are situated on chromosome 16, are reduplicated, equipping each diploid cell with four copies. The potential for genetic heterogeneity is proportionately great, as is illustrated by the quantitative depressing effect of α gene deletions in α-thal syndromes on the production of β chain variants in double heterozygotes (Table 9-2).

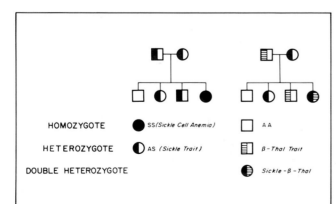

HOMOZYGOTE	● SS(Sickle Cell Anemia) □ AA
HETEROZYGOTE	◑ AS (Sickle Trait) ▤ β-Thal Trait
DOUBLE HETEROZYGOTE	◕ Sickle-β-Thal

FIGURE 9-1

Pedigrees showing inheritance of β chain alleles. Sickle cell anemia occurs in one of four offspring of parents both of whom have sickle cell trait (left). As shown on the right, one in four children of parents having β-thal trait and sickle cell trait, respectively, will be doubly heterozygous for both traits. (From Jandl JH: Chapt 13, in Blood: Textbook of Hematology. Boston, Little, Brown and Company,1987.)

TABLE 9-2

Effect of α-thal on the proportion of β chain variant in red cells from patients heterozygous for Hbs S, C, and E

	Average percent variant Hb in hemolysate		
α Chain genotype	AS	AC	AE
Normal ($\alpha\alpha/\alpha\alpha$)	41	44	30
$\alpha\alpha/\alpha-$	35	38	27
$\alpha-/\alpha-$ or $\alpha\alpha/--$	28	32	22
$\alpha-/--$ (Hb H)	17	—	15

Source: From Bunn HF and Forget BG: Hemoglobin: Molecular, Genetic and Clinical Aspects. Philadelphia, WB Saunders Company,1986.

HEMOGLOBIN S AND THE SICKLE CELL SYNDROMES

Hb S is the most prevalent and serious of abnormal Hbs. Inheritance of two β^S genes sentences most patients to a lifelong debilitating malady dominated by vasoocclusive crises and chronic hemolytic anemia.

Historically the β^S gene has been most concentrated in two primary regions of west central Africa: the overall β^S gene frequency in these primary regions is 0.14, indicating (in accordance with the Hardy-Weinberg law) that 24% of newborns are AS heterozygotes. The Hb S gene is also concentrated in Saudi Arabia and east central India. It has been spread extensively from Africa by migration to the Americas; the gene frequency among North and South American blacks is about 0.04 and prevalence of the AS and SS genotypes among American blacks is 8.60% and 0.14%, respectively. Whether the extensive geographic occurrence of sickle cell disease can be explained by a single origin of the mutation or whether it stemmed from multicentric origins has been examined by analysis of restriction fragment length polymorphisms (RFLPs) linked as haplotype packets to the β^S globin gene. The geographic distribution of β^S haplotypes in the Old World indicates that Hb S emanated from at least two separate seminal foci: a major

source centered in west Africa and the southwestern Arabian peninsula, and an independent Asian source centered in eastern Saudi Arabia and India and corresponding to a milder clinical phenotype [3].

The sustained high incidence of β^S genes in tropical and subtropical regions historically endemic for malaria is explained by the protective effect of Hb S against *P. falciparum* in heterozygotes (Chapter 8). Sickle cell trait is estimated to confer a 20% improvement in fitness during the first 5 years of life, a gain that more than offsets selection against the homozygous state. The protective effect of the sickle gene is a paradigm of balanced polymorphism; based on the calculated relative

FIGURE 9-2

(A) Electron micrograph of crystal growth in stirred solution of deoxy Hb S; the herringbone pattern is created by three adjacent antiparallel double strands of polymerized Hb S. (B) Electron density of a single double strand. Nubbins of increased density represent superimposition of α_2 and β_2 subunits. (From Bunn HF and Forget BG: Chapt 11, in Hemoglobin: Molecular, Genetic and Clinical Aspects. Philadelphia, WB Saunders Company,1986.)

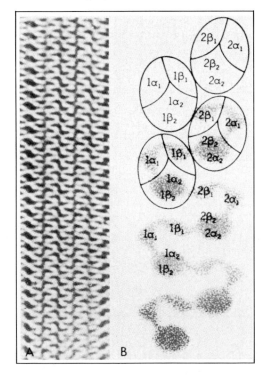

fitness conferred by the β^S gene, it has been estimated that a heterozygote frequency of about 32% would be reestablished within 40 generations (about 1,000 years) if the selection process in tropical Africa had to start anew [4].

PATHOPHYSIOLOGY

Polymerization of DeoxyHb S

Substitution of the hydrophobic valine residue for glutamate in the sixth position of the β chain permits intermolecular bonding of contiguous molecules when Hb S is in the deoxy conformation. Interaction between $\beta6$ valine residues with hydrophobic regions on neighboring β chains initiates intermolecular bonding

by other hydrophobic residues, strengthened by apposed electrostatic forces. Polymerization is initiated by homogeneous nucleation and proceeds with fiber growth to form stacks and then helical filaments which pair off in antiparallel fashion to form twisted double filaments (Figure 9-2) [5]. A growing rope of entwined double filaments is formed that eventually forms a cable composed of 14 densely packed strands (7 pairs of antiparallel polymers) that are gradually rotated about the core axis (Figure 9-3) [6]. With time the aligned 14-stranded polymers bundle together into macrofibers or fascicles—thick, ropey, rigid structures averaging 50 nm across, several μm long, and possessing a right-handed helical pitch of about 1 μm (Figure 9-4) [7]. The natural artistry of macrofibers is enhanced by entasis.

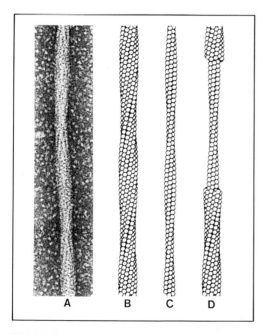

FIGURE 9-3

(A) Electron micrograph of negatively stained fiber of deoxy Hb S. (B, C, D) Reconstructed fibers represented in facsimile as ball models, each ball representing a Hb S tetramer. Models are presented as the outer sheath (B), inner core (C), and a combination of inner and outer filaments (D). (From Edelstein SJ: Structure of the fibers of hemoglobin S. Texas Rep Biol Med 40:221,1980.)

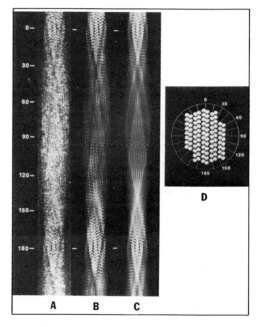

FIGURE 9-4

Images of macrofibers in lateral projection (A through C) and in cross-section (D). (A) Electron micrograph. (B) Fourier filtered image. (C) Computed model of macrofiber based on reconstructed cross-section and axial shift data. (D) Model of macrofiber cross-section with 0 to 180° projection angles. Scale at left indicates degrees of twist between two successive narrow regions 475 nm apart. (From Bluemke DA et al: Chapt X, in Pathophysiological Aspects of Sickle Cell Vaso-Occlusion, Nagel RL, Ed. New York, Alan R. Liss, Inc.,1987.)

Red Cell Sickling

The rate of initiation and growth of deoxyHb S polymers is exquisitely dependent upon Hb S concentration. The velocity of aggregation of deoxyHb S varies as the fifteenth power of Hb concentration, and when solutions of deoxyHb are concentrated above 20 g/dl, polymer growth propagates viscous paracrystalline arrays termed "tactoids." When the PO_2 in an intact red cell containing Hb S is reduced below a critical point, the earliest event is patchy aggregation (nucleation) of Hb. Within 1 or 2 seconds short polymers of Hb S are visible by EM, and simultaneously the Hb S undergoes sol:gel transformation and stiffening. These early pregelation steps occurring within 3 seconds cause vascular impedance and are capable of precipitating vasoocclusive crises. The formation of dense macroscopic bundles long enough to create the sickle-shaped deformity is a later event, consummated only after 1 to 2 minutes; sickling consolidates vascular obstruction, but gelation initiates the "vicious viscous sickle cycle." The relationship between kinetics of gelation, polymer formation, and red cell deformation of sickle cells are schematized in Figure 9-5 [8].

If obstructing wads of sickled cells are rammed through the microvasculature by arteriolar pressure, they are reoxygenated and most strands depolymerize within a few seconds. Recovery of cell shape lags behind depolymerization, however, and sustained or rapidly repeated hypoxic sickling subjects the membrane to bending forces that loosen the cytoskeletal assembly, causing shedding of membrane vesicles and clustering of glycophorins into sticky patches. Prolonged hypoxic exposure increases the leak rate for cations with a net loss of cell water and desiccation that is intensified by a volume-dependent K^+

FIGURE 9-5

Kinetics of gelation and morphology of sickle cells following various rates of deoxygenation. (A) Dependence of delay time in polymer formation on concentration of Hb S. (B, C, D) Kinetic progress curves for samples having different delay times. As shown in the schematics on the right, a slow rate of polymerization causes formation of well-aligned fibers growing out from a single domain to form the classic "sickle deformity." In more rapidly polymerizing cells numerous smaller domains of short aligned fibers form to create a "holly leaf" pattern. If deoxygenation is instantaneous large numbers of tiny domains form randomly oriented short fibers, generating a rigid "granular" discoid cell. (From Eaton WA and Hofrichter J: Hemoglobin S gelation and sickle cell disease. Blood 70:1245,1987.)

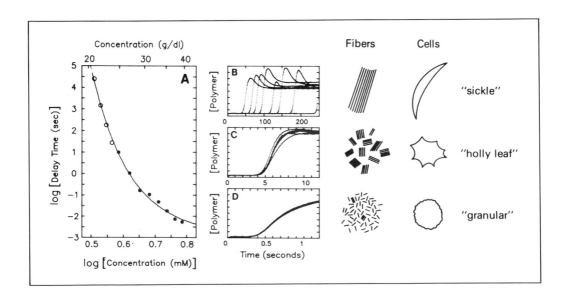

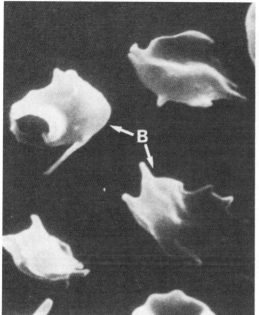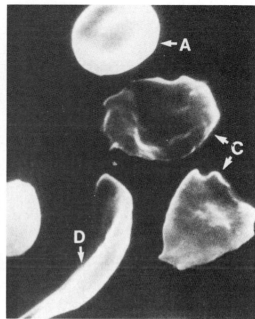

FIGURE 9-6

Scanning EMs of deoxygenated red cells from a patient with sickle cell anemia portray several major subpopulations. (A) A cell rich in Hb F is protected from sickling and retains a smooth discoid shape. (B) Reversibly sickled cells have multiple sharp spicules. (C) Dense unsickleable cells are irregularly contracted and show granular contours. (D) Irreversibly sickled cells appear flattened, fusiform, and fishlike. (From Kaul DK et al: Vaso-occlusion by sickle cells: evidence for selective trapping of dense red cells. Blood 68:1162,1986.)

transport mechanism unique to Hb S (and Hb C) red cells. Hb polymerization is potentiated, the initial delay phase of sol:gel transformation is shortened, and the dense, desiccated product is transformed into an irreversibly sickled cell (ISC) incapable of recovery despite reoxygenation (Figure 9-6) [9]. ISCs are more rigid than normal but not sufficiently to cause them to lodge in systemic capillaries when oxygenated. Cellular dehydration is primarily responsible for the rigidity of the intact cells and induces rhythmic oscillations in flow velocity through capillary beds that are likely to initiate episodes of vasoocclusion. Cells that enter the microcirculation containing partly polymerized Hb S will cause vasoocclusion only if deoxygenation occurs rapidly and passage is delayed beyond about 3 seconds; after that the deoxygenated and deformed cell, however rigid, is at liberty to commute back to the lungs and regain its supple shape.

Hb F Blocks Sickling

DeoxyHb S molecules copolymerize with (in decreasing order) Hbs C, D, O-Arab, A, J, and F. Hb F is not excluded from Hb S polymers, but its inclusion blocks further polymer growth. Inhibition of polymer growth by Hb F is due to its incorporation in an orientation *trans* to the subunit having the hydrophobic $\beta 6$ contact site. Coexistence of Hb F with Hb S in red cells of patients with sickle cell anemia ameliorates severity of the disease in direct proportion to the concentration of Hb F and to the extent Hb F is distributed uniformly among red cells. Concentrations of Hb F in excess of 10% protect against end-organ damage (stroke or avascular necrosis), and the episodic painful crises and pulmonary complications of sickle cell anemia are prevented by Hb F levels of 20% or more. The doubly heterozygous state for Hb S plus HPFH is harmless despite Hb S concentrations of 70% because fetal Hb is evenly allocated among red cells (pancellular distribution). Hb F levels are haplotype-linked, accounting for differences in the severity of Hb S disease among individuals with mild but comparable elevations of Hb F. In most individuals a subpopulation of red cells denoted "F cells" persists as a relic of fetal erythropoiesis, and in anemic patients this subpopulation may expand and provide partial protection against vascular occlusion. Several protocols have been devised (on shaky premises) to encourage the production of Hb F by administering cytotoxic drugs (azacytidine and later hydroxyurea) to patients with sickle cell anemia: significant rises in Hb F have been induced, but stimulation of γ chain synthesis has been confined to the amplified F cell population, with no overall S to F switching. This is analogous to exchange transfusing a sickle cell patient with Hb F–rich cells, and clinical benefit is unlikely unless heterocellular Hb F levels can be maintained above 20% [10].

Sickle Cell Trait

In sickle cell trait, the heterozygous state for the β^A and β^S genes, each red cell contains both Hbs A and S in proportions averaging 60% and 40%. Ordinarily sickle trait is innocuous because AS cells do not sickle until O_2 saturation falls below 40%, a level found only beyond the narrows of the microcirculation. Although the AS phenotype is not associated with any acknowledged actuarial disadvantage, sickle cell trait may be associated with an increased risk of unexplained sudden death accompanying strenuous physical exertion [11] and with an increased morbidity from renal papillary necrosis.

Diagnosis and Screening Tests

Sickle cell trait individuals have normal blood counts, and red cell morphology is normal or shows a sparse scattering of target forms. Diagnosis can be made by combined use of a sickling test using sodium metabisulfite plus either Hb electrophoresis or thin-layer isoelectric focusing on acrylamide gel. To be effective and accepted, screening programs must be coupled with educational programs and with care to ensure confidentiality. A major purpose of screening programs is to make genetic counseling available to adolescents and young adults at risk.

Sickle Cell Anemia

The natural history of homozygous sickle cell anemia (Hb SS disease) is characterized by the triad of chronic hemolytic anemia, vasoocclusive crises, and vulnerability to infection. The most commanding and disheartening of these are the vasoocclusive crises, which gradually consume the patient, organ by organ, through the destructive and debilitating effects of cumulative infarctions.

Chronic hemolytic anemia   Chronic hemolytic anemia is fully expressed within 3 to 6 months, and moderate to severe anemia—punctuated by spells of aplastic crises—persists for life. Blood Hb concentrations average 8 ± 2 g/dl, and blood smears reveal fusiform, crescentic, and cigar-shaped ISCs amidst a larger mixture of target forms and polychromatophils (Figure 9-7). Numerous ISCs in the absence of microcytosis rule out the most common simulators of sickle cell anemia: Hb S-β-thal; Hb S-Lepore; and Hb SC disease. Hemolytic anemia can be severe in patients with very low levels of Hb F, particularly during early childhood when the spleen is transiently enlarged and may even foment splenic sequestration crises; thereafter the spleen is destroyed by infarction ("autosplenectomy") and less volatile hepatic sequestration predominates.

In the steady state, anemic hypoxia does not dominate the disease. Ironically, patients who maintain relatively high concentrations of hemoglobin (Hb levels above 8.5 g/dl) are most subject to the wracking torment of painful crises.

Acute Vasoocclusive Syndromes

Acute episodes of musculoskeletal pain and organ infarction caused by vascular destruction due to sickled cells persecute victims of sickle cell anemia with relentless repetition. In their lifelong calendar of suffering, sickle cell patients must endure an assortment of maladies so various as to defy generalization.

Painful crises   Acute, episodic, spreading musculoskeletal pain is the most prominent and pitiful symptomatic manifestation of sickle

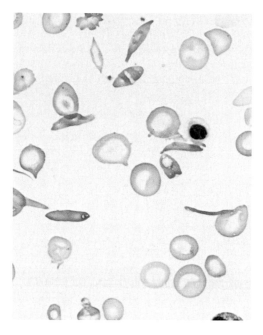

FIGURE 9-7

Blood smear in sickle cell anemia. Eye-catching crescentic and cigar-shaped ISCs are commingled with target forms, teardrops, and large smooth polychromatophils. Hypochromia of target cells is illusory, reflecting dense packing of the poorly soluble Hb S. Note the nucleated red cell, an indicator of splenic inactivity. (Photo by CT Kapff.)

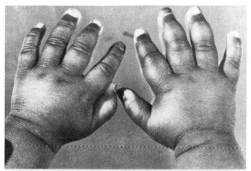

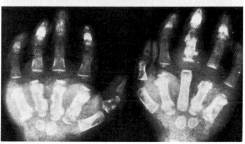

FIGURE 9-8

Dactylitis in an infant with sickle cell anemia. (Above) Both hands are tensely swollen, reddened, and very tender. (Below) By radiogram soft tissue swelling, areas of bone destruction, and regions of new bone formation are evident. The hand bones are floating in edema. (From Serjeant GR: Sickle Cell Disease. Oxford, Oxford University Press,1985; and Bohrer SP: Bone changes in the extremities in sickle cell anemia. Semin Roentgenol 22:176,1987.)

cell anemia and accounts for most hospital admissions. In children, attacks commonly are associated with infections, but in adults most painful crises are unheralded and unexplained. Painful crises appear to represent spells of muscular ischemia initiated by plugging of arteriolar beds by entangled sickled cells, but no anatomic or metabolic basis for their surging, tidal nature has been elucidated. In adult patients with less than 2% Hb F, mild bouts of short duration may occur every few weeks or months, interspersed with agonizing attacks lasting 5 to 10 days: the average adult "sickler" suffers about 4 severe attacks yearly. Many patients develop a tranquil stoicism that helps them pull through these punishing spells without becoming drug dependent; others are demoralized by these unpredictable attacks

and are unable to complete schooling or hold jobs.

Hand-foot syndrome The usual prelude to painful crises in sickle cell disease is the hand-foot syndrome, a form of dactylitis that damages the small bones of hands and feet. Dactylitis usually strikes within the first 24 months of life, when blood supply to growing bones is marginal. The typical triad is fever, pallor, and symmetrical swelling of hands and feet (Figure 9-8) [12, 13].

Bone and joint crises Bone or joint crises occur sporadically throughout life; most frequently involved sites are the marrow of the humerus, tibia, and femur. Acute bone infarction must be differentiated from acute osteomyelitis—particularly salmonella osteomyeli-tis, which is similarly prone to extend to multiple sites in long bones. Infarction of vertebral arteries damages the central weight-bearing growth plates, which demineralize and soften. The intervertebral discs are forc-ibly pressed into the bodies, which acquire a fishmouth or "H" deformity evident on anteroposterior radiologic views.

The proximal epiphyses of the femurs are highly vulnerable to ischemic damage because blood supply to the femoral head depends solely on the end artery of the ligamentum capitis femoris. Aseptic (avascular) necrosis is the major cause of crippling in adult sicklers. The femoral head becomes flattened as it collapses and is jammed into the joint space (Figure 9-9).

FIGURE 9-9

Advanced aseptic (avascular) necrosis of the femoral head in an adult man with sickle cell anemia. The joint is impacted and fused, the femoral neck is angulated, and gross coarsening of the trabeculae and radiolucent patches are ap-parent. (From Jandl JH: Chapt 13, in Blood: Textbook of Hematology. Boston, Little, Brown and Company,1987.)

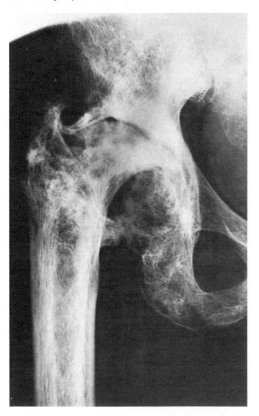

Neurologic damage   Vascular occlusions by sickled cells, possibly in conjunction with pro-gressive endothelial proliferation and secon-dary thrombosis, are capable of causing sei-zures, transient ischemic attacks, and abrupt cerebral aberrations, the most feared of which is stroke. Children are particularly prone to cerebral infarction; the majority survive but most of these will have recurrent strokes with permanent motor disabilities and IQs of less than 70. This melancholy progression can be forestalled by using transfusion therapy to improve cerebral rheology. Stroke had been underdiagnosed in sickle cell disease until the advent of MR imaging, which reveals lesions inapparent on CT scanning (Figure 9-10) [14].

Genitourinary complications   Red cells per-fusing the renal medulla are subjected to a low pO_2, acid pH, and hypertonicity, a milieu uniquely conducive to dehydration of sickle cells and polymerization of sickle hemoglobin. The consequences of vasoocclusion within the vasa rectae system include impairment of renal tubular concentrating function, ischemia of the medullary papillae, and almost complete oblit-eration of the fine vessel system (Figure 9-11) [12]. Sludged, sickled cells are highly destruc-tive to the renal medulla, and among their many trials Hb SS patients are prone to suffer bouts of gross hematuria caused by papillary necrosis with cavitation. Bleeding from ulcer-ated papillary infarcts may be a recurrent problem, sometimes necessitating transfusion, in patients with sickle cell trait as well as those with homozygous disease. Frank renal failure preceded by a nephrotic syndrome is uncom-mon but unrelenting and can only be corrected by renal transplantation.

Recurrent attacks of priapism are common, mortifying, and sometimes so excruciating that needle aspiration of the congested corpora may be required to achieve detumescence.

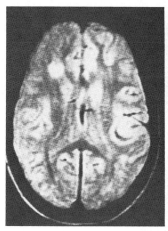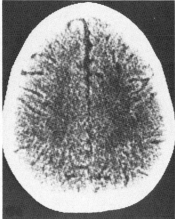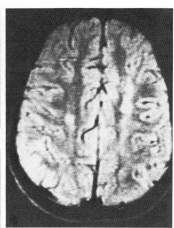

FIGURE 9-10

Bilateral deep infarcts of cerebral white matter in a 6-year-old patient with sickle cell anemia and sudden right monoparesis. (Center panel) Axial CT shows no abnormality. Axial MR imaging shows deep white matter infarcts involving left frontal lobe (left panel) and right parietal lobe (right panel). (From Zimmerman RA et al: MRI of sickle cell cerebral infarction. Neuroradiology 29:232,1987.)

Pulmonary and cardiovascular damage Pulmonary crises (acute chest syndrome) usually start with pulmonary infarctions that commonly become infected secondarily. With time, multiple lung infarctions cause pulmonary congestion, and intrapulmonary shunting creates a serious ventilation-perfusion mismatch with resultant arterial hypoxemia. This morbid collusion of forces hostile to cardiopulmonary function ushers in the final phase of cardiac failure.

Every organ is at risk in sickle cell disease and included in the legion of afflictions are

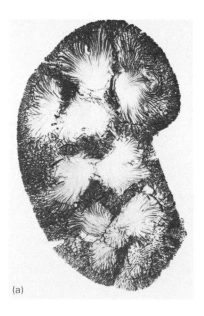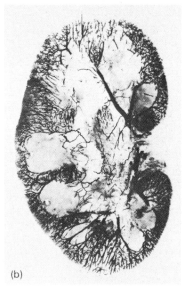

(a) (b)

FIGURE 9-11

Microradioangiographic comparison of normal renal vascular pattern (a) and the grossly abnormal vasculature in a 15-year-old patient with sickle cell anemia (b). Vascular occlusions in (b) have obliterated the vasa rectae system. (From Serjeant GR: Sickle Cell Disease. Oxford, Oxford University Press,1985.)

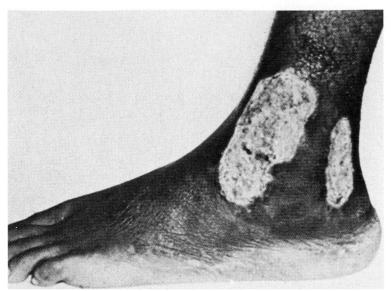

FIGURE 9-12

Characteristic deep un-
dermining leg ulcers in
a young adult man with
sickle cell anemia.
(From Barnhart MI et
al: Sickle Cell. A Scope
Publication. Kalama-
zoo, The Upjohn Com-
pany,1976.)

abdominal (visceral) infarctions, hepatic crises, pigment gallstones, retinopathy, and glaucoma. Ulcerations of the skin over the malleoli and distal portions of the leg are among the most galling and common complications of sickle cell anemia, occurring in 75% of patients at some time in their lives. Leg ulcers are unusually obstinate, tending to spread and erode deeply as long as the patient is ambulatory (Figure 9-12) [15]. Deep, infected, stubborn ulcerations that threaten to encircle the leg may yield only to a combination of plastic surgery and transfusions sufficient to lower the Hb S proportion below 50%.

Management

Treatment of sickle cell anemia and related syndromes is primarily palliative, and particular measures have been noted briefly in context with the various individual problems. There is no specific prophylaxis against painful crises or anemic crisis apart from the mixed blessings of narcotics and transfusions. Rational therapies under investigation include use of agents that inhibit Hb S polymerization, manipulation of osmolality, and chemotherapeutic efforts to activate the S to F switch. None of these has had lasting success at this writing.

Marrow transplantation carries more risk than the disease, but in time this procedure may become the therapy of choice for managing the most severely affected patients.

Prevention

If both marital partners are known to be AS heterozygotes, they may elect to avoid the 25% chance that any of their offspring will have sickle cell disease. This is a charged and sensitive issue, and the counselor must present pertinent information in such a manner that prospective parents can make a rational decision, free of guilt. An important aid in dealing with this critical dilemma is the availability of unequivocal antenatal testing.

As noted in Chapter 3, two restriction enzymes (*Mst* II and *Dde* I) cleave normal DNA specifically at the normal β6 Glu site but fail to cut the β6 Val site of β^S DNA (Figure 3-24). Two tactics have been perfected that permit rapid identification of the fetal β globin genotype on samples of fetal amniocytes containing less than 1μg of genomic DNA. The first involves a primer-mediated enzymatic amplification through the polymerase chain reaction of specific β globin target sequences. In the second stage, β^A and β^S alleles are identified directly by use of end-labeled synthetic oligonucleotide probes. Gene analysis of fetal DNA can be performed within 16 weeks of gestation by amniocyte analysis and within 10 weeks by biopsy of chorionic villi.

Doubly Heterozygous Sickling Disorders

Several doubly heterozygous states for the β^S gene and other structural genes involving the β gene locus feature to some degree the stigmata of sickle cell anemia. The most prevalent of these are Hb SC disease and Hb S–β-thalassemia.

Hemoglobin SC Disease

Hb SC disease is caused by inheritance of a Hb S gene from one parent and a Hb C gene that codes for the $\beta6$ Glu $\rightarrow$ Lys mutation from the other. Hb SC disease resembles mild sickle cell anemia. Life expectancy is shortened only slightly and vasoocclusive complications are less frequent and less disabling. Aseptic necrosis of the femoral head and renal medullary infarctions are about half as common. In contrast to Hb SS disease, splenomegaly is usually prominent in Hb SC disease and persists into adulthood in about 60% of patients. Hemolytic anemia is moderate, and red cell indices are normal except for a slight but influential rise in MCHC. Red cells appear dense on smear, about half are targeted, and some contain rhomboidal crystals of Hb. Hb SC is diagnosed by Hb electrophoresis, which reveals about equal amounts of Hb S and the slower-moving Hb C, which comigrates with Hbs E and O-Arab.

Hb S–β-Thalassemia

The most common cause of the sickle syndrome in patients of Mediterranean descent is double heterozygosity for Hb S and β-thal (microdrepanocytic or sickle–β-thal disease). In black Americans Hb S–β-thal has a gene frequency of about 0.01. Hemolytic anemia is generally severe and patients may experience the entire gamut of sickling disabilities. Unlike Hb SS disease, splenomegaly is prominent and persistent, accounting for the paucity of ISCs in unsplenectomized patients. The blood smears show marked hypochromia, microcytosis, tar-

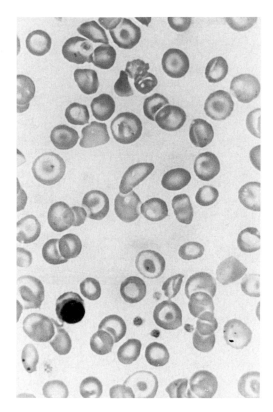

FIGURE 9-13

Blood smear in Hb S–β-thal disease is dominated by hypochromia, microcytosis, and conspicuous targeting, but small numbers of crescentic (rarely full-fledged ISCs) are the clue to diagnosis. The nucleated red cell, Howell-Jolly bodies, and large platelets intimate prior splenectomy. (Photo by CT Kapff.)

geting, teardrop deformities, basophilic stippling, and very occasional elongated cells (Figure 9-13).

About 90% of doubly heterozygous patients have Hb S–β^+-thal; as some Hb A is produced in this variant, the finding of 10 to 30% Hb A in a sickler with splenomegaly and thalassemic morphology virtually clinches the diagnosis. The differentiation of Hb SS disease and Hb S–β^0-thal is more difficult, because Hbs S, F, and A_2 account for all the Hb in both disorders. The issue is resolved most simply by family studies, for one parent will have sickle cell trait and the other β-thal minor.

Hemoglobin C Disease

Hb C (β6 Glu → Lys) occurs almost solely in blacks, the mutant structural gene having originated in Northern Ghana and nearby Upper Volta regions. In the Western hemisphere Hb C is second only to Hb S; among black Americans 2.4% are heterozygous for Hb AC and 0.02% have Hb CC disease.

Patients homozygous for Hb C have mild hemolytic anemia and splenomegaly but are spared the calamities of sickling or thalassemia. As in all chronic hemolytic disorders, aplastic crises and pigment gallstones may occur, but growth, vitality, and fertility are uncompromised.

Hemolysis of Hb C red cells in the spleen is the synergic consequence of two processes that render the cells rigid in the oxygenated state. Hb C is much less soluble than Hb A, forming crystals at Hb concentrations in excess of 35 g/dl. The diminished solubility of liganded Hb C is explained by the fact that three of the four β6 lysines of the mutant molecules engage in stable intermolecular contacts that rapidly generate platelike crystals; these form two-dimensional sheets that stack into decks like playing cards. Unlike Hb S polymers, Hb C crystals are formed of oxyHb; the crystals melt when the cells become deoxygenated, which aids their escape from the microcirculation. Hb C would probably not cause a disease were it not for the complicit activity of a unique K^+ pumping pathway that expels cation and water and so desiccates the cells, promoting precipitation of the poorly soluble Hb. Circulating cells appear small, shrivelled, darkly spheroidal, and boldly targeted. The singular appearance of octahedral Hb C crystals thinly cloaked by membrane seals the morphologic diagnosis (Figure 9-14). Desiccation stiffens Hb C cells and ordains their conditioning and eventual entrapment within splenic cords.

Diagnosis is established by the finding that Hb C accounts for most red cell Hb, Hb A being absent. Splenectomy is unnecessary except in patients with ruptured spleens, for the modest anemia is largely counterbalanced by a rightward shift in the O_2 dissociation curve.

Hemoglobin E Disease

Hb E (β26 Glu → Lys), the second most prevalent Hb variant, originated in Southeast Asia, where an estimated 30 million inhabitants are heterozygous for Hb E and 1 million have Hb E disease. This high prevalence in Southeast Asians implies that the E variant somehow improves fitness, but it does not do so by protecting against *P. falciparum*. Hb E is now a common variant in the United States as the result of resettlement in the aftermath of consecutive wars and other disasters.

Hb E disease is mechanistically analogous to β^+-thal, for the base substitution at codon 26 introduces a faulty splicing mechanism resulting in unstable mRNA and deficient synthesis of unstable β^E subunits. The result of these additive processing errors is an imbalance in α:β biosynthetic ratios. Hb E disease causes a mild symptomless anemia having little or no ill effects on health or longevity. The red cells are very small (av. MCV: 67 fl) and display uniform targeting (Figure 9-15). Absence of symptoms in this mildly hemolytic disorder is ex-

FIGURE 9-14

Myriads of small, boldly targeted red cells in the company of pyknotic spherocytes, some of which appear cracked, are characteristic of Hb C disease. The presence of an occasional brick-shaped Hb crystal (upper right) is pathognomonic. (Photo by CT Kapff.)

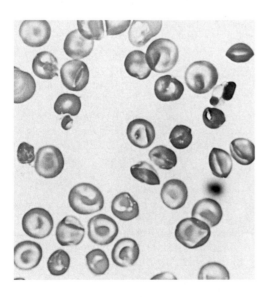

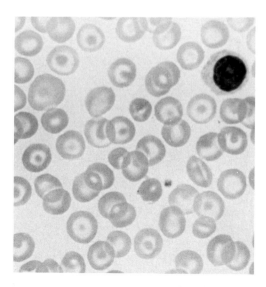

FIGURE 9-15

Monotonous microcytosis and targeting characteristic of Hb E disease. Smallness of the red cells is evident by comparison with the lymphocyte nucleus at upper right. (Photo by CT Kapff.)

plained by the right-shifted O_2 dissociation curve, which favors O_2 unloading to tissues.

REFERENCES

1. Bunn HF and Forget BG: Chapt 10, in Hemoglobin: Molecular, Genetic and Clinical Aspects. Philadelphia, WB Saunders Company,1986

2. Jandl JH: Chapt 13, in Blood: Textbook of Hematology. Boston, Little, Brown and Company,1987

3. Kulozik AE et al: Geographical survey of β^s-globin haplotypes: evidence for an independent Asian origin of the sickle-cell mutation. Am J Hum Genet 39:239,1986

4. Vogel F and Motulsky AG: Chapt 6, in Human Genetics. Problems and Approaches, 2d ed. Berlin, Springer-Verlag,1986

5. Bunn HF and Forget BG: Chapt 11, in Hemoglobin: Molecular, Genetic and Clinical Aspects. Philadelphia, WB Saunders Company,1986

6. Edelstein SJ: Structure of the fibers of hemoglobin S. Texas Rep Biol Med 40:221,1980

7. Bluemke DA et al: The three-dimensional structure of sickle hemoglobin macrofibers, in Pathophysiological Aspects of Sickle Cell Vaso-Occlusion. Nagel RL, Ed. New York, Alan R. Liss, Inc.,1987

8. Eaton WA and Hofrichter J: Hemoglobin S gelation and sickle cell disease. Blood 70: 1245,1987

9. Kaul DK et al: Vaso-occlusion by sickle cells: evidence for selective trapping of dense red cells. Blood 68:1162,1986

10. Noguchi CT et al: Levels of fetal hemoglobin necessary for treatment of sickle cell disease. N Engl J Med 318:96,1988

11. Kark JA et al: Sickle-cell trait as a risk factor for sudden death in physical training. N Engl J Med 317:781,1987

12. Serjeant GR: Chapt 16, in Sickle Cell Disease. New York, Oxford University Press,1985

13. Bohrer SP: Bone changes in the extremities in sickle cell anemia. Semin Roentgenol 22:176,1987

14. Zimmerman RA et al: MRI of sickle cell cerebral infarction. Neuroradiology 29:232, 1987

15. Barnhart MI et al: Sickle Cell. Kalamazoo, The Upjohn Company,1976.

10

Granulocytes

☐

Granulocytes are a picturesque family of mobile endstage cells formed by unipotential colony forming units (CFUs) in marrow. Specific glycoprotein hormones—the colony stimulating factors (CSFs) elaborated by macrophages, vascular endothelium, and T cells—direct low-echelon stem cells to generate either neutrophils, eosinophils, or basophils. The steady state is dependent on the idling rate set by master control molecules such as IL-3, which are secreted locally at low levels by marrow endothelium and fibroblasts. Most CSF genes are quiescent until they receive a signal from T cells that have been activated by intrusive antigens or toxins. Under the alert guidance of the T cell network, antigen-aroused lymphocytes prod macrophages into generating tumor necrosis factor (TNF) and IL-1, and these cytokines in turn trigger production of GM-CSF, G-CSF, and M-CSF by marrow macrophages and by peripheral populations of endothelial and mesenchymal cells [1]. The release of this barrage of CSFs has a broad range of clonogenic potential as the result of differences in surface receptor numbers on the individual subsets of granulocyte progenitors. The main agitators in the acute inflammatory response are the cytokines, GM-CSF and G-CSF, and their main function is to generate and mobilize neutrophils. Neutrophils are the infantry of host defense. They guard the barriers, police the barricades, and fling themselves on noxious invaders. Neutrophils are suicide troops; in fulfilling their mission to search and destroy, they are expendable.

MATURATION AND MORPHOLOGY

Neutrophils, eosinophils, and basophils arise from similar cytokinetic patterns of proliferation, differentiation, and division. They differ greatly in relative numbers and in their assigned functions. The turnover and production rate for neutrophils is prodigious (16×10^8/kg/24 h), lifespan is brief ($t_{1/2} = 7$ h), and their task is to patrol the bloodstream and barrier tissues and to congregate at sites of infection. Eosinophils are produced and destroyed at about 1% this rate, and their mission is to leave the bloodstream at first opportunity to search out entrenched deep-tissue antigens. Basophils are the least common of the granulocyte family, representing less than 0.1% of nucleated blood cells, and their defensive role is somewhat enigmatic. Presentation of the morphologic sequence in granulocyte generation is restricted here to an explication of neutrophil formation.

Morphology of the Myeloid Pedigree

Maturation and division of proliferating myeloid cells are associated with stepwise reductions in nuclear and cellular volume, progressive condensation of chromatin into inactive heterochromatin, and the sequential appearance of prominent primary (azurophilic) granules and small secondary (specific) granules.

The first three generations in the myeloid pedigree are the myeloblasts, promyelocytes, and myelocytes. Later myeloid stages cannot divide but continue to differentiate into morphologically distinctive forms: this postmitotic sequence consists of metamyelocytes, band form neutrophils, and segmented neutrophils.

The Myeloid Mitotic Compartment

The youngest identifiable progeny of the CFU-Gs are the myeloblasts. Myeloblasts are medium-sized cells, having large slightly oblong nuclei surrounded eccentrically by a thin rim of blue cytoplasm. Most myeloblast nuclei contain two or more pale punched-out nucleoli. Emergence of coarse red-purple primary granules and cytoplasmic expansion signify graduation to the promyelocyte stage, during which nucleoli begin to fade and nuclear chromatin grows increasingly granular. Toward the conclusion of the promyelocyte stage, synthesis of primary granules ceases and the first small secondary granules appear. The myelocyte stage is marked by an accumulation of secondary granules, which impart a blush to the belly of the cell as the nucleus is displaced, reduced, and slightly flattened (Figure 10-1).

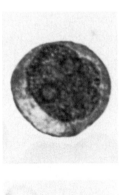
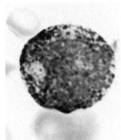
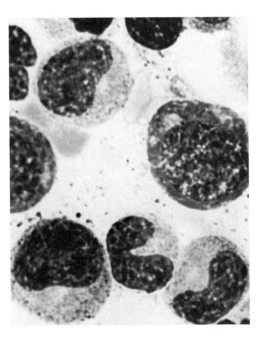

FIGURE 10-1

A triptych of early myeloid forms. (Upper left) Normal marrow myeloblast. (Lower left) Normal marrow promyelocyte. (Right) The two large cells on the left with granular cytoplasm are myelocytes at different levels of maturation, in the company of two smaller metamyelocytes (below) having deeply indented nuclei. The large, dark agranular cell (right center) is a basophilic erythroblast. (Photo by CT Kapff.)

The Myeloid Postmitotic Compartment

The issue of terminal myelocyte division is the metamyelocyte, a smaller cell with a gently indented or bean-shaped nucleus, lacking nucleoli, that is embedded eccentrically in finely mottled pink cytoplasm. Nuclear condensation leads to a cell known as the band form (or less aptly the "stab" form) that has achieved its final dimensions and possesses a sausage- or horseshoe-shaped nucleus. Nuclear chromatin is aggregated into heavy clumps, and the specific granules now outnumber the larger darker primary granules by 10 to 1. Band forms are the youngest neutrophils found in normal blood, constituting 1 to 5% of the differential white cell count. The end product of myeloid maturation-division is the segmented neutrophil, recognized readily by the assembly of nuclear chromatin into about three (two to five) lobes strung together in series by short filaments of chromatin. The predominant secondary granules are so fine and dispersed that only a faint lilac freckling may be apparent on Wright-Giemsa stain, and few if any primary granules remain. Nuclear segmentation of polymorphonuclear neutrophils ("polys" in laboratory idiom) is artfully designed to enable these mobile defenders to worm their way through endothelial gaps in response to chemo-attractant signals emanating from troubled tissues (Figure 10-2).

Eosinophils

Eosinophils cannot be differentiated from neutrophil precursors by light microscopy until they reach the myelocyte stage. Eosinophil granules are much larger than those of neutrophils and appear as refractile red-orange chunks on Wright-Giemsa–stained smears. By EM the granules are seen to contain a dense crystalloid core embedded in a peroxidase-positive matrix (Figure 10-3) [2].

Eosinophils are motivated to divide, differentiate, and become reactive by the 36,000 M_r dimer, IL-5, alias Eo-CSF; their principal targets are persistent antigens on alien objects too large to engulf. Eosinophils are armed with receptors for epitopes of the Fc region of IgG and IgE and for complement components. Release by macrophages, mast cells, and platelets of eosinophil chemotactic factor of anaphylaxis and of prostaglandins D_2 and E_2 lures eosinophils into deep inflammatory sites, inciting hypersensitivity reactions. Eosinophils participate very early in antigen recognition, accumulating in local lymph nodes within minutes to hours after sensing antigen, and they become reactively phagocytic and cytotoxic in the presence of antibody and chemotactic components of complement, particularly C5a. When, as in the case of schistosomes, the sheer bulk of antibody-coated invaders precludes phagocytosis, eosinophils flatten against the object and fire a fusillade of granules rich in hydrolytic enzymes. This nautical strike is most effective against large foreign structures in the presence of complement and T cell–derived perforins (Figure 10-4). When eosinophilic inflammatory reactions are intense and protracted, as occurs in chronic allergic and parasitic diseases, the site of battle becomes

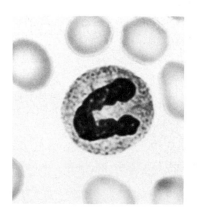 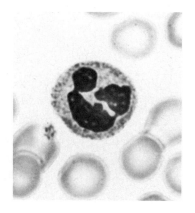

FIGURE 10-2

(Left) Horseshoe-shaped nucleus characteristic of a normal band form neutrophil. (Right) Normal three-lobed mature neutrophil. The terminal lobes are characteristically asymmetric, one being ovoid and the other scalloped. (Photo by CT Kapff.)

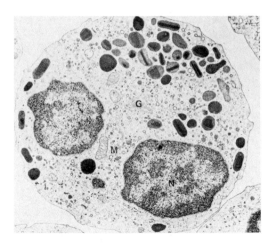

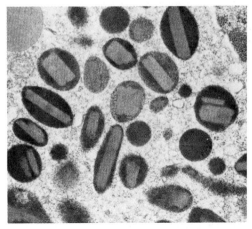

FIGURE 10-3

EMs of normal mature eosinophils. (Left) Low-power view reveals typical two-lobed nucleus (N), Golgi body (G), and mitochondria (M). Most granules display a central crystalloid. (Right) At higher power the biconvex lozenge shape of the granules is shown to result from squeezing of the matrix by the expanded planar crystal. (From Zucker-Franklin D: Eosinophil function and disorders, in Stollerman GH et al, Eds. Advances in Internal Medicine, Volume 19. Copyright © 1974 by Year Book Medical Publishers, Inc., Chicago.)

littered with needle-shaped and hexagonal bipyramidal bodies (Charcot-Leyden crystals) composed of crystalline lysophospholipase.

Basophils

Basophils are descended from the bipotent progenitor of both eosinophils and basophils. Like eosinophils, newborn basophils circulate briefly before they migrate into barrier tissues such as skin, mucosa, and serosa, where they play a role in immediate hyersensitivity reac-

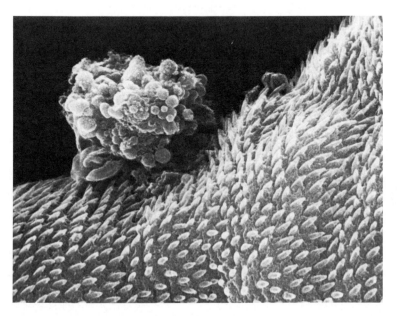

FIGURE 10-4

An intrepid David assaulting a spiny Goliath. Scanning EM of an eosinophil adhering to the surface of a larval schistosome that had been coated with IgE and IgG antibodies. Within 2 minutes the eosinophil had started to degranulate, discharging cytotoxic enzymes into its heavily armored enemy. (Photo courtesy of JD Caulfield.)

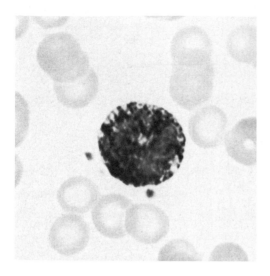

FIGURE 10-5

Normal blood basophil. The coarse metachromatic granules obscure the lumpy shape of the large, lobular (usually unsegmented) nucleus. (Photo by CT Kapff.)

tions. Basophils are readily distinguished from other granulocytes by their cargo of huge purple-black granules (Figure 10-5).

The prominent cytoplasmic granules of basophils—and of their distant, sessile cousins of connective tissue, the tissue mast cells—contain an arsenal of phlogistic mediators of acute inflammation, including histamine, serotonin, leukotrienes (the slow reactive substances of anaphylaxis), plasminogen activator, and an assortment of proteases. Basophils and mast cells are equipped with receptors for the Fc domain of IgE. If IgE molecules attached to the membrane are bridged by specific antigens, the cells degranulate, discharging histamine and other granular contents that provoke many of the manifestations of immediate hypersensitivity reactions; among these are anaphylaxis, urticaria, allergic rhinitis, and certain kinds of bronchial asthma.

NEUTROPHIL FUNCTIONS

Neutrophils form the front line of host defense and are the first cells to arrive at sites of pyogenic infection. In an acute inflammatory response, neutrophils adhere to and crawl over the luminal surface of endothelial cells, eel their way between and through the leaflets of the endothelium, and move through connective tissue toward the site of damage. Having arrived and stopped moving, neutrophils then engage in phagocytosis or secrete hydrolytic enzymes to digest large foreign objects. The first stages of this complex response require changes in shape, orientation, adhesiveness, and motor properties; the late stages are marked by explosive metabolic activation. At each step, neutrophil responses are governed by graded interactions between soluble or particulate ligands and various membrane receptors.

Receptors and Transduction Mechanisms

Neutrophils require much more sophisticated control systems than, for example, neurones, which stay in one place and make yes-or-no responses to familiar signals. In responding to urgent chemical messages emanating from remote inflammatory sites, neutrophils must undertake a voyage analogous to driving to work in Boston during rush hour—an exquisite test of signal-response coupling. In general, the binding of ligand molecules to receptors initiates enzymatic reactions that modify effector molecules such as cytoskeletal and contractile proteins or the NADPH oxidase enzyme complex responsible for the so-called "respiratory burst." In the case of the best-studied chemotactic peptides, occupancy of formylated tripeptide receptors leads to sequential modification of a G-protein, phospholipase C, and one or more types of protein kinase (Chapter 1). Calcium is redistributed by activation and inactivation of calcium channels and calcium binding proteins. Phosphorylation of effector molecules by protein kinase C alters their conformational state and enzymatic activity, enabling them to direct cell behavior. Low levels of the formylated tripeptide, formyl-methionyl-leucyl-phenylalanine (fMLP) elicit shape changes, alter the G/F-actin equilibrium, and stimulate directional movement, whereas high concentrations trigger metabolic activation and terminal degranulation. The movement and steering of neutrophils toward chemoattractants emitted at sites of infection is clearly dependent on gradient perception.

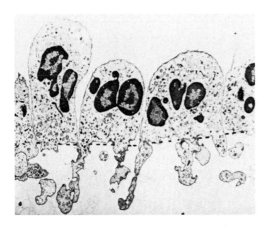

FIGURE 10-6

EM showing neutrophils perched like octopuses, reaching ineffectually toward the chemical source of attraction. The chamber contains a micropore filter (interrupted horizontal line) that bars the crowd of lunging cells (above) from the chemoattractant (below). (Reproduced from the Journal of Cell Biology, 1977, 75:666 by copyright permission of the Rockefeller University Press.)

FIGURE 10-7

Scanning EM of a neutrophil fixed while in the locomotor mode. The sticky pseudopod (PP) is advanced in the direction of travel and adheres to the surface; this causes the "neck" to arch up (white arrow), creating an undulating convex aspect (interrupted arrow), followed by a concave dent (black arrow) marking the perimeter of the nuclear bulge. Pseudoflagella (PF) known as microspikes extend from the trailing uropod. (From Senda N et al: The mechanism of the movement of leucocytes. Exp Cell Res 91:383,1975.)

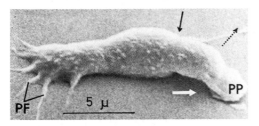

Chemotaxis

Chemotactic factors are generated by bacteria (fMLP), by macrophages and neutrophils at the site of infection (the leukotriene, LTB_4), or by activation of serum complement with release of C5a or C5a-desarg. That neutrophils sense these alluring molecules and move toward them can be demonstrated by automated cell tracking systems or by use of porous flow chambers (Figure 10-6) [3]. When neutrophils encounter a chemotactic gradient, those surface receptors closest to the source of savory emanations are occupied, serving to orient the cell; neutrophils respond directionally to as little as a 1% difference in concentration of chemotactic substances across their lengths.

Locomotion and Adhesion

As neutrophils crawl forward guided by their chemotactic compass, they move like inchworms, repetitiously pushing forward broad adhesive lamellipods, and then hiking up the nucleus and trailing uropod (Figure 10-7) [4]. Moving cells exhibit a fanlike shape created by the spreading glassy veil of the anterior lamellipod (the hyaline cortex), which is flung forward in the path of movement like a sticky cape.

Neutrophils could not advance toward their prey without having the power to regulate their adhesiveness suitably, thus providing an appropriate amount of traction for locomotion and of gluing power for phagocytosis. To enable their translocation from the circulation to vascular walls and the extravascular space, neutrophils are equipped with receptors for several kinds of adhesion molecules conferring various degrees of stickiness. Receptors for laminin, fibronectin, and the complement components are stored in or on the specific granules; when the neutrophil is stimulated by chemotactic signals, these granules fuse to the cell membrane, causing expression of the traction and adhesion receptors. During degranulation these adhesion proteins are translocated from the specific granules and expressed on the cell surface; this causes neutrophils to stop in their tracks and adhere to bacteria or stalk them by crawling through the subendothelium. The activity and appetite of neutrophils when in hot pursuit of interlopers are whetted by the cytokine GM-CSF. GM-CSF does not encourage adhesion to endothelium, which would interrupt the chase, but it stimulates agitated motion (cytokinesis), sharply upregulates receptors for adhesive proteins, and causes neutrophils to extend long sticky projections that facilitate both seizure of organisms and aggregation of neutrophils at the site of invasion (Figure 10-8) [5].

The mechanics of movement   Neutrophils are capable of purposeful locomotion, phagocytosis, and exocytosis. All of these movements depend upon coherent waves of assembly and dispersal of actin and myosin. Actin is a 42,500 M_r globular monomer (G-actin) that assembles into filaments (F-actin) by head-to-tail alignment to form rigid double-helical cables. The polymerization and depolymerization of actin is governed by a family of actin-binding, Ca^{2+}-dependent proteins that includes profilin, gelsolin, and acumentin. Proteins that block or reverse polymerization induce the liquidity necessary for movement and function of granules and organelles. Those that favor polymer growth and a sol-gel transformation are responsible for the propulsive posture and momentum of the hyaline cortex. The contraction necessary for "bringing up the rear" depends on interaction with myosin.

Nonmuscle myosin is an ATPase composed of a pair of rodlike strutures (200,000 M_r each) to which are attached cigar-shaped heads of heavy meromyosin. When phosphorylated by ATP, heavy chain heads bind to actin and the heads cock forward; this cocking movement acts as a winch, causing the actin fibers to slide toward one another. In the presence of regenerated ATP, myosin disengages from actin, reattaching at a new site where it again flexes its head, giving the filament another nudge in the direction of actin polarity. Decoration of actin filaments with cocked myosin beads creates an arrowhead appearance, aimed in the direction of movement (Figure 10-9) [6].

Phagocytosis, Degranulation, and Secretion

When a neutrophil encounters its target the actin-rich lamellipod flows around the quarry, its extensions fuse, and the particle or microbe is engulfed within a phagosomal chamber into

FIGURE 10-8

Activation and aggregation of neutrophils by GM-CSF. At rest (above) neutrophils are spheroidal and slightly roughened but appear unruffled. When activated by GM-CSF (below) neutrophils become excited and adhesive, extending long filopodia that cause them to aggregate in a manner favoring entrapment of noxious particles. (From Golde DW and Gasson JC: Hormones that stimulate the growth of blood cells. Sci Am 259(1):62,1988. Copyright © 1988 by Scientific American, Inc. All rights reserved.)

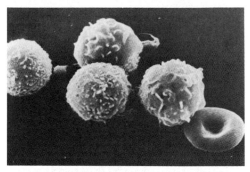

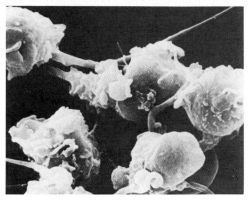

which granules are discharged. Once the phagosome is sealed, the pH within the chamber is lowered to 5.68, sufficient to marinate most captives and facilitate their digestion by peptidases. The adjacent hyaline cortex thins out and parts, leading to fusion of the phagosome with secondary (specific) granules, which spill their contents into the phagosome within 30 seconds, and with primary (azurophilic) granules, which release their poisonous products more slowly. Secretion of specific granules is crucial in mobilizing mediators of inflammation, for these particles contain activators of the complement cascade that generate

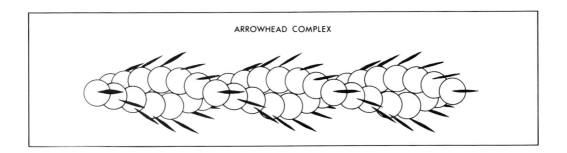

ARROWHEAD COMPLEX

FIGURE 10-9

Diagrammatic representation of the actin-myosin assembly in the "arrowhead" conformation. The helical actin duplex is portrayed by the white balls, and the cigar-shaped barbs of heavy meromyosin are shown cocked inward, indicating that the assembly is moving toward the left. (From Zucker-Franklin D: Chapt 10, in Atlas of Blood Cells, vol. 2, Zucker-Franklin D et al., Eds. Milan, Edi. Ermes s.r.l.,1988.)

the chemoattractant, C5a, and the opsonin, C3b. Specific granules also contain chemotaxins for monocytes and some components of the electron transport chain utilized in the respiratory burst. Azurophilic granules contain potent digestive enzymes and broad-spectrum antimicrobial peptides called defensins. An inventory of neutrophil granule constituents is listed in Table 10-1 [7].

TABLE 10-1

Neutrophil granule constituents

Constituent	Primary (azurophilic) granules	Secondary (specific) granules
Microbicidal enzymes	Myeloperoxidase Lysozyme	Lysozyme
Neutral serine proteases	Elastase Cathepsin G	
Metalloproteinases	Proteases	Collagenase
Acid hydrolases	N-Acetyl-glucuronidase Cathepsin B Cathepsin D β-Glucuronidase β-Glycerophosphatase α-Mannosidase	
Others	Defensins Antibacterial cationic proteins Kinin-generating enzyme C5a-inactivating factor	Lactoferrin Vitamin B_{12} binding proteins Cytochrome b_{558} Histaminase Complement activator Monocyte-chemoattractant Plasminogen activator Protein kinase C inhibitor fMLP receptors C3bi receptors

Source: Abbreviated from Boxer LA and Smolen JE: Neutrophil granule constituents and their release in health and disease. Hematol Oncol Clin North Am 2:101,1988.

The arsenal of host defense weaponry is built up nonsynchronously during neutrophil maturation. Primitive defensive capabilities (Fc receptor activity and phagocytosis) appear during early differentiation, but more evolved behavior such as chemotaxis is not expressed strongly until maturation is almost complete (Figure 10-10) [8]. The most celebrated and explosive device in the neutrophil armory is acquired late in maturation and is responsible for much of the self-inflicted damage of the inflammatory response: it involves reduction of O_2 into toxic free radical metabolites.

The Respiratory Burst

The term "respiratory burst" refers to an abrupt spurt of oxidative metabolism occurring within 2 to 3 seconds of receptor-agonist coupling at the neutrophil surface. The transductional mechanisms (including protein kinase C, through which surface contact and chemoattractant-receptor complexes excite neutrophil respiration) act through a surface enzyme known as respiratory burst oxidase. In resting cells this membrane-bound enzyme is dormant, but when neutrophils are activated the enzyme springs to life, catalyzing the single-electron reduction of O_2 to O_2^-, with the help of cytochrome b_{558} and at the expense of NADPH, according to the following stoichiometry:

$$2O_2 + NADPH \rightarrow 2O_2^- + NADP^+ + H^+$$

Most O_2^-, the superoxide anion, is converted rapidly and harmlessly to H_2O_2 by dismutation. Two colliding superoxide radicals interact so that one anion is reduced and the other oxidized, leading to formation of H_2O_2 and O_2, a reaction hastened by the metalloenzyme, superoxide dismutase:

$$O_2^- + O_2^- + 2H^+ \rightarrow H_2O_2 + O_2$$

The H_2O_2 thus generated is scavenged by catalase and, by a series of coupled reactions linked to the hexose monophosphate (HMP) shunt, by GSH, GSH peroxidase, and GSSG reductase. The increased conversion of NADPH to NADP$^+$ accelerates G6PD-mediated oxidation of glucose by the HMP shunt, with replenishment of NADPH.

Although both products (O_2^- and H_2O_2) produced by partial reduction of O_2 are potentially microbicidal, O_2^- is fleeting and relatively innocuous and H_2O_2 is well defended against by most microorganisms and other cells. Instead, the true microbicidal agents are products of further reactions involving O_2^- and H_2O_2. Two classes of microbicidal oxidants are formed in these reactions: highly oxidant free radicals and oxidized halogens.

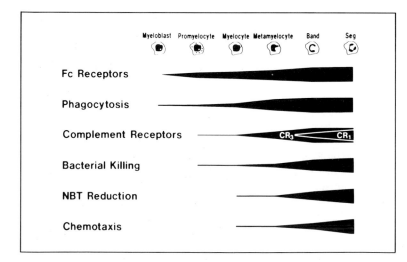

FIGURE 10-10

Schematic representation of relative expression of neutrophil functions at successive stages of differentiation. NBT (nitroblue tetrazolium) dye reduction is a cytochemical measure of respiratory burst activity. (From Glasser L and Fiederlein RL: Functional differentiation of normal human neutrophils. Blood 69:937, 1987.)

Although molecular O_2 is strongly oxidative with respect to its fully reduced form (H_2O), its oxidative potential is held in check by kinetic restrictions imposed by its two unpaired spin-parallel electrons. Consecutive univalent reductions yield the following sequence, with the reaction potentials shown [9]:

$$O_2 \xrightarrow{-0.33V} O_2^- \xrightarrow{+0.94V} H_2O_2 \xrightarrow{+0.38V}$$

$$HO\cdot + H_2O \xrightarrow{+2.38V} H_2O$$

Each of these reduced metabolites is exempt from the spin restriction and is thermodynamically proficient at monovalent electron changes. There are no natural mechanisms for containing the indiscriminate OH· (hydroxyl) free radical; it is an extraordinarily powerful and promiscuous oxidant, which is thought to be responsible for most of the oxidative damage by ionizing radiation. This hydroxyl species is produced by the metal-catalyzed Fenton, or Haber-Weiss, reaction; in this, Fe^{3+} is reduced to Fe^{2+} by O_2^-, and then oxidized to Fe^{3+} by H_2O_2, with production of the instantly reactive OH· radical. The sources of iron in this reaction appear to be lactoferrin and ferritin [10].

Oxidized halogens (Clorox is an example) are potent antimicrobial agents that are produced in neutrophils by peroxidase-catalyzed reactions in which H_2O_2 oxidizes either Cl^- or Br^- to the corresponding hypohalous acids (HOXs). In neutrophils the green heme enzyme, myeloperoxidase, enters the phagosome cavity together with H_2O_2 and Cl^-, generating HOCl; this in turn reacts with ambient amines to form microbicidal chloramines, which are highly effective in destroying bacteria, viruses, mycoplasmas, fungi, and tumor cells.

INFLAMMATION: THE PRICE OF NEUTROPHIL DEFENSE

During their brief sojourn in blood, neutrophils divide their time randomly between the axial stream and the plasma sheath bathing vascular walls. While in midstream they are merely passengers within the "circulating granulocyte pool," and when tumbling along and policing the endothelium they are said to be in the "marginal granulocyte pool." Whether the stimulus causing neutrophils to migrate into tissue is generalized or local, the initial step involves binding of marginalized neutrophils (and later of monocytes) in capillaries to subjacent endothelium in response to hormonal instructions issued by lymphocytes and macrophages. The chemotactic commands causing neutrophils to stick to focal areas of capillary endothelium are complex and include GM-CSF, IL-1, and tumor necrosis factor (TNF). Responding neutrophils promptly cease locomotion and display several sticky glycoproteins, beginning with a family of adhesives that includes Mo1 (CD11b) and LFA-1 (leukocyte function-associated antigen, or CD11a). At the same time, underlying endothelial cells are stimulated to secrete both IL-1 and TNF (Figure 10-11), project receptors for these biological

FIGURE 10-11

Adhesion of neutrophils to endothelium in response to IL-1 is shown in an experimental facsimile of early inflammation. Neutrophils normally do not stick to vascular endothelium but roam randomly on its surface (top). During inflammation IL-1 stimulates endothelial cells to synthesize and display endothelial-leukocyte adhesion molecules (Elam-1) that promote congregation of neutrophils on the vessel surface. (Courtesy MA Gimbrone, Jr.)

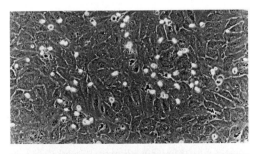

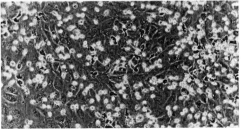

glues, and loosen their intercellular junctions. The combination of stickiness and loosening of the endothelial fabric enables adherent neutrophils to wriggle through the gaps, crawl purposefully along the chemotactic gradient, and gather (aggregate) at the target site. The participants in this focused assault on invading organisms are depicted schematically in Figure 10-12. As neutrophils charge valiantly to the site of invasion, recognition of the enemy is facilitated by coating of particulate invaders by proteins known collectively as "opsonins" (from the Greek, meaning "to prepare for dining"). Although the adhesive protein Mo1 (C3bi) is opsonic, it is less appetizing than IgG or C3b, and maximal phagocytosis requires the presence of both antibody and complement. Neutrophils experience a feeding frenzy when they encounter microorganisms garnished with opsonins, and, although their degradative enzymes and O_2 metabolites are segregated away from the central cytoplasm, the focal accumulation of these lethal secretions eventually kills friend and foe alike. In the presence of complement (C5a), IL-1, and tumor necrosis factor, the neighboring endothelial cells also become injured or destroyed by the neutrophil secretions. However painful to the host, the resultant vascular necrosis and disruption of blood flow serves to confine the area of combat. Vascular shutdown induced by neutrophil-mediated killing may also be important in ischemic isolation and destruction of tumor cells. In sacrificing themselves to save the host, the amassed neutrophil casualties are converted ignominiously to pus.

Neutrophilia of Acute Inflammation

Diapedesis and congregation of neutrophils at inflammatory sites is a very early event, followed in order of motility by arrival of monocytes, eosinophils, basophils, and lymphocytes, which appear in numbers determined by the nature of the noxious agent. If the lesion is large or infection becomes systemic, the concentration of blood neutrophils may fall momentarily and the IL-1–directed pyrogenic and phase responses are inaugurated. Neutrophil losses sustained in line of duty are offset temporarily by mobilization of marrow reserves of neutrophils and band forms, and this in turn sends a proliferative shiver throughout the stem cell hierarchy. Goaded by IL-3 and GM-CSF, the stem cells launch an exuberant and more sustained counterattack: for every multipotential stem cell

FIGURE 10-12

Cytokine-directed neutrophil emigration (diapedesis) from capillary lumen to the site of the tissue infection. (From Cannistra SA and Griffin JD: Regulation of the production and function of granulocytes and monocytes. Semin Hematol 24:173,1988.)

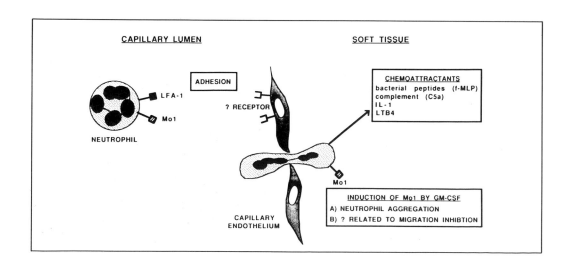

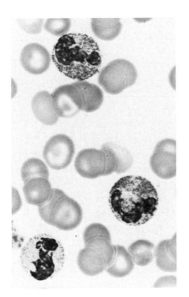 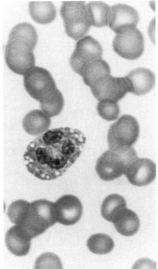 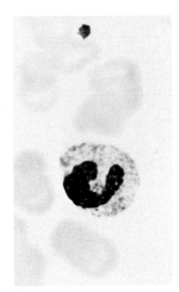

FIGURE 10-13

Blood neutrophil anomalies found during infection. (Left) "Toxic neutrophils": the coarse "toxic" granules are abundant in the cell at top, numerous but patchy in the cell below it containing phagocytized diplococci, and sparse in the spent neutrophil at bottom. (Center) Neutrophil containing vacuoles—holes left by exploding granules. (Right) The smooth comma-shaped inclusion at the upper left margin of the cytoplasm of this band form is a Döhle body. (Photos by CT Kapff.)

stimulated to differentiate, 10 CFU-GMs are generated, and each of these precursors is capable of spawning 500 to 1,000 mature neutrophils and monocytes. A healthy response to pyogenic infection usually elicits a neutrophilia ranging from 15,000 to 30,000 cells/μl.

Morphologic Changes in Neutrophils during Infection

As part of the kinetic adaptation to neutrophil losses at the "front," younger recruits (band forms and some metamyelocytes) are sent forth. Within hours this shift to immaturity ("leftward shift") in the differential white count is accompanied by telltale morphologic changes.

Toxic granulation, Döhle bodies, and toxic vacuolation: the indices of infection Toxic granulation of neutrophils, a trademark of infection, reflects rushed maturation. In the haste of mobilization, freshly enlisted neutrophils enter the bloodstream still laden with metachromatic primary granules. Another mark of precipitous cytokinetics during infection is the presence of Döhle bodies. These small (1 to 3 μm across) cerulean cytoplasmic puddles (on Wright-Giemsa) tend to locate near the periphery of neutrophils; they represent remnant patches of rough endoplasmic reticulum and are a dependable indicator of infection. Döhle bodies are particularly numerous in systemic infections and are often associated with cytoplasmic vacuoles—phagosomal cisterns into which lysosomal ingredients have been imploded. These three morphologic indices of infection are shown in Figure 10-13.

INHERITED DISORDERS OF NEUTROPHIL FUNCTION

Most of what has been learned of neutrophil function has come from studies of patients

TABLE 10-2

Hereditary disorders of neutrophil function

Disorder	Cellular defect	Distinguishing features
CD11/CD18 glycoprotein deficiency	Adherence; chemotaxis; ingestion	Omphalitis Leukemoid reactions, autosomal recessive
Hyper IgE (Job's) syndrome	Variable chemotaxis, decreased antistaphylococcal IgG, increased antistaphylococcal IgE	Increased IgE (>2500 IU/mL), eosinophilia, atypical eczema, cold abscesses, coarse facies, autosomal recessive
Specific granule deficiency	Abnormal or absent specific granules, chemotaxis, excessive O_2^-, markedly reduced defensins	Neutrophils with bilobed nuclei, alkaline phosphatase absent histochemically, extremely rare
Juvenile periodontitis	Chemotaxis	Early severe gingivitis, capnocytophaga infections of the gums, occasional systemic infections
Chédiak-Higashi syndrome	Giant granules, chemotaxis, degranulation, neutropenia, markedly reduced neutral proteases, decreased natural killer cell function	Oculocutaneous albinism, central and peripheral neuropathies, increased bleeding time, accelerated (lymphomalike) phase develops later in the disease, autosomal recessive
Myeloperoxidase deficiency	Absent myeloperoxidase, bactericidal (delayed)	Autosomal recessive, clinically silent unless with another defect (for example, diabetes mellitus)
Chronic granulomatous disease	Bactericidal (catalase-positive microbes)	Failure to generate superoxide and reduce nitroblue tetrazolium (NBT), multiple granulomata, X-linked and autosomal recessive forms

Source: Reproduced, with permission, from Curnutte JT: Chronic granulomatous disease: Clinical and genetic aspects, in Lehrer RI et al: Neutrophils and host defense. Ann Intern Med 109:127,1988.

whose problems (usually recurrent infections) stem from inherited defects of neutrophil adherence, chemotaxis, or microbicidal activity. By convention many of these rare disorders are classified as "leukocyte anomalies," even though some are life-threatening. The best-defined hereditary disorders of neutrophil function are characterized succinctly in Table 10-2 [11]. The most instructive of these functional disorders is chronic granulomatous disease.

Chronic Granulomatous Disease

Chronic granulomatous disease (CGD) comprises a group of at least three rare genetic disorders in which neutrophils and macrophages ingest but cannot kill catalase-positive microorganisms. Beginning in early childhood, this defect in host defense leads to recurrent purulent infections that stimulate chronic inflammatory reactions and granuloma formation and may threaten life. Inheritance is usually X-linked but in two variants the disease is transmitted by autosomal recessive genes. Neutrophils from all three subtypes of CGD are incapable of launching a respiratory burst in response to bacterial or particulate stimulation. In most X-linked kindreds the patient's phagocytes lack spectrally detectable cytochrome b_{558}, a heme protein that functions as a terminal component of the NADPH oxidase system required for generating free radical O_2 metabolites—hence the failure to respond with a "burst." Molecular cloning of the X-CGD gene, located on the short arm of the X-chromosome (at Xp21.1), has revealed an

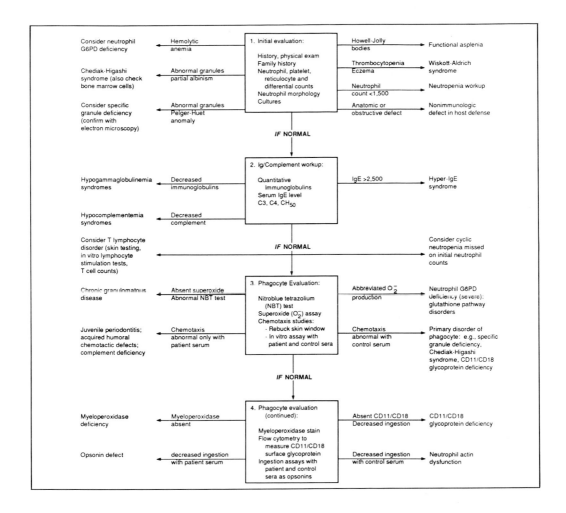

FIGURE 10-14

Algorithm for the work-up of a patient with recurrent infections. G6PD = glucose-6-phosphate dehydrogenase; Ig = immunoglobulin; NBT = nitroblue tetrazolium; O_2^- = superoxide. The units for the neutrophil count (box 1) are neutrophils/μl. (Reproduced, with permission, from: Curnutte JT: Chronic granulomatous disease: clinical and genetic aspects, in Lehrer RI et al: Neutrophils and host defense. Ann Intern Med 109:127,1988.)

assortment of thalassemialike defects that interfere with transcription. Neutrophils from most patients with autosomal recessive disease contain normal cytochrome b_{558} but lack a soluble cytosol factor essential to activation of the cell membrane oxidase. Both kinds of defect abrogate the respiratory burst, and both malfunc-

tions are readily detectable for they nullify NBT dye reduction in stimulated neutrophils. The deficit in synthesis of cytochrome b_{558} (and of its cofactor) in CGD can be overcome partially by periodic injection of the macrophage activator, gamma interferon (IFNγ). IFNγ coerces developing neutrophils, monocytes, and macrophages to manufacture sufficient oxidase activity to restore oxidative killing and correct this lethal congenital defect in host resistance.

An Algorithm for the Evaluation of Patients with Recurrent Infections

An algorithm for assessing patients with recurrent infections has been constructed by J.T. Curnutte (Figure 10-14) [11] and can be advocated as an orderly logic system for differentiating malfunctions of the phagocytic and immune systems.

REFERENCES

1. Cannistra SA and Griffin JD: Regulation of the production and function of granulocytes and monocytes. Semin Hematol 24:173,1988

2. Zucker-Franklin D: Eosinophil function and disorders. Adv Intern Med 19:1,1974

3. Marmont AM et al: Chapt 4, in Atlas of Blood Cells: Function and Pathology, vol. 1, Zucker-Franklin D et al, Eds. Milan, Edi. Ermes s.r.l.,1988

4. Senda N et al: The mechanism of the movement of leucocytes. Exp Cell Res 91:383, 1975

5. Golde DW and Gasson JC: Hormones that stimulate the growth of blood cells. Sci Am 259(1):62,1988

6. Marmont AM et al: Chapt 10, in Atlas of Blood Cells: Function and Pathology, vol. 1, Zucker-Franklin D et al, Eds. Milan, Edi. Ermes s.r.l.,1988

7. Boxer LA and Smolen JE: Neutrophil granule constituents and their release in health and disease. Hematol Oncol Clin North Am 2:101,1988

8. Glasser L and Fiederlein RL: Functional differentiation of normal human neutrophils. Blood 69:937,1987

9. Imlay JA and Linn S: DNA damage and oxygen radical toxicity. Science 240:1302, 1988

10. Babior BM: The respiratory burst, p. 132 in Lehrer RI et al: Neutrophils and host defense. Ann Intern Med 109:127,1988

11. Curnutte JT: Chronic granulomatous disease: clinical and genetic aspects, in Lehrer RI et al: Neutrophils and host defense. Ann Intern Med 109:127,1988

11

Monocytes, Macrophages, and the Mononuclear Phagocyte System

☐

Monocytes and their differentiated tissue forms, the macrophages, collectively comprise the mononuclear phagocyte system. Certain macrophages that reside in vascular and lymphatic sinuses elaborate a reticulin network that provides housing for functionally specialized subsets of the macrophage family such as professional phagocytes. In the spleen, liver, marrow, and lymph nodes, sessile macrophages (reticulin cells) and endothelial sinuses (endothelial channels having perforate basement membranes) integrate to form unique and sizeable organic structures. The term "reticuloendothelial system" (RES) for this alliance between macrophages and endothelium has become obsolescent, in recognition of the primogeniture status of macrophages. Macrophages are aboriginal cells essential to metazoan life. Without macrophages, organs would go unmodelled, wounds unmended, senescent cells would stagnate in leaking vessels, and swarming microbes would feast upon the defenseless host [1]. The pervasive distribution and manifold differentiated forms generated by the "mononuclear" stem cell are indicated in Figure 11-1 [2].

REGULATION OF MONOCYTES AND MACROPHAGES

Macrophages are monocytes that have undergone transformation after leaving the circulation. Monocytes are generated by CFU-Ms, and these in turn are the progeny of the bipotential stem cell, CFU-GM. CFU-GM is driven to spawn monocytes preferentially by M-CSF, whereas bacterial lipopolysaccharides stimulate expression of the G-CSF gene. Coordination of monocyte and granulocyte production is achieved by feedback regulation involving the two opposing CSFs and by a balanced synergy between IL-1 and TNFα (Chapter 1).

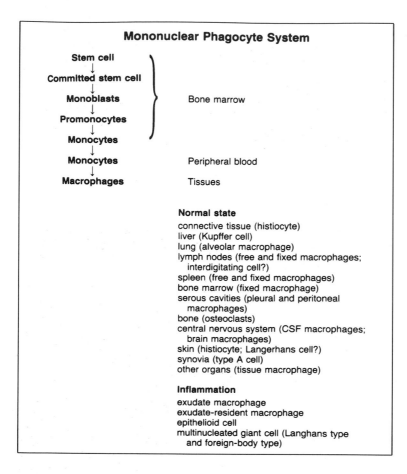

FIGURE 11-1

Mononuclear phagocyte
system. (From van
Furth R: Current view
on the mononuclear
phagocyte system.
Immunobiology 161:
178,1982.)

As macrophages are the major source of both CSF-M and CSF-G, they are capable of regulating their own production.

Maturation, Morphology, and Kinetics of Monocytes

The first identifiable offspring of CFU-Ms are monoblasts, which divide and give birth to promonocytes, the parents of blood monocytes. Monoblasts are nonmotile, medium-sized blasts having deep blue, clear cytoplasm on Wright-Giemsa staining. The bulky nucleus is indented or even folded centrally, and one or two large nucleoli are embedded in its speckled chromatin. Generation of promonocytes by monoblasts requires two concatenated divisions yielding a large cell capable of labored locomotion and possessing surface receptors for IgG and complement. Mature monocytes are the largest blood cells (diameter: 16 to 18 μm) and represent 3 to 8% of circulating white cells, ranging in concentration from 200 to 800 cells/μl. They possess abundant gray-blue cytoplasm peppered unevenly with red or purple granules that are only dimly visible on Wright-Giemsa. The lumpy, lobular, or reniform nucleus is located centroidally, and the nuclear chromatin is arrayed as a lacy fretwork decorated with small chromatin clumps. Figure 11-2 is a pastiche portraying monocyte maturation.

Monocyte Kinetics and Function

The transit time in marrow from first precursive monoblast to mature monocyte is about 6 days, there being no marrow reserve comparable to that for neutrophils. Within several days of release into circulation, selected monocytes (in obedience to IL-1 and TNF signals) display surface adhesive, bind to endothelium, and gain

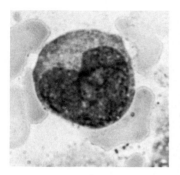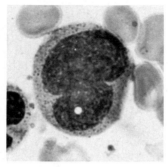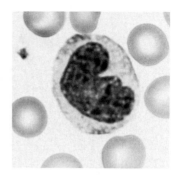

FIGURE 11-2

Portraits of monocytes at various stages of maturation: (left) monoblast, (center) promonocyte, and (right) mature monocyte. (Photos by CT Kapff.)

extravascular passage in much the same manner as neutrophils (Chapter 10). During their slower and more awkward diapedesis, monocytes transiently downregulate receptors linked to phagocytic, respiratory, and secretory functions as they emigrate toward tissue locations designated by chemotactic signals. Within 20 to 30 minutes after traversing the vascular barrier, extravascular (tissue) monocytes quickly regain their functional virtuosity and in the ensuing hours they transform to macrophages in response to surface activation, with prodding by gamma interferon (IFNγ) [3].

Monocytes travel in the marginal pool nearly 80% of the time, making them readily available for transudation at the behest of cytokines released from sites of inflammation. Monocytes are equipped with a multitude of signal receptors that enable them to navigate slowly but with resolute accuracy along chemotactic gradients. As compared with the speeding neutrophils, monocytes are sluggish and slower to appear at inflammatory sites, arriving in appreciable numbers in a matter of hours to days rather than minutes to hours. The topography of a blood monocyte lumbering toward a chemoattractant emitter, as can be observed through "skin windows" over abraded skin and on artificial filters, closely resembles that of a neutrophil in the locomotor mode (Figure 11-3) [4]. During inflammation

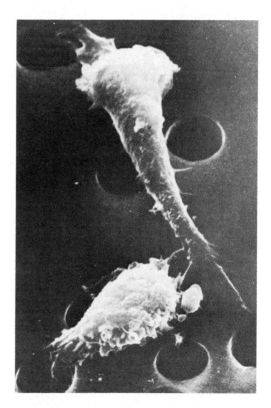

FIGURE 11-3

Scanning EM of two monocytes crawling through and upon a polycarbonate filter having pores 5 μm across. The head (cortical) end of the lower cell had just emerged en route to the chemotactic source. The monocyte above had traversed the channel and displays an advancing lamellipod (top), followed by cephalic ruffling and lateral microspikes on the trailing end (below). (From Snyderman R and Goetzl EJ: Molecular and cellular mechanisms of leukocyte chemotaxis. Science 213:830,1981. Copyright 1981 by the AAAS.)

the rate of monocyte transudation is increased, and monocytopoiesis is enhanced through the auspices of M-CSF and autocrine release of IL-1. Unlike neutrophils, monocytes are metabolically designed to withstand prolonged extravascular tours and some are capable of reentering the circulation for duty elsewhere. Blood monocytes can be subdivided into several subsets by differences in cytochemical characteristics and responsiveness to cytokines. Immature monocytes affect the languor of youth, have fewer Fc receptors, and are reluctant to phagocytize; nevertheless they are rich in granular peroxidase and possess the same arsenal of hydrolytic and oxidative enzymes as do neutrophils, plus the unique esterase, α-naphthyl butyrate (by which monocytes can be identified). As they mature, monocytes package and secrete fewer granules into the cytoplasm, additional primary granules made by circulating cells are often empty, and secondary granules formed during late maturation lack any peroxidase activity. Apart from age-dependent differences, only one of two major subsets of monocytes migrates toward the chemoattractant fMet-Leu-Phe (Chapter 10) and has receptors for C5a and Fcγ, while the other lacks these attributes.

Transformation in tissues   In the absence of inflammation, monocytes of all sorts escape the vasculature in a random fashion, showing no indication that they are programmed or predestined to play specialized roles. Once in the tissues, monocytes undergo transformation into tissue macrophages having morphologic and functional properties that are characteristic for the tissue in which they reside. When billeted appropriately, unstimulated tissue macrophages survive approximately 3 months; collectively these "resident macrophages" of various guises outnumber blood monocytes by over 100-fold. During early monocyte-macrophage transformation, the cells enlarge dramatically, spread out, and acquire numerous vacuoles, starting within several hours. While transformation proceeds, peroxidase-laden granules disappear as the metamorphosed macrophage converts from an indolent cell to a high-energy form briskly engaged in protein synthesis, production of added mitochondria, lysosomes, and respiratory enzymes. The cell is now geared for

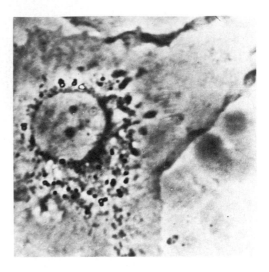

FIGURE 11-4

Monocyte transformed into a macrophage by incubation in a plastic Petri dish for 24 h and viewed by phase contrast microscopy. During incubation, the cell enlarged its cytoplasmic area 6-fold and extended thick pseudopods. The major features of transformation are evident: abundant cytoplasm filled with phase-dense granules and cytoplasmic inclusions and a rounded nucleus containing prominent nucleoli. (Photo courtesy G. Roth.)

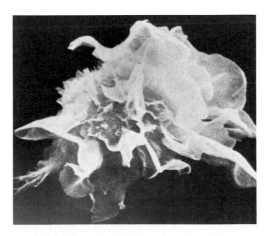

FIGURE 11-5

Scanning EM view of an activated macrophage, showing ruffles and waves of diaphanous but deadly veils. (From Warfel AH and Elberg SS: Macrophage membranes viewed through a scanning electron microscope. Science 170:446, 1970. Copyright 1970 by the AAAS.)

more active glycolysis, pinocytosis, phagocytosis, and cell division. Within 24 to 48 hours out of circulation, the pudgy monocyte has converted to a very large cell (25–50 μm across) loaded with cytoplasmic inclusions formed by invagination of the plasma membrane (Figure 11-4). Given the right instructions, this cell is prepared for war.

Macrophage Activation

The most dramatic behavioral change in resident macrophages is the cytokine-driven conversion to a state of irascible agitation known as activation. Activated macrophages enlarge and spread out further, grow stickier, become hypermotile, and release an arsenal of noxious secretions, including both oxidative and nonoxidative metabolites. The most constant feature of macrophage activation is the launching of an intense and sustained oxidative burst. Aroused macrophages become physically as well as temperamentally ruffled: the membrane surface is thrown into a tumble of intricate folds, veils, and fanlike processes that enable the cell to "mantle" and then ingest its quarry (Figure 11-5) [5]. Macrophage motions include endocytosis, exocytosis, and locomotion; as in neutrophils, all of these movements depend on manipulation of the actin-myosin assembly (Chapter 10) and are directed by chemotactic factors, cytokines, and other recognition signals that direct and propel the macrophage to its target. When the cell comes within grappling distance, various receptors concentrated on the crests of the ruffles seal the attachment sites, and the prey is either trapped or engulfed. Killing is accomplished by close-range bombardment of the enemy by a bewildering multitude of dangerous lysosomal ingredients that are toxic for most microorganisms but not for the macrophage. Macrophages, unlike the suicidal microphages (neutrophils), are designed to survive combat. An inventory of secretory products released by activated macrophages exceeds 100 kinds of molecules, many of them microbicidal; an abbreviated list of functions and secretions exploited by macrophages in host defense is given in Table 11-1 [6]. If intruders survive this noxious brew, the macrophage may either eat them alive or impound them by forming giant-cell granulomas.

TABLE 11-1

Functional changes in macrophages during activation

Microbicidal activity (↑)
Tumoricidal activity (↑)
Chemotaxis (↑)
Phagocytosis (varies with particle)
Pinocytosis (↑)
Glucose transport and metabolism (↑)
Phagocytosis-associated respiratory burst (↑)
Antigen presentation (↑)
Secretion
  Lysozyme (NC)*
  Prostaglandins, leukotrienes (↓)
  Apolipoprotein E and lipoprotein lipase (↓)
  Elastase (↓)
  Complement components (↑ or NC)*
  Acid hydrolases (↑)
  Collagenase (↑)
  Plasminogen activator (↑)
  Cytolytic proteinase (↑)
  Arginase (↑)
  Fibronectin (↑)
  Interleukin-1 (↑)
  Tumor necrosis factor-cachectin (↑ when stimulated)
  Interferon α and β (↑)
  Angiogenesis factor (↑)

*NC = no change.

Source: From Johnston RB Jr: Monocytes and macrophages. Reprinted, by permission of The New England Journal of Medicine, 318:747,1988.

Phagocytosis

Phagocytosis of foreign or denatured particles can occur by direct contact activation of macrophages even in the absence of opsonins, but the rate and vigor of ingestion is fervently intensified when the particles are buttered with such condiments as IgG and C3b, which trigger receptor-mediated endocytosis. In immune phagocytosis macrophage Fc receptors move freely in the plane of the ruffled surface membrane to encircle adherent cells, and occupied receptors gather together to form a ligating ring. Adhesion is strengthened and crosslinked by receptors to Arg-Gly-Asp (RGD) sequences expressed by fibronectin, vitronectin, and other adhesives secreted by macrophages and fibroblasts. As the coated cell is engulfed, Fc receptors and adhesive molecules are interiorized transiently along with it. Particle ingestion is accompanied by a sharp acceleration of the hexose monophosphate (HMP) shunt and explosive release of free radical forms of O_2, including OH· and hypohalous acids (Chapter 10). Within the phagosome these promiscuous oxidants are joined by acid hydrolases, neutral peptidases, and products of at least three enzyme cascades to aid in liquidation of the transgressor.

Some pathogens enjoy living in macrophages

The intensity of microbicidal response to infection is stimulated by IFNγ and subdued by prostaglandin E_2 (PGE_2), secretory products of T cells and of macrophages themselves that respectively enhance and suppress activation. Some organisms can resist the deadly potential of the secretory response by selectively stimulating PGE_2 secretion by both cell types, thereby quenching both O_2-dependent and O_2-independent antimicrobial mechanisms. Included among pathogens that are constitutively capable of surviving and even of replicating within macrophages are such diverse intracellular organisms as *Mycobacterium avium intracellulare*, *Histoplasma capsulatum*, various protozoa, and the human immunodeficiency virus (HIV) responsible for AIDS [7]. Lymphocytes from patients with some of these infections are immunocompromised and unable to secrete enough IFNγ to activate macrophage host cells, a defect that can be overcome by administration of either recombinant IFNγ or inhibitors of prostacyclin synthesis such as indomethacin. In the case of protozoa, macrophages actually provide sanctuaries essential to protozoan survival.

Role of Macrophages in Immunity

During phagocytosis of microbial protein antigens, part of each antigenic molecule is shielded from proteolysis and made accessible for recognition by T cells. Immunity rests upon a bicellular mechanism in which T cells act as inducers and macrophages act as accessory cells which process and present segments of antigen. For this macrophage–T cell collaboration to work, the two cells must share genetic identity at an appropriate portion of the major histocompatibility complex (MHC) (Chapter 12). The MHC genes code for two families of cell surface proteins termed class I and class II. Class I molecules are found on the surfaces of all cells, but class II (alias Ia) molecules are found only on the surfaces of the extended macrophage family (which includes Langerhans, interdigitating, and dendritic cells) and on B cells. Macrophages display class II antigens only during inflammation on instruction by IFNγ.

Immune responsiveness that depends on interplay between cells is called cell-mediated immunity. In the presence of processed antigen and of histocompatibility-linked gene products on both cell surfaces, T cells bind firmly to macrophages to form "immune recognition units" (Figure 11-6) [8]. Activation of T cells during this interaction requires participation by IL-1. IL-1 plays a dual role in the immune response: in its membrane form it is necessary for cell-cell interaction during antigen presentation; as a hormone in its secreted form it both induces T cell receptors for IL-2 and stimulates IL-2 production. This sets up a vigorous autocrine cycle that causes antigen-activated T cells to synthesize DNA and undergo clonal proliferation.

Macrophage Responses to Infection and Inflammation

Tissue responses to infection can be segregated into purulent and granulomatous kinds. Purulent infections are described in Chapter 10 and are marked by an acute course in which neutrophils predominate. Bacteria that cause purulent infections are classified as "extracellular," a category that includes cocci and gram-negative rods. Bacteria that elicit granulomatous responses thrive in neutrophils and may survive for days within macrophages because of the slowness of the T cell response. Such organisms are called facultative intracellular bacteria and include *M. tuberculosis*, *M.*

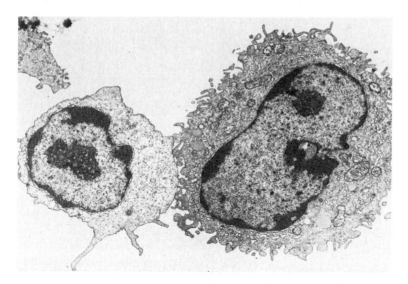

FIGURE 11-6

TEM view of an immune recognition unit, in which a T cell (left) bearing the CD4 marker makes momentary contact with an MHC class II–identical macrophage (right) presenting part of an antigenic protein. (From Rosenthal AS: Regulation of the immune response—role of the macrophage. Reprinted, by permission of the New England Journal of Medicine, 303:1153, 1980.)

leprae, Treponema pallidum, and *Legionella pneumophila.*

Granuloma Formation and Inflammatory Giant Cells

As activated macrophages crowd around clusters or masses of poorly digestible substances such as keratin, cholesterol, silica, or mycobacteria, they incarcerate the noxious targets, forming a protective multicellular shell called a granuloma. At first, infective granulomas are formed by macrophages and lymphocytes, but within several days fibroblasts appear. Crowding within granulomas, which is enhanced by IL-4, favors incidental fusion of adjacent macrophage margins, leading to formation of multinucleated giant cells. When more than one macrophage is engaged in receptor-mediated endocytosis of the same target, the

polykaryon formed has diminished phagocytic capacity for materials already interiorized but retains a normal appetite for materials that react with other receptors (Figure 11-7) [9].

There are three main kinds of inflammatory giant cells. Macrophage polykaryons that de-

FIGURE 11-7

Schematic representation of fusion of two macrophages each of which possesses receptors for denatured material (∪) and for the Fc portion of IgG molecules (⊔). Simultaneous endocytosis of the denatured debris causes interiorization of most ∪ receptors and cell fusion but Fc receptors remain fully displayed. The reverse is true during fusion of macrophages induced by IgG-coated particles. (From Chambers TJ and Spector WG: Inflammatory giant cells. Immunobiology 161:283,1982.)

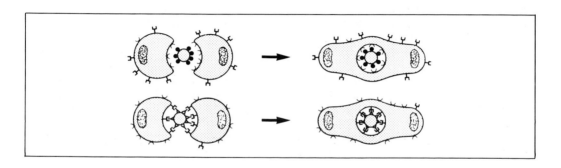

velop in response to lipids show foamy cytoplasm, an appearance resulting from long de-
marcating cytoplasmic processes that ensheath
lipid droplets, and the several nuclei are deployed around a central core of eosinophilic
cytoplasm (Touton giant cells). In foreign body
giant cells, nuclei are scattered haphazardly
throughout the cell. In the Langhans giant cells
that are a common (but not singular) feature of
mycobacterial infections, nuclei are arrayed in
a ring or horseshoe pattern surrounding the
amorphous, often necrotic pool of cytoplasm,
which may or may not contain intact acid fast
bacilli (Figure 11-8) [10]. During prolonged
and intense inflammation many granuloma
macrophages transform into nonadherent,
nonphagocytic epithelioid cells that lack Fc
receptors: these are large polygonal cells with
pale oblong nuclei and an abundance of
vacuolated cytoplasm. Epithelioid cell granulomas are a particular feature of tuberculosis,
tuberculoid leprosy, and syphilis. Secretory
epithelioid cells rich in rough endoplasmic
reticulum release fibroblast-activating factors
that stabilize granulomatous infiltrates and
promote fibrotic containment of these obstinate organisms.

Osteoclasts   Osteoclasts are physiologic multinucleated giant cells formed by fusion of
precursor cells descended from monocytes and
specially equipped to resorb bone. Osteoclasts
differ entirely in function and provenance
from mononuclear osteoblasts, creators of
bone and descendents of fibroblasts. Osteoclasts are very large cells (20 to 150 μm
across) containing from 2 to 50 evenly spaced
rounded nuclei. They are responsible for bone
resorption and are usually found nestled in
cavities on bone surfaces, where they display a
ruglike "ruffled border," with bristly processes designed to facilitate grooming and
resorption of bone under instructions by parathyroid hormone (Figure 11-9) [11, 12]. Normally osteoclast activity is controlled by antithetical actions of parathyroid hormone and
calcitonin. Malfunction or absence of osteoclasts leads to congenital malignant osteo-
petrosis, a disease curable by restoring CFU-
Ms through marrow transplantation.

FIGURE 11-8

Langhans-type giant cell containing a circle of
over 40 nuclei in a tuberculous granuloma.
(From Hill NS and Marx EJ: A 33-year-old
man with cough, fever, weight loss, and
pleuritic pain. Case 19-1988. Reprinted, by permission of The New England Journal of Medicine, 318:1257,1988.)

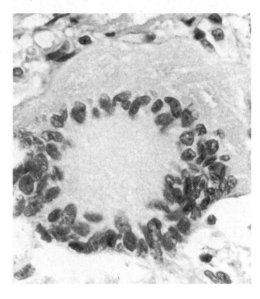

**Common Causes of Monocytosis and
Monocytopenia**

Chronic inflammatory and immune disorders
are associated with monocytosis, which is especially prominent in tuberculosis. *Mycobacterium* species and *Toxoplasma gondii* are able to
survive and multiply within macrophages for
years by their faculty for inhibiting cyclic
AMP–mediated formation of phagolysosomes.
Tubercule bacilli are extremely toxic and induce "high turnover" granulomas requiring
compensatory marrow proliferation and an IL-
1–driven exaggeration of monocytopoiesis.
Macrophages containing five or more tubercule bacilli are destroyed, and the coalescence of killed macrophages is responsible for
the central caseation characteristic of tuberculous granulomas. This necrotizing event is
spurred on by IFNγ, which, despite its good
intentions, induces focal release of tumor necrosis factor [13]. At the other extreme,

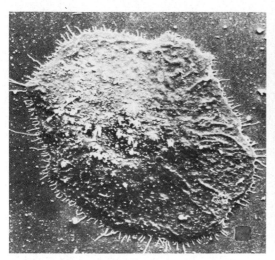 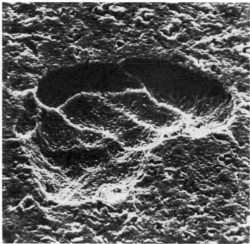

FIGURE 11-9

SEM showing an osteoclast (left) and the craters (right) that they create in intaglio while remodeling bone. (Left) Giant multinucleated osteoclast possesses a fringe of sticky processes containing lysosomes rich in acid phosphatase. (Right) Resorption-lacuna left behind after an osteoclast has eroded a crater. (Reproduced from the Journal of Cell Biology, 1985, 100:1592 by copyright permission of the Rockefeller University Press; and Boyde A et al: Optical and scanning electron microscopy in the single osteoclast resorption assay. Scan Electron Microsc 3:1259,1985.)

granulomas associated with *Salmonella* infections or sarcoid are of the "low turnover" type in which the causative agents possess low macrophage toxicity and acceleration of monocytopoiesis is unnecessary.

Prednisone and its glucocorticoid congeners induce a selective, often severe, monocytopenia, inhibit monocyte and macrophage responses to chemotactic factors, and suppress antimicrobial secretion by macrophages—actions opposite to those of IFNγ. Protracted suppression of monocytes and macrophages by glucocorticoids paves the way for opportunistic infections such as mycobacteriosis, listeriosis, and aspergillosis.

LIPID STORAGE DISEASES

Mononuclear phagocytes are victimized by an assortment of uncommon "storage disorders," most of which result from genetic deficiencies in enzymes necessary for lipid degradation. This catabolic defect and accumulation of indigestible lipids in macrophages results in the "constipated macrophage syndrome": marrow space is gradually encroached on by bloated and inert storage cells, and the spleen becomes enlarged by the surfeit of fat-filled forms. Splenomegaly may become massive and lead to increased splenic pooling of platelets, with thrombocytopenic purpura. The most prevalent cause of lipid engorgement in marrow and spleen is Gaucher's disease, caused by a genetic deficiency of lysosomal glucocerebrosidase, with accumulation in all macrophage populations of the sphingolipid, glucocerebroside. Very similar, but not identical, overloading of phagocytes with sphingoglycolipids occurs in protracted proliferative diseases such as chronic myelogenous leukemia (CML). The Gaucherlike cells appearing in CML marrow reflect massive overloading of phagocytes by membrane sphingolipid debris released by the enormous population of dying leukemic granulocytes. The sphingolipid hydrolases in macrophages of Gaucher's disease are nearly inert; those of CML are active but overwhelmed. Either way, the cerebroside-glutted macrophages display a

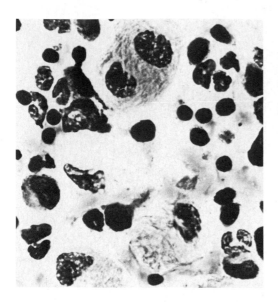
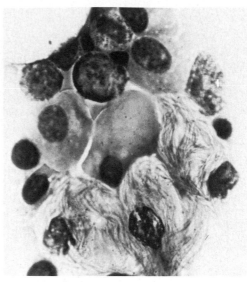

FIGURE 11-10

Gaucher cells in the marrow of a patient with the adult form of Gaucher's disease (glucosyl cera-mide lipidosis) (left) are indistinguishable by light microscopy from the huge storage macrophages, called pseudo-Gaucher cells (right), found in the marrow of many patients with chronic myelogenous leukemia. Gaucher cells of both kinds clog the parenchyma of marrow, spleen, and liver, and individual cells display cytoplasm crammed with pale tangled fibrils, conferring a distinctive ball-of-yarn appearance. (From Jandl JH: Chapt 17, in Blood: Textbook of Hematol-ogy. Boston, Little, Brown and Company, 1987.)

picturesque (however portentous) appearance (Figure 11-10) [14].

THE SPLEEN AND HYPERSPLENISM

Nowhere is vascular design so conducive to macrophage function as in the spleen, the lymph node and filter of the bloodstream. In the spleen, the architects of immunity and quality control—macrophages and lymphocytes—are so deployed that virtually all cells perfusing the organ are subject to scrutiny; imperfect cells are detained and either corrected or terminated.

Structure

In normal adults, the spleen weighs 135 ± 30 g and has a blood flow of 200 to 300 ml/min,

representing about 3 to 4% of cardiac output. The splenic artery penetrates the thick capsule of the spleen unaccompanied by afferent lym-phatics. Arterial vessels arborize and then subdivide into a trabecular spongework of connecting compartments that house the three structural components of splenic tissue: the centroidal white pulp, the surrounding red pulp, and the intervening marginal zone.

White Pulp Is Home for Lymphocytes

As branching "central" arteries penetrate the parenchyma they are invested with a cylindri-cal cuff of packed lymphocytes called the periarterial lymphatic sheath. Side branches of these arteries take off at right angles, enabling them to skim lymphocyte-rich plasma from the outer layer of streaming blood. Short branches deposit skimmed lymphocytes in the periarterial sheath, displacing cells vacation-ing there and bumping them back into circula-tion. This alternation of rest and recreation periods, interrupted briefly by tours of duty in the bloodstream, is characteristic of lympho-cytes, fewer than 1% of which are in circula-tion at a given moment. Lymphoid plasma in the longer branches is returned to the blood-stream via the sinuses of the surrounding red pulp, where red cells, plasma, and lympho-cytes are reunited. Prior to this reunion, as the terminal central arteries taper into arterioles, the axial blood becomes increasingly thickened with red cells ("hemoconcentrated"), and in this viscous state the red cells are dumped into and percolate through the maze-like vascular baffle called the marginal zone (Figure 11-11) [15].

Recirculating T cells and B cells follow different pathways in the spleen   T cells return to the periarterial lymphatic sheath where they rest up for 4 to 6 h before returning to the circulation on scouting sorties. B cells enter the sheath in smaller numbers but remain to form spherical foci called primary follicles. Later-arriving B cells that have encountered the antigen of their destiny home in on these follicles and stimulate stem cells located at the heart of primary follicles to proliferate as large, pale germinal center cells. Splenic nodules with germinal centers are termed "secondary follicles," and the progeny of germinal center cells (which are engaged in flat-out proliferation) gather around the follicle, forming the mantle layer. The entire follicular structure is embedded in the richly vascular spongiform red pulp (Figure 11-12) [15].

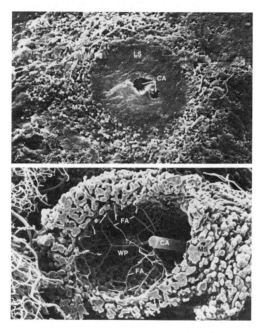

FIGURE 11-11

Cross-sectional views of the splenic white pulp (WP), showing the central artery (CA), the periarterial lymphatic sheath (LS), and the webby marginal zone (MZ). (Above) SEM of a cryofractured cross section reveals dense packing of lymphocytes in the lymphatic sheath and the extreme vascular complexity of the marginal zone. (Below) SEM of a microcorrosion cast after all parenchymal cells have been removed by alkaline hydrolysis bares small follicular arterioles (FA) and capillaries that traverse the vacated lymphatic nodule to drain into the marginal sinuses (MS), which in turn feed through the marginal zone into the red pulp. (From Tissues and Organs: A Text-Atlas of Scanning Electron Microscopy. By Richard Kessel and Randy Kardon. Copyright © 1979 by W.H. Freeman and Company. Reprinted with permission.)

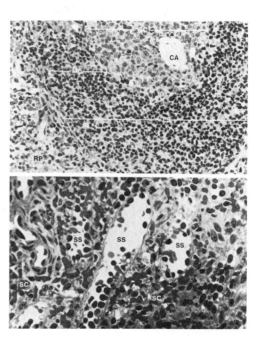

FIGURE 11-12

(Above) Germinal center (GC) cells bud off from the central artery (CA) of the lymphatic sheath (LS). Progeny of germinal center cells populate the outer shell or mantle layer (ML), and the entire lymphoid structure is embedded in red pulp (RP). (Below) Red pulp is shown to consist of alternating splenic sinuses (SS) and splenic cords (SC). (From Tissues and Organs: A Text-Atlas of Scanning Electron Microscopy. By Richard Kessel and Randy Kardon. Copyright © 1979 by W.H. Freeman and Company. Reprinted with permission.)

The Marginal Zone Is the Filter

The junctional tissue separating white pulp (lymphocytes) from red pulp (sinuses and cords) is called the marginal zone. The marginal zone is composed of perforate layers of pale oblong endothelial cells interlaced spaciously to form a reticular lattice placed perpendicular to the capillary current. It forms a living filter that acts as a brake on the heavy, confused traffic pouring in from the central artery and its tributaries. It is here that unnatural particles or defective cells are arrested for later disposal by wolfish macrophages, which move in from adjacent red pulp (Figure 11-13) [16].

Red Pulp Is Macrophage Country

Red pulp is composed of two alternating structures, the splenic sinuses and the splenic cords, which correspond to the major and minor hemodynamic compartments of the spleen.

The sinus compartment   The sinuses are broad and capacious avenues, 15 to 40 μm across. The sinus lining cells positioned along the axis of flow are long, fusiform, and tapered, crosslinked periodically side-by-side by tight junctional complexes. Between junctions,

endothelium is separated by slits, beneath which is the fenestrated screenlike basement membrane. These apposed vascular apertures enable sufficiently supple cells to squeeze and sideslip their way from the adjacent cords through the fenestrations and shingles of the sinus to reenter the bloodstream (Figure 11-14) [15]. Over 95% of blood entering the spleen passes directly through the broad boulevards of the splenic sinuses that empty their copious contents into trabecular veins, which then drain into the splenic vein. Normally about 20% of portal flow is contributed by the splenic vein.

Splenic cords   Splenic cords are discontinuous, often collapsed, endothelial structures that are sandwiched between sinuses, from which they are separated merely by the fenestrated basement membrane. Cords normally are packed with macrophages that dangle into the lumen and commingle with cordal lymphocytes and plasma cells. Less than 5% of blood cells traversing the mantle zone enter cordal openings; to escape these culs-de-sac and return to sinuses, they must jostle their way past obstructive macrophages and eel through the fenestrated sinus floor (Figure 8-3). Passage from cord to sinus is the ultimate test of size,

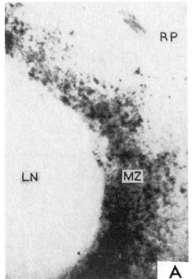 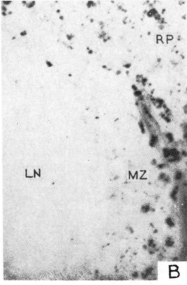

FIGURE 11-13

Filtration of particulate matter at the marginal zone and red pulp. (A) Within minutes of infusion, particles are trapped intercellularly between nonphagocytic marginal zone (MZ) cells surrounding the lymphatic nodule (LN). (B) Eight hours later, the particles have been carted into the red pulp (RP) by neighboring macrophages. (Reproduced from Snook T: Studies on the perifollicular region of the rat's spleen. Anat Rec 148:149,1964.)

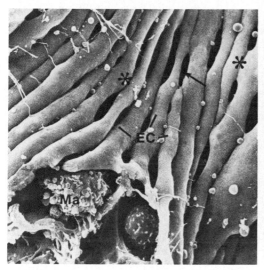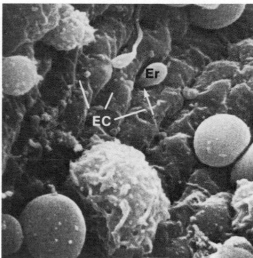

FIGURE 11-14

SEM interior views of splenic sinuses. (Left) Splenic sinuses are broad channels lined with fusiform endothelial cells (EC) that are joined at intervals by junctional complexes (*). Macrophages (Ma) can be seen lurking beneath the discontinuous basement membrane (not shown). Endothelial slits (black arrow) are numerous. (Right) Normally sinuses are crowded with perfusing blood cells, but most have fallen out during preparation. Small numbers of red cells (Er) can be seen slipping through tight endothelial slits (white arrow) to enter the sinus lumen from an adjacent cord. (From Tissues and Organs. A Text-Atlas of Scanning Electron Microscopy. By Richard Kessel and Randy Kardon. Copyright © 1979 by W.H. Freeman and Company. Reprinted with permission.)

shape, compliance, and stretch. Reticulocytes, being larger and less deformable than mature red cells, are detained for about 1 day in splenic cords; there they undergo final remodeling and are relieved by macrophages of attached debris or surplus membrane, and culled of inclusions such as Howell-Jolly bodies, intracellular vesicles ("pits" or "pocks"), siderotic granules, Pappenheimer bodies, or Heinz bodies, and of offensive organisms including protozoa. Cordal quality control is particularly evident in filtering out spherocytes. Spherocytes in hereditary spherocytosis or autoimmune hemolytic anemia (Chapter 8) lack the

membrane redundancy necessary for cordal passage. Being unable to "suck in their bellies," spherocytes become trapped in cords, causing hemolytic anemia—a problem rectified by surgical removal of the spleen.

Hemodynamic Features of Normal and Enlarged Spleens

Kinetic analyses indicate that the transit time for blood flowing through the normal spleen averages between 30 and 60 seconds, a rate only slightly slower than that of other major organs. The volume of blood that enters the sluggish cordal compartment is indiscernibly small in normal individuals, but hemodynamics are profoundly altered in patients with splenomegaly.

Red Cell Pooling

In most patients with splenomegaly (Table 11-2) [17] a large fraction of splenic arterial blood is diverted into the slow-moving, enlarged cordal compartment, wherein transit time may be prolonged to 60 minutes or longer. In massive splenomegaly, the content of red cells in this commodious exchangeable pool may represent up to 50% of the total red cell mass and cause a spurious dilutional anemia. In addition, red cells that by random misfortune wander into splenic cords are subjected to

TABLE 11-2

Common causes of splenomegaly

| Category | Magnitude of splenomegaly, size | | Representative disorders |
	Cm below left costal margin	Weight, g	
Normal	0	100–200	———
Slight	0–4	200–500	Infections
Moderate	4–8	500–2,000	Congestive splenomegaly Hemolytic anemia Infectious mononucleosis
Marked (massive)	>8	>2,000	Chronic myelogenous leukemia Idiopathic myelofibrosis Polycythemia vera Malignant lymphoma Chronic malaria (tropical splenomegaly) Kala-azar

Source: From Jandl H: Chapt 14, in Blood: Textbook of Hematology. Boston, Little, Brown and Company,1987.

packing, substrate depletion, acidosis, and other adverse conditions that disturb volume control and cause partial loss of membrane lipids and surface area. These changes are reversible on return to the nutrient circulation, but subpopulations of red cells subjected by chance to repetitive cordal pooling sustain additive metabolic insults, become spheroidal, and eventually are destroyed. Hence the dilutional anemia of splenomegaly is associated with mild to moderate hemolysis in the stagnant chambers of the spleen.

Massive splenomegaly and portal hypertension Splenomegaly may become truly massive (spleen weight: 20 to 30 times normal) in patients with chronic malaria ("tropical splenomegaly syndrome"), idiopathic myelofibrosis, chronic myelogenous leukemia, or visceral leishmaniasis. In such patients splenic regional blood flow may exceed 10 times normal, increasing total portal flow 2- to 4-fold. This voluminous torrent may overload the capacity of the splanchnic vasculature and lead to portal hypertension with variceal bleeding.

Platelet Pooling

Red cell pooling in normal spleens is negligible, but about 30% of platelets entering the spleen are diverted reversibly into the blind alleys and devious passages of the cordal compartment. The small size of platelets enables them to wander back and forth between cords and sinuses as they traverse the red pulp: like smaller molecules in a Sephadex column, smallness explains their retarded progress. If spleen blood flow is 4% of cardiac output and the average platelet spends 6 to 7 minutes in transit, about 24 to 28% of the total platelet population would be in transit within the spleen at a given instant. The intrasplenic platelet transit time is unaffected by spleen size, but the size of the splenic pool for platelets is roughly proportional to both splenic blood flow and spleen size (Figure 11-15) [18]. Platelet pooling serves a reservoir function, being greatest during tranquility or sleep; during adrenergic stimulation or excitement, platelets are expelled into the bloodstream from the cordal compartment and the exchangeable pool is closed temporarily. Splenectomy eliminates this adrenergic response. In splenomegalic states the splenic pool may contain 80 to 90% of the platelet mass, with very little damage to the viability of these ATP-rich minicorpuscles. Marrow stem cells appear not to sense compartmental diversion of platelets, suggesting that platelet formation is governed by signals reflecting total platelet mass.

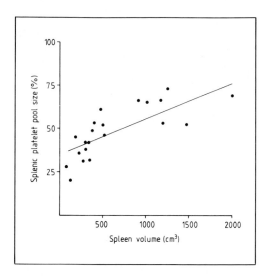

FIGURE 11-15

Relationship between spleen volume and the size of the exchangeable splenic platelet pool. Splenic blood flow (not shown) and splenic pooling was assessed by infusing ^{111}In-labeled platelets, and spleen size was determined by imaging after infusing ^{99m}Tc-labeled colloid. (From Wadenvik H et al: Splenic blood flow and intrasplenic platelet kinetics in relation to spleen volume. Br J Haematol 67:181,1987.)

Filtration, Phagocytosis, and Immunity

By virtue of its unique vascular structure the red pulp of the spleen is singularly proficient in sensing and destroying circulating cells having abnormalities that may escape detection in hepatic or marrow sinuses. Red cells exposed in vitro to IgG antibodies, oxidant drugs, heat, or sulfhydryl inhibitors in amounts insufficient to cause measurable morphologic or metabolic damage are nonetheless cleared rapidly and almost exclusively by the spleen following their infusion (Figure 11-16) [19]. Collectively, kinetic studies such as that portrayed in Figure 11-16 and perfusion studies performed ex vivo indicate that the potential efficacy of splenic clearance exceeds 50%. Thus nearly all clearance and destruction of damaged red cells perforce takes place in the spleen sinuses rather than in the low-flow cords—a conclusion borne out by histologic examination of spleens from patients with acquired hemolytic anemias. In immunohemolytic anemias, trapping and phagocytosis is initiated by macrophage Fc receptor binding of antibody-coated cells, a process that can be thwarted temporarily by intravenous IgG (Chapter 8). Other macrophage adhesives appear to mediate splenic

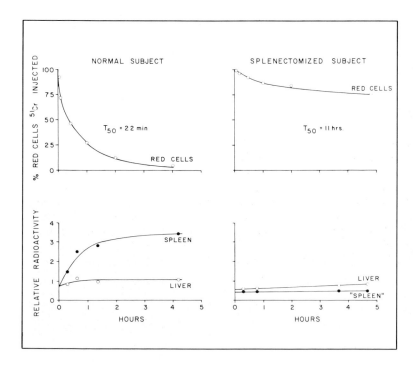

FIGURE 11-16

Selective splenic clearance of ^{51}Cr-labeled red cells exposed briefly to low concentrations of a sulfhydryl-blocking agent. (Left) In a normal subject clearance is a first-order process, with trapping of 3% of infused cells per minute. (Right) In splenectomized individuals, as exemplified here, clearance of identically damaged cells is extremely slow (half-time: 11 h). (Reproduced from the Journal of Clinical Investigation, 1962, 41: 1514, by copyright permission of the American Society for Clinical Investigation.)

clearance of cells damaged by nonimmune mechanisms [20], but the molecular basis of binding is poorly defined.

Splenic architecture is artfully designed for an integrated response to particulate antigens such as microorganisms. This compact arrangement consists of a trap (marginal zone and red pulp), antigen-coding cells (T cells and B cells) in the marginal and follicular mantle zones, and an adjoining source of stem cells and memory cells (germinal center cells). Splenectomized or asplenic individuals respond well to soluble antigens, but have depressed responses to intravenous particulate antigens.

Postsplenectomy and Asplenic States

Splenectomized or asplenic patients are quite vulnerable to first-encounter infections by certain encapsulated bacteria, namely *Streptococcus pneumoniae, Haemophilus influenzae,* and *Neisseria meningitidis.* Because of this limited bacterial spectrum, asplenic patients can be protected by appropriate polyvalent vaccine. Host resistance to alien organisms that directly infect red cells (e.g., plasmodia, babesia) is very difficult to bolster by vaccines in the absence of a splenic filter.

Absence of a functional spleen is associated with a set of harmless but telltale anomalies. After splenectomy red cells become flatter and broader as the result of gains in membrane lipids, and a minority of lipid-rich cells develop

wrinkles (become acanthocytes). Howell-Jolly bodies are removed during cordal transit, and their appearance (often accompanied by Pappenheimer bodies) is a trusty indication of splenic absence or hypofunction.

The spleen may be absent as a developmental disturbance originating in fetal life and associated with transpositions or malformations of the great vessels and viscera ("asplenia syndrome"). More often loss of splenic function is the consequence of splenic rupture and surgical extirpation. Blunt impact or crushing of the rib cage (as in road accidents) can tear the splenic capsule or create tumescent intrasplenic hematomas that eventually expand and dissect through the taut capsule. Either immediate or delayed intraabdominal bleeding must be dealt with by either splenectomy or splenorrhaphy. Recent awareness of the hazard

FIGURE 11-17

Growth and enhanced function of a splenulus (accessory spleen) in a patient with ITP recurring 6 years postsplenectomy, as shown by radionuclide splenic imaging. Splenic activity in the splenule is demonstrated by phagocytosis of ^{99m}Tc sulfur colloid (arrows). The large image of the liver is evident on the left of each panel. (A) Anterior oblique projection. (B) Left lateral projection. (From Sty JR and Conway JJ: The spleen: development and functional evaluation. Semin Nucl Med 15:276,1985.)

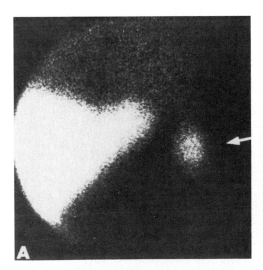
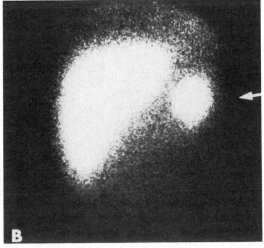

of overwhelming sepsis in patients splenectomized for trauma has inspired surgical techniques for salvaging a portion of intact spleen in cases when the hilum is intact: these include subtotal (segmental) splenectomy and splenorrhaphy, reinforced by omental patches and biologic adhesives. Among the remote complications of splenectomy are intraperitoneal seeding and autotransplantation of splenic fragments released during surgery (splenosis), and growth of small splenuli (accessory spleens) that were overlooked at surgery. Unlike splenotic autotransplants, which disseminate throughout peritoneal surfaces, splenuli occur commonly as one or two bits of embryologically misplaced tissue that may be stimulated to grow in patients with hemolytic anemia or immune thrombocytopenic purpura (ITP). Hemolytic anemias seldom relapse from regrowth of metaplastic splenic tissue, but postoperative resurgence of splenic function in patients splenectomized for ITP may restore sufficient platelet filtration to cause relapse of the purpura (Figure 11-17) [21]. The total circulating platelet mass normally is less than 10 ml, a quantity easily disposed of in ITP by a 20- to 30-g, born-again spleen.

REFERENCES

1. Nathan CF: Secretory products of macrophages. J Clin Invest 79:319,1987

2. van Furth R: Current view on the mononuclear phagocyte system. Immunobiology 161:178,1982

3. Nathan CF et al: Identification of interferon-γ as the lymphokine that activates human macrophage oxidative metabolism and antimicrobial activity. J Exp Med 158:670,1983

4. Snyderman R and Goetzl EJ: Molecular and cellular mechanisms of leukocyte chemotaxis. Science 213:830,1981

5. Warfel AH and Elberg SS: Macrophage membranes viewed through a scanning electron microscope. Science 170:446,1970

6. Johnston RB Jr: Monocytes and macrophages. N Engl J Med 318:747,1988

7. Murray HW: Survival of intracellular pathogens within human mononuclear phagocytes. Semin Hematol 25:101,1988

8. Rosenthal AS: Regulation of the immune response—role of the macrophage. N Engl J Med 303:1153,1980

9. Chambers TJ and Spector WG: Inflammatory giant cells. Immunobiology 161:283, 1982

10. Hill NS and Marx EJ: A 33-year-old man with cough, fever, weight loss, and pleuritic pain. Case 19-1988. N Engl J Med 318:1257,1988

11. Oursler MJ et al: Identification of osteoclast-specific monoclonal antibodies. J Cell Biol 100:1592,1985

12. Boyde A et al: Optical and scanning electron microscopy in the single osteoclast resorption assay. Scan Electron Microsc 3:1259, 1985

13. Rook GAW: Role of activated macrophages in the immunopathology of tuberculosis. Br Med Bull 44:611,1988

14. Jandl JH: Chapt 13, in Blood: Textbook of Hematology. Boston, Little, Brown and Company,1987

15. Kessel RG and Kardon RH: Chapt 2, in Tissues and Organs. A Text-Atlas of Scanning Electron Microscopy. New York, WH Freeman and Company,1979

16. Snook T: Studies on the perifollicular region of the rat's spleen. Anat Rec 148:149,1964

17. Jandl JH: Chapt 14, in Blood: Textbook of Hematology. Boston, Little, Brown and Company,1987

18. Wadenvik H et al: Splenic blood flow and intrasplenic platelet kinetics in relation to spleen volume. Br J Haematol 67:181,1987

19. Jacob HS and Jandl JH: Effects of sulfhydryl inhibition on red blood cells. II. Studies in vivo. J Clin Invest 41:1514,1962

20. Sills RH: Splenic function: physiology and splenic hypofunction. CRC Crit Rev Oncol Hematol 7:1,1987

21. Sty JR and Conway JJ: The spleen: development and functional evaluation. Semin Nucl Med 15:276,1985

12

Lymphocytes and Immunity

☐

ymphocytes are responsible for immunity. They protect against the universe of foreign antigens by marshalling two defensive strategies. Some lymphocytes produce humoral antibodies that bind specfically to the antigen that induced them; antibody binding then tags antigenic intruders for destruction by phagocytes. Lymphocytes genetically equipped to produce antibodies are designated B cells—a multiple entendre derived from the birthplace of B cells, which in birds is the bursa of Fabricius and in mammals is bone marrow. The other major mechanism for recognizing and destroying nonself antigens is allotted to a second and larger population of lymphocytes that are derived from the thymus, and hence termed T cells. T cells both regulate and participate in cell-mediated immune responses; this means that T cells are designed to respond to antigen that is presented to them by macrophages or B cells acting as "accessory cells."

Antigens Are Recognized by Membrane Receptors

B cells recognize antigens as such, with or without accessory cells, for in their formative stages they display unique single species of membrane immunoglobulins that serve as receptors for specific antigens. When activated by antigens for which they are genetically programmed, B cells transform into robotic antibody-secretory cells known as plasma cells. T cells recognize the antigen of their destiny through unique and integral membrane antigen receptors known in jargon as T cell receptors (TcRs or TCRs). Recognition requires that antigen (or parts of the antigen) is displayed by an accessory cell that is identical at the major histocompatibility (MHC) locus, for the TcR is a dual recognition complex that binds to both antigen and (by complementarity) to the MHC protein product; the TcR is a T cell antigen–MHC receptor. Once antigen is formally presented to a T cell, the cell undergoes transformation and, with the aid of cytokines, clonal proliferation. Thus both B cells and T cells are endowed with antigen-specific membrane receptors, and receptor occupancy leads each cell type to differentiate and clonally expand to launch an efficient immune response.

In addition to antigen-specific defenses, a more primitive generic effector response exists that is designed mainly to eliminate virus-infected or malignant cells. This line of defense is assigned to a special cadre of large granular lymphocytes known as natural killer (NK) cells.

MORPHOLOGY AND DIFFERENTIATION OF LYMPHOCYTES

The life history of B and T cells can be divided into two sequential stages: a primary antigen-independent phase and a secondary antigen-dependent one. During primary differentiation stem cells proceed through a series of concatenated divisions and differentiation steps that generate myriads of clones of B or T cells, each of which expresses on its surface an antigen receptor with novel specificity. For B cells these

FIGURE 12-1

Normal marrow lymphoblast (left) and mature blood lymphocyte (right). Normal lymphoblasts are round or oblong cells having a narrow rim of deeply basophilic cytoplasm, purple chromatin, and one or two boldly outlined nucleoli. Mature lymphocytes have a compact, rounded or slightly notched nucleus, chunky but blurred masses of chromatin, and scant blue cytoplasm lacking granules. (Photos by CT Kapff.)

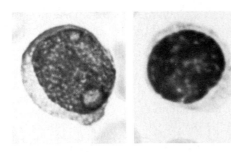

events take place in the fetal liver and adult marrow. For T cells similar events are initiated in these primary organs but are concluded during late fetal life in the T cell–specific primary differentiation organ, the thymus.

During differentiation of lymphoblasts into mature resting B and T cells, their DNA is packed tightly into dense heterochromatin masses and exhibits little transcriptional activity. The nucleus of these small cells is surrounded by a thin rim of clear agranular cytoplasm; in effect the resting lymphocyte is a vector for transporting inert genetic information to all parts of the body, prepared on appropriate stimulation to loosen up its packaged DNA for transcriptional activity. The morphology of lymphoblasts and mature resting lymphocytes of both B and T cell sorts are identical by light microscopy (Figure 12-1).

Lymphocyte Traffic

Even resting (antigen-independent) lymphocytes are restless. Maturing lymphocytes circulate continuously throughout the body, fulfilling their sensory role as scouts engaged in immune surveillance. The mobility of lymphocytes enables them to surprise invaders, explore various microenvironments, and interact with other lymphocyte subsets. Blood lymphocytes migrate into tissues and fluids by recognizing and adhering to regionally specialized high endothelial cells of the postcapillary venules (HEVs). Trafficking of the various lymphocyte subsets through venules is dependent on a turnstile mechanism in which 90,000 M_r homing receptors on lymphocytes attach to regional binding sites on endothelium, which provide specific portals of exit from the circulation to peripheral lymph nodes, mucosa-associated lymphoid tissues, and barrier tissues.

Migration versus Locomotion

Migration refers to compartmental redistribution of lymphocyte populations, whereas locomotion refers to the active crawling upon, over, or around other cell surfaces in response to complex traffic signals that arouse curiosity and chemotaxis. Lymphocyte locomotion is fundamentally similar to that of neutrophils and monocytes. Mature lymphocytes are driven by curiosity to cross physiological sur-

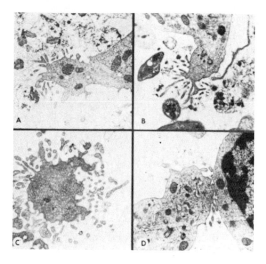

FIGURE 12-2

EM views of lymphocyte uropods. (A and B) Bristly structure of microvilli and microspikes extending from the macelike ends of uropods. (C) Cross-sectional view. (D) A uropod tip is attached by its talons to the outer aspect of another lymphocyte. (From McFarland W and Schecter GP: The lymphocyte in immunological reactions in vitro: ultrastructural studies. Blood 35:683,1970.)

faces at rates in excess of 20 μm/min, utilizing alternating propulsive and retractile movements involving rearrangements of the 3-D actin-myosin assembly. When in the locomotor mode lymphocytes assume a hand-mirror configuration. In addition any stimulus that induces locomotion or stimulates cell division causes lymphocytes to extend a unique trailing protuberance having a macelike tip known as the uropod.

Uropods are probing devices The uropod is a unique posterior proboscis used by an activated lymphocyte to explore strange objects and communicate with other lymphocytes. When a lymphocyte bumps into a macrophage or another activated lymphocyte with its anterior (cortical) end, its several tiny pseudopodal engines back the lymphocyte away and steer it into a reversed position that permits attachment of the uropod to the target. This long protuberance is studded with microvilli and smaller microspikes designed for grappling (Figure 12-2) [1].

B CELLS, PLASMA CELLS, AND ANTIBODY SYNTHESIS

B cells are lymphocytes genetically designed to recognize virtually all potential antigens and programmed to transform after antigen contact into antibody-secreting cells known as plasma cells.

B Cell Maturation and Replication

Release of immature B cells from marrow occurs prior to their antigen-dependent conversion to secretory forms. Antigen-independent maturation of B cells in marrow involves several divisions during which these small immature forms acquire early membrane markers, μ chains, and later light chains. Those cells lacking surface immunoglobulin (sIg) are called "pre B cells"; postmitotic pre B cells then acquire the capacity to synthesize light chains, which combine with heavy chains to form sIgM molecules capable of acting as antigen receptors. These immature, virgin B cells also express sIgD molecules having identical variable domains and hence identical antigen-binding specificities. They enter the circulation where they segregate into circulating and migratory classes; arrival of virgin B cells in B cell zones of lymphoid tissues provides a continuous source of fresh, genetically programmed (antigen-specific) B cells available for antigen-induced activation, clonal expansion, and maturation to plasma cells. Most virgin B cells never encounter the antigen for which they are intended and die within a few days, their mission unfulfilled. This prodigal waste may be an important strategem for ensuring constant replenishment with young receptive cells possessing the full repertoire of antigen specificities.

Immunoglobulin Gene Rearrangements and Expression

Genes encoding the heavy and light chains of antibodies are situated on three separate chromosomes: heavy (μ) chain, κ chain, and λ chain genes are located as discontinuous segments of chromosomes 14, 2, and 22, respectively. The singular mobility and rearrangements of genetic material within the B cell genome explain the nearly infinite diversity of antibody generation; the immunologic dogma of clonal selection can be explained by the capacity of B cells to rearrange multiple immunoglobulin gene segments prior to transcription. The multiple exons that encode for the variable (V) region genes must be rearranged from their original germline configuration before transcription can commence. During initial differentiation of B cell precursors the rearrangement cascade starts with selection of a heavy chain V region gene from the vast library of V_H coding segments. The initial recombination event involves movement of one of the 20 or more diversity (D) genes into juxtaposition with one of the six joining (J_H) genes, and the DNA between the two transposed genes is deleted (step 1). Next, one of the 50 or more (possibly over 300) V_H genes on one of the two allelic chromosomes is translocated to form a continuous VDJ_H gene complex encoding the entire variable region of the heavy chain (step 2). This brings a promoter sequence located 5' to the leader sequence of the transposed V_H under the influence of a transcriptional enhancer, which is located between the J_H and the invariable, or constant, $C\mu$ genes (Figure 12-3) [2].

Sequential Activation of Light Chain Genes

After V_H, D, and J_H exons have been spliced correctly, the next step in the gene rearrangement cascade is the simpler V to J joining on chromosome 2 (Figure 12-3); when the VJ_H splice is in an appropriate reading mode, the RNA transcript can be processed to form mRNA for κ light chain production. This step in gene rearrangement is quite error-prone; failure of one or both parental κ alleles to rearrange correctly occurs in about one-third of μ^+ pre B cells. When this happens, λ gene light chain rearrangements are initiated by default on chromosome 22, and if effective these lead to a μ, λ-bearing B cell. If such rearrangements are also aberrant, the cell is frozen in the pre B stage, unable to form antibody. If light chain formation is successful, the light chains match up with μ heavy chains of the same specificity, and the completed IgM molecules are transported through the Golgi region en route to the cell surface.

FIGURE 12-3

Sequential rearrangement of immunoglobulin genes encoding the variable regions of heavy (A) and kappa light (B) chains. The encircled numbers indicate the consecutive steps in gene rearrangement by DNA excision. C (constant) region exons for each Ig isotype are indicated within the white boxes, and black circles denote H chain isotype switch sequences. Not shown are promoter and enhancer sequences and the lambda gene light-chain rearrangement on chromosome 22. (From Cooper MD: B lymphocytes. Normal development and function. Reprinted, by permission of The New England Journal of Medicine, 317:1452,1987.)

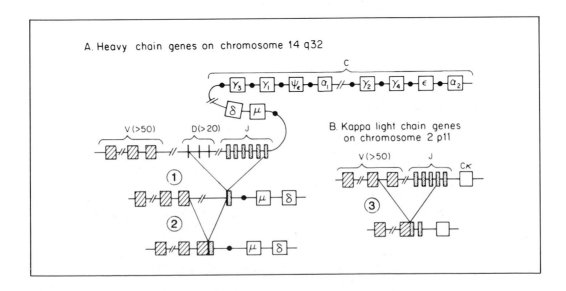

Membrane and secreted forms of IgM   The first antibodies made by newly matured B cells are not secreted but are firmly anchored by hydrophobic bonds to the cell membrane where they serve as receptors for antigen. Through alternative sites of polyA addition and RNA splicing, B cells then acquire different mRNAs containing either the secreted or the membrane-bound peptides (Figure 12-4) [3]. In its secreted form, IgM formed by the union of μ and light chains is a pentamer composed of five IgM monomers assembled in a starfish configuration.

Isotype Switching

B cells of any given clone can switch Ig production from IgM to antibodies of different heavy chain classes (isotypes), but all antibodies will have the same variable region sequence and each individual cell will express only one light chain and one heavy chain allele—a phenomenon known as allelic exclusion. Young B cells coexpressing IgM and IgD may undergo a class switch as a final step in the cascade of Ig gene rearrangements, thereby becoming B cells that express membrane-bound IgG, IgA, or IgE and

ultimately transforming to plasma cells that secrete IgG, IgA, or IgE (Figure 12-5) [3]. Isotype switching is accomplished by cutting off repetitive DNA sequences in a switch (S) region upstream of the $C\mu$ gene to be expressed. To switch from IgM to IgG3, the intervening DNA including $C\mu$, and $C\delta$ exons are extirpated, bringing the $C\gamma 3$ gene in line for transcription by placement next to the VDJ complex (Figure 12-6) [2].

Nonimmunoglobulin Receptors

Prior to their activation by antigen, maturing B cells arm themselves with numerous surface

FIGURE 12-4

Schematic reprise of the organization of the μ heavy chain gene and its secreted and membranous products. Both secreted and membranous forms of μ chains precursive to IgM are derived from a single constant μ region locus. (From Waldmann TA et al: Chapt 8, in The Molecular Basis of Blood Diseases, Stamatoyannopoulos G et al, Eds. Philadelphia, WB Saunders Company, 1987.)

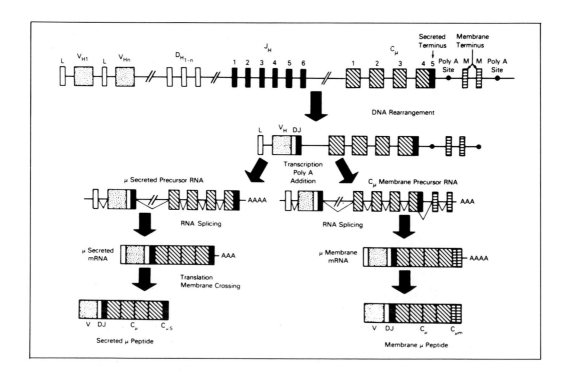

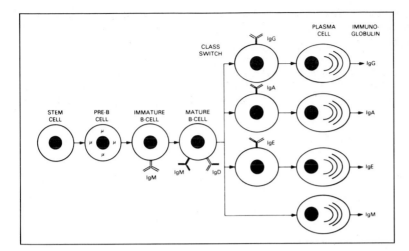

FIGURE 12-5

Differentiation of B cells and plasma cells. (From Waldmann TA et al: Chapt 8, in The Molecular Basis of Blood Diseases, Stamatoyannopoulos G et al, Eds. Philadelphia, WB Saunders Company, 1987.)

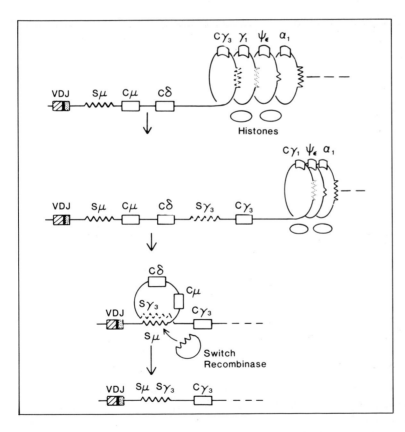

FIGURE 12-6

Mechanism of immunoglobulin isotype switching by DNA deletion during B cell differentiation. Immunoglobulin genes are indicated by boxes and switch sequences by serrated lines. (From Cooper MD: B lymphocytes. Normal development and function. Reprinted, by permission of The New England Journal of Medicine, 317:1452,1987.)

receptors, in addition to sIg, readying them to receive environmental signals that help guide their complex immune responses. Pre B cells transiently display terminal deoxynucleotidyl transferase (TdT), which acts as a somatic mutagen vital to generation of Ig gene diversity, after which the MHC antigens, HLA-DP and HLA-DR, surface to serve as self-recognition signals necessary for dealing with class II antigens. After acquisition of sIgM, B cells express surface receptors for the Fc portions of IgG, IgM, IgA, and IgE, followed by emergence of receptors for C3b (CR1) and C3d (CR2) (Chapter 8). After activation, growth and differentiation of B cells are modulated by upregulation of receptors for transferrin, IL-2, and for B cell growth factors IL-4 and IL-6 and their inhibitor, IFNγ.

Clonal Diversity Redux

Before describing their response to antigen activation, homage is due to the power of B cells for identifying antigen. Just as one can create a library of books from 26 letters used in different combinations, B cells utilize rearranged variable, diversity, and joining region gene elements to generate at least 1 billion different potential antibody-forming clones from combinations and permutations of only a few hundred different genetic elements in embryonic DNA.

B Cell Activation and Differentiation

Antigen selects from the repertoire of resting B cells, each expressing only one of the countless variable regions of Ig on its surface. Upon receptor occupancy by the complementary antigen, B cells are aroused from G_0, enlarge, increase RNA synthesis, and initiate transmembrane signalling, calling forth second messengers including cyclic AMP, GMP, and ion-channel effectors and inciting hydrolysis of phosphatidyl inositol lipids [4]. Activation causes B cells to begin DNA synthesis and to divide every 20 h for 5 to 15 divisions. Antigen molecules that bind to sIg receptors are internalized and partially digested. Antigen fragments are then recycled to B cell surfaces and expressed in association with class II molecules of the MHC. This presentation of antigen fragment and complementary class II molecule on the B cell surface is recognized by helper T cells (T_H cells) by means of their antigen receptors, causing release of T cell factors that promote proliferation and differentiation. Helper T cell stimulation and IL-1–secreting macrophages collaborate with antigen in prompting each successive wave of daughter cells to continue to replicate (Figure 12-7) [5]. After several cycles of proliferation, B cells are eventually induced to undergo terminal differentiation as plasma cells that produce thousands of antibody molecules per second before

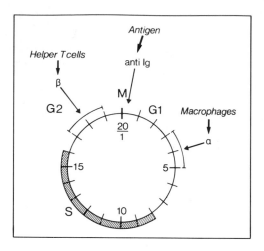

FIGURE 12-7

Cell cycle control of activated B cells. Cycling is initiated by antigen (or anti-Ig), and entry into subsequent cycles depends upon cytokines released at restriction point α (in G_1) by macrophages and at point β (in G_2) by helper T cells. (Reproduced, with permission, from the Annual Review of Immunology, Vol. 4. © 1986 by Annual Reviews Inc.)

their demise a day or so later [2]. Some activated B cells only divide once or twice before entering the memory cell pool—perpetuated clones of B cells that remember the antigen (Figure 12-8) [6]. Memory B cells immortalize the gene rearrangements which code for the antigen at issue. They mainly generate plasma cells that secrete IgG or IgA and proliferate very rapidly during second encounter with the antigen. Memory cells account for the ability of the immune system to storm back within a few days in response to reinfection by an organism and to secrete antibodies better fitted by addition of refined mutations to react with recalled antigens on the organism ("affinity maturation"). In patients whose lymphatic follicles are populated by memory B cells, the antibody response to antigen on second encounter is not only more prompt but several magnitudes greater (Figure 12-9) [6]. During the primary response, initial antibody is of the IgM subclass, but an isotype switch to IgG occurs in the second week and IgG antibodies dominate the magnified secondary response.

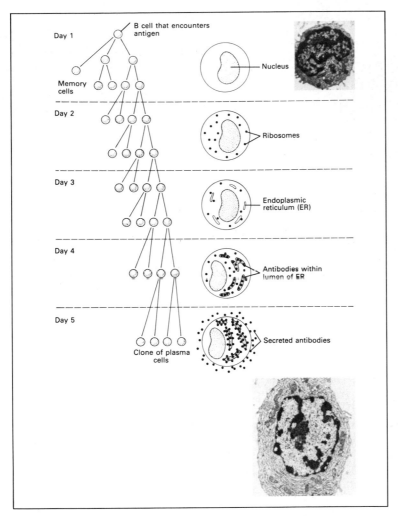

Day 1
B cell that encounters antigen

Memory cells

Nucleus

Day 2

Ribosomes

Day 3

Endoplasmic reticulum (ER)

Day 4

Antibodies within lumen of ER

Day 5

Clone of plasma cells

Secreted antibodies

FIGURE 12-8

Antigen activation of a B cell (EM at upper right) leads to proliferation and morphologic differentiation to create a populous clone of antibody-secreting plasma cells (EM at lower right). A minority of activated cells proliferate only briefly but survive as long-lived memory cells (upper left). (From Darnell J et al: Molecular Cell Biology. New York, Scientific American Books, 1986.)

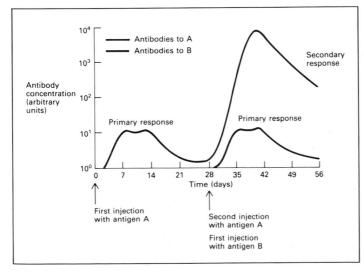

Antibodies to A
Antibodies to B

Secondary response

Antibody concentration (arbitrary units)

Primary response

Primary response

Time (days)

First injection with antigen A

Second injection with antigen A

First injection with antigen B

FIGURE 12-9

Antibody responses to initial and later injections of antigen. The secondary response to injection of antigen A at 28 days was faster and far greater than the primary response, whereas the response to an unrelated antigen (B) given at the same time showed the expected primary pattern. The enhancement of the secondary response is, accordingly, specific and reflects the amplified number of memory B cells. (From Darnell J et al: Molecular Cell Biology. New York, Scientific American Books, 1986.)

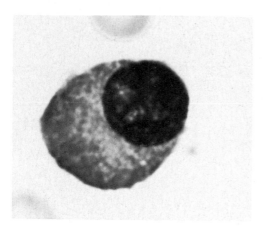

FIGURE 12-10

Normal plasma cell, containing a condensed rounded eccentric nucleus, which has been pushed aside by the bulky, floccular, dark gray-blue accumulation of Ig secretory elements in the cytoplasm. On Wright-Giemsa the cytoplasm is mottled, often vacuolated, and swollen with antibody. (Photo by CT Kapff.)

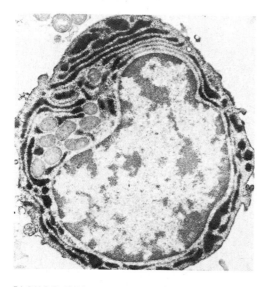

FIGURE 12-11

Ultrastructural localization of cytoplasmic Ig. In mature and "postmature" plasma cells the immunoglobulin (black rivulets and puddles) is channeled within convolutions of the dilated RER cisternae. (From Grossi CF et al: Chapt 9, in Atlas of Blood Cells: Function and Pathology. Zucker-Franklin D et al, Eds. Milan, Edi. Ermes s.r.l.,1988.)

Plasma Cells

Metamorphosis of an activated B cell to an endstage secretory plasma cell is obvious by light microscopy. The inactivated nucleus has become pyknotic and displaced to one side by the abundant cytoplasm, which occupies 80% of the cell and is turgid with ribosomes and secretory vacuoles filled with cytoplasmic Ig (Figure 12-10). The proliferative response to antigen yields multiple clones of the nonreplicating, terminally differentiated secretory cells. Polyclonal amplification generates plasma cells individually programmed to manufacture any one of the eight classes and subclasses of Ig having a common antigen specificity. Over 80% of transitional and mature plasma cells secrete IgG, 15% produce IgA, fewer than 5% make IgM, and only traces of IgD and IgE are elaborated. The large Golgi apparatus of plasma cells packages antibody made by rough endoplasmic reticulum (RER), transiently choking the dilated RER cisternae (Figure 12-11) [7], but eventually immunoglobulin droplets wend their way to the cell surface where they are secreted as free antibodies.

Idiotype–Anti-Idiotype Interactions: The Idiotypic Network

Being novel structures, antibodies themselves are immunogenic. The unique folds, crevices, and protrusions that make up the configuration of the variable region contain many individual antigenic determinants (idiotopes) that in the aggregate constitute the private antigenic profile, or idiotype, of an antibody. Thus the variable region of an antibody molecule not only constitutes its antigen combining site but also its serologic signature (idiotype), and the immune system responds by generating anti-idiotypes. Consider two lymphocytes—B cell$_1$ and B cell$_2$—whose complementary surface Igs represent an idiotype–anti-idiotype pair; the antibodies they secrete can be called antibody$_1$ and antibody$_2$. The idiotype of antibody$_1$ can bind to the variable region of the sIg of B cell$_2$, stimulating production of a corresponding anti-idiotype. The combining site of antibody$_1$ is complementary to a structure on the immunizing antigen, and the combining site of antibody$_2$ contains an internal image component that mimics the shape of the original antigen. This imaging is so faithful that anti-idiotypic antibodies can be used to prepare vaccines to corresponding antigens; antigen (ligand) mimicry also can cause anti-idiotypic antibodies to react with ligand receptors on cell membranes, which has inspired their trial use in the immunotherapy of B cell neoplasms (Figure 12-12) [8]. Anti–anti-idiotypes have also been found during the immune response, but there the network circuitry usually ends because of the resemblance of antibody₃ to antibody₁.

The presumed purpose of the anti-idiotype network is to help terminate the immune response after antigen has been eliminated. Similar principles and rules appear to apply to both B cells and T cells, and there is evidence of interactions between B cell idiotypes and the T cell idiotypes resulting from comparable rearrangements in the variable regions of TcRs. As T cells can be of either the helper-inducer or suppressor variety, the idiotypic network has global immunoregulatory powers.

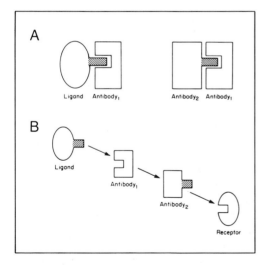

FIGURE 12-12

Ligand mimicry by anti-idiotypic antibodies. Part A depicts the complementary relation between antibody₁ and antibody₂ (anti-idiotype). Part B shows that antibody₂ both simulates the original antigenic ligand and can bind to the receptor for that ligand. (From Burdette S and Schwartz RS: Idiotypes and idiotypic networks. Reprinted, by permission of The New England Journal of Medicine, 317:219,1987.)

Major Histocompatibility Complex (MHC) and Its HLA Antigens Identify Self and Nonself

Knowledge of how the immune response (Ir) genes equip us to discriminate between self and nonself was not obtained from experiments of nature but rather from experiments of physicians performing organ transplantation. These revealed that successful transplantation requires a matchup between "histocompatibility antigens" of donor and recipient. The Ir genes are components of the MHC, a supergene complex that codes for the polymorphic HLA (human leukocyte-associated) antigens found on all nucleated cells in the body. In their diversity and ubiquitous expression, these MHC-generated proteins confer individuality and are responsible for private attributes ranging from body odor to autoimmunity. MHC genes are located on the short arm of chromosome 6 and are inherited in codominant haploid packets, except in rare instances of meiotic crossing over. As complete parental histocompatibility is rare, the likelihood that any two siblings will be HLA identical is 25%, in accordance with mendelian principles.

MHC Genes Produce Two Major Classes of Membrane Antigens

The loci of the MHC and their cell-surface protein (HLA) products can be divided into two principal classes. Class I glycoproteins, present on all nucleated cells, are encoded by HLA-A, -B, and -C genes, and each molecule is composed of a 45,000 M_r heavy chain coupled noncovalently to a β_2 microglobulin encoded on chromosome 15. The remarkable diversity and multiplicity of class I glycoproteins (which number in excess of 80 by microlymphocytotoxicity assay and nearly 200 by other techniques) is somewhat mysterious, as each individual inherits only a single allele at each locus from each parent. An uplifting explanation is that individuality provides survival advantages, in defiance of societal trends; a more mechanistic one is that heterozygosity for class I antigens sharpens the cognitive powers of cytolytic T cells in their obsessive search for minor alterations in self antigens caused by viruses, aging, or neoplasia.

Class II antigens are encoded mainly by three families of loci referred to as HLA-DR, -DQ, and -DP. These are expressed on cell surfaces as $\alpha\beta$ dimers which play crucial roles in the immune response. Class II MHC products are termed alternatively "Ia" antigens. Constitutive expression of class II genes is restricted to mature B cells, macrophages, activated T cells, and thymic epithelial cells, but their expression can be induced by IFNγ, IL-4, or prostaglandin in endothelial cells and fibroblasts.

MHC Restriction and the Immune Response

The central step in the immune response to proteins and peptides is the clonal selection and activation of helper T cells expressing the CD4 antigen. CD4-positive T cells (T4 cells) recognize proteins only when protein is presented formally by activated macrophages or B cells that bear identical MHC class II antigens. Hence the MHC imposes a restriction on recognition. Actual identification of the antigen requires dual recognition of both the MHC molecules on the accessory cell and the foreign antigen itself. In this pivotal process, B cell reactivity (antibody synthesis) can be against the protein in its native configuration, whereas T cells respond to sequences of amino acids displayed on the surface of HLA-identical cells after the antigen has been denatured and pro-cessed by endosomes in the accessory cell (Figure 12-13) [9]. Identification of presented peptides of foreign antigen depends upon expression of the clonally unique T cell antigen-MHC receptor.

T CELLS AND THE T CELL NETWORK

T cells are responsible for cell-mediated immunity. Unlike B cells, which can recognize antigen as such with or without T cell help, T cells recognize antigen only when it is presented in conjunction with class I or II HLA molecules. Cellular immunity is elicited by diffusible products released from microorganisms, tumors, or tissue grafts and is characteristically delayed in onset for many hours by the need to select and activate T cells genetically endowed with the

FIGURE 12-13

Diagrammatic scheme of how antigen processed and presented by a macrophage promotes attachment of a helper T cell that is identical at the HLA-D (Ia) locus. (From Alberts B et al: Molecular Biology of the Cell. New York, Garland Publishing, Inc.,1983.)

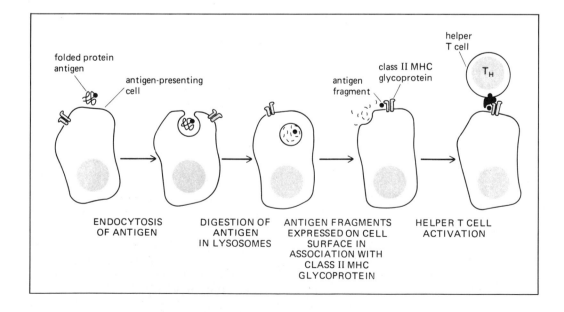

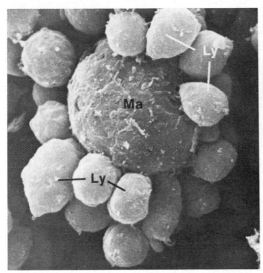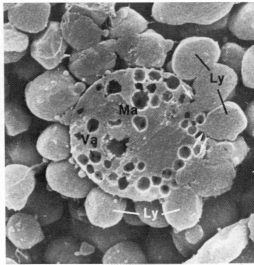

FIGURE 12-14

SEMs of thymic cortex showing extensive binding and destruction of T lymphocytes (Ly) by macrophages (Ma). (Left) Many lymphocytes are tightly attached to a single macrophage, forming a rosette. (Right) Cryofracture through a similar rosette reveals inspissation and phagocytosis of lymphocytes; phagocytized lymphocytes leave behind digestive vacuoles (Va) as the tombs of their liquidation. (From Tissues and Organs. A Text-Atlas of Scanning Electron Microscopy. By Richard Kessel and Randy Kardon. Copyright © 1979 by W.H. Freeman and Company. Reprinted with permission.)

appropriate antigen receptor; the antigen-activated T cell then summons resting T cell recruits to the scene and stimulates their proliferation by releasing IL-2 and other immune cytokines (lymphokines). The magnitude of the clonal response then depends on the extent of T cell proliferation in response to the IL-2–IL-2 receptor system. The prototype of cell-mediated immunity is the "delayed hypersensitivity reaction" to intradermal tuberculin.

Young T Cells Do or Die in the Thymus: Thymic Selection and Sorting

Large lymphoid stem cells (CFU-Ls) migrate from marrow to thymus beginning in early embryonic life and continuing into infancy.

Before its involution, this lymphoepithelioid organ provides a microenvironment that either matures thymocytes to lymphoblasts and lymphocytes or kills them. The majority of cortical lymphocytes die in situ, possibly by not meeting MHC (self) standards. Macrophages are widely distributed in both the thymic cortex and medulla, and function in selectively removing developing lymphocytes that either express forbidden differentiation markers, or fail to display correct differentiation markers such as CD2. The selection process guarantees that each matriculated T cell will react with a product of the MHC but will not react with self antigens, assuring both self-recognition and self-tolerance. Thymic selection leads to massive lymphocyte carnage; the execution of objectionable lymphocytes is performed through destructive binding of at least 95% of young thymocytes and lymphocytes by resident macrophages (Figure 12-14) [10].

T Cell Ontogeny

As the surviving cells mature in the thymus they display on their surfaces a programmed series of peptides denoted by the initialism CD (for clusters of differentiation numbers assigned by international workshops). In stage 1, large thymic lymphoblasts in the cortex express terminal deoxynucleotidyl transferase

(TdT) and brandish the adhesive CD2 (T11) antigen, a T cell lineage marker that incidentally is a receptor for sheep erythrocytes and is responsible for the E-rosetting phenomenon. Shortly afterward the maturing (stage 2) thymocytes become equipped with the CD3 (T3) antigen and the surface-mounted T cell antigen receptor (TcR) complex, sometimes called the T3-Ti complex. The most mature (stage 3) surviving thymocytes then penetrate into the medullary compartment where they transiently coexpress both the 62,000 M_r CD4 (T4) and the 76,000 M_r CD8 (T8) peptides. Mature T cells emerging from the thymus possess either the T4 or the T8 phenotype, but not both. When these mature subsets arrive at peripheral nodes, they are sorted out: in the paracortical T cell areas of nodes, T4 cells of helper and inducer type are embraced by interdigitating cells, while T8 cells of cytotoxic and suppressor type collect in intervening niches. T cell ontogeny is recapitulated in Figure 12-15 [11].

T Cell Subsets

Three functional classes of mature T cells have been defined. The T4 subset encompasses the majority of helper-inducer cells and represents about two-thirds of blood T lymphocytes. T4 cells help out and induce B cell activation and comprise virtually all lymphocytes that proliferate in response to antigen presentation and produce IL-2. The T8 subset, accounting for about one-third of blood T lymphocytes, includes the majority of both the suppressor and cytotoxic (cytolytic) T cells. Suppressor T8

cells are functionally antithetical to helper T4 cells, and the activation signal for cytolytic T8 cells consists of binding to antigenic epitopes in conjunction with HLA class I molecules on the target cell itself. The CD4 and CD8 glycoproteins on T4 and T8 cells are invariant structures, and their role appears to be to bind to invariant regions of class II and class I molecules, respectively, thereby facilitating reaction with target cells by promoting cell-to-cell contact. All T cell functions involve reactions on the surfaces of cells.

The number of cell surface markers that have been identified on immunocytes and other blood cells is bewildering—exceeding 50, not counting alternative synonyms, metonyms, and phenomenologic labels. Table 12-1 provides an abbreviated listing of the most significant surface marker molecules on lymphocytes, as cited in the international CD registry.

FIGURE 12-15

Expression of cell surface molecules on thymocytes and maturing lymphocytes. The adhesion molecule, CD2, is first to appear, followed by acquisition of the T cell antigen receptor linked to CD3 and then both the CD4 and CD8 molecules. Cells released to peripheral lymphatics display only CD4 or CD8. In some instances the "double positive" (CD4-CD8) stage may be bypassed (interrupted arrowlines). (Modified from Bierer BE et al: T-cell activation: the T-cell erythrocyte receptor (CD2) and sialophorin (CD42). Immunol Allergy Clin North Am 8:51,1988.)

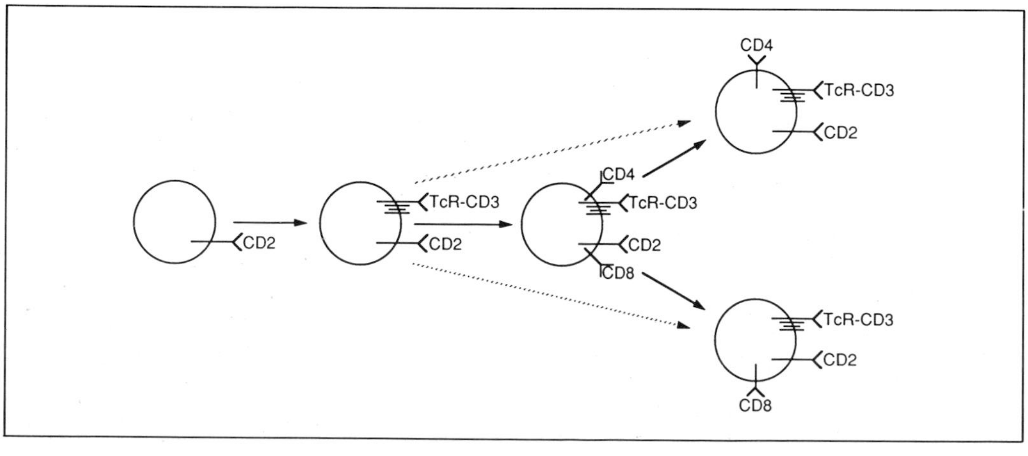

TABLE 12-1

Abridged listing of several important CD antigens found on lymphocytes

Antigen	Aliases	Distribution	Functional identity
CD2	T11, Leu5	T cells; also on many NK cells	Pan-T antigen; alternative activation pathway; sheep erythrocyte receptor; ?thymic credential
CD3	T3, Leu4	T cells	Pan-T antigen; associated with T cell antigen receptor (TcR)
CD4	T4, Leu3	T cell subset	Marker of helper-inducer subset of T cells; involved in recognition of class II MHC molecules; receptor for human immunodeficiency virus (HIV)
CD5	T1, Leu1	Most T cells and a subset of B cells	?Coactivation and proliferation signal
CD8	T8, Leu2	T cell subset	Marker of suppressor-cytolytic (cytotoxic) subset of T cells; involved in recognition of class I MHC molecules
CD16	Leu11	NK cells	Natural killer cells
CD19	B4, Leu12	B cells and pre B cells	Early pan-B antigen
CD20	B1, Leu16	B cells; follicular dendritic macrophages	Later pan-B antigen

T Cell Antigen Receptor (TcR)

T cell antigen receptors, like immunoglobulin genes, are assembled from separate clusters of germline DNA by novel rearrangements and deletions. Two distinct CD3-associated TcR (Ti) structures have been identified on blood T cells. The first structure, $TcR_{\alpha\beta}$, is found on most T cells and is responsible for antigen-specific MHC-restricted binding. This antigen receptor is a clonally unique 90,000 M_r disulfide-linked heterodimer, consisting of a 50,000 M_r α chain encoded by genes located on chromosome 14 band q11.2 and a 40,000 M_r β chain encoded by genes situated on chromosome 7 band q34. A second receptor structure, $TcR_{\gamma\delta}$, is expressed on a minority (1 to 10%) of T cells as well as on thymocytes and some natural killer (NK) cells. The antigens and restricting elements recognized by these lymphocytes are unknown but may be associated with constitutive NK activity. TcR_γ genes are situated on band p15 of chromosome 7, and TcR_δ genes are nested within the TcR_α gene coding region on chromosome 14, band q11; thus TcR_α gene rearrangement leads to deletion of the corresponding TcR_δ locus, accounting in part for the predominance in mature blood T cells of $TcR_{\alpha\beta}$ receptors.

TcR and Ig Gene Rearrangements Are Analogous

All four receptor chains are encoded by Ig-like gene segments that undergo deletions and rearrangements to form functional units during T cell differentiation in the thymus. The TcR_α locus is composed of approximately 50 variable (V) segments, 50 joining (J) segments, and a single constant (C) region; it lacks a diversity (D) segment. The TcR_β locus is comprised of about 70 V segments, 2 D segments, 13 J regions, and 2 constant genes. Germline diversity—combinatorial and imprecise V-(D)-J joining, random insertion by TdT of nongermline-encoded nucleotides (called N segments) between the rearranging VJ or VDJ

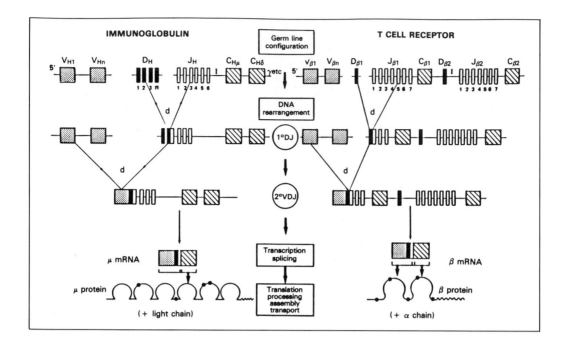

FIGURE 12-16

Organization and rearrangements pattern of the TcR$_\beta$ chain genes (right) is compared with that of immunoglobulin H chain genes (left). Both depend on highly analogous stepwise rearrangements, deletions, and splicings. TcR gene rearrangements take place exclusively in the thymus, whereas Ig gene rearrangements occur in marrow B cells. d = deletion, I = intronic sequences between coding exons (later spliced out); n signifies uncertainty as to the exact number of gene segments. (From Greaves MF et al: Chapt 9, in Atlas of Blood Cells: Function and Pathology. Zucker-Franklin D et al, Eds. Milan, Edi. Ermes s.r.l.,1988.)

elements, and combinatorial association of α and β polypeptides—collectively assures a repertoire quite sufficient to deal with a universe of antigens. The mechanism of combinatorial rearrangements underlying TcR diversity relies upon selective deletions, as is true of Ig rearrangements (Figure 12-16) [12]. For analogical comparison, the structure of the intact TcR-T3 complex and membrane-associated immunoglobulin structure are posed side-by-side in Figure 12-17 [12].

As with Ig genes there is a temporal hierarchy in the rearrangements of both TcR$_{\alpha\beta}$ and TcR$_{\gamma\delta}$ genes. TcR$_{\gamma\delta}$ genes are rearranged and expressed first in the subpopulation of thymic T cells involved. The TcR$_\gamma$ locus is composed of only six or seven V segments, five J segments, and two C regions; however, there are two D$_\delta$ elements in tandem and joining is both imprecise and associated with extensive incorporation of random N nucleotides. This permits unprecedented variability in the junctional region and in the antigen-coding potential of the TcR$_{\gamma\delta}$ genes.

T Cell Activation: Antigen Drives and IL-2 Amplifies the T Cell Response

T cell activation and proliferation occur as the result of a well-orchestrated series of events beginning with chance encounters between a resting T cell possessing a unique antigen-specific TcR and an antigen-presenting cell (APC) bearing a peptide segment of the corresponding antigen. Considering the likelihood

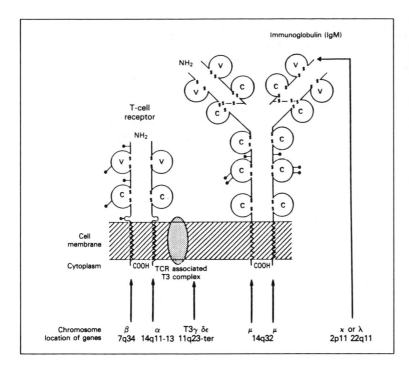

FIGURE 12-17

Skeletal structure of T cell receptor is similar in basic design to that of membrane-associated immunoglobulin. (From Greaves MF et al: Chapt 9, in Atlas of Blood Cells: Function and Pathology. Zucker-Franklin D et al, Eds. Milan, Edi. Ermes s.r.l.,1988.)

that only one in a million or so T cells is receptor primed for the antigen being newly presented, the only explanation for the success of immune responsiveness is that, in the crowded and tumultuous trafficking of lymphocytes and macrophages in spleen and lymph nodes, there is a considerable amount of accidental bumping. T cells are equipped with accessory molecules, the CD2, CD4, and CD8 receptors, which are adhesion molecules (as well as signal transducers) reactive with widely distributed cell surface ligands such as the lymphocyte function–associated antigens (LFAs), LFA-1 and LFA-3. Conjugation of CD2 to LFA-3 ligands, as an example, facilitates nonspecific adhesion of T cells to APCs, and in doing so helps promote both antigen recognition and T cell activation. The interaction of CD4 or CD8 with MHC proteins also contributes to the tightness with which appropriate T cells subsets bind to APCs or target cells. After adhesion, T cell recognition by the TcR and APC binding through MHC complementarity stimulates lymphocyte effector func-

tions (such as cytolysis or lymphokine production), after which the effector T cell detaches from the APC, creating a vacancy for additional untutored, antigen-coded, resting T cells.

Amplification of Activated T Cells

After the T cell receptors are occupied and triggered by antigen and a cognate MHC molecule, the number of surface TcRs is immediately downregulated, and the sensitized T cell is spurred to bare IL-2 receptors within a few hours. Display of IL-2 receptors is accompanied by endogenous induction and secretion of IL-2 molecules, which then occupy IL-2 receptors on the same cell. This initiates a self-regulated autocrine growth cycle. Expression of IL-2 receptors is pivotal to the success or failure of the T cell response. Once a critical number of these receptors has been occupied by IL-2 molecules, DNA synthesis, blastic transformation, and clonal proliferation follow. The ability of the CD2 structure to trigger T cell activation independent of antigen may be an important means of recruiting nonclonal resting T cells, thereby amplifying the immune response.

IL-2 is a network helper factor responsible for activating helper T cells that subsequently propel the B cell response to class II antigens. IL-2 also represents the second activation signal directing cytolytic T8 cell responses to foreign HLA antigens, viral antigens, and haptens.

Signal transduction in activated T cells   Stimulation of T cells by occupancy of the TcR (Ti) or ligation of CD2 (T11) by LFA-3 leads to synergistic signalling via the inositol-phospholipid pathway, which transmits information through a G protein that eventuates in the release of a set of second messengers: inositol triphosphate and diacyl glycerol (Chapter 1). This causes protein kinase C to migrate to the outer leaflet of the cell membrane, where it activates the Na^+-H^+ antiporter and opens the membrane Ca^{2+} channel. These modifications cause nuclear genes to transcribe IL-2, launching the T cell response described earlier (Figure 12-18) [13].

Helper and Suppressor T Cells

T cells do not secrete antibody but T4 cells provide help in inducing T-T, T-B, and T-macrophage interactions. T4 cells are at the heart of the T cell network. In primary re-

FIGURE 12-18

Circuitry of T cell activation. (T3 − Ti = TcR; T11 = CD2. C represents protein kinase C.) (From Royer HD and Reinherz EL: T lymphocytes: ontogeny, function, and relevance to clinical disorders. Reprinted, by permission of The New England Journal of Medicine, 317:1136,1987.)

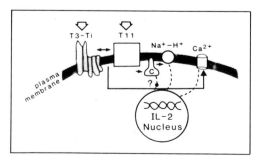

sponses, T4 cells require production of IL-1 by macrophages for activation, and elaboration of IL-2 for proliferation and amplification. Helper T cells are also instrumental in enabling cytolytic and suppressor T cells to respond to antigen in the shadow of class I determinants, with the aid of IL-2 as a second signal. Apart from their role in lysing virus-infected target cells, the effector functions of T8 cells are not well defined.

Demonology in the immune response   At this writing most of the workings of the T cell network are demonologic and seem shrouded in magical conjurations. The purposeful and vengeful behavior of cytolytic T cells and NK cells is more open to observation.

Cytolytic T Cells

As cytolytic (cytotoxic) T8 cells brush by objects in the circulation or lymphatics they are promptly activated on discovering viral, tumoral, or other foreign antigens on cell membranes bearing identical HLA class I molecules. Activation by TcR-MHC binding transforms the benign-looking lymphocyte into a uropod-probing killer cell that clings to the target by elaborate interdigitations of the two cell membranes at the contact region. Binding of target cell antigens by cytolytic T cell antigen receptors may involve thousands of intermolecular complexes, creating membrane folding forces that engage up to 10^5 effector-target cell linkages. Unlike other T cells, cytolytic T cells contain small electron-dense secretory granules in the trans Golgi region of cytoplasm. After receptor-mediated adhesion, the effector T cell rearranges its cytoplasm so that the Golgi, granules, and other components of the secretory apparatus polarize toward the clasped target. Actual slaying of the quarry is accomplished by firing a deadly mix of cytolytic buckshot directly into the body of the victim—with no danger to innocent bystanders or to the effector cell itself. Professional killer T cells assassinate discriminately by confining their secretions to cavitary spaces formed between the cells.

Granules isolated from killer T cells lyse tumor targets without specificity and do so by producing circular lesions having an internal diameter of about 16 nm. In the presence of

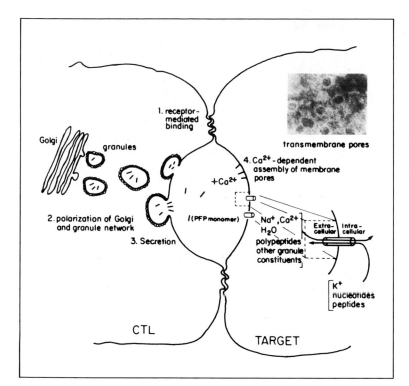

1. receptor-mediated binding

Golgi

granules

2. polarization of Golgi and granule network

3. Secretion

transmembrane pores

4. Ca²⁺-dependent assembly of membrane pores

+Ca²⁺

1 (PFP monomer)

Na⁺, Ca²⁺
H₂O
polypeptides
other granule
constituents

Extra-cellular | Intra-cellular

K⁺
nucleotides
peptides

CTL

TARGET

FIGURE 12-19

Stepwise binding and perforation of a target cell by a cytolytic T lymphocyte (CTL). PFP stands for the 70,000 M_r pore-forming protein, alias perforin. (From Young JD-E and Cohn ZA: Cell-mediated killing: a common mechanism? Cell 46: 641,1986.)

Ca^{2+}, the lytic pore-forming proteins, or perforin monomers, are polymerized into sealed cylindrical structures that penetrate glycoprotein domains in the lipid bilayer and cause an abrupt leakage of water, salts, nucleotides, and proteins. Further membrane damage is inflicted by injection of serine active proteases, serine esterases, and nucleases into the punctured cell. The consecutive steps by which target cells are apprehended by cytolytic T cells and then riddled with holes are recapitulated in Figure 12-19 [14].

After target cell destruction, cytolytic T cells detach from their prey and live to kill again. They are homicidal, not suicidal.

Natural Killer (NK) Cells

NK cells are a heterogeneous subset of lymphocytes capable of constitutive cytotoxicity against generic targets without prior sensitization or encounter. NK cells share many functional properties with cytolytic T cells (K cells),

and these two professional killer populations may also have overlapping origins, both lines being equipped with cytolytic secretory granules as their primary weapon for enforcing immunologic law and order. Unlike cell killing by cytolytic T cells, cytolysis by NK cells is unrestricted by MHC antigens, is not dependent upon rearrangement and expression of TcR genes, and is markedly enhanced by all three interferons. Most NK cells bear high-avidity Fcγ receptors, which help them to recognize opsonized particles, but they are incapable of phagocytosis (or even of adhesion to inert surfaces), relying instead upon bombardment with cytolytic granules. NK cells can be identified by a specific surface glycoprotein, CD16, recognized by Leu11 antibody, but their most singular feature is the cytoplasmic cargo of large azurophilic granules.

Large azurophilic (primary) granules are the rubric of NK cells NK cells are unusually large, oblong lymphocytes with abundant faintly blue

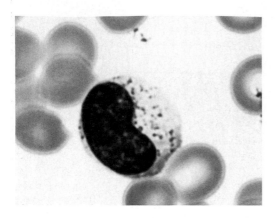

FIGURE 12-20

NK cell (large granular lymphocyte) in normal blood. Note the eccentric, oblong, smoothly indented nucleus and the numerous bold granules congregated in the Golgi (belly) region. NK cells are often tabulated mistakenly as atypical lymphocytes. (Photo by CT Kapff.)

cytoplasm containing one to two dozen prominent red-purple (azurophilic) granules, by which they were first identified as "large granular lymphocytes" (Figure 12-20). NK cells make up about 10% of normal lymphocytes, but their numbers increase during viral infections and certain immune responses.

Target Cell Recognition and Lysis

NK cells are professional killers engaged constantly in xenophobic surveillance without need for antibody or T cell help. NK clonal subpopulations are programmed for generic targets such as tumor cells, infected cells, and immature or imperfectly matured cells including fetal cells, immature thymocytes, and neoplastic or marrow cells that retain inappropriate fetal antigens. NK activity is upregulated by IFNγ, IL-2, and several ill-defined recognition proteins. NK cells driven to frenetic overactivity by exposure to foreign HLA antigens may yield to subsets of NK cells having natural suppressor function; some pre-NK cells possess partial veto power over harmfully zealous immunologic responses such as autoimmune or graft-versus-host diseases.

Target cell destruction   NK cells are precise and deliberate killers of cells having foreign, immature, or novel surfaces. In their innate animosity, NK cells bind to foreign cells through receptor-mediated ligation to receptor epitopes on the target surface, after which their primary granules migrate to the site of engagement and are discharged at close range. Lysis appears to be signalled by cyclic nucleotides, which trigger vectorially oriented exocytosis of granules and release of their payload of perforins and lymphotoxins; this culminates in large-hole hits, causing the target to explode its contents. After an NK cell dispatches its target, it dissociates from the dead cell and quickly recovers its killing power: like wasps, NK cells can sting repeatedly. Direct observation of the hit-and-run tactics of an NK cell are presented in Figure 12-21 [15].

Resistance to infection   NK cells are responsible for natural resistance to viral infections and to many microbial and protozoan organisms. NK cells contribute to the outraged immune response to the EB virus of infectious mononucleosis, in which the picturesque proliferation of NK and cytolytic T cells may upstage other manifestations of the disease.

INFECTIOUS MONONUCLEOSIS

Infectious mononucleosis (IM) is an acute sporadic viral infection, ubiquitous in all populations and communicated horizontally. It is characterized by fever, pharyngitis, lymphadenopathy, splenomegaly, and atypical lymphocytosis. IM is spread by virions containing the Epstein-Barr virus (EBV) genome, a double-stranded linear DNA molecule. In young children primary infection is nearly silent and infection is a blessing, conferring lifelong immunity. If primary infection is delayed to adolescence or beyond, as is the case with about 20% of young adults in affluent societies, the malaise and fever may prostrate the patient for 2 to 3 weeks, occasionally becoming complicated by severe immunohemolytic anemia, thrombocytopenic purpura, or hematosuppression. Unlike children, young adults can be infected only by intensive exposure;

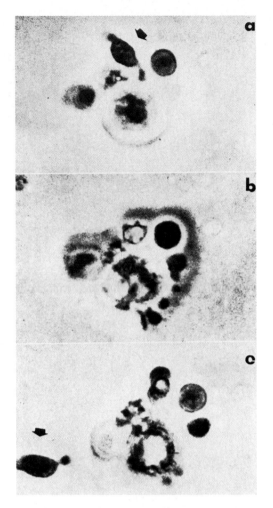

FIGURE 12-21

Time-lapse cinematographic views showing destruction of a lymphoma cell by an NK cell (arrow). (A) A fusiform NK cell attaches by its uropod to the large lymphoma cell. (B) The target explodes, scattering debris that obscures both cells. (C) The same NK cell, trailing its uropod, serenely cruises on, searching for the next victim. (From Ebina T et al: Time-lapse microcinematographic analysis of the natural cytotoxicity of murine lymphocytes: morphology of living natural killer [NK] cells. Microbiol Immunol 26:1095,1982.)

most often virus is bulk-transmitted in the course of prolonged and impassioned osculation, during which a seropositive carrier shedding virus passes large quantities of the virion while exchanging buccal fluids with a susceptible and cooperative acquaintance.

Pathogenesis

On entering the mouth of an antibody-negative person, EBV binds to cells that express CR2, a receptor that binds the C3d component of complement, now designated CD21. At first EBV binds to CD21 glycoprotein on oropharyngeal epithelium, but as these cells are desquamated EBV transfers to lymphoid tissue of the tonsils and Waldeyer's ring, where the density of CD21 molecules on resting B cells is the highest in the body. Occupancy of the B cell CD21 receptors drives the B cell out of quiescence, causes it to secrete a B cell transforming factor (CD23), which through autocrine stimulation induces blast transformation and proliferation. Once the B cell is activated, bound virus blocks further differentiation so that infected B cells are committed to immortalized proliferation [16].

Most "atypical mononuclear" cells in IM are cytolytic T8 cells and NK cells   Dissemination of infected B cells into circulation during the first week of illness precipitates the full fury of the T cell network. Hordes of activated T cells, most of them suppressor and cytolytic T8 cells, begin to flood the bloodstream and storm all affected lymphoid outposts, for the infected B cells are literally presenting the obnoxious viral antigen to T cell TcRs. Cytolytic T cells in league with virus-obsessed NK cells destroy infected B cells as fast as they emerge; most atypical lymphocytes that are so dramatic a morphologic feature of infectious mononucleosis during the second to fourth weeks of illness are cytolytic T cells and NK cells. Once thought to be "non-HLA-restricted," the colorful mixture of T8 cells that constitute the bulk of "atypical lymphocytes" in IM are polyclonal products expressing multiple HLA class I–dependent cytotoxicities [17].

Morphology of IM lymphocytes   Early in the disease large granular lymphocytes, and their degranulated battle-scarred compatriots, are a constant feature: the former cells are indistinguishable from normal NK cells (Figure 12-20). A second variety of atypical lymphocyte appearing at the peak of illness resembles a mitogen-transformed blastoid T cell (Figure 12-22). A third subpopulation of T8 cells that emerges during the immune response to EBV infection consists of large, pale, ameboid cells whose propensity to adhere to portions of neighboring red cells has inescapably elicited the sobriquet "kissing cells" (Figure 12-23). In producing kissing cells, nature imitates art and provides a pathogenetic clue.

The T cell response to EBV antigens presented by infected B cells is not morphologically pathognomonic but is an exaggerated version of similar T cell aberrations induced by most viral infections, tuberculosis, toxoplasmosis, mycoplasma pneumonia, and most hypersensitivity reactions to drugs.

IMMUNODEFICIENCY DISORDERS

All immunodeficiency disorders stem from defects in lymphocyte function. Failure to generate B cells occurs in the rare inherited malady, X-linked agammaglobulinemia. B cells either are not produced or are unresponsive to T cell signals, reflecting a genetic inability to translocate V_H region gene products during early B cell differentiation. Agammaglobulinemic male children possess normal T cell functions and are capable of homograft rejection and delayed hypersensitivity reactions but are highly vulnerable to pyogenic infections. The deficit in humoral antibody synthesis can be offset only by a systematic replacement program of injections of immune serum globulin. In congenital thymic aplasia (Di George's syndrome) the absence of the thymic anlage leads to deficient T cell function. These infants become infected by organisms normally controlled by cell-mediated immunity; hence they are mortally susceptible to viruses, acid-fast bacilli, and fungal diseases, and generally die of overwhelming sepsis in the first year of life. In hereditary severe combined immunodeficiency (SCID), both B and T cells are absent and affected infants generally succumb to recurrent bacterial, viral, and fungal infections within

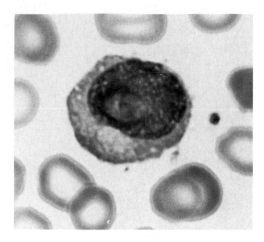

FIGURE 12-22

Large blastoid (transformed) T cell in the blood of a patient with IM. Cytoplasm is abundant, agranular, and darkly basophilic at the margins. The nucleus of this atypical lymphoblast contains a pair of large deformed nucleoli darkly rimmed with chromatin. (Photo by CT Kapff.)

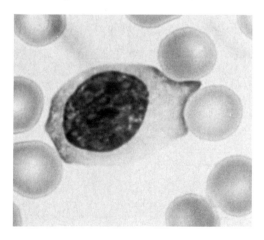

FIGURE 12-23

Large ameboid lymphocyte in the blood of a patient with infectious mononucleosis. Ameboid cells are quite large, appear hyperdiploid, and possess voluminous pale cytoplasm having dark-margined projections that "kiss" neighboring red cells, sometimes promiscuously. (Photo by CT Kapff.)

the first 2 years. The only rational therapeutic recourse for patients with thymic aplasia or SCID is marrow transplantation.

Fortunately, most genetic or congenital immunodeficient states are quite rare. Since the early 1980s, however, the public has been terrorized by the explosive spread of a murderous plague caused by a communicable retrovirus having destructive tropism for helper T4 cells. The resulting acquired immunodeficiency syndrome (AIDS) predisposes the host to death from repetitive opportunistic infections and tumors.

AIDS

Acquired immunodeficiency syndrome (AIDS) is caused by a communicable retrovirus known as human immunodeficiency virus (HIV). HIV is a T4-lymphotropic virion transmitted horizontally through intense, intimate exposure to blood, tissue, or secretions that contain the virus particles. In 90% of cases HIV infection occurs through anal intercourse or by intravenous drug abuse, the remainder of infections resulting from exposure to transfused blood or blood products or from mother-to-child transmission during the perinatal period. These risk factors explain the age distribution pattern for male and female AIDS patients (Figure 12-24). First described in 1981, AIDS has since reached epidemic proportions in the United States, with about 80,000 cases diagnosed by 1989, a cumulative case total projected to reach 365,000 by the end of 1992, and a fatality rate well in excess of 50%. The prevalence of covert HIV infection in 1989 as ascertained by routine serologic screening tests was over 2,000,000; of these seropositive individuals, 10% are expected to develop AIDS sooner or later. HIV kills by destroying its host cells, the helper T4 lymphocytes, thereby causing severe immunosuppression that renders the patient vulnerable to opportunistic infections and neoplasms.

HIV Is Tropic for T4 Cells and Macrophages

HIV is a spherical RNA retroviral particle, wrapped in a lipid bilayer envelope, about 100 nm across. As seen by electron microscopy it possesses a characteristic dense cylindrical nucleoid containing core proteins, genomic RNA, and the reverse transcriptase (RNA-dependent DNA polymerase) that qualifies it as a retrovirus. The 10-kb HIV proviral genome includes flanking long terminal repeat (LTR) sequences, which contain regulatory segments for HIV replication, plus the *gag*, *pol*, and *env* genes that code for core proteins, reverse transcriptase, and envelope glycoproteins, respectively. Of five additional genes, the *tat* gene is vital to transactivation and amplification of viral replication and the *trs/art* gene upregulates HIV synthesis through a trans-

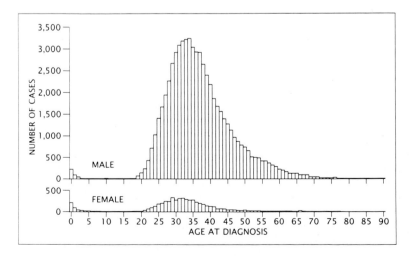

FIGURE 12-24

Age distributions for AIDS patients in the U.S. show that the vast majority are men between the ages of 25 and 45. Distinct peaks at the far left represent small, but growing numbers of pediatric cases in offspring of infected women. (From Heyward WL and Curran JW: The epidemiology of AIDS in the U.S. Sci Am 259(4):72, 1988. Copyright © 1988 by Scientific American, Inc. All rights reserved.)

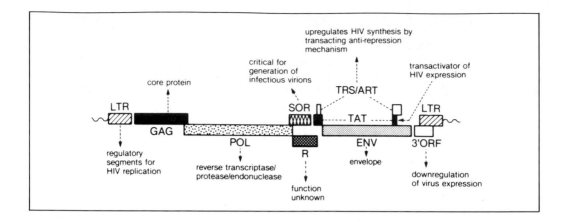

FIGURE 12-25

HIV proviral DNA genome and the known functions of its component parts. LTR = long terminal repeats. ORF = open reading frame. (From Fauci AS: The human immunodeficiency virus: infectivity and mechanisms of pathogenesis. Science 239:617,1988. Copyright 1988 by the AAAS.)

acting antirepression mechanism (Figure 12-25).

CD4 is the receptor for HIV   CD4 molecules densely displayed on T4 cell membranes project as spikes of serially linked immunoglobulinlike domains, the outermost of which possess loops containing the HIV binding site. Binding of the 120,000 M_r viral envelope glycoprotein, gp120, to a CD4 receptor, exposes a hydrophobic envelope protein, gp41, which initiates fusion to the outer lamina of the lymphocyte bilayer; this is followed by receptor-mediated endocytosis, uncoating of the virus, and injection of the viral core. The core includes two identical strands of viral RNA plus several enzymes essential to later steps in the cell cycle. Once internalized, genomic RNA is transcribed to DNA. DNA polymerase first makes a single-strand DNA copy of the viral RNA; an associated ribonuclease destroys the original RNA, and then the polymerase makes a second DNA copy using the first as template. (The polymerase and ribonuclease working together are called reverse transcriptase.) The double-stranded DNA product ("proviral DNA"), which can exist in a linear or circular form,

migrates to the nucleus and becomes integrated into the host cell's own DNA. After its integration, the provirus may remain latent for months or years, with restriction of the life cycle until the secretly infected T4 cell is activated. With activation, the integrated proviral DNA can command cellular mechanisms to transcribe viral genomic RNA. The transcribed RNA and translated viral proteins are then assembled into new virions that bud from the cell membrane and infect other cells (Figure 12-26) [18].

Mechanisms of Cytopathic Effect: The HIV Paradoxes

The early course of HIV infection is met by a flood of antibodies that are generated by an outraged polyclonal B cell response to the foreign antigen and associated with diffuse lymphadenopathy. This attack is joined for a time by cytotoxic T cells, always wary of helper T4 cells bearing novel offerings. NK cells, monocytes, and macrophages participate in the power struggle, responding to cytokine distress signals. As the apparent result, an immunologic standoff may halt progression of HIV infection for from 2 to 10 years.

HIV is a moving target   There are many explanations for the delayed progression of HIV infection, creating suspicion that none of them is adequate. Indeed, very little cell-free virus can be found in infected, seropositive individuals, and during evolution of infection less than 0.01% of circulating lymphocytes express de-

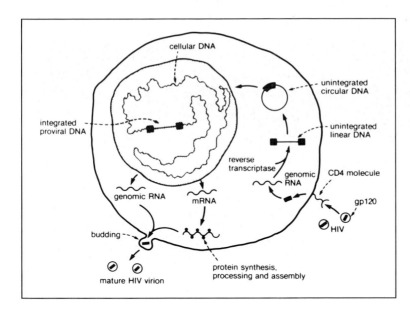

FIGURE 12-26

HIV replication cycle in T4 cells. (From Fauci AS: The human immunodeficiency virus: infectivity and mechanisms of pathogenesis. Science 239:617,1988. Copyright 1988 by the AAAS.)

FIGURE 12-27

Disintegration of a T4 cell by replicating HIV particles. This cultured cell contains chambers engorged with perfidious particles having characteristic disc-shaped cores. Similar virions are seen in vesicles, and some naked particles have been shed into the medium. (EM by H Gilderbloom of Robert Koch Institute in Berlin. From Haseltine WA and Wong-Staal F: The molecular biology of the AIDS virus. Sci Am 259(4):52,1988.)

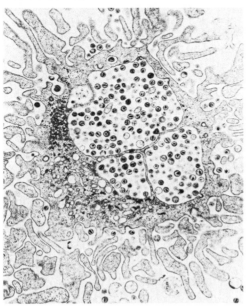

tectable HIV mRNA. The halting progression of AIDS appears to result from several independent mechanisms that account for the slow but certain virulence of this obstinate retrovirus. The viral envelope genes mutate at a rate millions of times faster than occurs in eukaryotic cells, theoretically helping the virion to evade immune control; antigenic shiftiness may also be explained by error-prone reverse transcription, for both the DNA and RNA polymerases lack the editorial enzymes that correct faulty transcripts in eukaryotes. HIV also has tropism for some monocytes and for most macrophages and their relatives in the central nervous system. Entry of virus into macrophages does not require CD4-mediated endocytosis for it can also occur through phagocytosis; macrophages are resistant to the cytolytic effect of HIV, granting sanctuary from the immune response, and yet serving as a lifelong reservoir that trickles lymphotropic particles back into the bloodstream.

In all likelihood T4 cells in AIDS fall upon their own swords, for only when HIV-infected T4 cells are activated while responding appropriately to secondary infections is replication of latent virus triggered. HIV replication in activated T4 cells can be devastating (Figure 12-27) [19]. Near-absence of HIV-infected T cells in the blood of patients with AIDS is

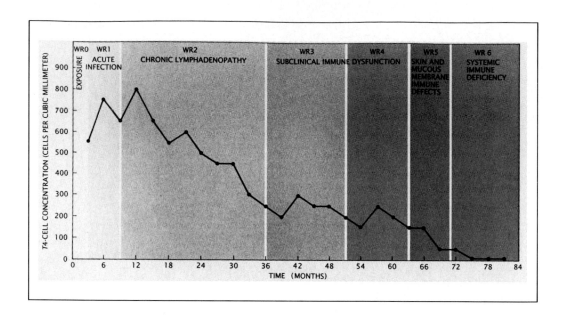

Decline in T4 cell count correlated with characteristic disease progression in a young man with AIDS. Numbers following initials WR denote stage of disease according to the Walter Reed classification system. (From Redfield RR and Burke DS: HIV infection: the clinical picture. Sci Am 259(4):90,1988. Copyright © 1988 by Scientific American, Inc. All rights reserved.)

apparently due to the rapidity of their lysis when virus-laden cells are activated by cytokines. Whatever the mechanism, the most conspicuous and constant measure of HIV infection is the attrition of T4 lymphocytes (Figure 12-28) [20].

Description

Infection by AIDS virus first appears as an acute mild, evanescent illness—a flulike syndrome of fever, swollen lymph nodes, and fleeting rashes, which resembles infectious mononucleosis. This viral prodrome vanishes within a few weeks, giving no hint of murderous portent. In the ensuing months or years the patient but sinister virus quietly continues its work, slowly but steadily destroying T4 cells. For most patients the first clue that something is amiss is the appearance of chronic painless lymphadenopathy, but general health is unaffected until the T4 count drops to levels that

preclude cell-mediated immunity, gradually engendering symptoms of overt anergy in the form of recurrent viral or fungal infections of skin and mucous membranes. Within 1 to 2 years of onset of those premonitory maladies, AIDS patients fall prey to relentless and recurrent parades of opportunistic infections. The most common "marker" infections causing morbidity in AIDS patients as they succumb to their immunodeficient fate are *Pneumocystis carinii* pneumonitis and dissemination of any of several mycobacterial strains including *M. avium intracellulare*. Patients are progressively enfeebled by the collective havoc of multiple infections and by a merciful mental wasting disease called AIDS encephalopathy. The immunologically defenseless host is also a target for opportunistic neoplasms, most common of which are Kaposi's sarcoma and high-grade B cell lymphomas. In its melancholy progression, AIDS and its complicating infections and tumors cripple all vital functions and patients die pitifully. Efforts to halt this modern scourge have fallen short. Unless given very early, antiretroviral drugs (such as 5'-azido-3'-deoxythymidine: AZT) appear to be temporizing and palliative, not curative, and strategies to block CD4 receptor function or to immunize against viral components have not been successful.

REFERENCES

1. McFarland W and Schecter GP: The lymphocyte in immunological reactions in vitro: ultrastructural studies. Blood 35:683,1970

2. Cooper MD: B lymphocytes. Normal development and function. N Engl J Med 317: 1452,1987

3. Waldmann TA et al: Chapt 8, in The Molecular Basis of Blood Diseases, Stamatoyannopoulos G et al, Eds. Philadelphia, WB Saunders Company,1987

4. Cambier JC et al: Transmembrane signals and intracellular "second messengers" in the regulation of quiescent B-lymphocyte activation. Immunol Rev 95:37,1987

5. Melchers F and Andersson J: Factors controlling the B-cell cycle. Annu Rev Immunol 4:13,1986

6. Darnell J et al: Molecular Cell Biology. New York, Scientific American Books,1986

7. Grossi CE et al: Chapt 9, in Atlas of Blood Cells: Function and Pathology. Zucker-Franklin D et al, Eds. Milan, Edi. Ermes s.r.l.,1988

8. Burdette S and Schwartz RS: Idiotypes and idiotypic networks. N Engl J Med 317:219, 1987

9. Alberts B et al: Molecular Biology of the Cell. New York, Garland Publishing, Inc.,1983

10. Kessel RG and Kardon RH: Chapt 2, in Tissues and Organs. A Text-Atlas of Scanning Electron Microscopy. New York, WH Freeman and Company,1979

11. Bierer BE et al: T-cell activation: the T-cell erythrocyte receptor (CD2) and sialophorin (CD42). Immunol Allergy Clin North Am 8:51,1988

12. Greaves MF et al: Chapt 9, in Atlas of Blood Cells: Function and Pathology. Zucker-Franklin D et al, Eds. Milan, Edi. Ermes s.r.l.,1988

13. Royer HD and Reinherz EL: T lymphocytes: ontogeny, function, and relevance to clinical disorders. N Engl J Med 317:1136,1987

14. Young JD-E and Cohn ZA: Cell-mediated killing: a common mechanism? Cell 46:641, 1986

15. Ebina T et al: Time-lapse microcinematographic analysis of the natural cytotoxicity of murine lymphocytes: morphology of living natural killer [NK] cells. Microbiol Immunol 26:1095,1982

16. Thorley-Lawson DA: Basic virological aspects of Epstein-Barr virus infection. Semin Hematol 25:247,1988

17. Heyward WL and Curran JW: The epidemiology of AIDS in the U.S. Sci Am 259(4): 72,1988

18. Fauci AS: The human immunodeficiency virus: infectivity and mechanisms of pathogenesis. Science 239:617,1988

19. Haseltine WA and Wong-Staal F: The molecular biology of the AIDS virus. Sci Am 259(4):52,1988

20. Redfield RR and Burke DS: HIV infection: the clinical picture. Sci Am 259(4):90,1988

13

Hematopoietic Malignancies

☐

Leukemias and lymphomas are cancers caused by unregulated and pointless proliferation of cellular clones derived from mutant hematopoietic stem cells. Individual cells of malignant clones are not programmed to differentiate fully or function adequately; in their cytokinetic torpor these incompetent cells divide slowly and linger in useless abundance, their mission unfulfilled. Because most tumor cells are sickly and frail some die from overcrowding, and when infiltrates or tumors become extensive they may outgrow their vascular supply and many cells succumb to ischemic necrosis. Consequently the doubling time of tumor masses may be greatly protracted beyond that predicted by the cell cycle time (Chapter 2). Acute myelogenous leukemia (AML) cells have an average cycling time of 7 days (as compared with the normal period of 18 h), but the population doubling time may exceed 10 times that long. This cytokinetic lethargy does not prevent the eventual displacement of normal resident cells, for the clonal progeny are indifferent to feedback signals. In leukemias accumulation of a lethal burden of tumor cells (about 5×10^{12} cells, or 1.5 kg) is usually achieved within 40 to 80 doubling times over a period ranging from 2 to 8 years. Leukemias and lymphomas are not hyperproliferative disorders; these cancers kill not because malignant cells divide too rapidly but because they never stop dividing.

Clonal overgrowth usually arises from an acquired chromosomal derangement that causes arrest at some stage in the maturation of blood cell precursors. Leukemia and lymphoma cell phenotypes are not perfect replicas of normal cell counterparts, but most are frozen as immortalized relics of an early stage of normal differentiation. The defective ancestral founder cell of malignant clones is emancipated from control by growth regulators. It is directly or indirectly activated to manufacture mutant, robotic progeny by one or more of a heterogeneous family of transforming genes known as oncogenes.

ONCOGENES AND MULTISTEP CARCINOGENESIS

Normal cells bear the seeds of their own destruction in the form of genes that are highly conserved components (cellular or proto-oncogenes) of the normal genome. Over 30 different oncogenes have been characterized in human cellular genomes, 10 or more exist in the genomes of infective DNA tumor viruses such as papovaviruses and certain adeno-viruses, and several are transmitted by RNA transforming retroviruses and are responsible for rare forms of T cell leukemia-lymphoma. Cellular oncogenes (c-oncogenes) are evolutionary progenitors of retroviral (v-) oncogenes found in RNA tumor viruses of animals; among the many classes of viruses with RNA genomes, only retroviruses have neoplastic potential. During their own evolution RNA viruses acquire oncogenes by recombinatorial transactions between the genome of the infecting retrovirus and that of the host cell. Retroviral oncogenes are captured (trans-duced) cellular genes; study of these trans-duced genes and of the life cycle of retroviruses has provided the first clues as to how certain genetic disruptions—recessive and dominant point mutations, rearrangements of DNA, and gene amplification—distort genomic function and cause cancer.

Retroviruses: A 2-Minute Drill

Animal retroviruses differ from all others in containing an RNA genome that replicates through a DNA intermediate. Extracellular virus particles are composed of two identical subunits of the single-stranded RNA genome imbedded in a core of protein and surrounded by an envelope studded with glycoproteins derived from the membrane of a previous host cell (Figure 13-1) [1]. Some of these viruses encode only for genes necessary for their own replication: *gag,* group-specific antigen; *pol,*

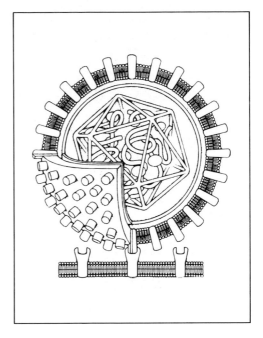

FIGURE 13-1

Schematic view of a retrovirus particle. The two identical single strands of viral RNA and the viral enzymes are packed within an icosahedral core. Binding of envelope glycoprotein to host-encoded cell surface receptor is shown below. (From Varmus H: Retroviruses. Science 240: 1427,1988. Copyright 1988 by the AAAS.)

reverse transcriptase; and *env,* envelope protein. These genes are under promotional control of specialized elements called long terminal repeats (LTRs) located at both ends of the virus, which are formed when the single-stranded RNAs of the diploid viral genome are transcribed into duplex DNA by reverse transcriptase. Viral DNA is then integrated into chromosomal DNA and the host cell uses its own machinery to express viral genes and their protein products. The DNA-integrated form of virus, called a provirus, replicates on demand but is not a transforming virus. Some retroviruses, however, are equipped with c-homologous transforming genes, or onco-genes, and these cause tumors in the infected host. Stripped-down representations of virus,

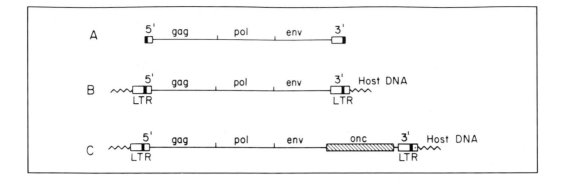

FIGURE 13-2

(A) Nontransforming RNA virus genome. (B) Integration of nontransforming provirus in host DNA. (C) Integration of transforming provirus containing an oncogene (onc) in host DNA. (From Brodeur GM: Molecular correlates of cytogenetic abnormalities in human cancer cells: implications for oncogene activation. Prog Hematol 14:229,1986.)

inserted provirus, and transforming provirus are shown schematically in Figure 13-2 [2].

Cancer Gene and Retrovirus: Sorcerer and Apprentice

The retrovirus life cycle presents two opportunities for the unleashing of cancer genes. First, integration of viral DNA is potentially disruptive to genomic function through the process known as "insertional mutagenesis," which can activate upstream cellular genes such as c-*myc*, even by a retrovirus that lacks oncogenes [3]. Second, recombination between retroviral and cellular genomes can implant cellular genes into exotic settings that incite functional growth genes to become dysfunctional oncogenes; genesis of retroviral oncogenes from cellular proto-oncogenes has been called "transduction." Transduced genes usually acquire mutations while en route from proto-oncogene to oncogene. Comparisons of retroviral oncogenes with their cellular counterparts have uncovered point mutations, deletions, and genetic substitutions in the viral allele. The recurrent theme that has arisen from the exhaustive studies of retroviral transduction in vitro and in animals is

that displacement, disorientation, or damage to otherwise sociable oncogenes releases them from allelic and allosteric controls or from recessively inherited regulatory elements that have been dubbed "anti-oncogenes." Anti-oncogenes, alias "emerogenes," can control cell maturation and may override the transforming action of highly expressed oncoproteins.

Cellular Oncogenes as Growth Factors and Growth Factor Receptors

The stubborn genomic conservation of cellular oncogenes (as proto-oncogenes) indicates that they are sufficiently advantageous to the host cell to offset their potential for mutation. Although there are about 30 proto-oncogenes and oncogenes (see Table 3, Chapter 1 for partial listing), they have been found responsible for only four categorical biochemical activities: protein phosphorylation, with tyrosine, serine, or threonine as the substrate amino acids; metabolic regulation by proteins that bind GTP in the manner of G or N proteins; control of gene expression by influencing biogenesis of mRNA; and participation in replication of DNA. These several mechanisms represent fundamental junction boxes in the circuitry for regulating cellular proliferation, for oncogene products include secreted growth and differentiation factors, transmembrane receptors, signal transducers, and regulators of nuclear proteins (Chapter 1). The temporal and spatial position of these components are recapitulated crudely in Figure 13-3 [4]. What we now know of oncogenes allows us to view their actions as "short circuits" in the junction boxes of cell cycle regulation [3].

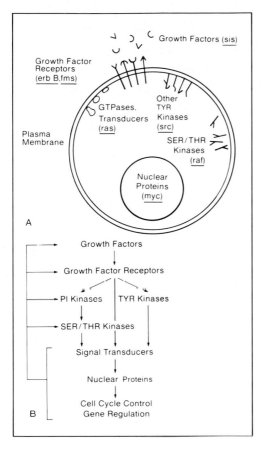

A

B

FIGURE 13-3

Local cellular actions of a selected repertoire of oncogene-coded proteins (A), demonstrating participation at consecutive points in cell cycle control (B). (From Varmus H: Chapt 9, in Stamatoyannopoulos G et al, Eds. The Molecular Basis of Blood Diseases. Philadelphia, WB Saunders Company,1987.)

Mechanisms of Activation of Oncogenes and Other Growth Factors

Three major types of lineage-specific structural chromosome abnormalities are microscopically visible in cytogenetic analyses of tumor cells. These include: translocations between (or inversions within) chromosomes; deletions affecting discrete regions of chromosomes; and amplification of large domains within intact chromosomes. In addition, whole chromosome gains and losses occur, but in general numeri-

cal changes are less specific and are catalogued under amplifications and deletions, respectively. Reciprocal translocations are the most common chromosomal aberrations associated with hematologic neoplasms. Four hematologic malignancies arise from unique translocations, and the remainder are associated with various shared defects involving over one dozen chromosomes.

Chromosome Translocations and Oncogene Activation

During reciprocal translocation between two chromosomes, one chromosome breaks at a specific site, releasing a "donor" fragment that somehow fuses to a breakpoint in a second, "recipient" chromosome; the second chromosome reciprocates by relinquishing a portion of its DNA to the breakpoint on the donor chromosome. This exchange of parts is known as a reciprocal translocation, whether or not it is balanced. Translocations can affect either the expression or the biochemical function of proto-oncogenes, depending on proximity of breakpoints to coding regions for oncogenes (or other growth factors) and on regulatory stability of the joined stump ends (Table 13-1) [5]. In many instances malignancies are associated with breakage at 1 of the 100 or more codominantly inherited "fragile sites" mysteriously present in the genome; fragile sites located near or within proto-oncogene coding regions appear to underlie 8 to 10 known translocations associated with hematologic malignancies. Breakpoints that interrupt genes that normally undergo rearrangements early in differentiation—namely, the immunoglobulin and T cell receptor gene loci—have a particularly sinister potential for poising an oncogene close to a transcriptional promoter. This has been borne out most clearly in studies of Burkitt's lymphoma and noted briefly in Chapter 2.

The Burkitt rearrangements cause c-myc deregulation
In the most common Burkitt's lymphomas, breakpoints are in bands 8q24 and 14q32; the resultant t(8;14)(q24;q32) translocation splits the distal end of the immunoglobulin heavy chain gene region on band 14q32 and attaches c-*myc* genes released from the amputated terminal limb of 8q. In the

TABLE 13-1

Chromosomal translocations in hematologic malignancies

Disease	Chromosome breakpoint	Gene(s) near breakpoint	Reciprocal breakpoint	Gene(s) near breakpoint	Percent of patients
Myeloid leukemias					
Chronic myelogenous leukemia	9q34	c-*abl**†	22q11	*bcr*†	95
Acute myelogenous leukemia (AML)					
M1	9q34	c-*abl**†	22q11	*bcr*†	5
M2	21q22	c-*ets*-2	8q22	c-*mos**	10
M3 acute promyelocytic leukemia	17q11	c-*erb*A Nerve growth factor receptor	15q22	?	100
M4 with abnormal eosinophils	16q22	Metallothionein	16p13	?	25
M4 and M5	11q23	c-*ets*-1	9p22	?	10
M6 erythro-leukemia	7q22	?	11p15	?	
	17q11	c-*erb*A Nerve growth factor receptor	16p13	?	
AML with basophilia	9q34	c-*abl**	6p23	*pim**	70
Lymphomas and lymphatic leukemias					
B cell neoplasms					
Burkitt's lymphoma	8q24	c-*myc**†	14q32	Ig H†	80
	8q24	c-*myc**	2p12	Ig kappa†	10
	8q24	c-*myc**	22q11	Ig lambda†	10
Chronic lymphocytic leukemia	11q13	*bcl*-1†	14q32	Ig H†	10
	2p13	?	14q32	Ig H†	
Follicular lymphoma	18q21	*bcl*-2†	14q32	Ig H†	20
T cell neoplasms	8q24	c-*myc**†	14q11–13	T cell receptor alpha chain†	?
	14q	*tcl*-1†	7q35	T cell receptor beta chain†	?
	11p13	*tcl*-2†	14q11-13	T cell receptor alpha chain†	25
	18q21	*bcl*-2†	14q32	Ig H†	?

Disease	Chromosome breakpoint	Gene(s) near breakpoint	Reciprocal breakpoint	Gene(s) near breakpoint	Percent of patients
Acute lymphatic leukemia					
L1, L2	9q34	c-*abl**	22q11	Ig lambda† or *bcr*†	10
L2	11q23	c-*ets*-1	4q21	?	5
L3 (B cell)	8q24	c-*myc**†	14q32	Ig H†	100

*Homologue of an established oncogene.
†Breakpoint interrupts the gene.
Acute leukemias are numbered according to the French-American-British (FAB) classification.

Source: Modified from Holt JT et al: Chapt 10, in The Molecular Basis of Blood Diseases, Stamatoyannopoulos G et al, Eds. Philadelphia, WB Saunders Company,1987.

variant translocations, seen in 10% of Burkitt's lymphoma cases, light chain gene loci are usually translocated oppositely to the c-*myc* locus on chromosome 8. The net result is the same: juxtaposition of a rearranging, transcriptionally tempestuous gene region in B cells and the normally stable c-*myc* gene locus (Figure 13-4) [2]. Joining c-*myc* to immunoglobulin genes causes rearrangement and deregulation of the proto-oncogene, which becomes truncated (decapitated) by excision of its first exon; this drives expression of c-*myc* to high levels, increases the stability and longevity of mRNA derived from the gene, and predisposes to various c-*myc* mutations that heighten their response to promoters. In addition, rearranged c-*myc* genes are aligned to immunoglobulin genes in opposite transcriptional directions. The exact molecular mechanism by which c-*myc* expression is thrown so wildly out of control by these rearrangements is still subject to debate, but disturbance of the mutant oncogene appears to be pivotal: in the t(14;18) translocation associated with a relatively benign follicular lymphoma, the chromo-

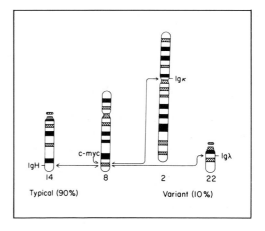

FIGURE 13-4

Representation of the three reciprocal translocations found in various patients with Burkitt's lymphoma. Regardless of the direction of exchange, an immunoglobulin-coding region is placed in proximity to the proto-oncogene, c-*myc*. (From Brodeur GM: Molecular correlates of cytogenetic abnormalities in human cancer cells: implications for oncogene activation. Prog Hematol 14:229,1986.)

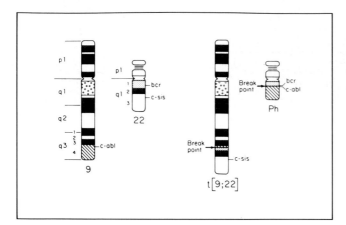

FIGURE 13-5

The t(9;22) rearrangement responsible for forming the minute Ph chromosome, showing the apposition of c-*abl* and *bcr*. During the exchange, the c-*sis* proto-oncogene is transposed to chromosome 9 but is too remote from the breakpoint to be disturbed (From Holt JT et al: Chapt 10, in The Molecular Basis of Blood Diseases, Stamatoyannopoulos G et al, Eds. Philadelphia, WB Saunders Company,1987.)

some 14 breakpoint is identical but the recipient chromosome lacks an oncogene.

Philadelphia chromosome: formation of a fusion gene with a robust protein product   The small but celebrated Philadelphia (Ph) chromosome that typifies the cells of chronic myelogenous leukemia (CML) results from an unbalanced translocation, t(9;22)(q34;q11), in which the bulk of the long arm of 22 is exchanged for a small but mischievous terminal piece of chromosome 9 containing part of the c-*abl* proto-oncogene. The unnatural transposition of the c-*abl* tyrosine kinase domain of chromosome 9 to the fractured genetic locus on 22q−, known for the moment as *bcr* (for "breakpoint cluster region"), creates a fusion gene composed of wedded elements of both c-*abl* and *bcr* (Figure 13-5). The c-*abl*-*bcr* genetic fusion causes CML cells to generate novel 8.2-kb *abl*-related RNA transcripts (in place of the two normal and smaller transcripts), and the hybrid transcripts in turn generate a 210,000 M_r chimeric protein possessing promiscuous tyrosine kinase activity far more vigorous than that of the normal gene product. This novel kinase has the properties of an oncogene growth factor, but the exact mechanism by which it induces expansion of the multipotential myeloid stem cell compartment and activates subordinate cell populations is unknown, as is its focus on myeloid proliferation and the ordained transformation to blast crisis (Chapter 15).

Chromosome Deletions and Recessive Cancer Genes

Over 15% of patients with acute myelogenous leukemia (AML) have recurrent defects, singly or in combination, that involve complete or partial deletion of chromosome 5 or chromosome 7. Cells monosomic for chromosomes 5 or 7 or those with chromosome 5 having an interstitial deletion are rendered structurally hemizygous for clusters of "hematopoietic genes," whether the defect is inborn or acquired.

The 5q− syndrome is caused by interstitial deletions of clustered genes coding for growth factors   The 5q− deletion occurring alone as a spontaneous event is associated with severe refractory anemia and an abundance of underlobulated or unilobular megakaryocytes exhibiting plentiful release of oversized platelets. These patients are at an increased risk of transforming to AML (5 to 10%)—an evolution usually associated with additional deletions of 7 (−7 and 7q−). In patients who acquire the 5q− syndrome by exposure to alkylating agents used in chemotherapy (see below) the incidence of leukemic transformation is much greater.

At least six genes whose protein products are colony stimulating factors, or their receptors, are encoded in the band q23 to q32 region of chromosome 5, and interstitial loss of these gene segments in one of the chromosome 5 alleles cuts production of the gene product by 50%. Among the growth factors (Chapter 1) known to be lost with this deletion are M-CSF, GM-CSF, IL-3, and IL-5, plus the neighboring DNA region (c-*fms*) coding for the receptor for M-CSF, and that coding for the PDGF (platelet-derived growth factor) receptor expressed on fibroblasts and macrophages (Figure 13-6) [5].

Recessive cancer genes   Deletions are the second most common type of cytogenetic abnormality associated with cancer cells, and it has been proposed that many cancers arise through a two-step process in which an individual is predisposed to cancer by inborn or acquired absence (or loss of function) of one of a pair of alleles, which may or may not be evident on cytogenetic analysis (e.g., in the case of a point mutation). Recessive deletions or mutations in proto-oncogenes or in other genes involved in cell growth would be silent in individuals with a normal allele, but would be conducive to delayed onset of cancer if a second change occurred in the surviving allele later in life. In familial retinoblastoma a defective RB-1 allele is transmitted through the germline, often as a deletion at 13q14.2. Tumors develop when a second change occurs during somatic development, nullifying the normal allele on the other

chromosome through deletion, rearrangement, or point mutation. Similar stepwise losses of recessive genes through deletion or mutation appear to account for the emergence of other embryonal tumors. Deletion of a recessive locus on chromosome 13 appears to foreshadow ductal breast carcinomas, and loss of an allele on chromosome 5 may presage colonic carcinomas [6].

Point Mutations

Point mutation in the c-*ras* oncogenes have been found in nearly 50% of patients with AML, including those of the M1, M2, M4, and M5 subclasses, and in about 20% of other human neoplasms. The *ras* gene family has three major branches, each with cellular alleles closely related to three prototype oncogenes: Ha-*ras*, N-*ras*, and Ki-*ras*. The *ras* gene products are small 21,000 M_r membrane-associated proteins that bind GTP, have ATPase activity, and, like G proteins (with which they are homologous), participate in transduction of signals from occupied membrane receptors. The transforming potential of *ras* proteins stems from point mutations in codons 12 or 13, in which the G to T transversion causes glycine to be replaced by valine or aspartic acid; *ras* proteins with these mutations have enfeebled GTPase activity, leading to ex-

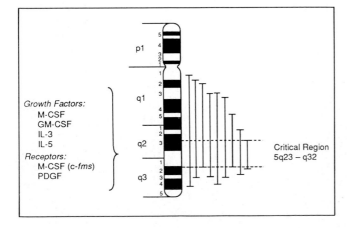

FIGURE 13-6

The 5q− chromosome, with the range of observed deletions defined by vertical lines on the right. The "critical region" of interstitial deletions extends from 5q23–q32, a busy coding strip containing genes for at least four hematopoietic growth factors and two growth factor receptors, as denoted on the left. (Modified and amended from Holt JT et al: Chapt 10, in The Molecular Basis of Blood Diseases, Stamatoyannopoulos G et al, Eds. Philadelphia, WB Saunders Company, 1987.)

tinction of the signal and deregulation of myelopoiesis.

Gene Amplification

Amplification is an unscheduled aberration that was first encountered in human cells as a mechanism by which leukemia acquires resistance to the chemotherapeutic agent, methotrexate. It then became clear that untreated cancer cells also can contain amplified DNA and that amplification can involve proto-oncogenes. Amplified proto-oncogenes are presumed to act through a gene dosage effect: the c-*myc* proto-oncogene, for example, is stably amplified 30 to 100 times in acute promyelocytic leukemia (APL), and c-*myc* or c-*myb* amplification occurs as a prelude to leukemic transformation in certain AMLs having myelomonocytic features.

Localized reduplication of DNA to produce as many as 100 copies of a given region usually spans hundreds of kilobases and disrupts the banding patterns of chromosomes. Amplified genes have been found in two peculiar chromosomal structures: double minute (DM) chromosomes that lack centromeres and segregate unpredictably during cell division, and homogeneously staining regions (HSRs) of centromeric chromosomes. DM chromosomes and HSRs are recurrent features of many malignancies,

including APL with amplification of c-*myc* and acute myelomonocytic leukemia with amplification of the Hu-*ets*-I oncogene. The most highly visible of these structures have been found in neuroblastomas associated with striking amplification of N-*myc* (Figure 13-7) [7].

Oncogenes as Growth Factors: Redux

Oncogene terminology has evolved through historical accidents and is actually a misnomer—but here to stay. It embraces genes that influence cell growth in many ways, both promoting and domesticating cell proliferation. Some cause transformation when they malfunction; others can overrule the transforming mutants. So-called oncogenes also supply factors indirectly necessary for the growth of tumors,

F I G U R E 13-7

Visible forms of DNA amplification as seen in neuroblastoma cells. (Left) HSRs stained for AT-rich regions (1) and GC-rich areas (2), and replicating regions during S phase (3). In each set of chromosomes, the leftmost one is a normal chromosome 1. (Right) Quinacrine-stained DMs appear as small paired dots, the large white structures being normal chromosomes. (From Darnell J et al, Eds.: Chapt 22, in Molecular Cell Biology. New York, Scientific American Books, Inc., 1986.)

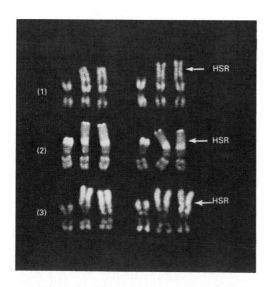

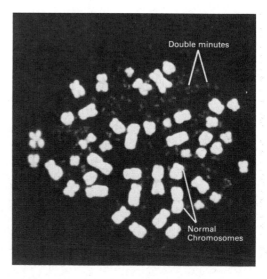

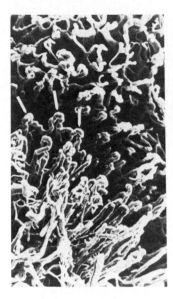 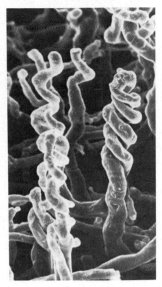

FIGURE 13-8

Border zone of a tumor richly nourished by ingrowth of capillary buds exposed to view by microcorrosion casts, with digestive stripping away of tumor cells. (Left) At tumor's border zone numerous capillary buds communicate with each other via vascular arcades (pointers). (Right) Closer view, showing corkscrew capillary loops resembling glomeruli present deeper in the tumor mass. (From Miodonski A et al: Scanning electron microscopic studies on blood vessels in cancer of the larynx. Arch Otolaryngol 106:321,1980.)

functioning as accessories after the fact. Examples of this include fibroblast growth factors and endothelial growth factors essential for angiogenesis. As noted early in this chapter, growth of solid tumors depends on formation of new nutrient blood vessels and supporting fibroblasts and other adventitial elements. The indirect but essential role of some oncogene products is to provide potent angiogenic agents (tumor angiogenesis factors) that foster growth of new blood vessels, nourishing tumor growth much as the placenta feeds the growing fetus (Figure 13-8) [8]. Tumor angiogenesis factors are encoded by a family of homologous proto-oncogenes that includes fibroblast growth factors and the angiogenic factors recoverable from Kaposi's sarcoma tumors of patients with AIDS. Clearly cancer is not caused by a single mutant oncogene run amok, but is a complicated multistep affair involving collusive participation of many growth and antigrowth genes, with commandeering by the founder clone of all of the supporting cast of factors required for any tissue growth.

Human T Cell Lymphotropic Retroviruses (HTLV)

For over 10 years identification of retroviruses was restricted to birds and several species of mammals, and not until 1980 were the first isolates of human T cell leukemia lymphoma virus (designated HTLV-I) recovered from patients with an uncommon but virulent lymphoproliferative disorder. HTLV-I is a type C human retrovirus etiologically associated with adult T cell leukemia (ATL) endemic to southwest Japan, Okinawa, the Caribbean, Central Africa, southeastern United States, and northeastern South America. The virus can be transmitted through sexual contact, intravenous drug use, breast milk, and blood transfusions. Although contagious, the virus is only feebly productive; even in endemic clusters areas such as Uwajima in Japan, the annual incidence of ATL per 1,000 seropositive individuals is less than 1, indicating that immunity ordinarily silences disease expression.

Pathophysiology of a Rogue Retrovirus

HTLV-I (and its rare sister retrovirus, HTLV-II) have the central structural features of conventional retroviruses, including the flanking LTRs and the *gag, pol,* and *env* genes, but they have proved to be curious agents, difficult to accept as pathogens for they fail to fulfill Koch's postulates [9]. Unlike the common oncogenic retroviruses of animals, the HTLVs neither carry host-derived oncogenes nor activate cellular proto-oncogenes by a specific pattern of insertion-mutation [1]. Instead their oncogenic action has been ascribed provisionally to an open reading frame, lying between the *env* gene and the 3' LTR, which encodes a unique 40,000 M_r "X protein" acting as a positive effector of transcription from the HTLV LTR and from certain cellular promoters. Models for tumorogenicity must also account for the very prolonged latency (HTLV is catalogued as a "slow virus"), infrequent occurrence of disease in infected people, dearth of viral gene expression in primary tumor tissue, and lack of an acute transforming gene. Cultured ATL cells do produce and release HTLV-I particles, but leukemic cells taken directly from patients contain few if any viral particles. Nevertheless HTLV-I proviral DNA can be demonstrated in leukemic cells by DNA amplification using the redoubtable polymerase chain reaction (PCR). Integration sites in leukemic blood cells are monoclonal (or oligoclonal): provirus is integrated into the same site in the DNA of any single infected individual, although the site of integration differs between individuals (no two patients sharing identical integration sites). This indicates that the leukemia is monoclonal with respect to integration and that the virus is in fact responsible for the disease.

Malignant transformation of T4 cells by HTLV-I
Productive retrovirus infection depends on binding of viral envelope determinants to receptors of T4 cell surfaces. Following receptor-mediated endocytosis, the *X* gene that encodes for the pX activator within the lymphocyte nucleus amplifies its expression in trans, enhancing the transcriptional activity of its own LTR as well as of other intracellular genes. HTLV-I infection immortalizes T cells and transforms them into Sézarylike lymphocytes having deeply indented, cerebriform nuclei (Figure 13-9) [10]. The leukemic T cells have clonally rearranged TcR genes, and cytogenetic studies show various nonrandom chromosome aberrations. Infiltrates or lymphomatous masses of these cells most often resemble large cell immunoblastic lymphoma.

Description   In both Japanese and American experience, the HTLV-I lymphoproliferative

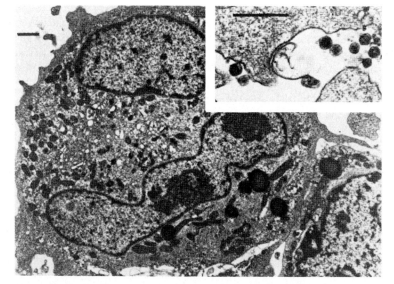

FIGURE 13-9

Deeply indented, lobulated nucleus of a T cell transformed by HTLV-I infection, as seen by EM. Inset shows the pathogenic type C virus particles released by budding from cultured cells. (From Sarin PS and Gallo RC: Human T-cell leukemia-lymphoma virus [HTLV]. Prog Hematol 13:149,1983.)

syndrome is characterized by lymphadeno-pathy, hepatomegaly, splenomegaly, cutaneous infiltration with lobulated lymphocytes, hypercalcemia, lytic skeletal lesions, and variable infiltration of marrow, gastrointestinal tract, and lungs, but with sparing of the mediastinum. The immunologic hallmarks are: lymphocytosis featuring pleomorphic cells with lobular nuclei; T4 membrane antigens; and prominent display of the IL-2 receptor. Most patients present with advanced-stage T cell lymphoma; 60% also present with leukemia, and nearly all terminate with acute T cell leukemia. Prompt treatment with combination chemotherapy brings remission in over half of patients, but responses are not durable, averaging about 12 months.

Chemical Leukemogens

The best documented chemical leukemogens are alkylating agents—alkyl (hydrocarbon) free radicals capable of substituting for hydrogen atoms. The efficacy of alkylators in chemotherapy is due to their propensity for modifying hydrogen bonding properties of purine and pyrimidine bases. As the result they have the potential for causing stable alterations and covalent crosslinkages that interfere with DNA replication and are capable of disrupting phosphodiester bonds, causing fragmentation of DNA strands. Most alkylating agents resemble their prototype parent compound, mechlorethamine (nitrogen mustard, alias HN_2) in the diffuseness of their cytotoxicity: among these nucleophilic compounds are cyclophosphamide, busulfan, melphalan, and chlorambucil—all of which react with the DNA of resting (G_0) cells as well as that of cycling cells. In general, alkylating agents induce AML (but no other types of leukemia), and immunosuppressive antimetabolites cause non-Hodgkin's lymphomas. The incidence of this dismaying side effect of well-intentioned chemotherapy varies with the nature of the primary disease being treated. Patients with multiple myeloma or Hodgkin's disease, for example, are innately predisposed to have secondary malignancies, possibly as the indirect result of compromised immunity. In patients with myeloma or polycythemia vera, the incidence of therapy-related

AML approaches 20% among those who survive 10 years. Treatment of ovarian carcinoma with alkylators incurs an 8 to 10% risk of AML within 10 years, and in Hodgkin's disease the incidence of this lamentable complication at 10 years ranges from 3 to 10% depending on the duration and intensity of therapy, jeopardy being increased by use of combined modality therapy. The pyrrhic nature of the victory of combined modality therapy over Hodgkin's disease is underscored by the even higher incidence of late-onset solid tumors.

Characteristic Features of Secondary (Therapy-Related) AML

Most cases of therapy-related AML (t-AML) emerge between 30 and 60 months after institution of alkylator chemotherapy, radiation therapy, or combinations of the two. Virtually all patients pass through a preliminary phase of refractory anemia or pancytopenia that rapidly progresses to trilineage myelodysplasia, with overt AML evolving within 1 to 3 years. Leukemias secondary to alkylator chemotherapy are predominantly of the M2, M4, and M6 types, a finding also reported in AML arising after prolonged, heavy exposure to benzene.

Hypodiploidy with deletions of chromosomes 7 and 5 are characteristic of secondary AML

Nearly 90% of patients presenting in either the myelodysplastic (see below) or overt AML phase of secondary leukemia have a hypodiploid karyotype, whereas hypodiploidy occurs in fewer than 15% of de novo cases of AML. Hypodiploidy is associated with clonal cytogenetic abnormalities in dividing marrow cells, with defects affecting chromosomes 7 and 5 occurring in two-thirds of these patients. Monosomy 7 (-7) predominates, with monosomy 5 and 5q— and 7q— deletions accounting for most of the rest (Figure 13-10) [11]. The commonest aberration of primary (spontaneous) AML, trisomy 8, is seldom encountered in secondary AML, and the unique translocations of primary AML such as t(15;17) of APL and t(8;21) of the M2 variant almost never occur as a consequence of chemical induction. Secondary AML also differs from the primary sort in being far less responsive to antileukemia

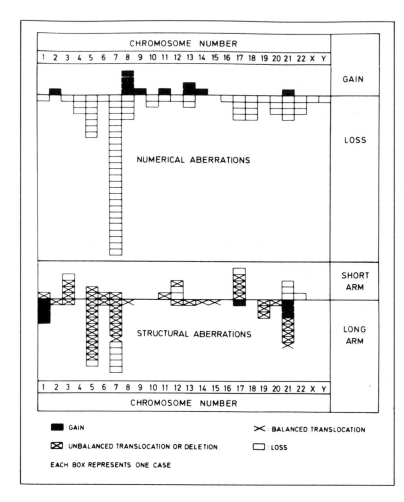

FIGURE 13-10

Numerical and structural aberrations observed in 61 cases of therapy-related AML. Most losses or deletions involve the long arms of chromosomes 7 or 5 (or of both); the third most frequently affected chromosome is 21. (From Pedersen-Bjergaard J and Philip P: Cytogenetic characteristics of therapy-related acute nonlymphocytic leukaemia, preleukaemia and acute myeloproliferative syndrome: correlation with clinical data for 61 consecutive cases. Br J Haematol 66:199,1987.)

chemotherapy, perhaps because alkylation was the culprit to begin with.

Leukemia Secondary to Ionizing Radiation

Ionizing radiation—radiation that removes electrons from atoms, creating free radicals capable of reacting as "nucleophiles" with DNA—can create an assortment of stable and unstable nuclear lesions that may either kill or mutate marrow cells. (See Chapter 5 for the physics of ionizing radiations.)

DNA Repair Mechanisms Defend against Carcinogens

Throughout our lives we are bathed in low-level ionizing radiation, usually without developing neoplasms from this, the "master" carcinogen. For radiant energy to initiate malignant transformation, sufficient sublesions must be created in DNA strands to overwhelm the proofreading capacity of cellular DNA polymerases. At least two kinds of DNA damage are difficult to repair correctly and can lead to stable mutation. If two or more sublesions affect a DNA duplex within a critical range of time and distance, double strand breaks occur in the DNA backbone. These can be repaired if the free ends of DNA can rejoin exactly, but without overlapping single-stranded regions there is no base-pair homology to catalyze correct rejoining. Incorrect joining of double strand fractures to broken segments of neighboring strands of DNA can cause translocation of pieces of DNA from one chromosome to another. Chromosome breaks that do not join, rejoin incorrectly, or that rejoin with breaks on other chromosomes to form exchange translocations—without causing the cell to die or cease replicating—are most apt to foment malignant transformation. A second circumstance in which repair of DNA may go astray occurs when cells resort hastily to postreplication repair, an error-prone system in which random nucleotides are inserted in place of the damaged ones in DNA. Hence radiation mutagenesis can be caused both by functional as well as by dysfunctional repair mechanisms. The importance of successful DNA repair enzymes in warding off cancer is brought out by the high incidence of cancers including leukemias in patients genetically deficient in these enzymes and mortally afflicted with chromosomal instability. Examples are Fanconi's anemia, Bloom's syndrome, and xeroderma pigmentosum.

Radiation Leukemogenesis and Dose-Response Projections

The dose-response aspect of leukemogenesis is a subject of rebarbative debate strongly flavored by contentious ideologies and shaky assumptions. The most definitive information stemmed from study of victims of the bombing of Hiroshima and Nagasaki, but in them exposure was instantaneous, leaving unanswered the question of whether dose-effect mathematics can be extrapolated to protracted low-dose cumulative exposures. It is astonishing how weakly leukemogenic penetrating radiations are when doses are highly fractionated, and there is no evidence that protracted exposures in the range 1 to 300 rem (1 rem = 1/100 J/kg) are leukemogenic. Indeed among 82,000 women treated for cervical cancer with fractionated x-radiation totaling between 300 and 1,500 rads (3 to 15 Gy), the relative risk of leukemia after over 600,000 woman-years of follow-up was barely significant [12].

Japanese survivors of atomic bombing A joyless byproduct of the nuclear holocausts of Hiroshima and Nagasaki in 1945 was the establishment of a Radiation Effects Research Foundation which followed the medical course of 82,000 atomic bomb survivors and 27,000 nonexposed controls. Leukemia was the earliest cancer to appear in excess, first becoming manifest in the third year, reaching a peak at 6 to 8 years, and declining gradually in the ensuing 20 years. Incidence of leukemia was directly proportional to magnitude of whole body irradiation dose at exposures exceeding 1 Gy. By all hematologic criteria, the leukemias engendered by this instantaneous overexposure were identical to de novo leukemias and were unpreceded by the preleukemic phase of trilineage myelodysplasia found in most patients whose leukemias were induced by alkylating agents. In Hiroshima most leukemias were classic AML or Ph-positive CML, with a minority of ALLs and no CLLs. In Nagasaki virtually all cases were AML. This suggests that CML may be neutron-dependent cancer, for the Hiroshima uranium detonation produced a substantial flux of both γ-rays and neutrons, whereas the "cleaner" Nagasaki plutonium bomb emissions were almost exclusively γ-rays. For both Japanese populations the induction period for radiation-induced leukemia was strongly influenced by the victim's age at the time of bombing (ATB) [13] (Figure 13-11). In children acute and chronic leukemias came on as a steep surging wave: this high incidence of acute leukemia was sustained for 20 years in older individuals, with latency (induction periods) prolonged proportional to age. With CML, however, the crest was almost unimodal, nearly independent of age. The induction of Ph-positive CML by a fugitive flux of neutrons means that all the multiple steps of leukemogenesis can occur simultaneously: concurrent hits to the DNA of a single founding stem cell can trigger the entire sequence of initiation, promotion, and progression necessary for expression of this complex disease.

Repetitious medical overexposure Over 13,000 persons were exposed to one or more courses (10 sessions each) of orthovoltage x-irradiation of the spine as a proposed remedy for ankylosing spondylitis in the period 1935–1954, when that ill-starred approach was fashionable. Appearance of excess leukemias (mostly AMLs) followed a wavelike pattern starting 2 years after first exposure and crest-

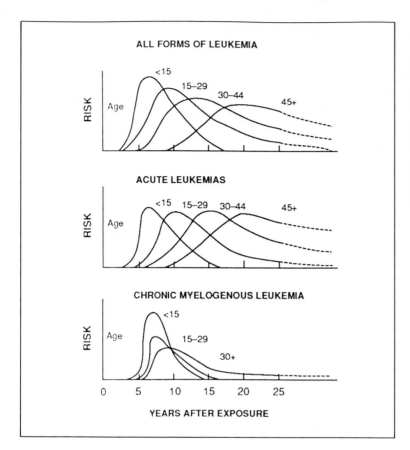

ALL FORMS OF LEUKEMIA

RISK

Age

<15

15–29

30–44

45+

ACUTE LEUKEMIAS

RISK

Age

<15   15–29   30–44   45+

CHRONIC MYELOGENOUS LEUKEMIA

RISK

Age

<15

15–29

30+

0   5   10   15   20   25

YEARS AFTER EXPOSURE

FIGURE 13-11

Influence of age ATB and calendar time on leukemogenic effect of radiation on heavily exposed survivors. (Redrawn from Land CE and Tokunaga M: Induction period, in Radiation Carcinogenesis: Epidemiology and Biological Significance, Boice JD Jr and Fraumeni JF Jr, Eds. New York, Raven Press, 1984.)

ing at 5 years. Unlike the leukemias observed after the Japanese bombings, these commenced with pancytopenia and trilineage myelodysplasia, with low levels of leukemic blasts entering the blood. The oligoblastic, myelodysplastic syndrome among irradiated spondylitics closely resembles that seen in AMLs occurring after alkylator therapy and shares the same relentless course and unresponsiveness to chemotherapy [14]. The atypical leukemias of heavy irradiation and of alkylator therapy both evolved following repetitious cytotoxic insults to the marrow, suggesting that fractionated or recurrent marrow damage may alter the expression of leukemia through the opposing effects of leukemogenic and antileukemic agents.

MYELODYSPLASTIC SYNDROMES AND PRELEUKEMIA

Marrow malfunction involving two or more blood cell lines that is refractory to physiologic hematopoietic factors and is commonly a prelude to overt AML has been labeled "preleukemia." Used prospectively, the term preleukemia is conjectural, for fewer than one-third of patients with the morphologic aberrations emblematic of preleukemia ever develop leukemia. Because they are appropriately ambiguous, connote pluralism, and skirt the stigma of preleukemia, the tongue-twisting expressions myelodysplastic syndromes (the current front runner), refractory dysplastic anemia (RDA), and dysmyelopoietic syndromes have gained broader acceptance in hematologic parlance. Myelodysplastic syndromes are characterized by blood cytopenias, ineffective hematopoiesis, and an anarchic but paradoxically hypercellular marrow pattern. On the basis of marrow morphologic criteria, five distinctive myelodysplastic syndromes have been sanctioned by the French-American-British (FAB) terminologists. This classification separates refractory anemias (RAs) into those without or with ringed sideroblasts (RA-S or RARS), those with a worrisome excess (5 to 20%) of blasts in the marrow (RAEB), and those with an alarming number of myeloblasts in the marrow (20 to 30%) and over 5% myeloblasts in blood— patients who appear to be "in transformation" to AML (RAEB-T); a fifth myelodysplastic syndrome having a flickering, unpredictable, often protracted course and varying numbers of myeloblasts and monoblasts in the marrow has been squeezed awkwardly into the category designated chronic myelomonocytic leukemia (CMMoL or CMML).

Myelodysplastic Syndromes Are Clonal Disorders

Myelodysplastic syndromes are insidious clonal disorders affecting all hematopoietic cell lines, implicating the multipotential stem cell or an immediate subordinate as the mutant clonal founder. Primary myelodysplasia usually affects the elderly, but therapy-related dysplastic syndromes may arise in patients of any age who received alkylators, radiotherapy, or both. The prognostic prospects for patients with primary myelodysplastic syndromes in these five FAB categories are given in Table 13-2 [15].

Myelodyssemantics   The canonical weight placed upon the magical number of 5% blasts and the sweeping inclusion of 20 to 30% myeloblasts as merely signifying a preleukemic entity is under assault by those (including this author) who believe these values indicate leukemia and nothing less. Bagby [16] has recommended a merciful reduction in myelodysplastic categories to three: preleukemic syndrome, with 5% or fewer blasts in marrow; oligoblastic leukemia, with 6 to 40% blasts in marrow; and AML with >40% blasts in marrow—with

T A B L E   13-2

Survival and leukemic progression in patients with primary myelodysplastic syndromes (MDS)

MDS subtype	% of total cases	Survival, months		Progression to AML, %
		Median	Range	
RA	28	50	10–64	12
RA-S	24	51	14– > 76	8
RAEB	23	11	7–16	44
CMMoL	16	11	9– > 60	14
RAEB-T	9	5	3–11	60

*Total number of cases classified = 1,081. Abbreviations are defined in the text.

Source: Reprinted by permission of the publisher from Report of the Third MIC Cooperative Study Group. Recommendations for a morphologic, immunologic, and cytogenetic (MIC) working classification of the primary and therapy-related myelodysplastic disorders. Cancer Genet Cytogenet 32:1, 1988. Copyright 1988 by Elsevier Science Publishing Co., Inc.

or without myeloblasts in the bloodstream. In this presentation, the "FAB 5" classification will be adhered to, with the caveat that more than 5 or 10% myeloblasts in marrow (expressed as a proportion of myeloid elements only) is almost always predictive of AML, especially when associated with evolution of cytogenetic abnormalities.

Chromosomal Abnormalities in Myelodysplasia

The clonal involvement of all hematopoietic cell lines in myelodysplastic syndromes has been certified by both G6PD isozyme analyses and cytogenetic studies. In primary syndromes, karyotypes usually reveal a single recurrent anomaly early in the course. The most common alterations involve chromosome 7 (either monosomy or partial loss of the long arm, $7q-$), chromosome 8 (trisomy), and chromosome 5 (monosomy and $5q-$). As stem cell instability worsens, additional subclones having complex defects emerge, presaging either progressive hematopoietic failure (the most common cause of death) or clonal escape with

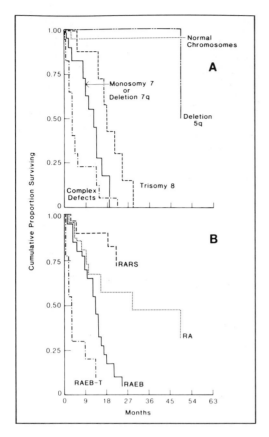

FIGURE 13-12

Survival of adult patients with myelodysplastic anemia as a function of (A) clonal chromosome abnormality and (B) FAB subgroup. RARS = refractory anemia with ringed sideroblasts. (From Yunis JJ et al: Refined chromosome study helps define prognostic subgroups in most patients with primary myelodysplastic syndrome and acute myelogenous leukaemia. Br J Haematol 68:189,1988.)

transformation to overt AML (Figure 13-12) [17].

Secondary therapy-related myelodysplasia
Chromosome changes observed in secondary myelodysplasia tend to be multiple at the outset and include the same group of abnormalities found in therapy-related AML: −7, 7q−, −5, 5q−, +8, 9q−, 11q−, 13q−, and 20q−, plus an assortment of translocations

such as t(1;3), t(2;11), and t(6;9). Complex rearrangements are omens of leukemic transformation both in preleukemia and in AML emerging de novo.

Myelodysplastic Morphology: A Sinister Pastiche

Suspicion that marrow failure represents a malignant myelodysplastic process is usually first aroused by the finding of any or several of a set of morphologic malformations—often bizarre, sometimes grotesque—in blood or marrow cells.

Dyserythropoiesis   Myelodysplastic processes are dominated by patterns of ineffective erythropoiesis, most common of which are megaloblastoid changes reminiscent of those in nutritional megaloblastic anemias. In patients with all subgroups of refractory anemia, ringed sideroblasts may be present, but when over 15% of orthochromatic erythroblasts possess perinuclear collars of prussian blue–positive siderotic granules (see Chapter 7, Figure 11), these sideroblastic cells signify the diagnosis of refractory anemia with ringed sideroblasts.

Dysgranulocytopoiesis   Blood and marrow neutrophils often appear agranular, a dysplastic marker easily overlooked; more blatant logos of preleukemia are the pseudo-Pelger-Huët and twinning anomalies (Figure 13-13). Nuclear-cytoplasmic maturation proceeds dyssynchronously in many ways, generating a cytologic bestiary of perverted forms.

Dysmegakaryocytopoiesis   Marrow megakaryocytes are deranged in many ways. Among the most characteristic morphologic abnormalities occurring in these normally polyploid cells are micromegakaryocytes ("dwarfs"), large mononuclear forms, and megakaryocytes having several separated nuclei. The presence of trinucleate ("pawn ball") nuclei is a curious cachet of preleukemic dysplasia (Figure 13-14).

Blast cells in myelodysplasia   The blast cells appearing overabundantly in myelodysplastic syndromes are jejune, locked in a state of maturation arrest. They resemble myeloblasts found in the M1 and M2 variants of AML, and

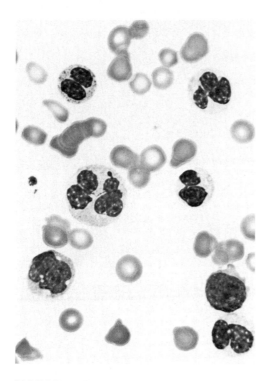

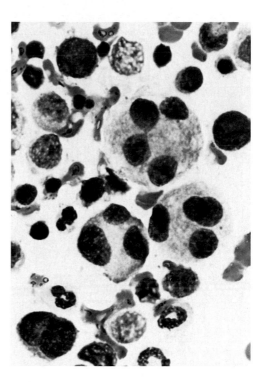

FIGURE 13-13

Pseudo-Pelger-Huët and twinning nuclear defor-mities in blood neutrophils of a patient with myelodysplastic syndrome. Pelger-Huët nuclear deformities are abundant and are comprised of bilobate (pince-nez) and mononuclear forms in which the chromatin is coarsely clumped into double or single masses. Oversized neutrophils containing two separated, lobulated, mirror-image nuclear chains (twinning deformity) are less frequent but indelible markers of myelodys-plasia. (Photo by CT Kapff.)

FIGURE 13-14

Dysplastic megakaryocytes in marrow of a patient with myelodysplastic (preleukemic) syn-drome. Normal megakaryocytes are multilobu-lated: the presence here of numerous multinu-clear and mononuclear forms is flagrant evi-dence of myelodysplasia. Note the unnatural and diagnostic "pawn ball" arrangement in the cell with three nuclei. (Photo by CT Kapff.)

their numbers are predictive of the pace of transformation.

Pathophysiology of Preleukemia: Coda

Dysplastic morphology affecting portions of all hematopoietic cell lines betrays the failure of mutant cells spawned by the clonal precur-sor to grow and function correctly. The out-come of their smoldering battle for survival depends upon whether the mutation has en-abled the clonal progeny—liberated from cytokine regulation—to compete successfully

with their normal counterparts for marrow space. The eviction by unprogrammed, defec-tive clonal cells of normal hematopoietic ele-ments represents a biological triumph of pathologic proliferation over physiologic differ-entiation. The implacable progression of failed differentiation and accumulation of blast forms in myelodysplastic syndromes is a sim-ple biological sequence, but the progression may be either stalled or lethally sidetracked in many ways, accounting for the heterogeneous evolution of these clonal disorders. The inexo-rable cell biology of preleukemic disorders following a leukemogenic event is matched

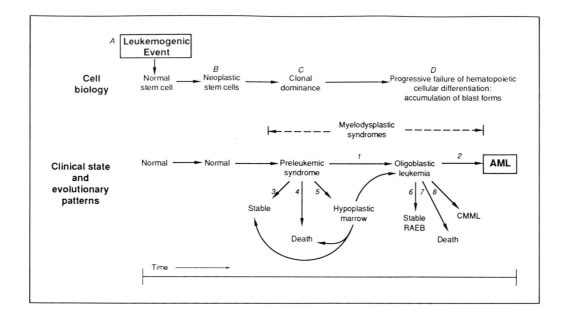

FIGURE 13-15

Schematic depiction of the biological progression following a leukemogenic event (upper sequence) and of the multiple potential digressions—some fatal, some halting—that may occur during clinical evolution (lower sequence). (Revised from Bagby GC Jr: The concept of preleukemia: clinical and laboratory studies. CRC Crit Rev Oncol Hematol 4:203,1986.)

with the alternative clinical patterns that may evolve along the way in Figure 13-15 [16].

Management: A Doctor's Dilemma

Diagnosis of myelodysplastic syndrome creates two dilemmas for the doctor. Informing the patient without precipitating panic requires a full and explicit exposition, but in patients in favorable subgroups (RA and RA-S) the scary word "preleukemia" is best avoided. The second dilemma is how and whether to administer myelodysplasia-producing drugs to patients dying of myelodysplasia. There is no settled therapeutic answer to the second quandary, but some durable remissions have been obtained in selected patients with the good for-

tune of having HLA-identical sibling donors available for marrow transplantation [18].

Do We Live in a Leukemogenic Environment? Is This the Cancer Century?

Since the turn of the century total production of chemicals in the United States has doubled approximately every 10 years, apart from some let-up since 1970. Between 1930 and 1985 the total production of organic chemicals has burgeoned from 1 to almost 200 billion pounds annually, as reported by the Federal Reserve Bulletins and the U.S. International Trade Commission. This 200-fold accumulation of synthetic or manhandled potential mutagens has been accompanied by a doubling of the annual death rate from cancer. A frightening perception prevails that we are being poisoned by our own technology, swimming and choking in a sea of environmental pollutants. Reduced to its essentials, the genomes of the Republic may be under assault by the collusion of corporate greed and public unawareness. Without denying the reality of both factors, it is mandatory that the epidemiologic evidence be scrutinized, for our lives depend on it.

Incidence of Leukemia, Lymphoma, and Other Cancers

Incidence and mortality may be presented in three ways: as crude rates in populations unadjusted for age distribution; as age-adjusted rates for a population whose age structure has been fitted to that of a given standard "index" population, as computed from census data; and as age-specific rates. Only age-adjusted or age-specific rates can be used for comparing populations and for determining secular trends, because crude rates are profoundly influenced by the age structure. Cancer is a disease of older age groups, with over half of all cases being diagnosed at age 65 and up (Figure 13-16) [19]. When cancer death rates are adjusted for age, factoring in the enormous impact of improved survival beyond age 65, it becomes evident that there has been no increase in the overall incidence of cancer between the years 1930 and 1985; the alarming magnitude of the upsurge in cancer of the lung has been offset by a pronounced and mysterious decline in cancers of the stomach, liver, and uterus. If cancer of the lung (largely a disease of cigarette smokers) is subtracted, it becomes clear that we do not face a general cancer epidemic: the incidence of most cancers is either stable or declining (Figure 13-17) [20].

Most leukemias and lymphomas are not caused by environment mutagens   Leukemias and lymphomas constitute 7 to 8% of all malignancies. Prior to 1960, the mortality from leukemia appeared to be edging upward, but in the subsequent 30 years age-adjusted mortality has leveled off and then declined slightly. The early increment during 1930–1960 undoubtedly represents in part improved diagnosis, for marrow aspiration and biopsy did not become routine procedures until the 1950s. Trends in recorded incidence are biased by improvements in the level of case ascertainment and registration, as is notably so of cancer of the breast. Despite the spacious assertions made by otherwise credible scientists that many or most leukemias and lymphomas are caused by chemical mutagens and are diseases of industrialization, there is no strong evidence supporting this view. Furthermore, there is no good evidence for any general increase in cancer occurring in response to environmental pollutants released

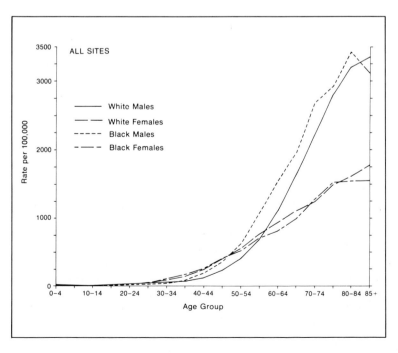

FIGURE 13-16

Average annual age-specific incidence of cancer at all sites combined, by race and sex, SEER program. SEER = Surveillance, Epidemiology, and End Results program of the National Cancer Institute. (From Young JL Jr and Pollock ES: Chapt 8, in Cancer Epidemiology and Prevention, Schottenfeld D and Fraumeni JF Jr, Eds. 1982. Courtesy of Charles C Thomas, Publisher, Springfield, Illinois.)

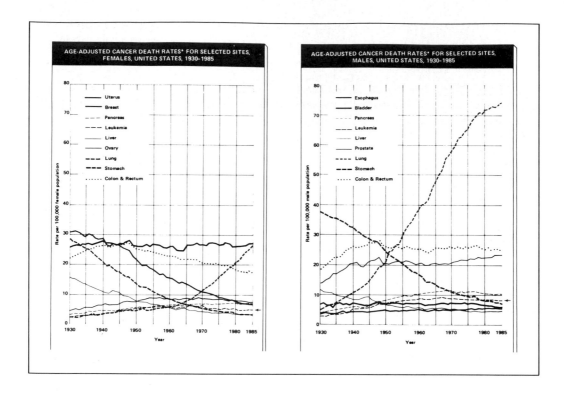

FIGURE 13-17

Trends in age-adjusted cancer mortality from 1930 through 1985, based on data compiled by the U.S. National Center for Health Statistics and the U.S. Bureau of the Census. Note the flattening of the leukemia mortality curves (arrows) and the frightful upsurge of cancer of the lung. *Adjusted to the age distribution of the 1970 US census population. (From Silverberg E and Lubera JA: Cancer statistics, 1988. CA 38:5,1988. By permission of the American Cancer Society, Inc.)

in the modern industrial world [21, 22]—a conclusion supported by contrasting the log growth of the chemical industry with the flat, trendless stability of collective cancer statistics.

Postscript: continue to fear the unknown The comforting perspective stated above is not grounds for complacency, for new causes of cancer (as from nuclear fallout) may at first be submerged in the high background level of de novo disease, and we should recognize de novo as signifying blank medieval ignorance, not

predestination. Absence of proof is not proof of absence, and until we can explain why some cancers are subsiding we should not abjectly accept those that persist, for if present rates continue 25% of us will die of cancer. Molecular biology is guiding us toward the fundamental mechanisms of malignancy, holding forth some promise for its eventual conquest.

REFERENCES

1. Varmus H: Retroviruses. Science 240:1427, 1988

2. Brodeur GM: Molecular correlates of cytogenetic abnormalities in human cancer cells: implications for oncogene activation. Prog Hematol 14:229,1986

3. Bishop JM: The molecular genetics of cancer. Science 235:305,1987

4. Varmus H: Chapt 9, in The Molecular Basis of Blood Diseases, Stamatoyannopoulos G et al, Eds. Philadelphia, WB Saunders Company,1987

5. Holt JT et al: Chapt 10, in The Molecular Basis of Blood Diseases, Stamatoyannopoulos G et al, Eds. Philadelphia, WB Saunders Company,1987

6. Klein G: The approaching era of the tumor suppressor genes. Science 238:1539,1987

7. Darnell J et al, Eds.: Chapt 22, in Molecular Cell Biology. New York, Scientific American Books,1986

8. Miodonski A et al: Scanning electron microscopic studies on blood vessels in cancer of the larynx. Arch Otolaryngol 106:321,1980

9. Duesberg PH: Retroviruses as carcinogens and pathogens: expectations and reality. Cancer Res 47:1199,1987

10. Sarin PS and Gallo RC: Human T-cell leukemia-lymphoma virus [HTLV]. Prog Hematol 13:149,1983

11. Pedersen-Bjergaard J and Philip P: Cytogenetic characteristics of therapy-related acute nonlymphocytic leukaemia, preleukaemia and acute myeloproliferative syndrome: correlation with clinical data for 61 consecutive cases. Br J Haematol 66:199,1987

12. Boice JD et al: Second cancers following radiation treatment for cervical cancer: an international collaboration among cancer registries. JNCI 74:955,1985

13. Land CE and Tokunaga M: Induction period, in Radiation Carcinogenesis: Epidemiology and Biological Significance, Boice JD Jr and Fraumeni JF Jr, Eds. New York, Raven Press,1984

14. Moloney WC: Radiogenic leukemia revisited. Blood 70:905,1987

15. Third MIC Cooperative Study Group: Recommendations for a morphologic, immunologic, and cytogenetic (MIC) working classification of the primary and therapy-related myelodysplastic disorders. Cancer Genet Cytogenet 32:1,1988

16. Bagby GC Jr: The concept of preleukemia: clinical and laboratory studies. CRC Crit Rev Oncol Hematol 4:203,1986

17. Yunis JJ et al: Refined chromosome study helps define prognostic subgroups in most patients with primary myelodysplastic syndrome and acute myelogenous leukaemia. Br J Haematol 68:189,1988

18. Appelbaum FR et al: Treatment of preleukemic syndromes with marrow transplantation. Blood 69:92,1987

19. Young JL Jr and Pollock ES: Chapt 8, in Cancer Epidemiology and Prevention, Schottenfeld D and Fraumeni JF Jr, Eds. Springfield, Charles C. Thomas, Publisher,1982.

20. Silverberg E and Lubera JA: Cancer statistics, 1988. CA 38:5,1988

21. Doll R and Peto R: The Causes of Cancer. Oxford, Oxford University Press,1981

22. Ames BN and Gold LS: Carcinogenic risk estimation [reply to letter by Epstein SS and Swartz JB]. Science 240:1043,1988

14

Acute Myelogenous Leukemia

☐

Acute myelogenous leukemia (AML) is a malignant clonal disorder originating from a deranged pluripotential stem cell in some cases and from a lower-echelon stem cell in most others. In AML of young adults and children the underlying mutation is confined to CFU-Gs and the neoplastic proliferation leads to relatively pure accumulations of myeloblasts or promyelocytes unprogrammed to differentiate further. In older adults surface marker, G6PD, and DNA probe analyses have shown the clonal lesion to occur one or two steps higher and include all cellular progeny of CFU-GEMM (Chapter 1), and thus the proliferative defect may be expressed by myeloid, monocytic, erythroid, or megakaryocytic lines, or combinations thereof [1]. The clonal lesion in CML (Chapter 15) occurs at a still higher level (ancestral multipotential stem cells are the founder cells), and the partial block in differentiation of malignant cells is capable of escalating during "blast crisis" to involve lymphoid as well as myeloid elements. The heterogeneous sites from which malignant clones emanate to generate the extended family of acute nonlymphocytic leukemias, as contrasted with the top-echelon defect responsible for CML, are indicated schematically in Figure 14-1 (2). Involvement of the erythroid or megakaryocyte lineages is particularly common in cases with preceding myelodysplastic syndrome.

In any of its many guises, neoplastic proliferations of defective myeloblasts, monoblasts, erythroblasts, or megakaryoblasts lead to a prodigious pileup of longlived cells that suffocate or dislodge normal marrow cells. The result is anemia, neutropenia, and thrombocytopenia; eventually relentless overproduction of leukemic cells causes them to spill into the bloodstream and flood the spleen, liver, lymph nodes, and most vital organs. A lethal burden of about 5×10^{12} tumor cells is generally accumulated within 2 to 8 years, the pace subject to factors discussed in Chapter 13.

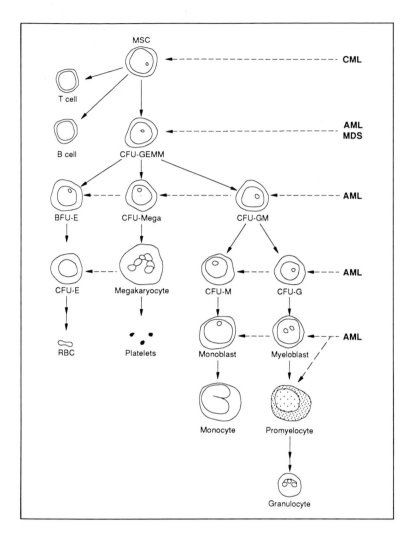

FIGURE 14-1

Cell of origin of AML is CFU-GEMM in some cases and stem cells lower in the heirarchy in others. "Classic" myeloblastic AML stems from progeny of committed CFU-Gs. MSC = multipotential stem cell. MDS = myelodysplastic syndromes. (Modified from Griffin JD and Lowenberg B: Clonogenic cells in acute myeloblastic leukemia. Blood 68: 1185,1986.)

Cytokinetics of AML: Leukemia Results from Maturation Arrest

Cell cycling of AML cells is either stalled or vastly prolonged, but numbers mount because maturation is frozen at some transient stage of early cell differentiation. Only a minor population of leukemic stem cells may be responsible for maintenance of neoplastic growth, most cells reposing in a dormant (G_0 or G_1) state, but as the replicating clones expand they become admixed with diminishing numbers of normal myeloid cells, creating an adversely shifting mosaicism. The malignant phenotype and multiplicity of leukemic syndromes encompassed by the term "AML" reflects the level at which maturation stops. In classic

AML the mutant cell line has been programmed to differentiate and replicate at the myeloblast level, but genetic instructions for further differentiation are lacking. If the genetic program codes for a single additional maturation-division, the progeny are promyelocytes and the arrested cells accumulate to cause acute promyelocytic leukemia (APL). In vitro, APL cells can be compelled to differentiate further by exposing them to a promoter or inducer (such as retinoic acid) that by brute force causes differentiation: this indicates that in APL, at least, the genetic apparatus for full differentiation is present but requires an added signal for differentiation to proceed—raising alluring hopes for new "induction" therapies. Most AML blasts are not perfect replicas of

TABLE 14-1

The French-American-British (FAB) classification of acute myelogenous leukemias

	Category	Abbreviation	Criteria
AML M1	Myeloblastic leukemia	AML	30% or more of nonerythroid marrow cells are myeloblasts; 3% or more of blasts stain for myeloperoxidase or for granule phospholipid (Sudan black).
AML M2	Myeloblastic leukemia with maturation	AML	30% or more of nonerythroid marrow cells are myeloblasts, > 10% are promyelocytes, and <20% are monocytic elements.
AML M3	Promyelocytic leukemia	APL	Most marrow cells are abnormal hypergranular promyelocytes; some may contain bundles of Auer rods.
AML M4	Myelomonocytic leukemia	AMML	30% or more of all nucleated marrow cells are blasts. Granulocytic elements make up >20% of nonerythroid marrow cells. A monocytic component is identified by: a. 5,000/μL or more monocytic elements in the blood and either (1) 20% or more cells of monocytic lineage in the marrow, or (2) A serum lysozyme level >3 times normal. b. If monocytic elements in the blood are <5,000/μL, recognition of 20% or more cells of monocytic lineage in the marrow with confirmation by cytochemical stains showing fluoride-inhibited nonspecific esterase activity or by elevated serum or urine lysozyme.
AML M5	Monocytic leukemia	AMoL	30% or more of all nonerythroid marrow cells are monoblasts, promonocytes, or monocytes. In subtype $M5_A$, 80% or more of all monocytic cells are monoblasts; in subtype $M5_B$, <80% of monocytic cells are monoblasts.
AML M6	Erythroleukemia	AEL	50% or more of all nucleated marrow cells are erythroid precursors, and 30% or more of the remaining nonerythroid cells are blasts.
AML M7	Megakaryoblastic leukemia	AMegL	30% or more of cells are of megakaryocytic lineage in a marrow aspirate. If aspirate is unobtainable because of marrow fibrosis, then identification may be made by: a. A marrow biopsy showing excess blasts and, often, increased numbers of maturing megakaryocytes plus b. Circulating megakaryoblasts. Megakaryocytic lineage of blasts should be confirmed by platelet peroxidase reaction on electron microscopy or immunologic identification with antibodies to platelet glycoproteins or von Willebrand factor.

Source: Modified from Rapaport SI: Introduction to Hematology, 2nd ed. Philadelphia, JB Lippincott Company, 1987.

early differentiation, some lines betraying lineage infidelity, and in many instances morphologic classification is difficult or impossible without the aid of special stains, phenotypic markers, and cytogenetic analyses.

Classification of AML Variants

Acute myelogenous leukemia, often identified by what it is not (acute nonlymphocytic leukemia, or ANLL), comes in seven major variant forms that share similar clinical features including a guarantee of death within several months after presentation if left untreated. Some variants are associated with unique clinical manifestations such as disseminated intravascular coagulation in APL, skin and gum infiltration in acute myelomonocytic (AMML) and acute

monocytic leukemia (AMoL), and malignant myelofibrosis in acute megakaryoblastic leukemia (AMegL). To aid prognosis, help tailor therapy, and permit comparison between therapeutic protocols, the French-American-British (FAB) classification was initiated and is undergoing refinements. The basic FAB classification depends upon marrow and blood morphology as illuminated by Romanowsky staining and supplemented by a limited battery of other staining reactions (Table 14-1) [3].

Special Cytochemical Stains

Routine use of certain cytochemical stains is often required in typing leukemic cells of blood and marrow. The most important of these are for myeloperoxidase, specific and nonspecific esterases, Sudan black B, PAS, and TdT (Table 14-2) [4].

TABLE 14-2

Special stains and assays used in classifying acute leukemias

Leukemia	Stain or assay					
	Peroxidase or Sudan black B	Esterases		PAS[c]	Murami-dase	TdT[d]
		Specific[a]	Nonspecific[b]			
AML-M1	+	+	−	−	−	− or +
AML-M2	+ to +++	++	−	−	+	−
AML-M3	+++	+++	−	−	+	−
AML-M4	++ to +++	+ to +++	+ to +++	−	++	−
AML-M5	+	−	+++	−	+++	−
AML-M6	−	−	−	+++	−	−
AML-M7	−	− to ++	− to ++ (punctate)[e]	++ (punctate)	−	−
ALL	−	−	−	+++	−	+++
Normal neutrophils	+++	+++	−	+++	+++	−
Normal monocytes	+	−	+++	+++	++	−
Normal lymphocytes	−	−	−	±	−	−

[a]α-Naphthol AS-D chloroacetate esterase.
[b]α-Naphthyl acetate esterase and α-napthyl butyrate esterase.
[c]Periodic acid-Schiff.
[d]Terminal deoxynucleotidyl transferase.
[e]Megakaryoblasts negative for α-naphthyl butyrate esterase.

Source: Prepared with the help of CT Kapff.

Phenotyping

Surface marker (antigen) analysis using immunofluorescent monoclonal antibodies has gained a place in cataloguing AML subtypes and in establishing the lineage of atypical or undifferentiated blast cells. Phenotyping is in a state of flux and is bedevilled by duplicative or supererogatory coding, a problem only partly resolved by employing the dauntingly extended CD (clusters of differentiation) system. Antibodies to surface antigens, expressed by AML cells, and their CD numbers, are correlated with the FAB classification in Table 14-3 [5, 6]. Immunophenotyping with the monoclonal antibodies cited in Table 14-3 should be performed in conjunction with typing for lymphoid antigens characteristic of cells of B lineage (CD19, HLA-DR, and TdT) and T lineage (CD3, TdT) (see Table 12-1). The combination of CD19, CD3 (or CD7), CD33, CD13, HLA-DR, and TdT should discriminate between the blasts of AML and those of acute lymphatic leukemia (ALL) in over 90% of cases [6]. Phenotyping fails or is puzzling in those ALL cases in which lymphoid surface antigens are lacking or in any leukemic cell lines that are guilty of lineage infidelity or that express bilineage markers.

Cytogenetics of AML

The percentage of AML cases associated with karyotypic abnormalities depends on the fervor and expertise of the cytogeneticists. Using standard techniques, with resolution of marrow mitoses at 150 to 320 bands per haploid set, chromosomal defects are seen in about 50% of cases. With extended high-resolution analysis of methotrexate-synchronized cells at the 400 to 1,000 G band level, marrow chromosome aberrations can be found in about 95% of AML patients. Over 30 categorical defects have been discovered, many of which represent single, recurrent, clonal defects that are considered specific (i.e., primary) and distinctive for morphological FAB subtypes (Figure 14-2) [7]. Two translocations are unique

TABLE 14-3

Immunophenotyping of AML variants

Monoclonal antibodies to	CD*	FAB classification						
		M1	M2	M3	M4	M5	M6	M7
HLA-DR		+	+	−	+	+	+/−	+/−
MY9, L4F3	CD33	+	+	+	+	+	+/−	+/−
MCS-2, MY7	CD13	+/−	+	+	+	+	−	NR†
Mo1, OKM1	CD11b	−	+	+/−	+	+	−	NR
Leu M1	CD15	−	+	+/−	+	+	+/−	NR
Mo2, UCHM1	CD14	−	+/−	−	+	+	−	NR
Glycophorin A		−	−	−	−	−	+	−
Glycoprotein IIb/IIIa	CDw41	−	−	−	−	−	−	+
Glycoprotein Ib	CDw42	−	−	−	−	−	−	+
von Willebrand factor (vWF)		−	−	−	−	−	−	+

*Clusters of differentiation number.
†Not reported.

Source: Derived and amended from Foucar K: Bone marrow examination in the diagnosis of acute and chronic leukemias. Hematol Oncol Clin North Am 2:567,1988; and Van den Berghe: Morphologic, immunologic and cytogenetic (MIC) working classification of the acute myeloid leukaemias. Br J Haematol 68:487,1988.

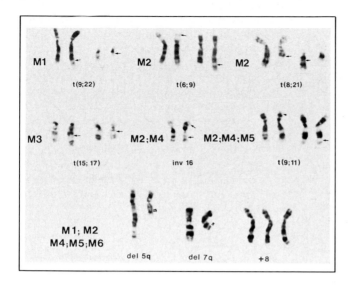

FIGURE 14-2

Selected G banded marrow chromosomes from patients with one of nine single distinctive chromosome defects found in de novo AML. Breakpoints are denoted by arrows and deletions by brackets. In del 5q the interstitial segments of bands q13–31 are missing, and in most cases del 7q involves loss of the distal segment, band q31–qter. (From Yunis JJ: Chapt 5, in Important Advances in Oncology 1986, DeVita VT Jr et al, Eds. Philadelphia, JB Lippincott Company,1986.)

and singular features of AML variants; one— the (15;17) translocation—is pathognomonic of APL. Several others are characteristic but shared by two or more FAB morphologic variants.

8;21 translocation is restricted to AML-M2   The M2 subset of AML, comprising almost 30% of AMLs and occurring primarily in children and young adults, often bears a unique chromosomal rubric, a balanced translocation with breakpoints occurring at 8q22 and 21q22. The 8q22 breakpoint exposes the coding region for

FIGURE 14-3

Schematic rendition of the 15;17 translocation pathognomonic of APL. (From Van den Berghe: Morphologic, immunologic and cytogenetic (MIC) working classification of the acute myeloid leukaemias. Br J Haematol 68:487,1988.)

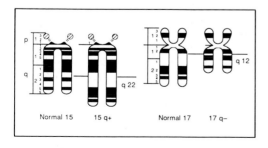

c-*mos* and it is presumed that the t(8;21) (q22;q22) rearrangement alters and somehow activates the c-*mos* oncogene. The 8;21 anomaly prophesies a comparatively good prognosis unless the anomaly is accompanied by loss or inactivation of a sex chromosome. Less often the M2 variant of AML is associated with a specific (primary) t(6;9) defect or with the various shared abnormalities portrayed in Figure 14-2.

t(15;17) is diagnostic of APL   The third (M3) variant of AML, acute promyelocytic leukemia, has a singular association with a 15;17 translocation (Figure 14-3) [6]. The chromosomal defect, t(15;17)(q22;q12), is in the same band as the oncogene c-*fes*, but subbanding suggests the relationship is casual, not causal. Demonstration of this diagnostic abnormality is important in certifying variants of APL in which the characteristic hypergranularity is invisible by light microscopy (microgranular APL), for management of this disorder requires adventurous use of plasma products and anticoagulation.

inv 16 is associated with good responses to standard chemotherapy   In myelomonocytic leukemia with an inv(16)(p13q22), the metallothionein gene cluster located at 16q22.1 is split during the inversion rearrangement, moving some of these genes to the short arm

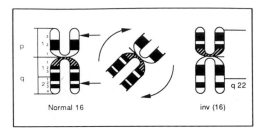

FIGURE 14-4

Inversion with breakpoints at p13 and q22 of a segment of chromosome 16 characterizes an M4 type of AML displaying marrow eosinophilia and unique staining anomalies. (From Van den Berghe: Morphologic, immunologic and cytogenetic (MIC) working classification of the acute myeloid leukaemias. Br J Haematol 68:487, 1988.)

(Figure 14-4) [6]. The plentiful marrow eosinophils in this treatable syndrome contain numerous large granules that stain magenta with Wright-Giemsa, and these dysplastic eosinophil precursors are anomalously positive for chloroacetate esterase and contain pointillistic patterns of PAS positivity.

The Philadelphia (Ph) chromosome also occurs in acute leukemias   Although the Ph chromosome signifying a t(9;22)(q34;q11) translocation is considered the cachet of CML, being found in over 95% of cases (Figure 13-5), this abnormality and the minute Philadelphia chromosome containing juxtaposed *abl* genes and *bcr* segments are also found in about 20% of cases of ALL and 1 to 2% of patients with AML. In Ph-positive ALL and AML, over half of cases fail to show rearrangement within the *bcr* locus, and breakpoints can occur anywhere between *bcr* and the C_λ regions of the lambda light chain cluster. In these cases the recombination of c-*abl* oncogene with a DNA segment upstream of the *bcr* region leads to generation of a unique mRNA that codes for a 190,000 M_r fusion kinase and not for the 210,000 M_r mutant protein of CML. That the 190,000 M_r chimeric protein product signifies acuteness irrespective of lymphoid versus myeloid lineage shows that the Ph chromosome in acute leukemias can accompany contradictory phenotypic and molecular expressions. In both AML and ALL, the Ph chromosome confers a dismal, forlorn prognosis.

Combined cytogenetic analysis and cell lineage phenotyping of AML variants have shown that dual or multiple cell lineage involvement is generically predictive of refractoriness to chemotherapy. In the society of cells, as well as of people, infidelity is punished. Lineage infidelity in AML is most often biphenotypic, and the poor survival in patients with biphenotypic leukemia is traceable to the site of clonal origin at the pluripotential, and even the multipotential, stem cell level.

Stem Cell Level of Clonal Disease Determines Response to Therapy

Morphological classification of leukemias has considerable practical value but has introduced confusion as regards the level of clonal transformation. Most AMLs, particularly those in early or middle adulthood, arise from transformation of committed stem cells, usually of GFU-GM or subordinate, nonreplicative blast cells. G6PD and cytogenetic analyses reveal that the leukemic clones are restricted, not involving red cells, megakaryocytes, or lymphocytes: the M2 variant with t(8;21) and the M3 variant with t(15;17) are exemplary of "low-echelon" leukemias, and such unipotential disorders of nonreplicative stem cells are responsive to chemotherapy. In some AMLs, particularly those occurring in later adulthood, the leukemic clone includes erythroid and megakaryocytic as well as myeloid lineages (and occasionally B cells are included). In these AMLs, of which Ph-positive leukemias and those with monosomy 7 or multiple chromosomal defects are examples, the clonal defect is higher up—traceable to the pluripotential and occasionally the multipotential stem cell level. In the first group, marrow becomes repopulated by normal polyclonal stem cells during chemotherapy-induced remission; in the second, the leukemic clone persists in the marrow even during hematologic remission. It follows (at least in theory) that "committed cell leukemias" [8] are chemocurable, but those leukemias devolved from high-echelon stem cells, however amenable at first, can be salvaged only by marrow replacement (transplantation).

DESCRIPTION

Prevalent complaints at presentation are fatigue, malaise, and unexplained but profound weakness worsening over a period of 2 to 3 months. Fever, night sweats, and easy bruising are often noted, but the traditional presenting features of cancer (weight loss and anorexia) usually are not early problems. Primary findings are the pallor and cardiovascular signs of hypovolemia, thrombocytopenic purpura, and various consequences of leukemic infiltrations including moderate splenomegaly in half and inconspicuous lymphadenopathy in about one-third of patients.

Hematologic Findings

The white count is elevated in half of patients at presentation and is normal or subnormal in the rest. Patients with elevated white counts generally have proportionately depressed levels of normal neutrophils, and infection is the bête noir that haunts patients with this depressing disease. The number of myeloblasts in the blood is not a good gauge of the total mass of leukemic cells, but blast counts exceeding 100,000 cells/μl signify terminal progression and pose an immediate risk of causing leuko-occlusions in small vessels of lungs and brain. Leukostatic plugging of CNS vessels by gummy accretions of sticky blasts can cause serious neurologic damage including fatal cerebral hemorrhage; this "hyperleukocytic syndrome" constitutes a hematologic emergency, best managed by leukapheresis followed by chemotherapeutic cytoreduction.

Blood and marrow morphology are essential to diagnosis and influence management. The several cytologic entities covered by the term AML are as picturesque as they are deadly and warrant individual portrayal.

Portrait Gallery of the FAB 7

AML without and with maturation   In AML without maturation (M1), representing about 20% of cases, myeloblasts show little individuality, most having small amounts of gray-blue cytoplasm and large plump nuclei containing one or more pale, punched-out nucleoli. The leukemic and dysplastic character of M1 myeloblasts is particularly evident in marrow preparations, for these include accumulations of

blasts so large and deformed that many never escape the marrow sinuses. In AML with (partial) maturation (M2), constituting about 30% of AMLs, the dominant myeloblast population is accompanied by 3 to 30% promyelocytes and lesser numbers of myelocytes. These cells have more cytoplasm, staining a darker blue, than do M1 myeloblasts; small numbers of primary granules may be present, and Auer rods—fused cylindrical stacks of dysplastic primary granules—are usually visible to a keen eye as red or purple needle- or splinter-shaped inclusions. That Auer rods are derived from coalescence of azurophilic primary granules is attested to by their staining for myeloperoxidase, α-naphthol AS-D chloroacetate, and PAS; they are found in the M2 and M4 variants and are particularly numerous and dysplastic in acute promyelocytic leukemia (Figure 14-5) [9]. Auer rods are the totem and

FIGURE 14-5

EM of an Auer rod, showing stacking of atypical primary granules to form tubular structures that align as fusiform bodies. (Horizontal scale bar = 250 nm.) (From Pearson EC et al: Ultrastructure and cytogenetics in seven cases of acute promyelocytic leukaemia (APL). Br J Haematol 63:247,1986.)

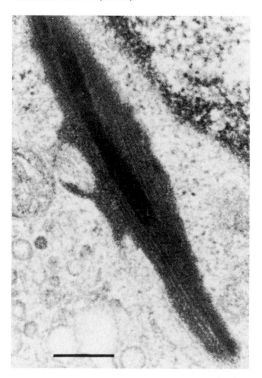

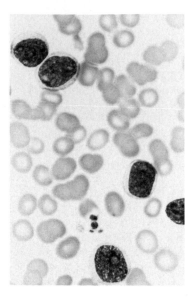 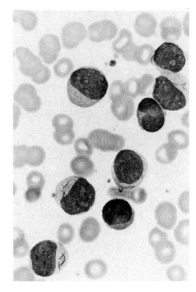

FIGURE 14-6

Myeloblasts in Wright-Giemsa–stained blood of patients with AML-M1 (left) and AML-M2 (right). The cells in AML-M1 are large, non-uniform, and display one or more pale, punched-out pleomorphic nucleoli. Cytoplasm is devoid of granules. The myeloblasts in AML-M2 possess voluminous cytoplasm containing (in four of the cells shown) multiple needle-shaped Auer rods that crisscross each other. (Photos by CT Kapff.)

mantra of AML, and time is well spent searching for them in any patient with acute leukemia. AML blasts without and with maturation are compared in Figure 14-6.

Acute promyelocytic leukemia (APL)   Diagnosis of APL (M3) is made when marrow contains more than 30% promyelocytes. Usually this is the most diagnosable of the AML family because the copious cytoplasm is stuffed with dark reddish lysosomal granules (azurophilic primary granules), often admixed with bundles of peroxidase-positive Auer rods simulating stacked twigs (Figure 14-7). Azurophilic granulation may be so heavy that the rounded or irregular nucleus (which may or may not contain nucleoli) is obscured, even in APL variants in which the granules are fine or dustlike. In 20% of APLs the granules are invisible by light microscopy (microgranular APL), but a telltale morphologic feature of this variant is that the exposed nucleus is bilobed or even binucleate and nucleoli are quite prominent. Diagnosis is certified by finding the pathognomonic t(15;17) translocation, unless cytogenetic analysis is hampered by the sluggish cytokinetics and fuzzy chromosome morphology characteristic of APL. It is essential that APL be recognized, for the myriads of cytoplasmic granules, large or small, are replete with procoagulants that leak out and initiate disseminated intravascular coagulation (DIC). This leads to bleeding, starting in skin and mucosal surfaces, which can progress to abrupt and often fatal pulmonary or cerebral hemorrhage. In patients with hypergranular APL and extreme leukocytosis, prophylactic heparin is warranted; the advent of severe DIC mandates intensive support with fresh-frozen plasma until the leukemia is brought under control by chemotherapy.

Acute myelomonocytic leukemia (AMML)   In AMML (M4), one of the commonest of the AML variants, the leukemic cell population is a variable mixture of myeloblasts and monoblasts (plus promonocytes and monocytes). These progeny of CFU-GM coexist in proportions ranging reciprocally from 20 to 80%, with the more agile monocytes predominating in blood, leaving a disproportionate number of myeloblasts languishing passively in the marrow. Marrow usually contains numerous dysplastic myeloblasts and promyelocytes intermingled with bulky ameboid cells, many of which have folded or bluntly notched nuclei betraying their monoblastic origin. As noted earlier, AMML associated with inv 16 is marked by admixture in the marrow of large monocytoid blasts and eosinophil precursors, some of which also contain basophilic granules and hence display granular chimerism.

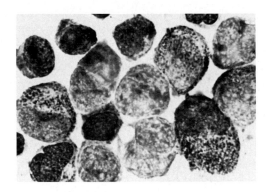

FIGURE 14-7

Hypergranular promyelocytes in the marrow of a patient with APL. Several promyelocytes at center stage are bursting with crisscrossed and fused Auer rods. (Photo by CT Kapff.)

FIGURE 14-8

Plummy infiltrates by AMoL blast cells, causing boggy gingival overgrowths prone to corruption (top) and lumpy violaceous tumors (middle) and nodular lesions (below) of the skin. (From Hoffbrand AV and Pettit JE: Clinical Hematology Illustrated. An Integrated Text and Color Atlas. Philadelphia, WB Saunders Company,1987.)

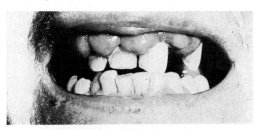

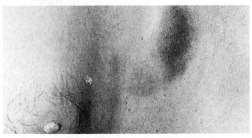

Acute monocytic leukemia (AMoL)   AMoL is a rapidly progressive leukemia characterized by very high white counts and a notorious propensity for the large ameboid leukemic cells to form gross focal accumulations in gums, skin, mucosa, lungs, larynx, and lymph nodes (Figure 14-8) [10]. Plasma and urinary muramidase is always elevated in AMoL, and in patients with extreme leukocytosis, glomerular filtration of lysozyme released from the dysplastic primary granules may suffice to cause a urinary "M component."

The leukemic blasts in AMoL are large, the basophilic cytoplasm is abundant, often containing agranular pseudopods and characteristically staining intensely for α-naphthyl butyrate esterase (Table 14-2), and the nucleus is either round, dented, or folded. In a poorly differentiated subset of AMoL ($M5_A$), large leukemic blast cells with rounded nuclei and very few azurophilic granules overwhelm blood and marrow, accompanied by very few promonocytes or monocytes. In AMoL with partial differentiation ($M5_B$), marrow is occupied by a mixture of monoblasts and promonocytes, and the blood soon swarms with indisputable monocytic forms having folded, twisted, or ameboid nuclei (Figure 14-9). Promonoblasts resemble monoblasts, but their less basophilic cytoplasm is freckled with fine pink granules. The leukemic monocytes in $M5_B$ blood are lightly laden with primary granules and may contain sparse Auer rods. Diagnosis of AMoL can be problematic but may be facilitated by use of monoclonal antibodies for the CD14 and CD11c markers and by demonstrating translocations involving band 11q23, particularly t(9;11)(p11q23), which inserts the Hu-*ets*-1 proto-oncogene into the IFNα coding cluster.

Erythroleukemia (AEL)   Acute erythroleukemia (AEL), alias Di Guglielmo's syndrome or the M6 variant of AML, represents only 4 to 5% of de novo AMLs but constitutes 15 to 20% of leukemias secondary to alkylator therapy, irradiation, or overexposure to benzene. This is a high-echelon clonal disorder of the pluripotential stem cell, and hence the disease may pursue a chameleon course, shifting its expression from erythroid dysplasia to overt myeloblastic leukemia; its malignant evolution is generally

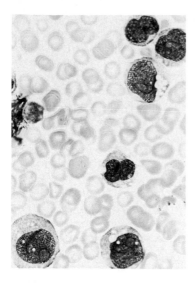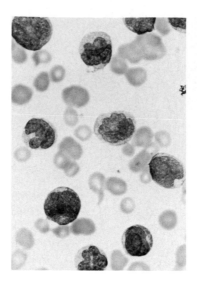

FIGURE 14-9

Blood smears from patients with AMoL. Undifferentiated M5$_A$ monoblasts (left) possess copious cytoplasm, and the folded nuclei contain finely dappled chromatin and large irregular nucleoli. In the more differentiated M5$_B$ subtype (right), monoblasts are admixed with promonocytes and monocytes having folded, twisted, and ameboid nuclei. (Photo by CT Kapff.)

refractory to chemotherapy. In the initial stages, sometimes termed "erythremic myelosis," the marrow is richly occupied by erythroid cells, of which most are dysplastic and many are megaloblastic; some displaying multinucleated gigantism can only be described as outré (Figure 14-10). Diagnosis is often delayed by befuddlement over whether the disease is megaloblastic, hemolytic, or myelodysplastic. Chunky PAS positivity of the cytoplasm and erythroid phenotyping with monoclonal antibodies to glycophorin A affirm erythroidhood, but this is recognizable with routine panoptic stains. The finding of multinucleated erythroblasts and the burgeoning population of M1-type myeloblasts soon dispels diagnostic doubts. If the patient does not succumb to thrombocytopenic purpura, anemia, and infection secondary to marrow replacement, myeloblastic expansion soon brings the course to a melancholy end.

Acute megakaryoblastic leukemia (AMegL)

Megakaryoblastic leukemia (AML-M7) is a fulminant and deadly disorder characterized by marrow infiltration by sheets or clusters of dysplastic megakaryocytes, with densely matted reticulin fibrosis, and delayed emergence into the blood of underdifferentiated polymorphic blast cells with dark nuclei reminiscent of lymphoblasts. Patients present with pancyto-

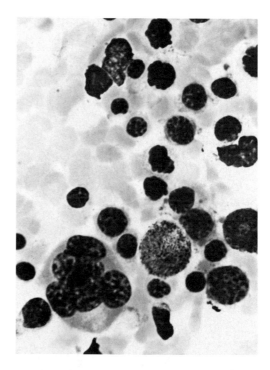

FIGURE 14-10

Marrow from a patient with acute erythroleukemia (AEL) and extreme erythroid hyperplasia. Most erythroblasts are dysplastic and many show megaloblastic changes and nuclear anomalies. Presence of the huge multinucleated erythroblast at bottom left is pathognomonic of AEL. (Photo by CT Kapff.)

penia, pallor, weakness, and petechiae, and diagnosis of acute leukemia is often foiled or delayed by low blood blast levels, absence of hepatosplenomegaly, and unsuccessful efforts to aspirate marrow ("dry taps"). Megakaryoblasts and megakaryocytes in patients with AMegL look something like lymphoblasts encountered in the "L2" variant of ALL (Chapter 16), but some are twice their size and many are adorned with cytoplasmic knobs and pseudopodal tassels containing granules. Some cells are dwarf mononuclear megakaryocytes or fragments of megakaryocytes; others are recognizable as differentiating megakaryocytes by

FIGURE 14-11

Acute megakaryoblastic leukemia cells ranging up to 20 μm across. Some resemble large lymphoblasts, but in several the cell origin is betrayed by earlike pseudopodal flaps and wreaths of shedding platelets. Very similar cells may emerge as a terminal event in some patients with CML. (Reproduced, with permission, from Bennett JM et al: Criteria for the diagnosis of acute leukemia of megakaryocyte lineage (M7). A report of the French-American-British Cooperative Group. Ann Intern Med 103:460,1985.)

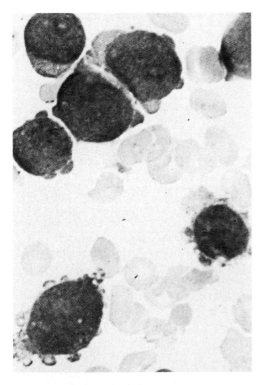

adherent streamers of platelets (Figure 14-11) [11]. In many instances it is impossible to distinguish the leukemic cells from atypical myeloblasts by routine morphologic or cytochemical criteria; definitive diagnosis can be made most expeditiously by use of fluorescent monoclonal antibodies against vWF or (more usually) platelet glycoproteins IIb-IIIa (CDw41). Like erythroleukemia, AMegL represents a cytokinetic disturbance of the penultimate stem cell and thus may pass swiftly through transitional stages from trilineage myelodysplasia through malignant myelofibrosis to terminal megakaryoblastic leukemia, often converting to myeloblastic leukemia in the process. The characteristic presentation with acute myelofibrosis can be attributed to local leakage by leukemic cells of platelet-derived growth factor and other mitogens that stimulate proliferation of fibroblasts.

THERAPY OF AML

Two basic sorts of therapy are capable of inducing remission in AML: combination chemotherapy and marrow transplantation. Combination chemotherapy has been the mainstay of management, but side effects are disheartening, remissions are seldom permanent, and the 10-year "cure" rate is well under 20% in most large series. Marrow transplantation induces permanent remission in a substantial minority of patients, but its use is restricted by the need for HLA-compatible donors and the sternly prejudicial influence of age in this aging-related disease.

Chemotherapy: Anticancer Pharmacology

Virtually all patients with AML should receive combination chemotherapy "up front" within 2 days of diagnosis. The objective of therapy is elimination of malignant stem cells without inflicting crucial losses on the normal marrow hierarchy. In the competition between normal and leukemic cell growth, normal cells have the advantage, for their sturdier stem cells are capable of orderly and spirited regeneration in response to casualties, whereas leukemic clones march along woodenly and recuperate slowly. The dose of cytotoxic drugs is limited by the need to ensure survival of between 1 and 10%

of normal multipotential cells. If the capacity for recovery of leukemic stem cells is one-tenth of that (a favorable kill ratio), a single course of therapy causing severe marrow hypoplasia nevertheless will spare about 0.1% of the leukemic stem cells; a second course given after normal hematopoietic elements have been replenished will still leave a leukemic stem cell residuum of battalion strength (roughly 10^3 cells). These calculations illustrate both the mathematical possibility of clonal eradication and the improbability of actually attaining it without obliterating normal hematopoiesis.

Remission Induction

The intent of chemotherapy in AML, as opposed to that in ALL (Chapter 16), is to induce reversible marrow hypoplasia. Countless cytotoxic agents have been evaluated for antileukemic effect; none is both antileukemic and innocent of hematosuppression, for they are designed to interfere with the synthesis or expression of DNA. Antitumor drugs can be grouped into five categories: alkylators, intercalating agents, metabolic inhibitors (antimetabolites), antimitotic agents, and a group of unlike drugs having undeciphered powers. Most antitumor agents only damage cells while they are in cycle (cycle specific) or in a particular phase of cycle (cycle phase specific); the latter confer the property of "schedule dependence," meaning that drug action is linked to the timing of its administration and full effect requires continuous administration.

Daunorubicin and Cytarabine: The "3 + 7" Regimen

The combination of an anthracycline (daunorubicin) and cytarabine (ara-C) is currently the cornerstone of remission induction chemotherapy, and the two drugs provide instructive examples of the mechanisms and benefit/harm aspects of anticancer pharmacology. Both daunorubicin and doxorubicin are anthracycline chromophores having planar 4-ring structures that intercalate between base pairs of the DNA duplex. This rigidifies DNA, inhibits DNA and RNA polymerases, and blocks DNA repair enzymes, making the crosslinkages and strand breaks irreversible. Daunorubicin is not schedule-dependent and can be given in spaced boluses for up to 3 consecutive days per course.

Like doxorubicin, it also damages mitochondria and interferes with $Na^+K^+ATPase$, resulting in dose-limiting cardiotoxicity.

Cytarabine, a synthetic analog of the pyrimidine nucleoside cytosine, must be given by continuous infusion because of its schedule dependence; it is cytocidal only during the S phase of cell cycle. For activation, cytarabine must be phosphorylated enzymatically to the corresponding antimetabolite, cytidine triphosphate, and cellular resistance to the drug has been linked to the exhaustion of oxycytidine kinase and to deamination of the antimetabolite. Very high doses of cytarabine can override drug resistance for, when given in gram quantities, it not only inhibits DNA polymerase during S phase but also blocks DNA repair during G_2, but this therapeutic bravado risks some intimidating side effects including irreversible cerebellar ataxia. The probability of achieving "complete remission" with "3 + 7" (daunorubicin by bolus infusion for 3 days; cytarabine by continuous infusion for 7 days) is about 60%. Once remission is achieved, further cytoreduction is required (postremission chemotherapy) to abort or eradicate residual leukemic nests and sanctuaries and thus forestall induction of drug-resistant cells. Usually this involves two to six additional cycles of cytarabine and 6-thioguanine, with or without daunorubicin.

Complete remission does not mean cure The expression "complete remission" is the opiate of oncology. Reduction of marrow blast numbers to the mystical level of 5% or less is an accepted but uncomfortably generous criterion for remission, and even restoration of blood counts and a normal karyotype does not assure eradication of the leukemic clone. G6PD isozyme analyses have shown that pathogenesis of AML usually occurs in two broad steps: one causes preleukemic clonal overgrowth; a second causes chromosomal abnormalities and proliferation of blasts. Intensive chemotherapy often reverses the second step but seldom the first. Of the 60% of AML patients who enjoy complete remission following induction chemotherapy, most relapse within 24 months and only a fortunate few (10 to 20%) survive disease-free beyond 5 years. Because of the dismal longterm results with chemotherapy, there has been an increasing trend toward use of marrow transplantation, especially in patients in first chemotherapy-induced remission.

Marrow Transplantation: Great Expectations

Cytogenetic and cell marker evidence that many AMLs represent malignant malfunction at the pluripotential stem cell level has spurred efforts to replace the stem cell pool during remission by ablating all marrow cell elements and rescuing the patient by transplanting normal marrow. This audacious approach necessitates: selection of an HLA-compatible donor; ablative "conditioning" of the patient's hematopoietic and immune systems; marrow replacement ("rescue") by infusing syngeneic, allogeneic, or cryopreserved autologous marrow cells; and control of graft-versus-host disease (GVHD) and other complications of the harrowing regimen required. Nearly 10,000 patients worldwide have received marrow transplants as of this writing, most of them for AML and ALL. Both the successes and failures have been rich in serendipity, clarifying such contentious pathophysiologic matters as the origins of osteoclasts and functions of T cell subsets.

Selection of Donors

Graft rejection and GVHD are the alternative reactions to unmatched grafts. The preferred candidate donor is an HLA-genotypically identical sibling, which narrows this option considerably and has led to use of marrow from HLA-matched related or unrelated donors—the latter becoming increasingly available through establishment of marrow donor registries—and, with less success, from related donors who are only haplotype-identical. In performance of the conventional allogeneic transplant, serological testing for HLA compatibility is less dependable than the mixed lymphocyte reaction (MLR), which has proved to be the best routine technique for predicting durable engraftment. An even more refined predictor of compatibility is the mixed epidermal cell–lymphocyte reaction which pits cytotoxic T cells of the donor against the minor antigens (and antigen-presenting cells) of recipient's skin.

How to Transplant Marrow

Pretransplant conditioning of AML recipients for marrow grafts has three objectives: ablation of resident hematopoietic cells to create intramedullary lodgings for the forthcoming donor cells, suppression of immunologic resistance, and eradication of malignant stem cells. To accomplish these goals, most conditioning protocols involve high-dose cyclophosphamide or cytarabine followed by single-dose or fractionated total body irradiation (7.5 to 15.0 Gy). Allogeneic marrow is secured via 100 or so aspirations from the iliac crests, which aspirates are pooled, suspended, and infused via a graduated filter into the patient's bloodstream. For adequate engraftment from 2 to 3 $\times$ 10^8 nucleated marrow cells are required to ensure that sufficient numbers (several thousands) of multipotential stem cells home to and become housed in recipient marrow spaces; fewer cells are needed in syngeneic or autologous transplants. During the ensuing months methotrexate or cyclosporine (cyclosporin A) are administered to prevent or tame GVHD (Figure 14-12) [12]. Donor marrow takes root

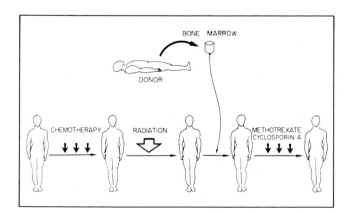

BONE MARROW

DONOR

CHEMOTHERAPY   RADIATION   METHOTREXATE CYCLOSPORIN A

FIGURE 14-12

Schematic reprise of the steps involved in marrow transplantation in AML or other cancers. (From Champlin RE and Gale RP: Role of bone marrow transplantation in the treatment of hematologic malignancies and solid tumors: critical review of syngeneic, autologous, and allogeneic transplants. Cancer Treat Rep 68:145,1984.)

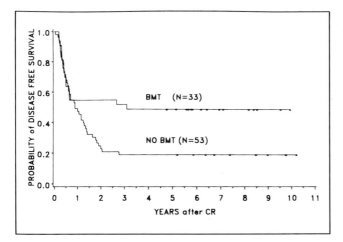

FIGURE 14-13

Probability (Kaplan-Meier product-limit estimates) of disease-free survival in AML patients receiving transplants from HLA-identical siblings (BMT) is compared with that in patients treated with chemotherapy alone (NO BMT). (From Appelbaum FR et al: Chemotherapy v. marrow transplantation for adults with acute nonlymphocytic leukemia: a five-year follow-up. Blood 72:179,1988.)

within 1 week, marrow cellularity is half-restored in 3 to 4 weeks, and within 2 months (barring misadventure) the recipient's entire hematopoietic and immune systems plus marrow stroma are composed of donor cells. Engraftment can be confirmed by blood cell phenotyping, karyotyping, and RFLP analysis.

In AML patients receiving allogeneic transplants during the first chemotherapy-induced remission, 10-year disease-free survival can be attained in almost 50% of cases, a considerable improvement over the survivorship for chemotherapy alone (Figure 14-13) [13]. Treatment failures are due to opportunistic infections, interstitial pneumonia, and leukemic relapse. Relapse occurs in 20 to 30% of AML patients after marrow transplantation. Most relapses are of host cell origin and occur within 1 to 2 years, signifying persistence of clonal stem cells. AMML and AMoL stem cells are particularly adept at surviving "marrow ablation" and are responsible for most early relapses [14]. In rare instances latencies are as long as 3 to 6 years, and the leukemic cells have been found to be of donor origin by sex chromosome or other markers such as RFLPs. This unforeseen phenomenon raises the possibility of leukemic induction of donor cells by oncogene transfection.

A set of rigorous qualifiers must be attached to the sunny summarization of the marrow transplant results in Figure 14-13: (1) In most centers transplants are available only to patients with HLA- and MLR-compatible do-nors, preferably sibling donors, lowering the transplant option to less than 20% of patients; (2) only patients under age 40 (or 45) are usually considered for marrow grafting, results being poor in older patients; and (3) median age for onset of AML is over 60 years. Factoring in these constraints, allogeneic marrow transplantation is a curative option in less than 10% of all patients with AML.

Autologous Marrow Transplantation: Purging of Leukemic Cells

For the older, desperate majority of AML patients lacking a compatible and altruistic sibling donor, one recourse is postablation rescue by use of cryopreserved autologous marrow secured during complete remission. Procedures have been improvised to exorcize the clonogenic stem cells concealed within marrow populations collected during remission. Selective immunotoxins have performed successfully in eliminating T cells from allogeneic marrow, but the use of toxins ligated to monoclonal antibodies against leukemia antigens has been frustrated by inadequate specificity. Recently immunotoxins constructed from anti-CD13 monoclonal antibodies armed with a ricin (ribosome-inactivating phytotoxin) warhead have proved effective in purging autologous marrow suspensions of myeloid leukemia progenitors, paving the way for clinical application. If this hurdle is cleared, autologous marrow transplants hold considerable promise for

AML therapy, for histocompatibility problems are circumvented and autologous stem cells have the wherewithal for total and permanent rescue.

Prevention and Treatment of GVHD

GVHD develops in 30 to 70% of AML patients transplanted with HLA-identical, MLR-compatible donor marrow and in nearly all recipients of histoincompatible marrow. Although a major obstacle blocking expanded

FIGURE 14-14

Skin and liver biopsies in grade III acute GVHD. (Above) Cutaneous lesions show epidermal vacuolar degeneration and inflammatory changes, necrosis of individual keratinocytes (arrow), and edema of the basal region. (Below) Liver biopsy 82 days postallograft shows atypia, necrosis, and occlusion of four prominent bile ducts (arrows). (From Thomas ED et al: Chapt 12, in Atlas of Blood Cells: Function and Pathology, vol. 1, 2nd ed, Zucker-Franklin D et al, Eds. Milan, Edi. Ermes s.r.l.,1988.)

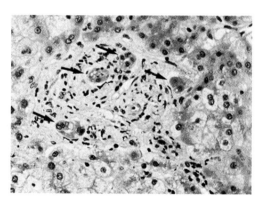

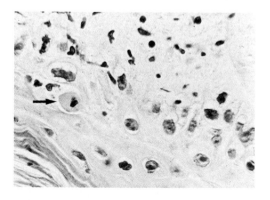

use of marrow transplants as primary therapy for AML, GVHD has served as an experimental model for exploring therapies for autoimmune disease and immune dysregulation of unknown origins.

Acute GVHD By definition, acute GVHD occurs within 100 days after transplantation. It is characterized by rapid onset of confluent exanthema simulating scalded skin, watery and bloody diarrhea, and hepatic malfunction associated with cholestasis resulting from bile duct atypia and degeneration, with epithelial obliteration (Figure 14-14) [15]. Acute GVHD is caused by cytolytic T cells from the donor, which, enraged by the foreign HLA antigens of recipient tissues, launch a frontal attack, supported by T cell–released effector cytokines including TNFα.

Chronic GVHD: exemplar of autoimmunity
Chronic GVHD, which usually evolves from the acute reaction, is a multisystem collagen-vascular type of autoimmune disorder associated with severe immunodeficiency and expressed maximally between 100 and 400 days postgraft. Clinical manifestations include alopecia, polyserositis, Sjögren's syndrome, and (most characteristically) lichen planuslike papules and papulosquamous plaques on the tongue, lips, and skin. Within the first year or so, the process envelops the patient in a casement of pain composed of scleroderma, joint contractures, epidermal fibrosis and atrophy, dysphagia, ocular siccus, atrophic enteritis, bronchiolitis, and assorted musculoskeletal problems (Figure 14-15) [16]. Donor-derived T cells of several subsets having specificity for class II histocompatibility antigens shared by donor and recipient are the responsible villains and hence are capable of igniting both acute and chronic GVHD even in grafts from identical twin donors, confirming that twins may be identical to the eye and by test but not to the immune system.

Management of GVHD T cells of the cytolytic and cytotoxic T8 phenotype are responsible for initiating GVHD and (in complicity with NK cells) for sustaining this iatrogenic autoimmune warfare. Combinations of cyclosporine and methotrexate or prednisone usually are

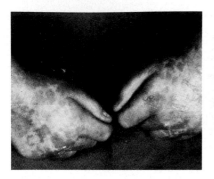 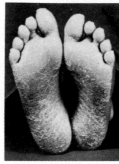

FIGURE 14-15

Skin and joint lesions in untreated chronic GVHD. (Left) Scleroderma-like contractures of the hands with glossy thickening and patchy pigmentation of overlying skin. (Right) Erythema and exfoliative dermatitis involving soles of the feet. (From Hoffbrand AV and Pettit JE: Chapt 6, in Clinical Hematology Illustrated. An Integrated Text and Color Atlas. Philadelphia, WB Saunders, 1987.)

effective in controlling or at least placating acute GVHD but are ineffective in chronic GVHD, suggesting that the pathophysiology of the two disorders may be fundamentally different. Nonetheless, removal of T cells by various techniques for purging donor cell suspensions can prevent acute, and mitigate chronic, GVHD. Unfortunately the risk of leukemic relapse and of opportunistic infections is increased by thus paralyzing immunity, and it remains to be determined whether T cell depletion improves survival.

REFERENCES

1. Fialkow PJ et al: Clonal development, stem-cell differentiation, and clinical remissions in acute nonlymphocytic leukemia. N Engl J Med 317:468, 1987

2. Griffin JD and Lowenberg B: Clonogenic cells in acute myeloblastic leukemia. Blood 68:1185, 1986

3. Rapaport SI: Introduction to Hematology. 2nd ed. Philadelphia, JB Lippincott Company, 1987

4. Jandl JH: Chapt 21, in Blood: Textbook of Hematology. Boston, Little, Brown, 1987

5. Foucar K: Bone marrow examination in the diagnosis of acute and chronic leukemias. Hematol Oncol Clin North Am 2:567, 1988

6. Van den Berghe: Morphologic, immunologic and cytogenetic (MIC) working classification of the acute myeloid leukaemias. Br J Haematol 68:48

7. Yunis JJ: Chapt 5, in Important Advances in Oncology 1986, DeVita VJ Jr et al, Eds. Philadelphia, JB Lippincott Company, 1986

8. Jasmin C: Leukemic stem cells and the curability of leukemias. Leuk Res 12:703, 1988

9. Pearson EC et al: Ultrastructure and cytogenetics in seven cases of acute promyelocytic leukaemia (APL). Br J Haematol 63:247, 1986

10. Hoffbrand AV and Pettit JE: Chapt 8, in Clinical Hematology Illustrated. An Integrated Text and Color Atlas. Philadelphia, WB Saunders Company, 1987

11. Bennett JM et al: Criteria for the diagnosis of acute leukemia of megakaryocyte lineage (M7). A report of the French-American-British Cooperative Group. Ann Intern Med 103:460, 1985

12. Champlin RE and Gale RP: Role of bone marrow transplantation in the treatment of hematologic malignancies and solid tumors: critical review of syngeneic, autologous, and allogeneic transplants. Cancer Treat Rep 68:145, 1984

13. Appelbaum FR et al: Chemotherapy v. marrow transplantation for adults with acute nonlymphocytic leukemia: a five-year follow-up. Blood 72:179, 1988

14. McGlave PB et al: Allogeneic bone marrow transplantation for acute nonlymphocytic leukemia in first remission. Blood 72:1512, 1988

15. Thomas ED et al: Chapt 12, in Atlas of Blood Cells: Function and Pathology, vol. 1, 2nd ed., Zucker-Franklin D et al, Eds. Milan, Edi. Ermes s.r.l., 1988

16. Hoffbrand AV and Pettit JE: Chapt 6, in Clinical Hematology Illustrated. An Integrated Text and Color Atlas. Philadelphia, WB Saunders Company, 1987

15

Chronic
Myeloproliferative
Syndromes

□

C hronic myeloproliferative syndromes are a diversiform family of acquired clonal disorders arising from malignant transformations of multipotential stem cells. Derangement of the founder stem cell leads to clonal expansion of the pluripotential compartment and overproduction of one or more of the subordinate cell lines. The most common myeloproliferative disorder—chronic myelogenous leukemia—is overtly leukemic from the outset; the others are variably predisposed to transform to leukemia spontaneously or in reaction to therapy. This variegate family includes chronic myelogenous leukemia, idiopathic myelofibrosis, polycythemia vera, and essential thrombocythemia.

CHRONIC MYELOGENOUS LEUKEMIA

Chronic myelogenous leukemia (CML) is a clonal myeloproliferative disorder originating from a single neoplastic multipotential stem cell and characterized by perpetual or resurgent overproduction of granulocytes and their precursors, most of which appear normal morphologically but are somewhat defective functionally. CML is uniquely characterized by a preordained triphasic course consisting of a long preliminary "chronic phase" of mounting granulocytosis, an interlude of "acute transformation" toward cellular immaturity, and a stormy climax known as "blast crisis" in which myelopoiesis is concentrated on manufacture of functionless blasts.

Pathophysiology

The fundamental defect in CML is a robotic expansion of the myeloid stem cell compartment due to incessant proliferation but slightly discordant maturation of neoplastic precursor cells. A vigorous rate of granulocyte formation is sustained despite prolongation of the stem cell cycle by reiterative divisions at the myelocyte and promyelocyte levels. The combination of stem cell expansion, redundant divisions, and protraction of lifespan of the defective leukemic cells leads to amplification of the total granulocyte pool by at least 100-fold.

That CML is a clonal disorder of the multipotential stem cell has been demonstrated by isozyme analysis using G6PD and adenylate kinase as cell markers and by X-chromosome DNA restriction fragment length polymorphisms. The cytogenetic hallmark of CML is the Philadelphia (Ph) chromosome, the minute but celebrated product of an unequal 9;22 translocation (Figure 13-5) found in over 95% of cases. Both isozyme and cytogenetic findings prove that the CML clone encompasses neutrophils, eosinophils, basophils, erythroblasts, platelets, monocytes, B cells, and some T cells—attesting to the high-echelon (multipotential) level of the mutation. The Ph anomaly has been observed to precede overt CML by up to 6 years, indicating that clonal cytogenetic translocation is an early event in the multiple steps involved in leukemogenesis.

Molecular Biology of the Ph Translocation

The crucial molecular error in Ph$^+$ CML is the 9;22 translocation, which results in fusion of the *abl* proto-oncogene of chromosome 9 with the interrupted end of the breakpoint cluster region (*bcr*) of chromosome 22.

The c-*abl* proto-oncogene is a 145,000 M_r tyrosine protein kinase (phosphokinase) which phosphorylates tyrosine and certain serine and threonine residues of intracellular proteins and is somehow involved in regulating normal cell growth. Cloning of c-*abl*, which resides on the long arm of chromosome 9, reveals that it contains two alternative 5' exons (1a and 1b) spliced to a common set of ten 3' exons. As the result of this genomic configuration, two major c-*abl* messages are transcribed (6 kb and 7 kb mRNAs) and all c-*abl* messages share a set of 3' exons starting from c-*abl* exon 2. The splice acceptor site is unusual in that it can accept a multiplicity of exon donor fragments; this promiscuity is pivotal to the tumorigenicity of this gene for it predisposes c-*abl* to fuse with non-*abl* sequences and become activated.

Unlike this potential variability in position of breakpoints near or within c-*abl* on chromosome 9, the breakpoints in chromosome 22 are clustered within a 5.8 kb DNA segment known as the *bcr* gene. In virtually all CML patients with the Ph chromosome, rearrangements of the *bcr* gene can be detected by molecular probing and shown to be unique to each individual patient—a molecular change that serves as a sensitive test for Ph$^+$ CML. The point of breakage within *bcr* usually occurs between exons 2 and 3 or 3 and 4; as the result of the reciprocal exchange between the long arms of chromosomes 9 and 22, c-*abl* proto-oncogene is transferred from band 9q34 to 22q11, whereas proximal 5' *bcr* gene exons including 1 and 2 (with or without exon 3) remain on chromosome 22. The end result is that the rearranged proximal *bcr* gene sequences are annealed to c-*abl* sequences in a head-to-tail fashion, forming the chimeric *bcr-abl* fusion gene located on chromosome 22 (Figure 15-1) [1].

The bcr-abl *fusion gene generates a hyperactive tyrosine kinase*   During transcription of *bcr-abl* the c-*abl* exon 2 skips splice donor sites in exons 1a and 1b, excluding them as it fuses with 5' splice donor sites of the juxtaposed *bcr* exons. The resultant novel 8.5 *bcr-abl* transcript codes for a chimeric protein (M_r, 210,000) having tyrosine kinase activity considerably greater than its normal 145,000 M_r counterpart. This novel kinase has the properties of an oncogene growth factor, but the mechanism by which it induces expansion of the senior stem cell compartments and the selective expansion of myeloid proliferation is unknown. As the Ph chromosome and its protein product are found early in the chronic phase and expression of the fusion gene is not consistently heightened during blast crisis, it is likely that *bcr* rearrangement paves the way but is not sufficient for later escalation of the leukemia.

Ph$^+$ acute leukemia redux   About 20% of adults with ALL and 1 to 2% of those with AML have a t(9;22) translocation indistinguishable cytogenetically from that found in

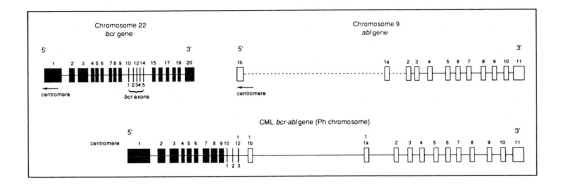

FIGURE 15-1

(Above) Normal *bcr* and *abl* genes. (Below) Chimeric *bcr-abl* fusion gene associated with CML. Numbered boxes and vertical lines represent exons, horizontal lines denote introns, and the long interrupted line connecting the first exons of the *abl* gene represents the extended region in which breakpoints occur. (From Kurzrock R et al: The molecular genetics of Philadelphia chromosome–positive leukemias. Reprinted, by permission of The New England Journal of Medicine, 319:990,1988.)

CML (Chapter 14). Molecular analysis, aided in some instances by polymerase chain reaction (PCR) amplification, has revealed that in over half of the ALL cases (and most of the few AML patients studied) the break in chromosome 22q11 occurs at the first intron of the *bcr* gene. Hence only the 3′ end of the first exon of the *bcr* gene is juxtaposed to the translocated c-*abl* gene and the fused protein product is smaller (M_r, 190,000) and lacks the *bcr* rearrangement characteristic of CML (Figure 15-2) [1, 2]. The p190^{c-abl} protein product in ALL is essentially a stripped-down version of the c-*abl* product and possesses potent tyrosine phosphokinase activity.

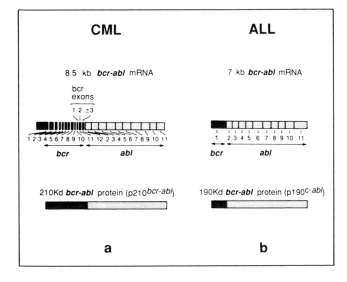

FIGURE 15-2

Hybrid mRNA and protein products in (a) CML and (b) about 50% of cases of Ph+ ALL. In CML the chimeric *bcr-abl* gene is transcribed as a hybrid 8.5 kb mRNA; the translated product is a 210 kd (210,000 M_r) protein elongated by the N-terminal substitution of rearranged *bcr*-coded sequences. In half of Ph+ ALL patients, *bcr* exon 1 alone is fused to c-*abl* exons 2 through 12, forming an unrearranged 7.0 kb mRNA. The translation product is a smaller 190 kd hybrid protein termed p190^{c-abl}. (From Kurzrock R et al. Reprinted, by permission of The New England Journal of Medicine, 319:990, 1988.)

Ph chromosome: consolation or curse The Philadelphia chromosome serves as a valuable asset in diagnosis of CML. The biologic significance of this diminutive marker chromosome is hard to assess, however, for the unleashed c-*abl* phosphokinase has no defined molecular target, and there is no known link between formation of either $p210^{bcr-abl}$ or $p190^{c-abl}$ and any specific cytokinetic event. The molecular mechanism propelling Ph^+ CML patients to blast crisis is unexplained, for the "blast-off" is unaccompanied by consistent quantitative or qualitative changes in *bcr* or *abl*. Furthermore Ph positivity usually signifies leisurely and delayed progression of CML, whereas Ph^- CML is a rapidly progressive disease from the start. In acute leukemias, on the contrary, Ph positivity (with or without rearranged *bcr*) confers a dismal prognosis. Synthesis of mutant c-*abl* transcripts somehow initiates proliferation, but the triphasic progression to blast crisis requires superimposed genetic driving forces. Additional cytogenetic aberrations occur in over 80% of patients with CML approaching blast crisis and are of remarkable consistency: doubling of the Ph chromosome (+Ph) and trisomy 8(+8) are most commonly observed, followed by isochromosome 17q [i(17q)], trisomy 19 (+19), and loss of the Y chromosome (−Y). Most of these secondary anomalies can be found in both myeloid and lymphoid blast crises, but the occurrence of a secondary t(15;17) or an i(17q) is unique to myeloid irruptions (the latter being associated with basophilic proliferation); lymphoid crises often display hypodiploidy with loss of chromosome 7, and most have clonal immunoglobulin or T cell receptor gene rearrangements [3]. In all blast crises, regardless of phenotype, cells derived from the new neoplastic clone have a survival advantage over both normal and chronic phase Ph^+ clones, and the malignant blast forms accumulate and dispossess cells with lesser maturational defects.

Advantages and Disadvantages of CML Cells

CML cells, although defective, possess several proliferative advantages that account for their capacity to displace normal stem cells. In the initial chronic phase, myeloid stem cells elaborate prostaglandin E and an acid isoferritin termed "leukemia-associated inhibitor," both of which selectively suppress normal colony-forming and pluripotential stem cells. These inhibitors account for the virtual absence of Ph-negative normal stem cell activity in CML marrow; in cell culture, quiescent normal stem cells arrested in G_1 are present but can only replicate when relieved of this suppression. Because of this competitive advantage in the expanding, turbulent marrow, the number of clonal CFU-GM and CFU-G progenitors extruded into the bloodstream is increased as much as 10,000-fold at diagnosis.

Despite their teeming abundance, circulating granulocytes are flawed by several functional defects. Prominent among these are the following: diagnostically low leukocyte alkaline phosphatase (LAP) activity; impaired adhesiveness to artificial or stromal surfaces; sluggish emigration to extravascular sites; and reduction in phagocytic and bactericidal activities and enzymes. Although low LAP activity is an independent variable, adhesiveness, phagocytic activity, and vigor of motility as measured by the skin window technique or passage through porous flow chambers (Chapter 10) appear to be linked properties, all of which are depressed in CML neutrophils. Consequently, most neutrophils remain trapped and unmotivated in circulation or in sinus structures of spleen, liver, and marrow, accounting in part for the profound leukocytosis and prominent splenomegaly in patients first presenting with CML. The lethargic movement of neutrophils explains the predisposition toward barrier infections and eczema in CML patients.

Description

CML is an insidious disorder in which the Ph^+ clone replaces myeloid stem cells before the white count is elevated. Clinical manifestations surface several years after clonal initiation, the slow pace of myeloproliferative progression reflecting the dilatory doubling time of 2 to 4 months. The greatest incidence of CML is at age 40 to 60, but nearly 20% present at an earlier age.

Features of the Chronic Phase

Elevations of the granulocyte count may go unrecognized for months or years, but chance discovery on routine examination may reveal

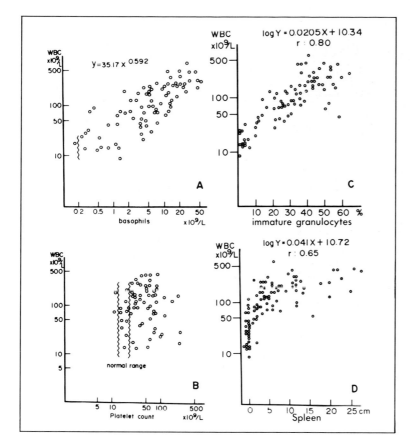

FIGURE 15-3

Clinical and laboratory
findings at diagnosis in
102 CML patients.
White counts are plot-
ted on the ordinate
against basophil levels
(A), platelet counts (B),
percentage of immature
granulocytes (C), and
spleen size (D). (From
Kamada N and Uchino
H: Chronologic se-
quence in appearance of
clinical and laboratory
findings characteristic
of chronic myelocytic
leukemia. Blood 51:
843,1978.)

an increase in basophils, a nearly symmetrical shift toward granulocyte immaturity, and a profound lowering of LAP scores. As the granulocyte count exceeds about 50,000 cells/μl the spleen becomes palpable and hypermetabolic symptoms may appear. Presenting symptoms of CML in the chronic active state include loss of energy, fatigue, anorexia and weight loss, and diminished exercise tolerance of several months duration. Splenomegaly is the commonest physical finding, sometimes gripping the patient's attention by becoming painfully infarcted. In over half of patients the spleen extends more than 5 cm below the left costal margin on admission, and in general the magnitude of splenomegaly correlates well with the blood granulocyte count, the proportion of immature granulocytes in the blood, and the blood basophil level (Figure 15-3) [4]. Splenomegaly is a gauge of the duration of

chronic phase CML, very large spleens being harbingers of acute transformation and blast crisis. The spleen in CML rivals that of tropical splenomegaly and may become so large that it extends across the midline and nestles its lower pole in the pelvis (Figure 15-4) [5].

Hematologic findings During the first several years in the chronic phase, leukocyte and platelet counts steadily rise, red counts gradually fall, and immature myeloid forms spill into the bloodstream. Most patients have white counts between 20,000 and 600,000/μl at the time of diagnosis, but leukocyte levels may climb to prodigious heights, causing the blood to look milky as counts approach 1,000,000 cells/μl (Figure 15-5) [6]. As white counts rise above 100,000 cells/μl the hazard of leukostatic vasoocclusions increases proportionately. The problem is particularly serious in

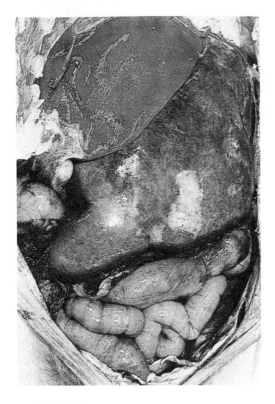

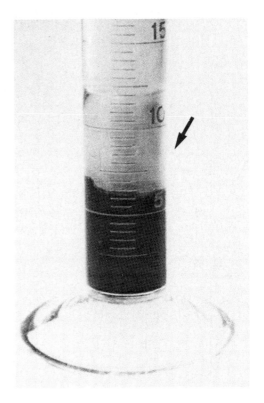

FIGURE 15-4

Massive splenomegaly at autopsy of a 54-year-old man with advanced CML. The grossly enlarged spleen extends toward the right iliac fossa. The central pale area is fibrinous exudate overlying a subcapsular splenic infarct. (From Hoffbrand AV and Pettit JE: Clinical Hematology Illustrated. An Integrated Text and Color Atlas. Philadelphia, WB Saunders Company, 1987.)

FIGURE 15-5

Illustration of the startling leukocrit or "buffy coat" (arrow) revealed when anticoagulated blood of a CML patient with extreme leukocytosis is allowed to settle. CML is usually characterized by much higher white counts than occur in AML. (From Marmont AM et al: Chapt 4, in Atlas of Blood Cells: Function and Pathology, vol. 1, Zucker-Franklin D et al, Eds. Milan, Edi. Ermes s.r.l.,1988.)

young patients, among whom 50% present with white counts in excess of 300,000 cells/μl, and in patients in transformation with burgeoning numbers of sticky blast forms. Sludging with gummy accretions of immature leukemic cells disturbs rheology, obstructs blood flow in small vessels, and may precipitate a busy assortment of alarming complications including CNS hemorrhages, digital gangrene, adult respiratory distress syndrome, and retinal papilledema and hemorrhage (Figure 15-6) [7].

Morphology in chronic phase CML Diagnosis of chronic phase CML is usually obvious on low-power examination of blood smears, for

all stages of myeloid differentiation are represented in approximate rank order, resembling therefore a thin smear of reactive myeloid marrow. The sum of metamyelocytes, myelocytes, and younger forms (including occasional myeloblasts) generally approaches that of bands plus segmented neutrophils, platelets are plentiful, and basophils are ominously numerous (Figure 15-7). Blood cell differential counts show the complete spectrum of granulocytic forms, as though marrow had leaked into the circulation, and differential counts reveal two signatures of CML: absolute basophilia and an anomalous increase in myelocytes (Figure 15-8) [8]. Nucleated red cells are found in the

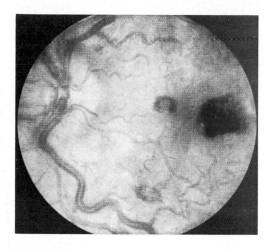

FIGURE 15-6

Left optic fundus at time of first diagnosis of
CML in a 28-year-old woman with a white
count of 600,000 cells/μl. Fundoscopy shows
damage by leukostasis: papilledema, venous obstruction, and widespread hemorrhages corresponding to field defects. (From Stainsby D et
al: Papilloedema in chronic granulocytic
leukaemia. Br J Haematol 55:243,1983.)

blood of nearly all CML patients, and all cell
lines display dysplastic changes, among which
pseudo-Pelger forms, hypogranular neutrophils, mononuclear megakaryocytes, and numerous smudge forms are notable. Cytochemical staining of blood smears in CML shows a
negative or weak LAP reaction, but all other
myelospecific reactions are strongly positive
(Figure 15-9) [6].

Marrow biopsy adds little surprising information, revealing hypercellularity due to exuberant myeloid proliferation, a conspicuous
shift toward immaturity, and an M:E ratio of at
least 10:1. In many CML patients sphingo-
lipid-glutted Gaucherlike cells may collect in

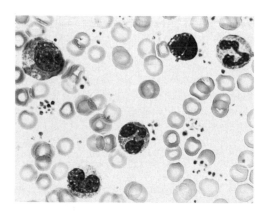

FIGURE 15-7

Blood smear from a patient with CML reveals
pronounced granulocytosis with a shift toward
immature myeloid forms and a surplus of platelets. Note the inappropriate presence of an early
myelocyte (upper left) and a metamyelocyte
(lower left), plus the partly degranulated
basophil (upper right-center). Basophils in overabundance are a marker of myeloproliferative
disorders. (Photo by CT Kapff.)

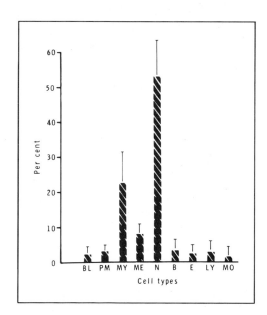

FIGURE 15-8

Histogram representing differential white count
in CML (mean white count: 225,000 cells/μl).
All granulocytic forms are represented, but
there is a unique excess of myelocytes (MY),
which are more numerous than metamyelocytes
(ME), and of basophils (B)—the cachet of
chronic myeloproliferative disorders. BL =
blasts, PM = promyelocytes, N = neutrophils,
E = eosinophils, LY = lymphocytes, and MO
= monocytes. (From Spiers ASD: The clinical
features of chronic granulocytic leukaemia. Clin
Haematol 6:77,1977.)

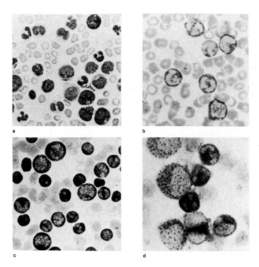

FIGURE 15-9

Blood cell cytochemistry in chronic phase CML. The following cytoplasmic reactions are all decisively positive: (a) peroxidase; (b) α naphthol AS-D chloroacetate esterase; (c) Sudan black; and (d) acid phosphatase. (From Marmont AM et al: Chapt 4, in Atlas of Blood Cells: Function and Pathology, vol. 1, Zucker-Franklin D et al, Eds. Milan, Edi. Ermes s.r.l.,1988.)

marrow and spleen, reflecting massive dumping of membrane lipid debris into macrophages. These storage cells are not lacking in sphingolipid hydrolase, but the enzyme is overwhelmed by an enormous daily load of membrane lipid released in situ by fragile, defective leukemic cells as they expire in their packed chambers. Another peculiarity of CML marrow that attests to the infirmity of leukemic cells is the leakage of free granules, which often clutter the background. Many leukemia cells display granular chimerism, showing both eosinophilic and basophilic granules admixed in the same cell (Figure 15-10) [9].

Acute transformation (accelerated phase) Eventually in all chronic phase CML patients, clonal growth undergoes malignant escalation, often explosively, and within several months there are progressive rises in myeloblast levels at the expense of more differentiated forms. As the burgeoning populations of unprogrammed blasts blindly usurp marrow space normal hematopoiesis is smothered and anemia, neutropenia, and thrombocytopenia ensue. Acute transformation may set in as soon as several weeks and as late as 20 years after diagnosis, but the average is 3.5 years; transformation is actually the prelude to a complete block in myeloid differentiation that precedes the final metamorphosis to blast crisis.

Blast crisis Blast crisis is a preordained sequel to chronic phase CML; it is inevitable regardless of prior responsiveness to therapy and is usually fatal within 3 months. Most patients (65%) experience myeloid blast crisis with a mixture of dysplastic myeloblasts and promyelocytes; a large minority (25%) enter a lym-

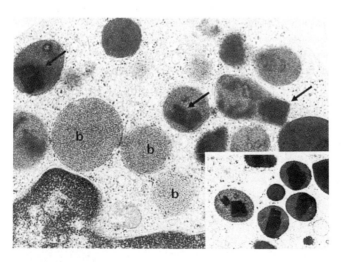

FIGURE 15-10

EM of a CML granulocyte displaying granular chimerism. The cytoplasm contains both secondary basophilic granules (b) and secondary eosinophilic granules with crystalloid inclusions (arrows). Inset shows secondary granules from a normal eosinophil. Even more prevalent (not shown) are basophils containing either mast cell granules or eosinophilic granules. (From Schmidt U et al: Electron-microscopic characterization of mixed granulated (hybridoid) leucocytes of chronic myeloid leukaemia. Br J Haematol 68:175,1988.)

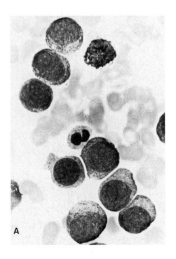 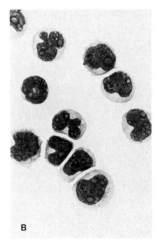

A   B

FIGURE 15-11

Blast forms in blood (A) and cerebrospinal fluid (B) of a CML patient during myeloid blast crisis. Dysplastic myeloblasts and promyelocytes constitute 80 to 90% of nucleated blood cells. Note in (A) the degranulated basophil near the top and the twin-lobed pseudo-Pelger neutrophil at center. In (B), cytocentrifuged preparation of spinal fluid from the same patient displays a pure population of myeloblasts (flattened somewhat by gravity), indicating meningeal involvement. (From Jandl JH: Chapt 22, in Blood: Textbook of Hematology. Boston, Little, Brown and Company,1987.)

phoid crisis dominated by Ph⁺ lymphoblasts usually of pre B cell phenotype, and the remainder of blast crises feature DiGuglielmo-type erythroblasts or megakaryoblasts, sometimes terminating with an admixed surge of myeloblasts. The variegate expression of blast crises, which may involve maturation arrest of any one or several of the hematopoietic cell lines often with biphenotypic or multilineage markers, affirms the prediction that malignant disturbances at the sovereign (multipotential) stem cell level can eventually cause maturation arrest of any cell lines within the clone. In AML the disease presents in "blast crisis" and all the multiple steps of leukemogenesis are simultaneous. In CML these steps occur sequentially in a deliberate march toward the finale.

Myeloid blast crisis   As blast crisis supervenes, arrested myeloblasts rapidly displace the more orderly ranks of differentiating cells and the stem cell activity is diverted almost entirely to production of myeloblasts and promyelocytes (Figure 15-11) [10]. The throngs of blasts admixed with fading remnants of normal differentiating cells inevitably lead to marrow failure, thrombocytopenic bleeding, and overwhelming infection.

Lymphoid blast crisis   The dominant cells during lymphoid blast crisis have lymphoblast morphology (sometimes intermingled with a

minor population of chronic phase myeloid cells) and in most cases are phenotypically similar to the pre B cells of common ALL. The cells are TdT and HLA-DR positive, express the cALL antigen, and contain cytoplasmic Ig μ chains and clonal immunoglobulin gene rearrangements. Most retain or even duplicate the Ph chromosome. In exceptional cases the blast cells bare the T cell phenotype and show clonal rearrangement of the T cell antigen receptor genes, indicating inclusion of T cells in the malignant clone. About half of patients with lymphoid blast crisis respond well, if briefly, to "anti-ALL" therapy (vincristine plus prednisone) and median survival is 6 months, as compared with only 2 to 3 months in chemotherapy-treated patients in myeloid blast crisis.

Treatment

Therapy of chronic phase CML is aimed at reducing the proliferating leukocyte mass and relieving problems created by hyperleukocytosis, thrombocytosis, and splenomegaly.

Conventional Therapy

Nearly all oral cytotoxic chemotherapeutic agents are effective in lowering the white count early in chronic phase CML. Among the many agents tried, oral alkylating agents (busulfan) and antimetabolites (hydroxyurea, 6-thioguanine) have been most extensively used. In the last 30 years busulfan (Myeleran) has been the most popular agent for controlling the chronic phase: on the usual dose of 4 to 8 mg p.o. daily the white count drops exponentially, enabling the therapist to predict when to stop medication so that the delayed nadir does not fall below 10,000 cells/μl. Busulfan acts on managerial (multipotential) stem cells, explaining its slow but lingering effect and its propensity to induce multilineage marrow aplasia. A single course of busulfan usually reduces the leukemic cell mass by 1 to 2 logs, but the response to successive courses diminishes, requiring increasing drug dosage with attendant complications by side effects. Hydroxyurea, a ribonucleotide reductase inhibitor, is a cell cycle-specific inhibitor of DNA synthesis that acts on subordinate (committed) progenitor stem cells. The dose of hydroxyurea is 2 to 10 g orally daily and its "debulking" action is more rapid but shorter lived: the annoyance of daily therapy and closer monitoring is offset by the selective sparing of normal hematopoietic cells, and hydroxyurea is gaining on busulfan as frontline conventional therapy. On either chemotherapeutic regimen the marrow usually remains Ph-positive even during apparent remission; a few cases of Ph-negative remission have followed busulfan-induced aplasia, but even then the normal-appearing blood cells retain their clonal identity, affirming that Ph positivity is not the seminal event. Neither therapy is effective in controlling blast crisis.

Combination chemotherapy   Cyclic courses of intensive chemotherapy, involving combinations of four or more agents having different mechanisms by cytotoxicity, have improved the duration of remission and of survival by 1 to 2 years, but the quality of life during remission is often sullied by the ills of myelosuppression. Patients with significant Ph mosaicism may respond for longer periods because the nonclonal hematopoietic cells are favorably selected to proliferate [11]. None of the patients is cured by chemotherapy, for the malignant multipotential stem cells require ablation and can only be securely replaced by postablatory marrow transplantation.

The inability to conquer CML by chemother-apy, even when treatment is initiated early in the chronic phase is demonstrated by Figure 15-12 [12]. Although blood findings often resemble those of de novo acute leukemia, CML in blast crisis is the most refractory form of leukemia and has defied every imaginable combination of chemotherapeutic agents. Regardless of chemotherapeutic strategies employed, median survival from onset of therapy is under 3 months, and fewer than 10% survive 1 year.

Because of the failure of chemotherapy and the brutal invasiveness and limitations imposed by marrow transplantation, several biological response modifiers have been incorporated into combined modality protocols. Among the most promising are α and γ interferons. Recombinant IFNα causes complete clinical remission in 60 to 70% of cases of chronic phase CML, and half of responders show partial cytogenetic remission. Remissions are decidedly longer than with chemotherapy alone, but interferons offer no reprieve from eventual relapse and death from blast crisis (or from its treatment).

FIGURE 15-12

Actuarial survival curve of 1,445 patients with Ph-positive CML treated with chemotherapy. Death rate is low (10%) during the first 2 years, but increases to 25% per year thereafter, as indicated by the straight-line decline on the semilogarithmic plot. The gain over untreated historical controls is modest. (From Sokal JE et al: Staging and prognosis in chronic myelogenous leukemia. Semin Hematol 25:49,1988.)

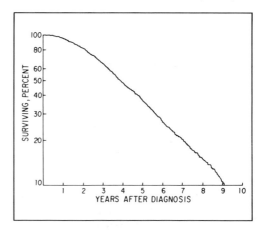

The inability of chemicals to tame blast crises and the ordained progression of all CML patients into blast crisis has forced recourse to the one means of eliminating the malignant multipotential clone: marrow ablation followed by transplant rescue.

Marrow Transplantion Offers the Only Hope of Curing CML

There is so little difference between the sensitivity of CML and normal stem cells that chemotherapeutic eradication of disease cannot be achieved without unacceptable damage to normal hematopoiesis. To cure the disease it is necessary to destroy all marrow elements—normal and malignant—with ablative doses of combined irradiation and chemotherapy followed by infusion of normal HLA-identical marrow; this ablate-and-rescue strategy is described in Chapter 14. Three sources of marrow have been utilized: autologous cryopreserved blood or marrow; syngeneic marrow from an identical twin; and HLA- and MLR-compatible marrow, preferably obtained from HLA-matched sibling donors. Virtually all cells from autologous marrow obtained during chronic phase or accelerated phase nonetheless are leukemic and Ph-positive. Thus the predictable result is that patients are merely returned to early chronic phase, and the marginal benefit achieved by this invasive meddling is to defer blast crisis.

With both syngeneic and allogeneic marrow transplants the objective is cure rather than palliation. In CML patients receiving marrow grafts from identical twin donors during chronic phase, nearly all achieve hematologic remission: one-third of these suffer leukemic relapse (despite putative marrow "ablation"), but the remainder sustain disease-free remissions that appear to represent permanent cures. Few patients transplanted while in blast crisis survive beyond 1 year.

Allogeneic transplants and catch-22   Nearly 1,000 CML patients have received transplants from HLA-identical siblings while in chronic phase, and overall 5-year remissions have been achieved in about 50% of patients. Successful engraftment and replacement of the Ph⁺ clone can be determined by immunologic, cytoge-

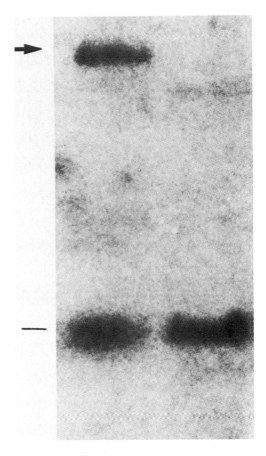

FIGURE 15-13

Southern blot analysis of *bcr* gene DNA in pre- and post-bone marrow transplant (BMT). Genomic DNA was digested with *Bam* HI and probed with a DNA probe for the *bcr* gene of chromosome 22. Pretransplant blood sample (left) shows both germline DNA (line) and the rearranged *bcr* fragment (arrow), but the posttransplant sample (right) shows only the unrearranged germline configuration (lower band). (From Miller WJ et al: Molecular genetic rearrangements distinguish pre- and post-bone marrow transplantation lymphoproliferative processes. Blood 70:882,1987.)

netic, or DNA analytic methods (Figure 15-13) [13]. Transplantation during chronic phase is associated with 20% mortality in the first 100 days and a 30% death rate within 1 year. The likelihood of disease-free engraftment thereafter is influenced by the ages of the patient and donor, and by the use or nonuse of preemptive purging of T cells to forestall graft-versus-host disease (GVHD). Best results are obtained in patients transplanted early in the chronic phase. Age of the patient (and consequently of sibling donors) is a major prognostic indicator; apparent cure is possible in nearly 70% of patients age 20 or younger, but in patients over 20 (the overwhelming majority), 5-year cure rates are under 50%. A graft-versus-leukemia effect mediated by T cells is instrumental in achieving cure, but this invites the intimidating problems of acute and chronic GVHD (Chapter 14). The catch-22 is that T cell depletion of donor marrow sufficient to prevent GVHD incurs a 30 to 40% risk of either leukemic relapse or failure to engraft [14, 15].

The need for universal donors The efficacy of marrow transplantation in CML is tightly restricted by limited availability of suitably matched sibling donors, the harsh prejudice of age in this age-dependent disease, and the Morton's fork of T cell purging and GVHD. Because observations in recent years indicated that HLA-matched, haplotype-matched, or HLA-near-matched marrow from unrelated donors can be used successfully in CML [16], a National Bone Marrow Donor Registry was established in the United States in 1987.

Representative results of allogeneic marrow transplantation and conventional chemotherapy of CML in chronic phase are compared in Figure 15-14 [17]. Proof that marrow transplantation can cure CML patients, provided they are not in acute transformation, has

prompted innovative approaches aimed at making transplants available to all patients presenting in chronic phase regardless of age, HLA identity, and family structure. Among creative prospects are conversion of autologous marrow to the Ph-negative state by IFNα and reinfusion of the marrow after treatment ex vivo with chemotherapeutic agents and selected cytokines.

IDIOPATHIC MYELOFIBROSIS

Idiopathic myelofibrosis (MF) is an uncommon chronic myeloproliferative disorder defined by five eclectic abnormalities: splenomegaly secondary to extramedullary hematopoiesis, leukoerythroblastic blood changes, teardrop-shaped red cells, megakaryocytic hyperplasia and atypia, and reticulin fibrosis of marrow. Isoenzyme and cytogenetic evidence indicates that the trilineage hematologic abnormalities reflect a neoplastic clonal disorder originating in a single pluripotential stem cell, but that marrow fibrosis represents a nonclonal fibrogenic reaction to products of the malignant clone, most notably to growth factors liberated from the dysplastic megakaryocytes. Observers who wish to emphasize the priority and impressive magnitude of extramedullary hematopoiesis employ the expression "myeloid metaplasia" (or the scholarly but ponderous term "agnogenic myeloid metaplasia"), in recognition that pronounced splenic hematopoiesis is not a physiologic process in people, even in response to extreme hypoxia. Those, including

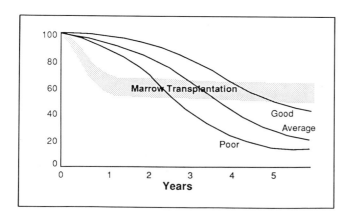

FIGURE 15-14

Survival results in CML treated with allogeneic marrow transplantation from HLA-matched donors versus standard chemotherapy (lines) in various prognostic groups. Results were brightened somewhat by selection of young patients for both therapies. (From Champlin RE et al: Bone marrow transplantation in chronic myelogenous leukemia. Semin Hematol 25:74,1988.)

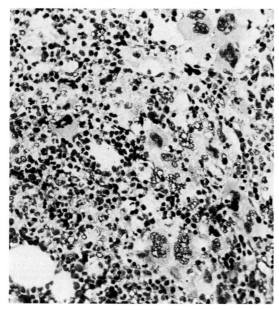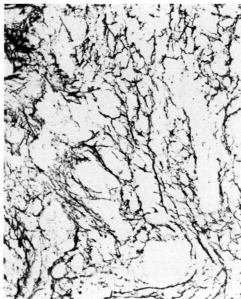

FIGURE 15-15

Marrow biopsy from a patient with myelofibrosis. (Left) Section stained with H & E displays hyperplastic clusters of megakaryocytes, many of which are dysplastic and multinucleated. (Right) The dense reticulin fibrosis in which hematopoietic cells are enmeshed is brought out by impregnating an adjacent section with silver for reticulin staining. The strands of reticulin fibrosis trap marrow cells, disturbing the marrow:blood barrier and foiling attempts at aspiration. (From Rappaport H: Tumors of the Hematopoietic System. Washington, DC, American Registry of Pathology. Armed Forces Institute of Pathology,1966.)

the author, who are more intrigued by the pathophysiologic role of megakaryocytic hyperplasia and dysplasia in engendering intramedullary fibrosis (and consequent eviction of hematopoietic elements) prefer the synechdochical brevity of the term "myelofibrosis."

Pathogenesis and Pathophysiology

Dysmegakaryocytopoiesis with overproduction of defective platelets is the most constant feature and occurs to a lesser extent in all chronic myeloproliferative disorders. Clusters of dysplastic megakaryocytes collect in vascular sinuses of marrow and spleen and gradually are imprisoned by a fibrotic webbing induced by their own sickly secretions (Figure 15-15) [18].

PDGF and the c-sis Oncogene

As the swarms of effete dysplastic megakaryocytes undergo death and dissolution within marrow sinus crypts, the fibroblast mitogen, platelet-derived growth factor (PDGF) is discharged into the parenchyma. PDGF is a 28,000 M_r transforming growth product of the c-sis oncogene located distally on the long arm of chromosome 22. PDGF released into the marrow environment binds to specific receptors on neighboring fibroblasts, thereby stimulating tyrosine phosphorylation, proliferation, and fibrogenesis. Normal enzymatic degradation of newly formed collagen is blocked by the simultaneous discharge from dying megakaryocytes of platelet factor 4, a cationic polypeptide of platelet α granules that inhibits collagenases of both neutrophils and fibroblasts. Normally the timely release by activated platelets of PDGF and platelet factor 4 is an essential step in wound healing, but when both factors continue to seep out from moribund megakaryocytes, the quantity of collagen and the ratio of

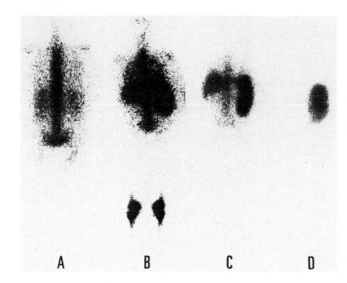

FIGURE 15-16

Distribution patterns of erythropoiesis in four patients with MF as determined by quantitative scanning after infusion of ^{52}Fe-labeled transferrin. (A) Normal medullary activity plus minor uptake in the spleen and liver. (B) Pronounced erythropoietic activity in the spleen and liver plus hematopoietic expansion into the long bones. (C) Most ^{52}Fe uptake is delimited to spleen and liver. (D) Erythropoiesis in this patient perseveres exclusively within the enlarged spleen. (From Ferrant A: Chapt 6, in Myelofibrosis. Pathophysiology and Clinical Management, SM Lewis, Ed. New York, Marcel Dekker, Inc.,1985. Reprinted by courtesy of Marcel Dekker Inc.)

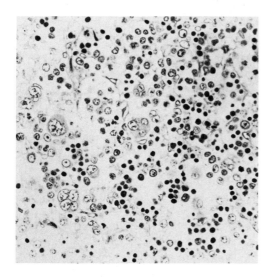

FIGURE 15-17

Trilineage hematopoiesis (myeloid metaplasia) in the removed spleen of a patient with MF. Note the abundant megakaryocytes—most of which are dysplastic multinuclear or mononuclear forms—and strong representation by megaloblastoid erythroblasts. Giemsa-stained section. (Courtesy DS Rosenthal.)

reticulin and fibronectin to collagen inexorably increases. This scarring distorts and disrupts the artfully designed exits of the marrow:blood barrier and permits escape into circulation of hematopoietic stem cells, which then lodge in the spleen and liver.

Myeloid Metaplasia

As clonal hematopoiesis in the marrow expands beyond the regions of reticulin fibrosis there may be patchy invasion of the long bones, but with time the marrow is impacted with stromal reticulin and variable amounts of collagen, and there is a progressive shift of hematopoiesis from marrow to spleen as can be visualized by ^{52}Fe scanning (Figure 15-16) [19].

Transplanted stem cells capable of self-replenishment flourish in the marrowlike sinuses of the spleen, and their burgeoning progeny may accumulate massively despite clonal infirmities, dysplastic features, and a high death rate. Splenic histology reveals trilineage hematopoiesis largely confined to the sinuses (Figure 15-17).

Pathogenesis of teardrop deformity   With time the clonal overgrowth in splenic sinuses spills into and distends the cordal compartments. This predicament traps and assures destruction of megakaryocytes but does not prevent emi-

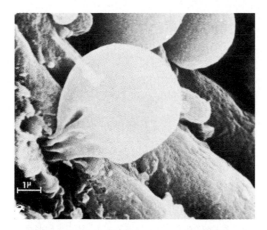

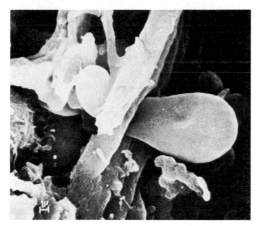

FIGURE 15-18

SEMs of red cells in the agonizing act of squeezing between interendothelial slits in the splenic cords (above) en route to a sinus. The cells are presumed to have been born in erythropoietic colonies located within cords; while tugging free into the venous sinuses (below) many acquire a tail, conferring the characteristic teardrop deformity. (From Leblond PF and Weed RI: The peripheral blood in polycythaemia vera and myelofibrosis. Clin Haematol 4:353,1975.)

gration of differentiated granulocytes or red cells. These limber forms can escape their cordal confines but only by slithering through slitlike apertures connecting cords to the outflowing sinuses (see Chapter 8). Lacking the compliance of normal red cells, the clonal cells of MF have difficulty negotiating this tight transmural passage, and while doing so their cytoskeletons are rearranged to form tailed,

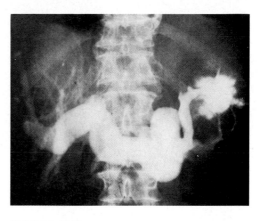

FIGURE 15-19

Splenoportagram demonstrating marked distension of the splenic and portal veins in an MF patient with massive splenomegaly and resultant increased portal blood flow. (From Geary CG: Chapt 2, in Myelofibrosis: Pathophysiology and Clinical Management, SM Lewis, Ed. New York, Marcel Dekker, Inc.,1985. Reprinted by courtesy of Marcel Dekker Inc.)

tapered, or teardrop conformations (Figure 15-18) [20].

Description

Clinical onset is insidious, patients presenting with symptoms and signs of anemia, weight loss, and left abdominal fulness with early satiety caused by encroachment of the enlarged spleen on gastric capacity. Splenomegaly develops in all patients, being marked in 50% and massive (weighing up to 7 kg) in about 10%. As a vascular adaptation to this hematopoietic tumor, splenic regional blood flow may exceed 10 times normal, overloading the capacity of the portal venous system and causing portal hypertension, bleeding varices, and ascites (Figure 15-19) [21]. Hematopoietic infiltration of the liver compresses the portal and hepatic venous return, aggravating portal hypertension and predisposing to mesenteric bleeding and thrombotic complications, including mesenteric artery thrombosis and Budd-Chiari syndrome. Bleeding and thromboses of systemic vessels are major causes of morbidity and mortality, arising in part from qualitative plate-

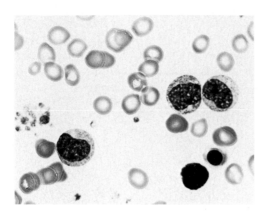

FIGURE 15-20

Blood morphology in myelofibrosis. Teardrop deformities of red cells (upper left) and leukoerythroblastic changes (anomalous presence of myelocytes, metamyelocytes, and a nucleated red cell) are the indicators of marrow infiltration. In this context, presence of a basophil (lower right) and of giant platelets implicates myelofibrosis as causing breakdown of the marrow:blood barrier. (Photo by CT Kapff.)

let defects. Osteosclerosis, often associated with bone pain, develops in about half of MF patients and may eventually obliterate the marrow cavity. The axial skeleton and proximal portions of long bones are most commonly affected, and x-ray films may reveal a "ground glass" appearance of involved bones due to merging of individual trabeculae. The finding of diffusely dense (but undeformed) bones and marked splenomegaly on routine radiologic examination is sufficient for a provisional diagnosis of MF.

Hematologic Findings

As MF progresses the combined morphologic consequences of infiltrative myelopathy and myeloid metaplasia emerge, revealing teardrop deformities, anomalous and premature release of nucleated red cells and early myeloid forms, and giant or bizarre platelets often accompanied by megakaryocyte fragments (Figure 15-20). Leukoerythroblastic changes and teardrop deformities are frequently associated with increased basophils, the insignia of chronic myeloproliferative disorders. In patients seen postsplenectomy, the

number of dysplastic erythroid, myeloid, and megakaryocytic elements in blood is magnified, but, as in thalassemia, the teardrop-shaped red cells lose their tails.

Blood counts in MF are nonuniform   Anemia is found in most patients at presentation and is of complex origin, representing the combined effects of dyserythropoiesis, shrinkage of the red cell mass, and hemodilution caused by expansion of the plasma volume. The neutrophil count is elevated in about half of patients but seldom exceeds 30,000 cells/μl, myelopoiesis being constrained by worsening dysmyelopoietic changes; as the result, neutrophil peroxidase activity and phagocytic function become impaired. In patients with markedly increased neutrophil turnover, excess leakage of cobalamin bound to transcobalamin I causes elevation of serum cobalamin levels as in CML, but unlike CML, LAP scores in MF neutrophils are normal or elevated in 85% of cases. Endstage MF often is associated with a pronounced shift toward myeloid immaturity, but only in about 5% of patients does MF terminate in flagrant AML.

Platelet levels are increased, often strikingly so, in about half of patients early in the disease, but with progression platelet counts decline, dysplastic forms emerge, and qualitative platelet defects predispose to excessive bleeding as well as to thrombotic complications.

Marrow fibrosis and "dry taps"   Attempts at marrow aspiration are frustrated in 90% of cases by reticulin fibrosis that locks in marrow contents—even in patients whose marrow is still hypercellular. Marrow biopsy is required for diagnosis: this usually reveals sheets of arid fibrosis, but medullary fibrosis often is patchy, and scanning of an adequate sample frequently reveals areas of marked hypercellularity, whether or not populated by the characteristic megakaryocytes described earlier [22].

Differential Diagnosis

In patients with myelofibrotic marrow the physician's foremost obligation is to exclude secondary forms of myelofibrosis, for these are managed by elimination of the underlying cause, whereas a diagnosis of primary (idiopathic) MF eventually mandates splenectomy, chemotherapy, or marrow transplantation. Nearly all forms of secondary myelofibrosis are caused by infiltrative disorders: metastatic carcinoma, lymphomas and leukemias, and disseminated tuberculosis. In secondary myelofibrosis the connective tissue reaction is ragged and marked by a high death rate among fibroblasts, whereas primary myelofibrosis, even when discontinuous, is well-knit and robust. Accordingly, fibrosis secondary to marrow infiltration is associated with increased excretion of hydroxyproline, whereas hydroxyprolinuria is not a feature of untreated primary MF.

CML, the spent phase of polycythemia vera, and essential thrombocythemia are the disorders most difficult to distinguish from MF.

These myeloproliferative processes have overlapping clinical and laboratory features, and occasionally patients present with findings so perplexingly intermediate that a generic diagnosis of chronic myeloproliferative disorder is the only taxonomic refuge. In the vast majority of cases, however, the characteristics listed in Table 15-1 suffice to segregate these four myeloproliferative syndromes [10].

Prognosis and Treatment

Predicting the natural history of MF can be difficult because of the impossibility of defining the starting time and because most patients present late in the course of the disease. Median survival after diagnosis is 5 years, but at least two subsets have been delineated having

TABLE 15-1

Differential characteristics of the chronic myeloproliferative syndromes

Observation	CML	Idiopathic myelofibrosis	Polycythemia vera	Essential thrombo-cythemia
Hemoglobin level	Usually ↓	Usually ↓	↑	Normal or ↓
White count/μl	Usually >50,000	Usually <30,000	Usually <25,000	Usually <25,000
Differential white count	Myelocytes and younger stages on presentation	Occasional immature myeloid cells of all stages	Moderate granulocytosis with shift to immaturity	Moderate granulocytosis
Basophilia > 1%	+	Usually +	±	±
Red cell morphology	Usually normal	Numerous teardrop poikilocytes	Normal to hypochromic, microcytic	Normal to hypochromic, microcytic
Nucleated red cells in blood	Common	Customary	Rare	Rare
Platelet count	Normal or ↑	Normal, ↑, or ↓	Normal or ↑	↑ ↑
LAP	↓ ↓	Usually ↑	Usually ↑	Normal
Bone marrow	Marked myeloid hyperplasia	"Dry tap," fibrosis	Hypercellular, ↓ iron stores	Hypercellular, ↑ ↑ mega-karyocytes
Special studies	Ph^1 chromosome	Marrow imaging	↑ RBC mass	———

Source: From Jandl JH: Chapt 22, in Blood: Textbook of Hematology. Boston, Little, Brown and Company, 1987.

2-year and 10-year mean survivorships, respectively. Favorable prognostic indicators are Hb concentrations above 10 g/dl and normal marrow cellularity, with or without patchy fibrosis. Negative indicators are Hb levels below 10 g/dl, marrow hypocellularity, megakaryocytic hyperplasia, and dense fibrosis and osteosclerosis. Some time may be bought with the combination of anabolic steroids and prednisone, but the responses are neither complete nor durable and are replete with side effects. MF is a capricious, often lingering disease that does not invite therapeutic audacity, but in selected patients medical or surgical intervention is inescapable.

Splenic Irradiation and Splenectomy

Splenic irradiation in daily fractions of 15 to 24 cGy is quite effective in palliating the distress and compressive problems of splenomegaly and in quelling splenic pain or tenderness. Improvement is usually temporary, and in patients dependent upon splenic hematopoiesis, radiodestruction of hematopoietic stem cells may worsen anemia and precipitate thrombocytopenia. Splenectomy is advisable in patients with massive splenomegaly, severe thrombocytopenia, unacceptably high transfusion requirements, or portal hypertension. Early postoperative mortality is high (about 10%) unless good risk patients are selected and amply supported by blood and platelet transfusion. Splenectomy does not extend survival but can improve the quality of life by eliminating problems created by the ponderous spleen (including the arteriovenous shunt effect on portal flow) and by raising blood counts. Regrettably, the manifestations used as criteria for selecting patients for splenectomy are identical to those forecasting excessive postoperative mortality.

Cytotoxic Chemotherapy

These fragile patients respond partially to judicious exhibition of single agent chemotherapy (busulfan, 6-thioguanine, or hydroxyurea), with reduction in spleen size, elevation of blood counts, and variable reversal of marrow and splenic fibrosis [23]. Results are unpredictable and impermanent, and the most valued role of chemotherapy in MF is for controlling hypermetabolic symptoms, hemostatic complications in patients with thrombocytosis, and

for invigorating patients deemed candidates for marrow transplantation.

Marrow Transplantation

Marrow transplantation following ablation of the malignant hematopoietic clone offers the only rational prospect for cure of MF, provided the grave risks entailed are justified by clinical, actuarial, and logistic considerations. As in CML associated with marrow fibrosis, transplantation of HLA-compatible marrow in selected patients is capable not only of eradicating malignant myeloproliferation but also leads to resolution of the accompanying myelofibrosis [24].

POLYCYTHEMIA VERA

Polycythemia vera (PV), or polycythemia rubra vera, is an insidious and insistent clonal disorder of pluripotential hematopoietic stem cells that is dominated clinically by senseless expansion of the red cell mass. Unlike polycythemias secondary to hypoxia, this "primary" polycythemia is characterized by trilineage hyperplasia involving granulocytes and platelets as well as red cells, and hence PV is a paradigmatic chronic myeloproliferative disorder. Evolution of PV occurs over many years, during which multitudinous malign complications of hypervolemia, hyperviscosity, thrombocythemia, and platelet dysfunction conspire to cause vascular accidents; ultimately the momentum of the hyperplasia may escalate into AML, or more often clonal exhaustion eventuates in a "spent phase" known as postpolycythemic myelofibrosis.

Pathophysiology

Increased production of red cells, granulocytes, and platelets in PV occurs in the absence of any recognizable extrinsic stimulus. Overproduction of all three cell lines is traceable by isozyme analysis to a mutation in a single pluripotential founder cell, and in some way this clonal derangement causes unceasing proliferation of subordinate unipotential stem cells. In normal marrow most pluripotential progenitors are quiescent, but in PV the majority of primitive hematopoietic stem cells are in a continuous state of cell cycling. PV cells of all involved lineages are equipped with at least three intracellular autocrine growth factors that collectively possess both mutagenic and transforming activity [25, 26]. In culture, normal CFU-Es stagnate without added erythropoietin (EP), but the CFU-Es of PV need little or no EP to prod them into dividing, conferring a competitive advantage. Overgrowth by erythroid members of the PV clone occurs because cell proliferation flourishes in the absence of hypoxia, is unsuppressed by hyperoxia, and is independent of the EP level. Autonomous proliferation of robotic PV erythroblasts generates sufficient red cells to suppress growth of normal EP-dependent cells through feedback inhibition and accounts for the competitive growth advantage of PV cells. This difference in EP dependence provides one diagnostic means (in cell culture) for distinguishing PV from the various secondary polycythemias. A more routine procedure for this differential diagnosis is radioimmunoassay for serum EP concentration: EP levels in PV (mean: 22 ± 7 mU/ml) are slightly below normal (30 ± 7 mU/ml), whereas serum EP in secondary polycythemia is elevated 2- to 3-fold.

Erythroid stem cell autonomy in PV is most faithfully represented by the vigorous feral growth of immature BFU-Es, which spread out from proximal marrow to colonize centrifugal stromal niches (free of hematosuppressive mononuclear cells) where their proliferative capacity is enhanced. This geographic appropriation sets the stage for morbid expansion of the red cell mass and the clinical sequelae.

Description

Most symptoms and signs of PV are the direct result of expansion or distension of the vasculature with voluminous, viscid, glutinous blood. Red cell mass increases to 2 to 4 times normal without an accompanying change in plasma volume. The vasculature accommodates the heavy burden of sluggish flow by generalized vasodilation, resulting in glowing rubor of the skin and mucous membranes, bloodshot eyes, and generalized ruddy plethora colorfully adorned by red splotches, intercurrent ecchymoses, and assorted skin eruptions encompassed by the term "acne rosacea." The high color of PV is not explained by the high hematocrit but by the volume of blood perfusing the skin. Attacks of maddening

pruritis, with severe burning pain, erythema, swelling, and warmth of the skin (erythromelalgia), are brought on by exposure to hot bath water; relief can be achieved by gentle cooling and administration of aspirin, and attacks can be prevented in some but not all cases by reducing the hematocrit. In occasional patients pruritis may obstinately persist despite venisections and the full catalog of dermal nostrums but may respond to photochemotherapy. The pathogenesis of this common, often infuriating complication is unclear: sluggish, intermittent blood flow may contribute, but there is evidence that perivascular dermal mast cells are overabundant in PV and leak prostaglandins and histamine when heated.

Circulatory disturbances of the CNS   Nearly half of PV patients present with headache, weakness, dizziness, visual disturbances, paresthesias, and various other problems attributable to hyperviscosity. Viscous retardation of cerebral and retinal blood flow predisposes to thromboses and hemorrhage, particularly in older patients. Transient ischemic attacks, cerebral infarction, and cerebral hemorrhage threaten all patients with uncontrolled PV but can be averted by phlebotomy plus isovolemic fluid replacement. The primary objective is not to improve O_2 carriage so much as to reduce the menace of viscous stagnation. The sluggish cerebral flow of PV may induce less dramatic neurologic changes, including fluctuating dementia and confusional states resulting from multiple small, deep cerebral infarctions [27] (Figure 15-21).

Other vascular misfortunes in PV   Peripheral venous thromboses, coronary thrombosis, and moderate hypertension are common products of viscous blood flow through increasingly noncompliant vasculature in older patients. Mesenteric thrombosis with ischemic infarction of the bowel and hepatic vein thrombosis eventuating in the Budd-Chiari syndrome are among the mortal hazards of PV in patients of all ages (Figure 15-22) [28].

Splenomegaly   Splenomegaly develops in over 90% of patients with PV and provides the simplest physical means for distinguishing PV from secondary polycythemias. Splenomegaly is not caused by extramedullary hematopoiesis

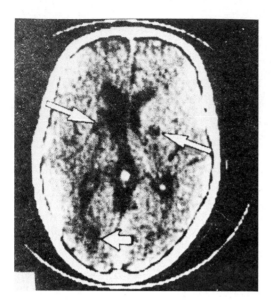

FIGURE 15-21

CT cerebral cut in a 66-year-old man with PV, showing lacunar infarcts (long arrows) in the right internal capsule and left caudate nucleus and an old occipital infarct (stubby arrow). (From Pearce JMS et al: Lacunar infarcts in polycythaemia with raised packed cell volumes. Br Med J 287:935,1983.)

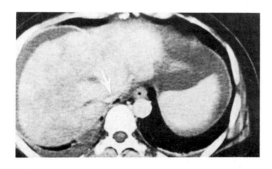

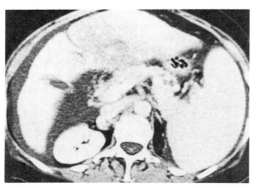

but by a marked expansion of the splenic red cell pool, an evident vascular accommodation to expansion of the red cell mass. In about 10% of patients splenomegaly becomes massive (with attendant risks of portal hypertension and bleeding varices) and signifies conversion from classic PV to postpolycythemic myelofibrosis.

Hematologic and Laboratory Findings

Red cell counts range from high normal to 10,000,000 cells/μl, and Hct levels are elevated proportionately. In flagrant plethora measurement of red cell mass is superfluous, but in borderline cases (Hct values below 55%) it is the final diagnostic arbiter. Initially red cells appear normal, but hypochromia and microcytosis are common in patients whose voracious expanding erythron has arrogated all available iron; iron-deficient changes are inevitable in patients who bleed extensively or who are managed by systematic phlebotomies. Leukocytosis with a moderate shift toward immaturity is customary, and basophil levels are increased in two-thirds of patients. Granulocytes in their plenitude release large amounts of the R-type cobalamin binding proteins, TC III and TC I, and neutrophils generally possess increased LAP activity. Thrombocytosis is usually moderate but can be profound and associated with platelet dysfunction and resultant thrombotic complications. The composite blood findings provide the basis for diagnostic criteria promulgated by a committee of PV mavens known as the Polycythemia Vera Study Group (Table 15-2) [29].

◀ **FIGURE 15-22**

CT scan (following iodinated contrast medium) of the upper abdomen in a 51-year-old woman with PV and Budd-Chiari syndrome. A section through the liver dome (top) fails to reveal a patent hepatic vein, and the inferior vena cava is narrowed to a slit (arrow). Ascites is evident. A lower section (below) shows an enlarged left hepatic lobe, a shrunken right lobe (which is drained by the caudate vein), and splenomegaly. (From Gollan JL et al: Progressive abdominal distention in a 51-year-old woman with polycythemia vera. Reprinted, by permission of The New England Journal of Medicine, 317:1587,1987.)

TABLE 15-2

Criteria for diagnosis of PV

Category A	Category B
A1 ↑ Red cell mass Male ≥ 36 ml/kg Female ≥32 ml/kg	B1 Thrombocytosis Platelet count >400,000/μl
A2 Normal arterial O_2 saturation ≥ 92%	B2 Leukocytosis >12,000/μl (No fever or infection)
A3 Splenomegaly	B3 ↑ Leukocyte alkaline phosphatase >100 ↑ Serum B_{12}(>900 pg/ml) or ↑ Unbound B_{12} binding capacity (>2,200 pg/ml)

Diagnosis acceptable if following combinations are present:
A1 + A2 + A3;
A1 + A2 + any two from category B

Source: Modified from Berk PD et al: Therapeutic recommendations in polycythemia vera based on Polycythemia Vera Study Group protocols. Semin Hematol 23:132,1986.

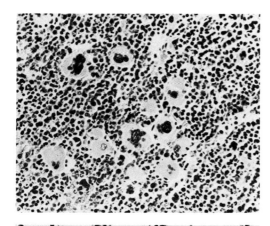
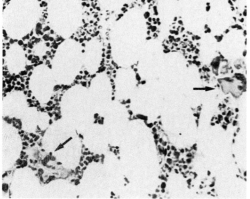

FIGURE 15-23

Marrow biopsies in two patients with untreated PV demonstrating cellularity ranging from 100% (above) to only 40% (below). Trilineage hyperplasia (above) is the rule, and megakaryocytes are numerous and prone to cluster (arrows). The abundant megakaryocytes are large but do not appear dysplastic. (From Ellis JT et al: Studies of the bone marrow in polycythemia vera and the evolution of myelofibrosis and second hematologic malignancies. Semin Hematol 23:144,1986.)

Marrow   It is no oversight that marrow findings are not included among diagnostic criteria for PV. Marrow hypercellularity and increased concentration of megakaryocytes are evident in 90% of cases, but cellularity can vary widely and there are no morphologic insignia unique to this disease. In the conventional "erythrocytotic" phase (i.e., prior to the delayed phase of "spent polycythemia") marrow shows trilineage hyperplasia and megakaryocytes are increased, voluminous, pleomorphic, and often clustered, but marrow cells do not display the striking atypia seen in MF and advanced stages of other myeloproliferative syndromes (Figure 15-23) [30].

Postpolycythemic myelofibrosis Postpolycythemic myelofibrosis—the spent phase of PV—occurs in about 15% of patients within 5 to 20 years of clinical onset, regardless of the therapeutic regimen employed. Postpolycythemic myelofibrosis is associated with splenomegaly, myeloid metaplasia, and leukoerythroblastic blood changes, making it indistinguishable from idiopathic MF.

AML in PV PV must be regarded as a clonal form of preleukemia, expression of which is markedly potentiated by alkylating agents or radiotherapy. The risk of AML (principally the M1, M2, M4, and M6 variants) developing in patients treated with chlorambucil is 14%, half the cases occurring within 5 years. In patients managed with ^{32}P the risk is almost as great (10%), but most cases occur between 6 and 10 years after initiation of therapy. The incidence of AML in patients treated with phlebotomy alone is considerably lower (1.5%) and largely confined to those with postpolycythemic myelofibrosis.

Diagnosis and Treatment

The finding of noncyanotic polycythemia in the context of trilineage hyperplasia and splenomegaly is virtually diagnostic of PV. In partially expressed or puzzling cases compli-cated by blood loss or other perturbations, an algorithmic diagnostic protocol is advised (Figure 15-24) [31].

Management

As the course of this disease is protracted and amenable to humane measures such as venisection, PV (unlike overt leukemia) is not a malignancy requiring heroic interventions such as marrow transplantation. The initial objective is to reduce the red cell mass by a condign regimen of phlebotomies until the Hct is brought to the low normal range. Patients presenting with hyperviscosity problems should be infused with plasma or dextran as phlebotomy is in progress. The selection of maintenance therapy once cytoreduction has been achieved must be guided by factors such as patient's age, activity, compliance, and phase of the disease of presentation. In patients with high phlebotomy requirements, each bleeding further excites hematopoiesis and increases production of dysfunctional,

FIGURE 15-24

Algorithm for evaluation of polycythemia. EPO = erythropoietin. (Modified from Erslev AJ and Caro J: Pure erythrocytosis classified according to erythropoietin titers. Am J Med 76:57,1984.)

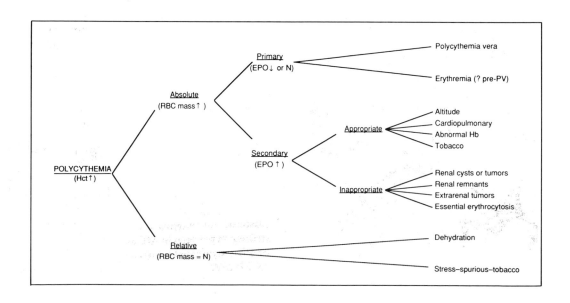

sticky platelets that account in part for the high hazard of thrombotic complications. In such patients the nonleukemogenic ribonucleotide reductase inhibitor, hydroxyurea, is effective in controlling PV following cytoreduction [32] and is especially effective in curbing platelet production.

ESSENTIAL THROMBOCYTHEMIA

Primary or essential thrombocythemia (ET) is an uncommon myeloproliferative disorder distinguished by pronounced thrombocytosis, phlegmatic progression, and episodes of thrombotic or bleeding problems. Most patients with ET have platelet counts between 1,000,000 and 3,000,000 cells/μl at diagnosis, but levels in excess of 10,000,000 have been reported.

Pathophysiology

Like polycythemia vera, with which it shares many features, ET is a proliferative disorder of pluripotential stem cells; the somewhat limited clonal family includes red cells, platelets, and granulocytes, but not monocytes or lymphocytes. Thrombokinetic studies have shown that in ET, platelet production and the total megakaryocyte mass are increased in tandem by up to 15-fold. The resultant surfeit of platelets remains a stable, symptomless anomaly early in the course, but with time the megakaryocytes become dysplastic and their teeming platelet progeny acquire numerous qualitative defects in membrane composition that may have opposing effects. The most salient flaws are deficiencies in α adrenergic receptors, loss of platelet coagulant activity, and various storage-pool lesions, which collectively account for episodic bleeding. Malfunctions antithetical to these include a reduction in platelet receptors for prostaglandin D_2 (PGD_2); by abrogating their response to PGD_2, this defect causes platelets to aggregate spontaneously and predisposes to serious, sometimes fatal, thromboembolic accidents.

As in PV, the overproduction of platelets in ET reflects unbridled proliferation of precursive megakaryocytes in the absence of colony stimulating factors. "Spontaneous" CFU-Meg colony formation takes place in semisolid media (and in some cases is associated with spontaneous erythroid colony growth) without requirement for serum growth factors, including EP, demonstrating independence of the ET clone from hormonal feedback regulation [33].

Description

The disease is manifest by an equal predilection for thrombotic and for bleeding problems that increase in frequency with age and as platelet counts rise above 1,000,000. Peripheral arteriolar occlusions are most common and cause ischemia, gangrene, acrocyanosis, and paresthesias of digits [34]. Of more concern are thromboses of major vessels including internal carotid, coronary, and renal arteries and hepatic and mesenteric veins. Painful postinfarction atrophy of the spleen occurs in 5 to 10% of patients, and silent infarcts may explain the relatively low incidence of splenomegaly (30%) in this proliferative disorder. Recurrent gastrointestinal bleeding and epistaxes afflict at least 50% of patients, and the clinical course is punctuated by episodes of spontaneous bleeding into skin or mucous membranes (Figure 15-25) [35].

Hematologic Findings

Platelet counts generally exceed 1,000,000 cells/μl, and the disorder may first be suspected by routine examination of the blood smear; in their abundance, platelets may form swarms and drifts (Figure 15-26) [10]. With disease progression giant platelets and megakaryocyte fragments enter the blood in increasing numbers. Chronic gastrointestinal or mucosal bleeding is responsible for the prevalent iron deficiency anemia in ET, and most patients have granulocytosis (median white count: 12,000; range: 6,000 to 40,000) as a variable reflection of the disturbed pluripotential stem cells.

Marrow cellularity is normal or moderately increased, but megakaryocyte proliferation is striking. During early evolution of ET, megakaryocytes, however numerous, appear normal or slightly enlarged. In more advanced ET, megakaryocytes tend to form sheets or clusters amidst windrows of platelets and some appear bizarre.

Leukemic transformation   Leukemic transformation occurs in less than 5% of patients, and

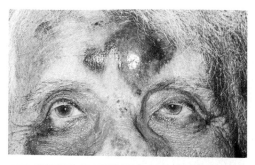

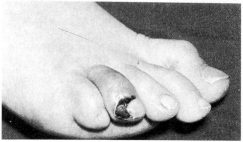

FIGURE 15-25

Antipodal misfortunes brought on by ET in a patient with a platelet count of 2,300,000. (Above) Spreading hemorrhages into soft tissues induced by trivial blunt trauma. (Below) Gangrene of left fourth toe. (From Hoffbrand AV and Pettit JE: Chapt 12, in Clinical Hematology Illustrated. An Integrated Text and Color Atlas. Philadelphia, WB Saunders Company,1987.)

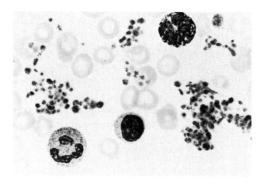

FIGURE 15-26

Swarms of platelets characteristic of thrombocythemia: most platelets are normal appearing, some are large, and one (upper right) qualifies as a giant form. Note the basophil—a myeloproliferative marker—and the hypochromic red cells, signifying iron deficiency from recurrent bleeding. (From Jandl JH: Chapt 22, in Blood: Textbook of Hematology. Boston, Little, Brown and Company,1987.)

most of these had been exposed to alkylator chemotherapy. There is, nonetheless, a modest excess of spontaneous transformation to AML, comparable to that in PV. A minority of patients with classic presentations of ET have been shown to have the Ph chromosome in their marrow karyotype; in Ph[+] patients the future is darker, for within several years most will experience precipitous transition to the accelerated phase of CML and die in blast crisis. Forewarning of this dire turn is provided by discovery of rising blood basophilia and of sheets or clumps of small atypical megakaryocytes in the marrow, both findings being signatures of CML [36].

Diagnosis and Therapy

Absent a specific diagnostic test for ET, the diagnosis is made by exclusion. The first and foremost issue is exclusion of thrombocytosis secondary to underlying disorders, many of which are correctable. The principal causes of secondary or "reactive" thrombocytosis are, in declining order of prevalence, solid tumors, iron deficiency, inflammatory or connective tissue diseases, myelodysplastic syndromes, and prior splenectomy (or splenic atrophy) in patients with unresponsive hemolytic anemia. If a platelet count in excess of 400,000 serves as the criterion, almost 40% of cases of thrombocytosis are secondary to malignant tumors, but counts seldom exceed 1,000,000 and then only in widely disseminated disease. Most patients with iron deficiency anemia have thrombocytosis, with counts commonly exceeding 600,000 and very occasionally reaching 2,000,000 cells/μl. A noteworthy feature of thrombocytosis secondary to iron deficiency is that platelet levels fall promptly during replenishment with oral iron. Unless there are added risk factors such as preexisting vascular disease, the various secondary thrombocytoses do not cause thromboembolic events, for the platelets, albeit numerous, are functionally well-behaved. Although myeloproliferative disorders account for only 5% of all cases of thrombocytosis (platelet counts exceeding 400,000), these disorders are responsible for the majority of patients in whom thrombocytosis persists above the 1,000,000 mark and is associated with "thrombohemorrhagic" complications. A set of criteria have been promulgated by the

TABLE 15-3

Criteria for diagnosis of essential
thrombocythemia

1. Platelet count $\geq$ 1,000,000/μl
2. Megakaryocytic hyperplasia in the
   bone marrow
3. Absence of identifiable cause of
   thrombocytosis
4. Absence of the Philadelphia chromosome
5. Normal red cell mass (male $\leq$ 36 ml/
   kg, female $\leq$ 32 ml/kg), or hemoglobin
   $\leq$ 13 g/dl
6. Presence of stainable bone marrow
   iron, or no more than 1 gm/dl increase
   in hemoglobin following 1 month of
   oral iron therapy
7. Absence of significant fibrosis (significant fibrosis defined as > ⅓ cross-
   sectional area of bone marrow biopsy)
8. No more than two of the following:
   (a) Mild fibrosis (defined as < ⅓ area
       of bone marrow biopsy)
   (b) Splenomegaly
   (c) Leukoerythroblastic reaction

Source: From Iland HJ et al: Differentiation between essential thrombocythemia and polycythemia
vera with marked thrombocytosis. Am J Hematol
25:191,1987.

PVSG for formulating algorithms useful in
differentiating ET from other myeloproliferative disorders associated with extreme thrombocytosis (Table 15-3). The most troublesome
differentiation is between ET and PV, and for
this specific purpose a logistic regression algorithm incorporating hematocrit, white count,
and spleen size has been espoused as being
92% accurate [37].

Management

Management of ET depends upon clinical
manifestations, stage of the disease, and age.
When extreme thrombocytosis is found in a
patient with hemorrhagic or thrombotic complications, immediate platelet pheresis can be
lifesaving; a 50% reduction in the number of
dysfunctional platelets can be achieved within
a few hours and generally this relieves symp-

toms, including many of those caused by
vasoocclusion. Marrow suppressive therapy is
begun concurrently, and the safest agent for
keeping platelet levels below 1,000,000 is
hydroxyurea. In patients plagued by thrombotic problems, even after cytoreduction, cau-
tious administration of antiaggregating agents
such as aspirin (500 mg on alternate days) is
effective; use of aspirin should be supervised,
however, for its unselective use in prophylaxis
introduces serious risk of precipitating bleeding. Agents that selectively suppress platelet
production (e.g., anagrelide) are under current
investigation.

REFERENCES

1. Kurzrock R et al: The molecular genetics of
   Philadelphia chromosome-positive leukemias. N Engl J Med 319:990,1988

2. Dreazen O et al: Molecular biology of chronic
   myelogenous leukemia. Semin Hematol 25:
   35,1988

3. Bernstein R: Cytogenetics of chronic myelogenous leukemia. Semin Hematol 25:20,
   1988

4. Kamada N and Uchino H: Chronologic sequence in appearance of clinical and laboratory findings characteristic of chronic myelocytic leukemia. Blood 51:843,1978

5. Hoffbrand AV and Pettit JE: Chapt 9, in
   Clinical Hematology Illustrated. An Inte-
   grated Text and Color Atlas. Philadelphia,
   WB Saunders Company,1987

6. Marmont AM et al: Chapt 4, in Atlas of
   Blood Cells: Function and Pathology, vol. 1,
   Zucker-Franklin D et al, Eds. Milan, Edi.
   Ermes s.r.l.,1988

7. Stainsby D et al: Papilloedema in chronic
   granulocytic leukaemia. Br J Haematol 55:
   243,1983

8. Spiers ASD: The clinical features of chronic
   granulocytic leukaemia. Clin Haematol 6:
   77,1977

9. Schmidt U et al: Electron-microscopic characterization of mixed granulated (hybridoid)
   leucocytes of chronic myeloid leukaemia. Br
   J Haematol 68:175,1988

10. Jandl JH: Chapt 22, in Blood: Textbook of
    Hematology. Boston, Little, Brown and Com-
    pany,1987

11. Talpaz M et al: Therapy of chronic myelogenous leukemia: chemotherapy and interferons. Semin Hematol 25:62,1988

12. Sokal JE et al: Staging and prognosis in chronic myelogenous leukemia. Semin Hematol 25:49,1988

13. Miller WJ et al: Molecular genetic rearrangements distinguish pre- and post-bone marrow transplantation lymphoproliferative processes. Blood 70:882,1987

14. Goldman JM et al: Bone marrow transplantation for chronic myelogenous leukemia in chronic phase. Ann Intern Med 108:806, 1988

15. Apperley JF et al: Bone marrow transplantation for chronic myeloid leukaemia in first chronic phase: importance of a graft-versus-leukaemia effect. Br J Haematol 69:239, 1988

16. Anasetti C et al: Effect of HLA compatibility on engraftment of bone marrow transplants in patients with leukemia or lymphoma. N Engl J Med 320:197,1989

17. Champlin RE et al: Bone marrow transplantation in chronic myelogenous leukemia. Semin Hematol 25:74,1988

18. Rappaport H: Tumors of the Hematopoietic System. Washington DC, American Registry of Pathology. Armed Forces Institute of Pathology,1966

19. Ferrant A: Chapt 6, in Myelofibrosis. Pathophysiology and Clinical Management, SM Lewis, Ed. New York, Marcel Dekker, Inc., 1985

20. Leblond PF and Weed RI: The peripheral blood in polycythaemia vera and myelofibrosis. Clin Haematol 4:353,1975

21. Geary CG: Chapt 2, in Myelofibrosis: Pathophysiology and Clinical Management, SM Lewis Ed. New York, Marcel Dekker, Inc., 1985

22. Wolf BC and Neiman RS: Myelofibrosis with myeloid metaplasia: pathophysiologic implications of the correlation between bone marrow changes and progression of splenomegaly. Blood 65:803,1985

23. Manoharan A et al: Ultrasonic characterization of splenic tissue in myelofibrosis: further evidence for reversal of fibrosis with chemotherapy. Eur J Haematol 40:149,1988

24. Dokal I et al: Allogeneic bone marrow transplantation for primary myelofibrosis. Br J Haematol 71:158,1989

25. Eid J et al: Intracellular growth factors in polycythemia vera and other myeloproliferative disorders. Proc Natl Acad Sci USA 84:532,1987

26. Cashman JD et al: Unregulated proliferation of primitive neoplastic progenitor cells in long-term polycythemia vera marrow cultures. J Clin Invest 81:87,1988

27. Pearce JMS et al: Lacunar infarcts in polycythaemia with raised packed cell volumes. Br Med J 287:935,1983

28. Gollan JL et al: Progressive abdominal distention in a 51-year-old woman with polycythemia vera. N Engl J Med 317:1587,1987

29. Berk PD et al: Therapeutic recommendations in polycythemia vera based on Polycythemia Vera Study Group Protocols. Semin Hematol 23:132,1988

30. Ellis JT et al: Studies of the bone marrow in polycythemia vera and the evolution of myelofibrosis and second hematologic malignancies. Semin Hematol 23:144,1986

31. Erslev AJ and Caro J: Pure erythrocytosis classified according to erythropoietin titers. Am J Med 76:57,1984

32. Kaplan ME et al: Long-term management of polycythemia vera with hydroxyurea: a progress report. Semin Hematol 23:167,1986

33. Juvonen E et al: Colony formation by megakaryocytic progenitors in essential thrombocythaemia. Br J Haematol 66:161,1987

34. Hehlmann R et al: Essential thrombocythemia. Clinical characteristics and course of 61 cases. Cancer 61:2487,1988

35. Hoffbrand AV and Pettit JE: Chapt 12, in Clinical Hematology Illustrated. An Integrated Text and Color Atlas. Philadelphia, WB Saunders Company,1987

36. Stoll DB et al: Clinical presentation and natural history of patients with essential thrombocythemia and the Philadelphia chromosome. Am J Hematol 27:77,1988

37. Iland HJ et al: Differentiation between essential thrombocythemia and polycythemia vera with marked thrombocytosis. Am J Hematol 25:191,1987

16

Acute Lymphatic Leukemia

□

Acute lymphatic leukemia (acute lympho-blastic leukemia; ALL) is a clonal malignancy usually arising in committed lymphopoietic stem cells of marrow. Malignant lymphoblasts initially remain and accumulate in marrow, but eventually variable numbers emerge and sometimes flood the bloodstream. About 20% of ALL cases are T cell leukemias (T-ALLs), and most of the remainder are neoplastic counterparts of normal pre B cells or their immediate antecedents (B-ALLs). The clonal abnormality does not usually involve the multipotential stem cell, but the frequency of ALL blasts possessing mixed lineage phenotypic markers indicates that in some cases origin of the founding mutation may be in the pluripotential lymphoid cell, and in some older patients coexistence of lymphoid and myeloid markers implicates multipotential cells. With a few exceptions (Chapter 13) the cause of ALL is unknown. High-level (> 100 cGy) total body irradiation, as in Japanese survivors of atomic bombing in 1945, increases the relative risk of ALL by over 25-fold, but there is no evidence that low-level irradiation is leukemogenic. Patients with inherited chromosome instability syndromes have a 100- to 200-fold relative risk of developing ALL, and the association of "null cell" ALL in infants with a 4;11 translocation involving a hereditary fragile site at band 11q23 suggests a possible genetic predisposition in this minor subset of ALL [1].

Incidence and Classification

ALL has a peak incidence between 2 and 6 years of age ("childhood ALL"), followed by a more gradual rise in frequency during adulthood. Childhood ALL is a disease restricted to clonal growth of unipotential lymphoid precursors and with the best therapy about 50% of this subset of ALL patients survive beyond 10 years and may be deemed cured. Older children, infants, and all adults have a less sunny outlook and more complex clonal lesions; longterm remission rates are highly age-dependent, ranging from 10 to 30% event-free survival at 7 years.

Morphologic Classification

Three morphologic subsets of ALL have been specified by French-American-British (FAB) criteria. In the L1 subtype, predominantly found in children 15 years of age or younger, lymphoblasts are uniformly small, nuclei are round to oval, and surrounded by a thin rim of deeply basophilic agranular cytoplasm. The L2 variant most commonly occurs in adults: lymphoblasts are heterogeneous but larger, cytoplasm is more abundant, and nucleoli are conspicuous. In the rare L3 (Burkitt's) variant, leukemic blasts are large, pleomorphic, and display numerous cytoplasmic vacuoles (Figure 16-1) [2].

Immunologic Classification

ALL can be subclassified into two principal categories based upon cell surface antigen profiles. About 75 to 80% of ALLs represent clonal expansion of B cell lymphoblasts arrested at various differentiation stages early in their maturation. In the most common stage of arrest ALL lymphoblasts express the HLA-DR (Ia) antigen, terminal deoxynucleotidyl transferase (TdT), the common ALL antigen (CALLA) or CD 10—a 100,000 M_r surface

glycoprotein having metalloendopeptidase activity [3] and expressed transiently during early differentiation, and the B cell lineage marker, B4 or CD 19. Hence the phenotypic profile of most B cell ALLs including L1 and L2 variants is Ia+, CD19+, CD10+, and TdT+ (Figure 16-2). A subset of ALL lymphoblasts (comprising about 10% of cases) are trapped so early in differentiation that they only express the HLA-DR antigen and are termed "null cells": most of these show ineffective H chain rearrangements (see Chapter 12 and below), but many also express T cell markers and appear to represent a block at the B:T branchpoint. Null cell ALL is predominant in infants and older adults [3].

T cell ALL accounts for about 20% of ALLs and results from a block in any of the consecutive thymocyte stages of T cell differentiation. Leukemic T cells are morphologically indistinguishable from those of common-type B cell

FIGURE 16-1

Three morphologic subsets of ALL. (Left) L1 subtype lymphoblasts are small, homogeneous, and have a high nuclear-cytoplasmic ratio, with indistinct nucleoli. (Middle) L2 lymphoblasts are more variable in size and shape, nuclear chromatin is coarser, and the one to three nucleoli are boldly outlined by chromatin. (Right) L3 blasts are bulky and vacuolated, and the nuclei are eccentric and often contain large dark nucleoli. (From Jandl JH: Chapt 23, in Blood: Textbook of Hematology. Boston, Little, Brown and Company,1987.)

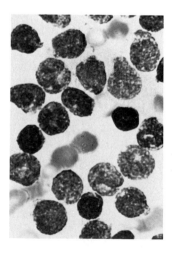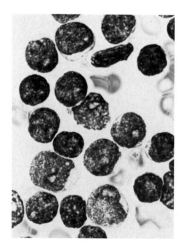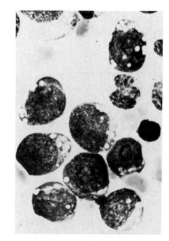

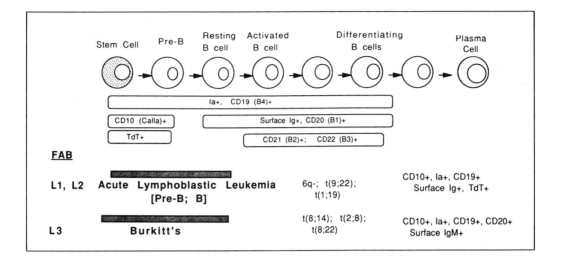

FIGURE 16-2

B cell ALL represents maturation arrest at various stages of early B cell differentiation. Common ALL is CD10+ and TdT+, but some more mature L2 variants and all L3 variants also display surface immunoglobulin and are CD20 (B1) positive. Note the association with certain recurrent chromosomal abnormalities. (Courtesy of BE Bierer.)

ALL, and those formed early in thymocyte differentiation are also TdT+. Primitive T-ALL lymphoblasts are distinctively marked by the early thymic antigen CD7 (Leu 9) and the pan-T marker CD2, and T-ALLs arising later in ontogeny acquire the emblems of cytotoxic/suppressor (CD8+) cells and helper/inducer (CD4+) cells (Figure 16-3).

FIGURE 16-3

T cell ALL represents maturation arrest at various stages of early T cell differentiation. The cell marker profile varies according to the stage at which mutation occurred. (Courtesy of BE Bierer.)

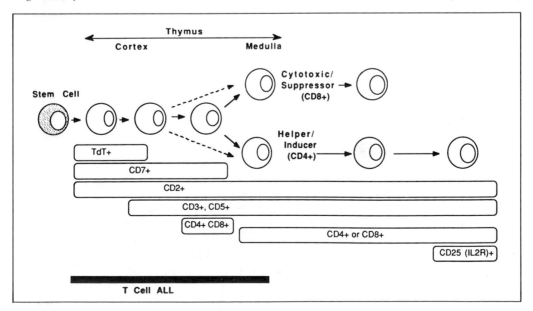

Pathophysiology

Lymphocyte progenitors are unique in undergoing diverse clonal rearrangements during ontogeny. This process is achieved by a complex sequence of recombination events, deletions, and somatic mutations to produce functional immunoglobulin genes and T cell antigen receptor (TcR) genes (Chapter 12). These rearrangements are facilitated by the presence in lymphoid precursors of TdT, which serves as a mutagen by random addition of nucleotides to DNA. Assembly of genes coding for receptors of both kinds (i.e., sIg and TcR) has a high failure rate, producing incomplete or faulty rearrangements and "sterile" transcripts that normally are proofread and eliminated by programmed thymic "suicide" genes. In ALL, the primitive leukemic cells execute incomplete or senseless gene rearrangements, implying that the surviving mutant clone is reprieved

from cell death by leukemic transformation [1] and acquires growth advantages. The high incidence of ALL during early life suggests that these rare immortalizing mutations represent mistakes in gene movement occurring as the immune system prepares to deal with the world of antigens. The upsurge in adulthood is unexplained but is characteristic of nearly all cancers.

In B Cell ALL, Ig Gene Rearrangements Are Frozen and Monoclonal

Normal B cell differentiation involves orderly acquisition of antigens linked by sequential, productive Ig gene rearrangements. B lymphoid stem cells with ineffectively arranged H chains are incapable of further maturation and the stalled rearrangement generates a malignant clone of null cells. Effective H chain gene

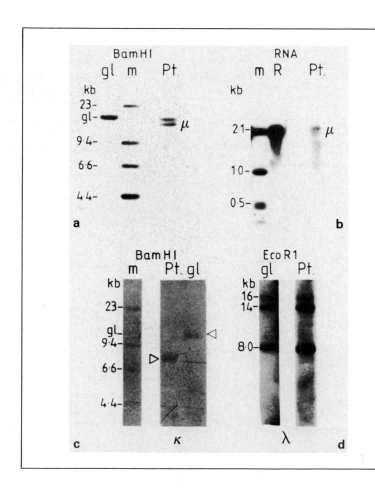

FIGURE 16-4

Southern blot restriction fragment analysis of DNA (a, c, and d) and northern blot analysis of mRNA (b) in a patient with CALLA+ ALL. Patient's cells have clonal rearrangements of μ gene (a) and κ chain (c) but not λ chain (d) genes. The μ chain clonal rearrangements are dimly reflected in the patient's RNA, and lymphoblast surface membranes (not shown) expressed CD10 and DR proteins, but not CD20. gl = germline position, m = molecular weight markers, Pt. = patient's leukemic cell DNA or RNA. (From Greaves MF et al: Differentiation-linked gene rearrangement and expression in acute lymphoblastic leukaemia. Clin Haematol 15:621, 1986.)

rearrangements, on the contrary, enable sequential induction of μ chain genes, and these in turn stimulate light chain genes to rearrange and code for κ chains. Ineffective κ chain rearrangement blocks consummation of light chain formation by aborting subsequent λ chain synthesis (Figure 16-4) [4]. If H chain gene rearrangements are productive and κ or λ genes are activated, the leukemic cells acquire a more mature gene phenotype, with surface Ig and CD21 markers (Figure 16-2); these leukemic cells have the morphology, phenotype, and vigorous growth characteristic of the uncommon L3 (Burkitt's) variant of ALL.

In T Cell ALL, Frozen TcR Rearrangements Evince Monoclonality

The T cell antigen receptors are heterodimeric molecules designated by their component peptides as $\alpha\beta$ and $\gamma\delta$ receptors, respectively (Chapter 12). In adults T cells bearing the $\gamma\delta$ TcR are in the minority, for δ chain rearrangement occurs early and transiently in ontogeny. In pre T ALLs that are TdT+ and CD7+ but CD4− and CD8−, no common karyotype or T cell gene rearrangement pattern can be defined, and this variant of null cell ALL appears to represent malignancy of pluripotential stem cells [5]. Most T cell ALLs (and most T cell neoplasms) do express monoclonal T cell lineage gene rearrangements that are most flagrantly expressed by T_β chains. The size of the Eco RI fragment bearing the $C_\beta 1$ gene (10.5 kb in germline cells) is altered by virtually all rearrangements or deletions affecting TcR V, D, or J genes. All patients with leukemic

lymphocytes analogous to stage I and II thymocytes (CD7+, CD4+, and CD8+) show T_β gene rearrangements (Figure 16-5).

Crosslineage rearrangement of Ig and TcR genes   Nice distinctions between B and T cell ALL, and even the issue of clonality, are muddied by the disquieting discovery that clonal rearrangements of Ig heavy chain and TcR chain genes are not restricted exclusively to leukemias of B and T cell lineage, respectively. Rearrangement of TcR_β and TcR_γ genes occur in about 10% of B cell ALL, and Ig H chain rearrangements are found in an equivalent proportion of T cell ALL. DNA probe analysis of the J_α region of the TcR_α gene have demonstrated an even greater degree of lineage infidelity in B cell ALL [6]. It is possible that enzymes such as TdT that move Ig genes around may incidentally rearrange TcR genes in leukemic B cells. Most "inappropriate" rearrangements are incomplete (e.g., DJ rearrangement only) or are either sterile or very nearly unproductive. Productive rearrangements of TcR genes and Ig heavy plus light chains are lineage specific, but these quantitative considerations caution that composite phenotypy and gene analyses are both necessary for assigning lineage membership.

Cytogenetics in ALL: Favorable and Unfavorable Prognostic Indicators

High-resolution banding techniques have revealed clonal chromosomal abnormalities in over 90% of patients. Collectively three recur-

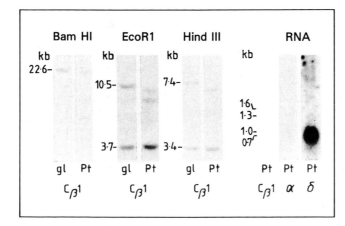

FIGURE 16-5

Molecular phenotypes of T cell precursor (early thymic cell) ALL. *Eco* RI restriction fragment analysis (midleft) uncovers two rearranged TcR ($C_\beta 1$) genes, and by northern blot TcR β and T3 δ but not TcR α messages are expressed. These ALL blasts exhibited CD7 and CD2 but not CD3 surface antigens. gl = germline position, Pt = patient. (From Greaves MF et al: Differentiation-linked gene rearrangement and expression in acute lymphoblastic leukaemia. Clin Haematol 15:621, 1986.)

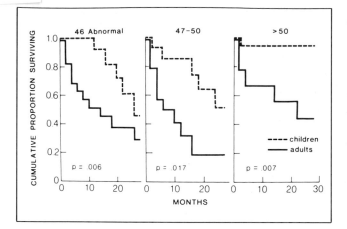

FIGURE 16-6

Comparison of survival of children and adults with ALL within karyotype groups based on modal number. (From Bloomfield CD et al: Chromosomal abnormalities and their clinical significance in acute lymphoblastic leukemia. Third International Workshop on Chromosomes in Leukemia. Cancer Res 43:868,1983.)

ring types of reciprocal translocations have been reported in about one-third of adult and one-fifth of childhood cases: t(9;22), t(4;11), and t(8;14). Patients with these chromosomal defects have a median survival of under 12 months as compared with the prospect of longterm remission or even cure in about half of patients without these translocations. In contrast, infants with the 6q− deletion and children with the 1;19 translocation respond better, although not permanently, to chemotherapy. About 30% of children and 8% of adults are hyperdiploid (modal number: 47 to 60 chromosomes) as determined both by cytogenetic and flow cytometric studies. Hyperdiploidy with more than 50 chromosomes is a strongly favorable prognostic indicator in children with B cell ALL (Figure 16-6) [7].

DESCRIPTION

Unheralded by preleukemic phenomena, leukemic spread is usually covert and diffuse, eliciting minimal tumoral signs even when marrow replacement has led to serious problems stemming from anemia, neutropenia, and thrombocytopenia. Skeletal pain and tenderness of the spine, hips, or sternum are common reflections of forceful infiltration of the marrow cavity by lymphoblasts. Presenting complaints almost always include fatigue, malaise, and fever, and ailing infants are touchy and irascible. Painless lymphadenopathy and splenomegaly are preva-

lent but seldom flagrant features. About 30% of patients present with painful bones and joints, and in children point tenderness may signify focal periosteal elevation (Figure 16-7) [8]. Patients with T cell ALL—a disease characterized by rapid progression, male predominance, and high numbers of circulating lymphoblasts—commonly present with infiltrative masses of the thymus or mediastinal nodes that may compromise the airway. (Figure 16-8).

Extramedullary ALL and Leukemic Sanctuaries

Two organs, the CNS and testes, offer asylum to leukemic cells: by providing protective barriers against chemotherapeutic agents these locations serve as secure sanctuaries for leukemic refugees and are major founts of relapse following systemic chemotherapy. CNS leukemia originates from small pockets of malignant blasts that survive by concealment behind the blood:brain barrier. From this privileged haven lymphoblasts eventually burst through the pia-glial membrane and congregate in subjacent CNS parenchyma or spill into the spinal fluid to cause "meningeal leukemia." Postremission CNS leukemia is a harbinger of systemic relapse, and CNS prophylaxis is a mandatory component of management.

Hematologic Findings

Anemia and reticulocytopenia are present in most patients at diagnosis, and in those

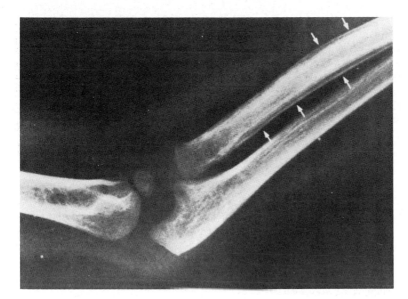

FIGURE 16-7

Subperiosteal new bone formation (arrows) encasing the radial shaft of a child with ALL. Periosteal elevation is caused by leukemic infiltrates that strip periosteum from the underlying bone. (From Clausen N et al: Skeletal scintigraphy and radiography at onset of acute lymphocytic leukemia in children. Med Pediatr Oncol 11:291, 1983.)

with marrow infiltration leukoerythroblastic changes with teardrop deformities may be found. Platelet counts are usually low at first presentation, often dangerously so.

If childhood and adult cases of ALL are combined, about 40% of patients present with white counts below 10,000 cells/μl, a comparable percentage have counts between 10,000 and 50,000, and an ill-starred 20% have counts in excess of 50,000. Because of the busy traffic between lymphoid organs and the bloodstream, white counts (principally reflecting lymphoblast numbers) usually correlate with the total tumor volume, but in many instances most of the blasts remain stuck in the marrow throughout the early course of disease. Tumor progression and prognosis are profoundly influenced by two factors: age and

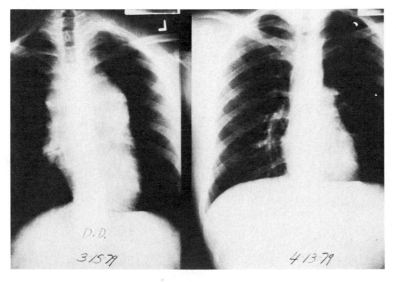

FIGURE 16-8

Chest radiographs showing bulky mediastinal and thymic involvement by T cell ALL before (left) and after (right) chemotherapy. Displacement of the mediastinum to the right and tightening encirclement of both main bronchi by tumor cells threatened to throttle this 17-year-old male, but the tumor masses melted away beginning within a few days of therapy. (Courtesy A. Skarin.)

white count at diagnosis. Older patients are predisposed to rapid progression, high white counts, organomegaly, nodal involvement, T cell disease, and mediastinal masses. Younger patients, particularly those with CALLA$^+$ blasts, have lower white counts and the pace of the disease is slower and much more amenable to cytotoxic therapy.

Cytochemical Profile

The cytochemical profile is useful not only for distinguishing lymphoid from myeloid leukemias (Table 14-2) but also aids in differentiating B cell and T cell ALL. The most helpful cytochemical markers for profiling ALL blasts are the PAS reaction, acid phosphatase, and antibodies to TdT, CALLA, HLA-DR (Ia), and surface or cytoplasmic immunoglobulins. ALL blasts characteristically display heavy granular or chunky red or pink aggregates on PAS staining, representing deposition of glycogen. Antibodies to TdT stain the nuclei of leukemic blasts of nearly all ALL sorts, including null cell ALL. Staining for the CALL antigen is diagnostic of the common early precursor B-ALL most prevalent in childhood (Figure 16-2). These three cytochemical talismans are displayed in Figure 16-9 [9, 10]. The prevalent CALLA$^+$ subset can be distinguished from the more mature pre B ALL variant by testing for cytoplasmic μ chains: CALLA$^+$ blasts lack cytoplasmic μ chains and IgM; pre B ALL is μ-chain positive; and the most mature (L3) variant displays surface Ig and is sIg$^+$. Absence of HLA-DR is a key feature for distinguishing T-

ALL from B-ALL, and the "T-ness" of ALL lymphoblasts with convoluted nuclei can be ascertained by demonstrating strong focal or unipolar concentrations of acid phosphatase (Figure 16-10) [10].

Marrow Biopsy Is the Key to Diagnosis

White counts may or may not be elevated, and leukemic blasts may be overlooked in the differential count—particularly if performed by machine. Marrow aspirate or biopsy invariably discloses rampant overgrowth by sheets of closely packed blasts displaying L1 or L2 (and rarely, L3) morphology of the sort portrayed in Figure 16-11.

FIGURE 16-9

A pastiche of ALL blasts identified by cytochemical stains. (Left) PAS reaction for glycogen shows coarse (red) granular deposits. (Middle) Immunofluorescent staining for TdT in blast nuclei is characteristic of all variants of ALL but occurs rarely in undifferentiated AML. (Right) Immunoperoxidase staining for the cell surface glycoprotein, CALLA, is characteristic of common-type childhood ALL. (From Greaves MF et al: Chapt 9, in Atlas of Blood Cells: Function and Pathology, vol. 1, Zucker-Franklin D et al, Eds. Milan, Edi. Ermes s.r.l.,1988; and Kass L and Elias JM: Cytochemistry and immunocytochemistry in bone marrow examination: contemporary techniques for the diagnosis of acute leukemia and myelodysplastic syndromes. A combined approach. Hematol Oncol Clin North Am 2:537,1988.)

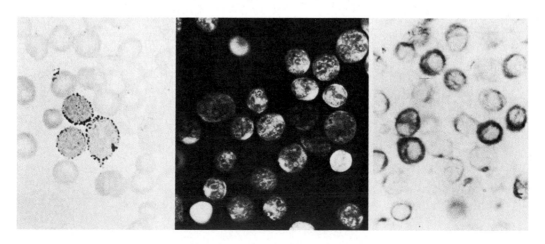

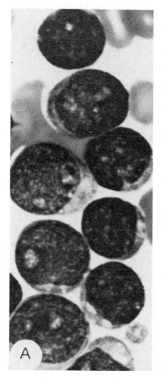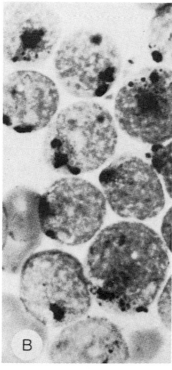

FIGURE 16-10

(A) Leukemic T cell blasts, some of which possess cleaved or convoluted nuclei and nucleoli boldly marginated by nucleoprotein (Wright-Giemsa). (B) Acid phosphatase reaction reveals intense unipolar localization in the Golgi system. Local paranuclear concentrations of acid phosphatase are characteristic of all T cell–derived malignancies including T cell lymphomas. (From Kass L and Elias JM: Cytochemistry and immunocytochemistry in bone marrow examination: contemporary techniques for the diagnosis of acute leukemia and myelodysplastic syndromes. A combined approach. Hematol Oncol Clin North Am 2:537,1988.)

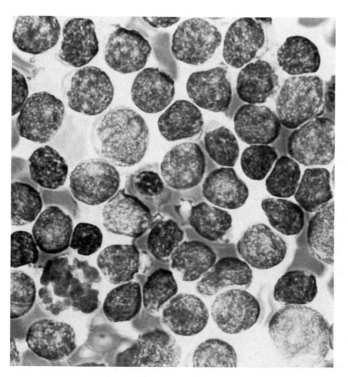

FIGURE 16-11

Replacement of marrow by lymphoblasts in an adult with ALL. The numerous large blast forms with plentiful cytoplasm and irregular nuclei having one or two prominent nucleoli are typical of the L2 subset of ALL, but many smaller blasts are evident having little cytoplasm and inconspicuous nucleoli (L1 morphology). By FAB criteria the presence in marrow of more than 25% large nucleolated lymphoblasts identifies this as the L2 variant of ALL. Except for a token two erythroblasts, the marrow is overrun by the leukemic cells. Wright-Giemsa–stained aspirates. (Photo by CT Kapff.)

MANAGEMENT

ALL treatment is divided into three parts. These are: remission induction and maintenance with combination chemotherapy, CNS prophylaxis, and marrow transplantation.

Combination Chemotherapy

The objective of induction therapy is to destroy as many leukemic cells as quickly as possible. Unlike the blasts of AML, those in ALL are selectively responsive to several agents (prednisone, vincristine, asparaginase, and antifolates), and thus longterm remissions are commonly achieved in ALL uncomplicated by the perils of generalized marrow hypoplasia. Treatment regimens are complex and multicyclic, and vary from one prognostic group to another and from one treatment center to another. Basically most regimens consist of an initial induction phase beginning with vincristine, prednisone, an anthracycline (in adults), and L-asparaginase, followed by a second cycle of the same combination plus cyclophosphamide. The recipes for consolidation, early and late intensification, and maintenance regimens are beyond the scope of this book, but an essential component of therapy is prophylaxis designed to obviate leukemic infiltration of the CNS and to destroy leukemic sanctuaries protected by the blood:brain barrier. The two modes of prophylaxis, and (if necessary) CNS therapy, are intrathecal methotrexate with intravenous

Leukovorin rescue and craniospinal irradiation, sometimes given together as "combined modality" measures. Although prophylaxis reduces the incidence of CNS leukemia, it has surprisingly little survival advantage and brings with it numerous sinister side effects in the form of arachnoiditis, leukoencephalopathy, myelopathy, and more ominously (particularly in older regimens used for children), a high incidence of subclinical cognitive malfunctions, learning disabilities, and even cortical thinning.

Remission Rates Are Governed by Age, Leukemic Cell Count, Phenotype, and Karyotype

Complete continuous remission rates in adults do not approach the level achieved in childhood ALL. In patients 16 years of age or younger, 10-year disease-free survival has been reported in 40 to 50% of patients given intensive combination chemotherapy. In patients over 16 years of age, overall survival is only 20%, with cure rates declining steeply above age 50. Hence evaluation of published success rates requires inclusion of the age structure of treatment groups. Among other factors adversely affecting survival are white counts above 30,000 cells/μl (counts below 15,000 granting a particularly favorable prognosis) and dislodgement of normal marrow by lymphoblasts. Adults with CALLA$^+$ lymphoblasts fare better than patients with null cell

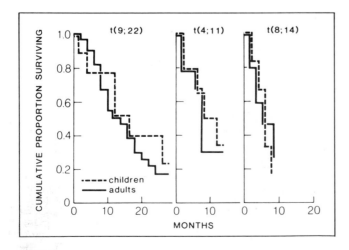

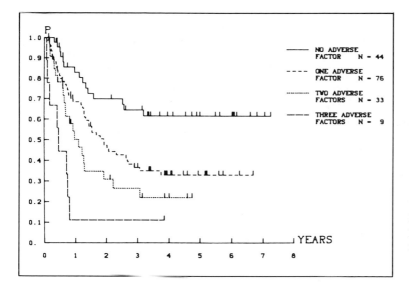

FIGURE 16-13

Probability of continuous clinical remission for patients having 0, 1, 2, or 3 adverse prognostic factors. Data was gathered in a prospective multicenter study of 368 ALL patients aged 15 to 65 years treated with intensified induction and reinduction chemotherapy. (From Hoelzer D et al: Prognostic factors in a multicenter study for treatment of acute lymphoblastic leukemia in adults. Blood 71: 123,1988.)

leukemia; recently it has been learned that the notorious T cell subset of adult ALL responds surprisingly well to aggressive chemotherapy, with longterm survivorships in excess of 50%. In older patients, blast cells in as many as one-third of ALLs express myeloid as well as lymphoid surface antigens; these biphenotypic cells signify a lesion at the senior stem cell level, heralding a poor prognosis and accounting in part for the melancholy impact of age. Prognosis is poorest in patients of any age with the following pseudodiploid translocations: t(9;22), t(4;11), and t(8;14) (Figure 16-12). Adverse factors such as age, mixed phenotype, and malign chromosomal translocations are additive in their impact, as illustrated in Figure 16-13 [11].

Marrow Transplantation

Children with conventional CALLA+ ALL and standard risk factors have a selectively good prognosis with chemotherapy and should not be considered for marrow transplantation while in first remission, and it is uncertain whether or not "favorable" cases of adult ALL are candidates for this therapy with all of the immediate and delayed dangers and debilitations of ablation and rescue strategems (Chapter 14). In patients of any age with refractory leukemia, those who relapse while receiving maintenance chemotherapy, and those in high-risk categories (WBC > 50,000; age > 35 years; unfavorable chromosome abnormalities), marrow transplantation is the last and best resort. About 4,000 transplants have been performed for patients with high-risk ALL, with results superior to those receiving intensive combination chemotherapy [12]. At first most transplants were from HLA-identical sibling donors and subject to the statistical limitations of availability, the high (>60%) actuarial rate of leukemic relapse in advanced disease, plus all the attendant horrors of graft-versus-host disease (GVHD). This has led to a drift toward use of autotransplants harvested and cryopreserved during chemotherapy-induced complete remission. The predictable proclivity of autotransplants to relapse can be countered by exorcizing the autotransplant ex vivo by addition of a cocktail of complement-fixing monoclonal antibodies such as anti-CALLA or ricin-armed antibodies to leukemia-associated antigens. Unequivocally the quality of life in patients rescued from marrow ablation with autologous marrow—with or without cytotoxic antibody-purging—is superior to that in patients receiving GVHD-prone allogeneic transplants and is preferable to the brutal complications of "salvage chemotherapy" (Figure 16-14) [13]. Autotransplantation shows promise in management of adult ALL, but a

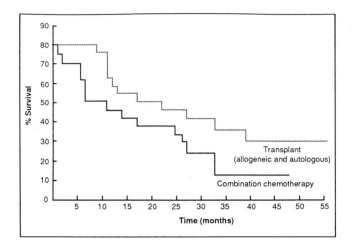

FIGURE 16-14

Actuarial relapse-free survival for high-risk adults receiving marrow transplants versus those treated with chemotherapy. Patients rescued with autologous marrow survived no better than those given allogeneic marrow, but the quality of life was much better. Note that in both groups 20% of patients failed to enter remission. (Modified from Proctor SJ et al: A comparative study of combination chemotherapy versus marrow transplant in first remission in adult acute lymphoblastic leukaemia. Br J Haematol 69:35, 1988.)

longterm success rate of only 20 to 30% underscores the need for further research.

REFERENCES

1. Greaves MF and Chan LC: Is spontaneous mutation the major 'cause' of childhood acute lymphoblastic leukaemia? Br J Haematol 64:1,1986

2. Jandl JH: Blood: Textbook of Hematology. Boston, Little, Brown and Company,1987

3. LeBien TW and McCormack RT: The common acute lymphoblastic leukemia antigen (CD10)—emancipation from a functional enigma. Blood 73:625,1989

4. Greaves MF et al: Differentiation-linked gene rearrangement and expression in acute lymphoblastic leukaemia. Clin Haematol 15:621,1986

5. Kurtzberg J et al: CD7+, CD4−, CD8− acute leukemia: a syndrome of malignant pluripotent lymphohematopoietic cells. Blood 73:381,1989

6. Hara J et al: Relationship between rearrangement and transcription of the T-cell receptor α, β, and γ genes in B-precursor acute lymphoblastic leukemia. Blood 73:500,1989

7. Bloomfield CD et al: Chromosomal abnormalities and their clinical significance in acute lymphoblastic leukemia. Third International Workshop on Chromosomes in Leukemia. Cancer Res 43:868,1983

8. Clausen N et al: Skeletal scintigraphy and radiography at onset of acute lymphocytic leukemia in children. Med Pediatr Oncol 11:291,1983

9. Greaves MF et al: Chapt 9, in Atlas of Blood Cells: Function and Pathology, vol. 1, Zucker-Franklin D et al, Eds. Milan, Edi. Ermes s.r.l.,1988

10. Kass L and Elias JM: Cytochemistry and immunocytochemistry in bone marrow examination: contemporary techniques for the diagnosis of acute leukemia and myelodysplastic syndromes. A combined approach. Hematol Oncol Clin North Am 2:537,1988

11. Hoelzer D et al: Prognostic factors in a multicenter study for treatment of acute lymphoblastic leukemia in adults. Blood 71:123,1988

12. Champlin R and Gale RP: Bone marrow transplantation for acute leukemia: recent advances and comparison with alternative therapies. Semin Hematol 24:55,1987

13. Proctor SJ et al: A comparative study of combination chemotherapy versus marrow transplant in first remission in adult acute lymphoblastic leukaemia. Br J Haematol 69:35,1988

17

Chronic Lymphatic Leukemia and Related Leukemias

☐

C hronic lymphatic leukemia (CLL), prolymphocytic leukemia (PLL), and hairy
cell leukemia (HCL) are acquired clonal
lymphoproliferative disorders, usually of B
cell lineage. The proportional incidence of
these three nonacute lymphatic leukemias is
approximately as follows: CLL, 80%; PLL,
10%; and HCL, 10%. Worldwide, CLL is the
most common form of chronic leukemia, accounting for 25 to 30% of all leukemias
encountered in white populations; the very
low incidence of CLL in Asians (10% as
great) is unexplained but is clearly genetic, for
the difference remains generations after emigration to non-Asian venues.

CHRONIC LYMPHATIC LEUKEMIA

Chronic lymphatic leukemia (chronic lymphocytic leukemia, CLL) is a languid lymphoproliferative disorder of late adulthood involving
slow but inexorable propagation of immense
numbers of small, uniform, immunologically
indolent lymphocytes. The disease is characterized by lymphadenopathy, hepatosplenomegaly, and relentless amassment of lymphocytes
in blood and tissues, with eventual choking off
of marrow function that paves the way for neutropenia and thrombocytopenia—and hence
infection and bleeding. The logarithmic link
between age and predisposition to CLL is very
likely the reduction in immune competence
associated with aging, a decline aggravated by
the disease itself.

Pathophysiology

The most convincing markers that certify CLL
as a monoclonal neoplasm exist in the variable
(V) domains of the Ig molecule and the rearranged gene segments that encode them.
During differentiation of pre B cells, genes of

heavy (H) and then light (L) chain V regions undergo sequential rearrangements, which endow their B cell progeny with distinctive V_H and V_L immunoglobulin regions that serve as antigen receptors. Consequently a clone of malignant B cells has a characteristic rearrangement pattern of H and L chain genes that are evident on Southern blot analysis, as well as unique idiotypic (Id) determinants in the V_H and V_L domains of immunoglobulins that can be identified by anti-idiotypic antibodies. These two approaches to clonal analysis of B cell neoplasms complement each other.

Ig Gene Analysis Revisited

To reprise Ig gene movements in early B cells (Chapter 12), recall that joining of heavy chain DJ gene occurs first and that VDJ assembly follows as a discrete event. As J_H is adjacent to the constant region C_μ, the intermediate prod-

uct (VDJ-C_μ) is able to produce only μ chains; in most cases of CLL, rearrangements are frozen at this level, abrogating the third (class switch) rearrangement. The preliminary VDJ rearrangements and joinings often misfire for reasons stipulated in Chapter 12, and as the result a cell containing one or more rearranged genes may not produce any Ig chain. Normally at each Ig locus there are two allelic genes on the homologous chromosomes, only one of which can be productive; this law of "allelic exclusion" prevents synthesis of hybrid antibody molecules having different specificity on each of the two Fab halves. Neoplastic monoclonal B cell populations may disobey exclusionary laws and can have at each Ig locus either one or both alleles rearranged.

Monoclonality by Southern blot analysis CLL cells of B lineage have surface B cell specific

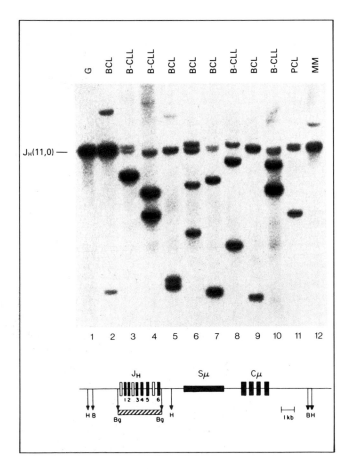

FIGURE 17-1

Southern blot analysis (above) showing immunoglobulin gene rearrangements in 11 patients with B cell neoplasms. DNA from blood cells was digested with *Bam* HI (B) and *Hind* III (H), electrophoresed, blotted, and then analyzed with a 3.2 kb *Bgl* II (Bg) DNA probe specific for the J_H band found in cells in the normal germline (G) configuration. In all patients with B-CLL, B cell lymphoma (BCL), plasma cell lymphoma (PCL), and multiple myeloma (MM), out-of-line clonal gene rearrangements are found. In most cases two rearranged bands are observed that represent alleles which have undergone one productive and one unproductive rearrangement. (Below) Restriction enzyme map of a 16.5 kb region spanning the human germline J_H-C_μ region. S_μ = heavy chain class switch exon. (From Greaves MF et al: Chapt 9, in Atlas of Blood Cells: Function and Pathology, vol. 1, Zucker-Franklin D et al, Eds. Milan, Edi. Ermes s.r.l., 1988; and Bertoli LF et al: Analysis with antiidiotype antibody of a patient with chronic lymphocytic leukemia and a large cell lymphoma (Richter's syndrome). Blood 70:45,1987.)

antigens detectable by monoclonal antibodies to class II HLA (Ia) antigens, B cell lineage antigens CD19, CD20, and CD21, and surface membrane immunoglobulins (sIg) (Figure 16-2). Unlike normal immature B cells, which boldly display surface IgM (and then both IgM and IgD) before losing sIg during matriculation to plasma cells, CLL B cells demonstrate very low-density sIg and impaired capping capability, signifying a weakened cytoskeletal structure. The monoclonality of sIg in B cell leukemias can be ascertained by demonstrating clonal immunoglobulin gene rearrangements by Southern blot analysis of affected cells (Figure 17-1) [1, 2].

Monoclonality by light chain analysis   B cell neoplasms that express only κ or λ chains are monoclonal by definition, and κ/λ analysis of cellular or of secreted immunoglobulins is commonly used as a determinant of monoclonality and by inference of malignancy. In B-CLL cases in which cells express membrane κ chains, no rearrangement of λ chains is observed, proving that neoplastic κ rearrangements are unproductive. Sole expression of λ chains in CLL indicates that genes encoding κ chains were abortively bypassed or deleted.

Clonal analysis with anti-idiotype antibody   Restriction enzyme analysis by Southern blot technology registers the DNA profile of whole populations of cells, and will include both clonal and nonclonal contributions. A direct means of identifying individual cell members of a neoplastic clone is accomplished by immunofluorescent monoclonal antibodies made against an idiotypic determinant of sIg molecules (Figure 17-2) [2].

B-CLL Cells Are Arrested at an Intermediate State of B Cell Maturation

In addition to displaying either μ (or μ plus δ) heavy chains on their surface, B-CLL lymphocytes also possess receptors for mouse red blood cells (mrbc+)—a marker for B cell immaturity—and for the Fc fragment of IgG (FcγR) and the C3bi receptor (CR3, CD11). They also carry HLA-DR (Ia) antigens, several B lineage antigens (B1 and B4) and express the T cell–associated 67,000 M_r CD5 antigens found on mature B cells. Moreover B-CLL cells are variably responsive to B cell mitogens, cytoplasmic Ig is often demonstrable by immunofluorescence staining, and secretion of small amounts of monoclonal Ig occurs in nearly 50% of patients, signifying the approach of terminal differentiation. Occasionally Ig crystals can be found in the cytoplasm of CLL cells by electron microscopy. Altogether these findings, a discordant mix indicating both maturity and immaturity, suggest either that the leukemic event traps cells guilty of unbalanced maturation or, less likely, that B-CLL is derived from a unique subset of normal B cells, possibly corresponding to those at the outer rim of lymph follicles.

FIGURE 17-2

Virtually all the lymphocytes in the blood of this 71-year-old woman with CLL glowed in the dark when exposed to fluorescein-labeled anti-idiotypic antibodies specific for the leukemic cell line sIg. The minority of nonclonal B cells present are not visualized. (From Bertoli LF et al: Analysis with antiidiotype antibody of a patient with chronic lymphocytic leukemia and a large cell lymphoma (Richter's syndrome). Blood 70:45,1987.)

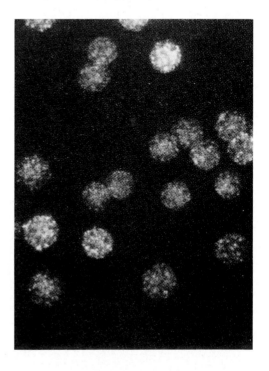

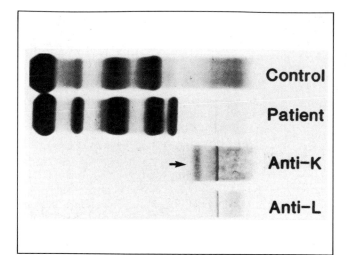

FIGURE 17-3

Hypogammaglobulinemia and free κ chains in the serum of a patient with CLL. On high-resolution agarose gel electrophoresis, normal (control) serum shows a broad polyclonal pattern, whereas the patient's serum is nearly bereft of tetrameric immunoglobulins. Immunofixation analysis of undiluted serum from the patient reveals a homogeneous monoclonal band (arrow) staining with anti-K (anti-κ) but not with anti-L (anti-λ). (From Deegan MG et al: High incidence of monoclonal proteins in the serum and urine of chronic lymphocytic leukemia patients. Blood 64:1207,1984.)

Hypogammaglobulinemia and Unbalanced Immunoglobulin Synthesis

Hypogammaglobulinemia develops early in about half of CLL patients. B-CLL cells have the curious property of secreting free light chains, usually κ chains, as their major Ig product, a biosynthetic imbalance due in large part to absence of the secretory mRNA required for heavy chain export. This disparity eventuates in a characteristic pattern on serum electrophoresis of a sharp monoclonal κ chain peak set off against a barren background in the Ig region (Figure 17-3) [3].

Surplus light chain secretion is a constitutive feature of neoplastic B cells regardless of phenotype, whereas the amount of cytoplasmic or surface immunoglobulin on CLL lymphocytes correlates directly with the level of phenotypic maturation achieved. In some patients with an early B cell phenotype, crystalline inclusions composed of monotypic light chains (usually λ chains) cause obstipation of RER-lined secretory channels (Figure 7-4) [4]. Ordinarily, as noted, CLL lymphocytes are incapable of secreting tetrameric immunoglobulins for lack of secretory mRNA. In CLL populations with unusually mature phenotype and plasmacytoid morphology, however, the cells secrete a fully assembled immunoglobulin, creating a prominent monoclonal Ig peak that contrasts sharply with the broad depressed plain of polyclonal immunoglobulins.

Most clinical manifestations of dysproteinemia stem from the shortage of normal polyclonal immunoglobulins (i.e., hypogammaglobulinemia), with the resultant failure of humoral immunity. Hypogammaglobulinemia, the nemesis of CLL patients, has an exaggerated negative impact on resistance to infection, for the nonclonal T cells have blunted or absent mitogenic and mixed lymphocyte responses and their T4:T8 ratios are inverted and decline further with advancement of the disease. Immunodeficiency problems are worsened by the native propensity of NK cells to downregulate B cell proliferations; affronted by the intrusion of myriads of "foreign" leukemic lymphocytes, patients' nonclonal NK cells fulfill their xenophobic role too well and (despite the best intentions) cause further reduction in polyclonal immunoglobulin synthesis [5].

Chromosome Abnormalities

Chromosome abnormalities are evident in about half of CLL patients. The most common is trisomy 12, an ominous prognostic indicator that warrants unusually early intervention with antileukemia therapy. The most frequent structural abnormality is 14q⁺, which

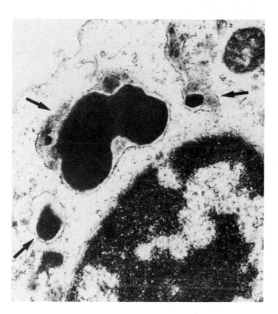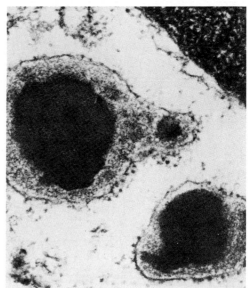

FIGURE 17-4

Ultrastructure of cytoplasmic inclusions of CLL lymphocytes. (Left) Most inclusions are compact, rounded or crystalloid masses (arrows) composed of monotypic λ chains, indicating a stage-specific defect in secretory function. (Right) Close-up reveals a two-layer enveloping membrane. (From Feliu E et al: Cytoplasmic inclusions in lymphocytes of chronic lymphocytic leukaemia. Scand J Haematol 31:510,1983. © 1983 Munksgaard International Publishers Ltd., Copenhagen, Denmark.)

often evolves late in the course of CLL and frequently foreshadows transformation to prolymphocytic leukemia. Chromosome 14 contains two or more regions that direct lymphocyte production. The notorious Burkitt's band, 14q32, contains rearranging Ig H chain genes, and translocations involving 14q32 similar to those found in Burkitt's and follicular lymphomas occur in about 10% of CLL cases (see Chapter 13). The unique combination of breakpoints leading to the t(11;14)(q13;q32) rearrangement found in many cases of CLL has been cloned, revealing that a DNA segment translocated from chromosome 11 contains a novel oncogene named bcl-1 that is rearranged when annealed to the J segment of the rearrang-

ing H chain loci. Since an immunoglobulin enhancer element is located between the J_H and switch regions of the μ gene, it has been proposed that the enhancer activates transcription of the juxtaposed bcl-1 gene, causing elaboration of B cell growth factors. As with most chromosomal rearrangements in neoplasia, the finding of unnatural encounters between unstable enhancers and oncogenes or other growth genes breeds expansive interpretations offering regrettably few specific conclusions.

Cytokinetics

The comparatively indolent course of CLL reflects the lengthened lifespan of the inert leukemia cells and the very low fractional production rate as determined by ^{3}H-thymidine incorporation. As a result of these factors, the tumor mass doubling time (Td) is vastly prolonged—in most cases exceeding 12 months. In over half of CLL patients lymphocyte doubling time is astonishingly protracted (mean: 67 ± 19 months), and patient survival probability in those patients without treatment rivals that of age-matched control populations. In the 44% of patients with Td values below 12 months (mean: 10 ± 2 months), average survival (despite antileukemia ther-

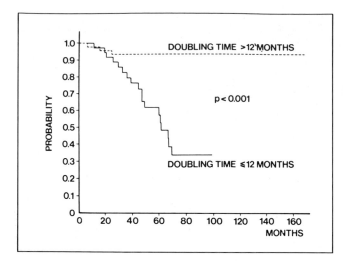

FIGURE 17-5

Survival probability in CLL as a function of lymphocyte doubling time. The total population of 100 patients includes all prognostic stages and treatment groups. (From Montserrat E et al: Lymphocyte doubling time in chronic lympho-cytic leukaemia: analysis of its prognostic significance. Br J Haematol 62:567,1986.)

apy) is only 5 years (Figure 17-5) [6]. Despite the languid cytokinetics of CLL, the obstinate constancy with which the expanded stem cell clone overproduces lymphocytes—as the result of prodding by a self-generated B cell growth factor—leads to massive numbers of circulating cells, with clogging of lymphoidal space and overflow into extravascular sites.

Description

The earliest clinical manifestations of CLL are fatigue and reduced exercise tolerance, which worsen in parallel with the rising lymphocytosis. Within a few years of the first sense of enervation, painless but growing lymphadenopathy becomes notable, involving (in order of frequency) cervical, axillary, bronchial, mesenteric, retroperitoneal, and inguinal regions. With nodal distention by crowds of small lymphocytes, adenopathy may impinge on strategic structures, sometimes causing upper respiratory or bronchial obstruction and parenchymal infiltration of the lungs, skin, central nervous system, and gastrointestinal tract. Nodal masses in the iliac or periaortic region may obstruct venous or lymphatic channels, and in advanced disease leukemic cells may penetrate the nodal capsules and compress or girdle vascular structures (Figure 17-6) [7]. Splenic enlargement occurs early in over 90% of patients, and with disease progression the spleen may extend deeply into the pelvis, becoming

frangible and prone to rupture, sometimes as a consequence of overzealous palpation. Splenic engrossment is commonly accompanied by extensive infiltration and enlargement of the liver, but severe liver functional impairment is uncommon.

Opportunistic Infections and Malignancies

At this writing CLL is second only to the HIV-induced AIDS syndrome as a cause of acquired immunodeficiency. In addition to predisposing to infection (the principal cause of death in CLL), this slow-paced leukemia and the attendant lapse in immunity subject the patients to a remarkably high risk of secondary, more impetuous malignancies. Most frequent are solid tumors of the colon or skin, but other B cell neoplasms such as multiple myeloma and B cell lymphomas occur at least 10 times more often in CLL than predicted by fortuitous association. One form of secondary neoplasm occurs with sufficient regularity in advanced CLL (10% of cases) as to be considered an evolutionary endphase of the disease, analogous to blast transformation: this malign metamorphosis is known as Richter's syndrome or Richter's transformation.

Richter's Syndrome

Richter's syndrome represents a built-in propensity of advanced stage CLL to transform to a poorly differentiated large cell lymphoma

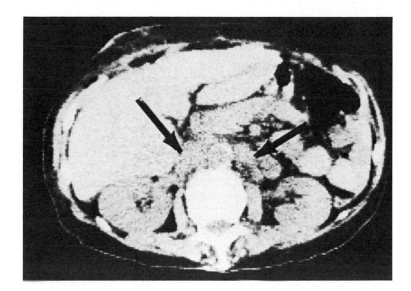

FIGURE 17-6

CT scan of the upper abdomen of a CLL patient with bilaterally enlarged coalescing periaortic lymph nodes (arrows) that have girdled the inferior vena cava, causing lymphedema below the obstruction. (From Gunz FW and Henderson ES: Chapt 11, in Leukemia, 4th ed, Gunz FW and Henderson ES, Eds. New York, Grune & Stratton, Inc.,1983.)

that originates in leukemic lymph nodes and rapidly spreads to neighboring organs. This atavistic transition begins with clonal evolution of "immature foci" of leukemic cells; these form focal aggregates of large round or angulated lymphoid cells that bear a bold sIg$^+$ B cell phenotype distinct from that of the antecedent CLL cells. These highly proliferative, fulminant "secondary clones" quickly coalesce into bulky tumor masses that occupy retroperitoneal nodes, marrow, liver, and (in-

variably) the spleen (Figure 17-7) [8]. Richter's transformation appears to be a preordained and dolorous epilogue to the leukemogenic event causing CLL. It is remarkably refractory to intensive chemotherapy.

Hematologic Findings

In normal persons, blood lymphocyte counts do not exceed 4,000 cells/μl, and a provisional diagnosis of CLL should be made in anyone

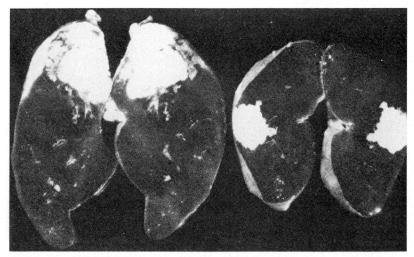

FIGURE 17-7

Sectioned surfaces of the spleen of a 63-year-old woman with a 15-year history of CLL and recent onset of abdominal pain. The prominent, pale, well-defined tumor masses represent large B cell lymphoma having some immunoblastic features. (From Kruskall MS and Harris NL. N Engl J Med 309: 297,1983. Reprinted by permission of The New England Journal of Medicine.)

with sustained levels in excess of 5,000. Most CLL patients present with lymphocytosis exceeding 10,000, and counts may mount gradually thereafter to as high as 1,000,000 cells/μl. CLL lymphocytes appear nearly normal but are slightly large and may burst during preparation of blood films, signifying their skeletal frailty (Figure 17-8). In patients with slow-paced disease, leukemic lymphocytes appear quite homogeneous both on blood smears and by electron microscopy (Figure 17-9) [9]. In more aggressive forms of CLL, lymphocytes may be pleomorphic (large, or small and bereft of cytoplasm) or may contain deeply cloven or cracked nuclei suggestive of follicular cell origin (Figure 17-10).

Anemia, Neutropenia, and Thrombocytopenia

Roughly half of CLL patients are anemic at presentation, and with preemption of marrow space by leukemic lymphocytes, precursors of neutrophils and platelets are gradually dislodged. Thrombocytopenia usually signifies irreversible marrow replacement, but in patients

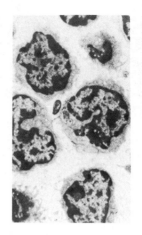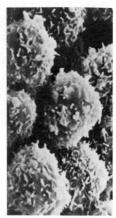

FIGURE 17-9

Ultrastructure of CLL lymphocytes as viewed by TEM (left) and SEM (right). By TEM the cells display slightly more pleomorphism than is evident on stained smears, and many nuclei are indented by nuclear fissures not obvious on spread smears. The cytoplasmic microvilli and lacey ruffles visible on SEM are characteristic of B cells. (From Sweet DL Jr et al: Chronic lymphocytic leukaemia and its relationship to other lymphoproliferative disorders. Clin Haematol 6:141,1977.)

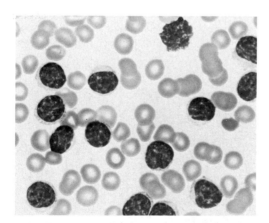

FIGURE 17-8

Blood lymphocyte morphology in patient with CLL and a white count of over 200,000 cells/μl. Most lymphocytes are slightly large and several have vacuolated cytoplasm, but otherwise they appear normal. The presence of several broken "smudge cells" is sufficiently suggestive of leukemia to warrant inclusion in the differential report. (Photo by CT Kapff.)

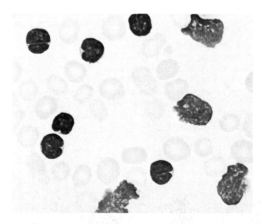

FIGURE 17-10

Numerous small lymphocytes with variously cleft nuclei and sparse cytoplasm in a patient with advancing CLL. The fevered imaginations of hematologists have generated many descriptive words for the nuclear cleavage: cracked, slotted, coffee bean, and buttock pattern are among them. Note the numerous smudge cells. (Photo by CT Kapff.)

with unusually large spleens, thrombocytopenic purpura of moderate severity may represent excessive platelet pooling, a compartmental shift that may be remedied by splenic
irradiation (Figure 17-11) [10]. Neutropenia is
seldom severe in CLL until terminal progression with extinction of all marrow elements.

Pure red cell aplasia in B-CLL   CLL patients are
vulnerable to self-limited but dangerous episodes of pure red cell aplasia that last 3 to 9
months, coming unannounced and without
obvious provocation or relationship to stage or
therapy. Some observations indicate that the
erythrosuppression is caused by T suppressor
cell prodding of NK cells, which switch off
BFU-E and CFU-E proliferation in a manner
analogous to indirect NK suppression of
polyclonal Ig synthesis. Among other mechanisms implicated in this curious complication
of B-CLL are IgG autoantibodies to EP and
erythroblast membranes, and intercurrent opportunistic infections by parvovirus and other
low-profile organisms that prey on immunosuppressed individuals.

*Autoimmune hemolytic anemia: a strange inter-
lude*   The course of B-CLL is punctuated by
an assortment of autoimmune events, among
which autoimmune hemolytic anemia is the
most obvious. Hemolysis is unpredictable in
onset, severity, and duration and is nearly
always mediated by warm-active IgG autoantibodies of low avidity and unknown objective.
CLL is the commonest pathologic process predisposing to Coombs-positive hemolytic anemia, a complication both capricious and potentially serious. Hemolytic anemia is managed in
the same manner as other immunohemolytic
anemias (Chapter 8) until the process vanishes
as mysteriously as it commenced.

Marrow Findings

Lymphocytic infiltration of marrow is a constant feature of CLL patients with blood lymphocyte levels exceeding 10,000 cells/μl and is
mainly a confirmatory finding. Normal marrow elements are crowded or displaced by
legions of lymphocytes, many of which appear
quite normal; others are too large and may
display a single prominent nucleolus (Figure
17-12). Early in CLL, leukemic lymphocytes

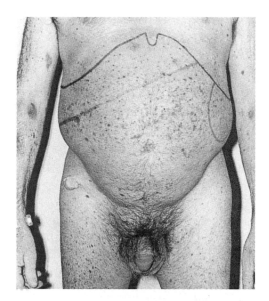

FIGURE 17-11

Thrombocytopenic purpura and abdominal distension in a 54-year-old man with CLL, a white
count of 250,000, and a platelet level of 35,000
cells/μl. The enlarged spleen and liver are outlined with ink. (From Hoffbrand AV and Pettit
JE: Chapt 9, in Clinical Hematology Illustrated.
An Integrated Text and Color Atlas. Philadelphia, WB Saunders Company,1987.)

FIGURE 17-12

Marrow aspirate from a patient with advanced
CLL, showing inundation by myriads of benign-
looking, but slightly large, lymphocytes, several
of which have one or more nucleoli. In this field
the only remnant of normal hematopoiesis is a
solitary young neutrophil at bottom-right.
(Photo by CT Kapff.)

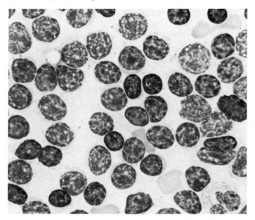

gather in nodular patterns, simulating well-differentiated lymphocytic lymphoma, but as infiltration advances, invasion of marrow space becomes increasingly widespread and diffuse, hematopoietic stem cells are displaced, and deepening pancytopenia forecasts hematopoietic extinction.

T Cell CLL

A minority of CLL cases (<5%) are chronic T cell neoplasms that are subdivisible into two heterogeneous groups.

T4-CLL

CLL of lymphocytes possessing the CD4 phenotype and helper-inducer behavior usually presents with moderately advanced disease, marked lymphocytosis (range: 30,000–70,000 cells/μl), gross adenopathy, extensive cutaneous involvement, a diffuse pattern of marrow infiltration, and a predilection for CNS invasion. Leukemic cells are small and mature, the nucleus is irregular, often convoluted, and scantily clothed with cytoplasm. Unlike B-CLL lymphocytes, T4-CLL cells display brazen focal acid phosphatase activity, receptors for mouse red cells, and do not undergo clonal Ig gene rearrangements. As with all T cell malignancies, Southern blot analyses of TcR α, β, γ, and δ chain genes reveal clonal rearrangements. Median survival of T-CLL patients treated with chemotherapy alone is between 1 and 2 years. Sporadic T-CLL must be differentiated from endemic adult T cell leukemia caused by HTLV-I (Chapter 13).

T8-CLL (Large Granular Lymphocyte Leukemia)

The term "large granular lymphocyte leukemia" (LGL leukemia) is used to encompass at least two phenotypic sorts of proliferation of large granular lymphocytes that cause a syndrome of neutropenia, recurrent infections, splenomegaly, and rheumatoid arthritis. The disease begins with relatively low white counts, progression is usually gradual and halting, and the cells have NK morphology (Figure 17-13) [11]. On the basis of immune phenotyping, LGL leukemias have been sorted into two discrete subsets: type A, having a CD2+, CD3+, CD8+ profile; and type B, dis-

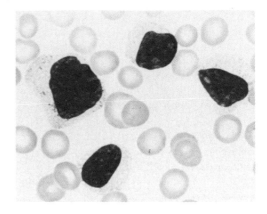

FIGURE 17-13

Blood lymphocytes in a 65-year-old patient with LGL leukemia display NK morphology. The cells have abundant cytoplasm with azurophilic granules or vacuoles and bulky dark oblong nuclei. (From Sheridan W et al: Leukemia of non-T lineage natural killer cells. Blood 72:1701,1988.)

playing CD2+, CD3−, CD8± surface markers. The CD3+ LDL proliferations have been found by Southern and northern blot analyses to undergo clonal gene and transcript rearrangements involving the TcR α, β, and γ chains; these are indicators of T cell lineage, and this category of T8-CLL is a leukemia of non-MHC–restricted cytotoxic T cells. The CD3− proliferations are less common and fail to show TcR β-chain rearrangements but do possess all the antigenic credentials of NK-ness; this rare look-alike disorder is actually a leukemia of "non-T lineage" natural killer cells (Figure 17-14) [11]. The ancestry of the NK variant of LGL leukemia remains obscured by phenotypic infidelities and the finding that in some cases showing no β chain rearrangements the TcR γ chains are rearranged [12]. Although NK (LGL) geneology remains murky, it does seem clear that these cells and cytotoxic T cells share a common ancestry. The corresponding leukemias differ in that the frank T cell (type A) subset is so indolent that harsh therapies are counterindicated, whereas the NK (type B) process—after idling for several years as a harmless lymphocytosis—eventually ignites into an aggressive malignant phase requiring intensive chemotherapy.

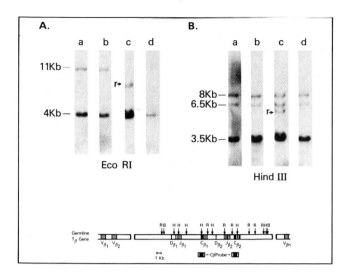

A.   **B.**

Eco RI

Hind III

FIGURE 17-14

Radioautographs of Southern blots, using a c-DNA probe for the constant (C) region of the TcR-β chain, show that some LGL leukemias are T cell proliferations (lanes c; r→ indicates clonal rearrangement) and some (lanes b) are not. Rearranged bands (r→) indicate T lineage. Lanes (a) and (d) represent controls. The schematic (below) of TcR β-chain gene organization indicates the sites of endonuclease cleavage: R = *Eco* RI; H = *Hind* III; and B = *Bam* HI. (From Sheridan W et al: Leukemia of non-T lineage natural killer cells. Blood 72:1701,1988.)

Management

The natural course of CLL is remarkably variable, as an apparent result of biological differences built-in at the moment of mutation. Some patients are predestined to die within a year of diagnosis, others live well beyond 10 years, and rarely miraculous deliverance occurs. Once a diagnosis of CLL is made, the decisions to consider are whether or not to treat the patient at all and, when intervention is indicated, how serious should it be?

In patients with mild or subclinical disease, restraint is the rule for there is no evidence that early intervention extends life. Prognostic factors include the number and locale of leukemic cells and the extent to which marrow function is compromised, factors weighed and incorporated in the Binet adaptation of the Rai clinical staging system for CLL (Table 17-1) [13, 14].

TABLE 17-1

Three stage prognostic classification of CLL

Stage	Findings at diagnosis	Percentage of patients	5-year survival after diagnosis (%)
A	Blood lymphocyte count 4,000 cells/μl or more, with 40% or more lymphocytes in marrow differential count; no anemia or thrombocytopenia; less than three involved areas*	66	80
B	State A plus three or more involved areas	30	40
C	Stage A plus anemia (Hb less than 10 g/dl) or thrombocytopenia (platelets less than 100,000/μl)	4	20

*Counting as one each the following areas: (1) axillary, cervical, and inguinal lymph nodes, whether unilateral or bilateral; (2) spleen; and (3) liver.

Source: From Binet JL et al: A new prognostic classification of chronic lymphocytic leukemia derived from a multivariate survival analysis. Cancer 48:198,1981; and French Cooperative Group on Chronic Lymphocytic Leukemia: Prognostic and therapeutic advances in CLL management: the experience of the French Cooperative Group. Semin Hematol 24:275,1987.

Important complications having a negative effect on survival are hypogammaglobulinemia, recurrent infections, and evidence of transformation to Richter's syndrome.

Survival of CLL patients has not been extended greatly by therapeutic measures, but amelioration with improved quality of life can be achieved in most patients in stages A and B. Corticosteroids, alkylators, combination chemotherapy, and total body irradiation when used judiciously can be very effective in controlling for a number of years the tumor mass and sustaining hematopoiesis. Apart from holding complications of CLL at bay until terminal progression sets in, the physician's greatest service to the patient is to educate him about this comparatively benign leukemia and (when appropriate) assure him that his chances are good for enjoying a long life relatively free of medical harassment.

PROLYMPHOCYTIC LEUKEMIA

Prolymphocytic leukemia (PLL) is characterized by pronounced splenomegaly and extreme leukocytosis (white counts usually exceed 100,000 at presentation), with little or no adenopathy. PLL is even more decidedly a leukemia of the elderly than CLL, with a maximum incidence in the eighth decade, and progression is more aggressive, median survival being 2 to 3 years. Although PLL and CLL are distinctive clonal entities, arising from mature and adolescent B cells, respectively, about 15% of CLL patients undergo prolymphocytoid transformation and the leukemic cells adopt the morphology of prolymphocytes.

Pathophysiology

The membrane phenotype and morphology of PLL cells indicate that they are the product of maturation arrest at a point midway between CLL and well-differentiated B cell neoplasms such as multiple myeloma. (The term "prolymphocytic" is unfortunate for it errantly implies that these cells are precursive rather than full-fledged B cells.) Unlike CLL cells, malignant prolymphocytes flaunt the full phenotypic credentials of maturing B cells: high-density sIg, downregulated mrbc receptors, strong reaction to monoclonal antibodies to B cell antigens,

and clonal rearrangements of both heavy and light chain Ig genes. These generalizations are admittedly violated by the fact that PLL can present while in transformation from CLL, and (worse) in nearly 20% of PLL cases the prolymphocytes lack sIg and bear the full blazonry of T cell lineage emblems: $CD2^+$, $CD3^+$, $CD4^+$ or $CD8^+$ (or both), and clonal TcR rearrangements. In terms of helper/inducer and suppressor/cytotoxic functional subsets, phenotypic and functional correlations in T-PLL are often scrambled.

Cytogenetics The most common abnormality in B-PLL is a marker chromosome $14q^+$ or the t(11;14) translocation described earlier in B-CLL. No specific chromosomal abnormalities have been reported, but deletions and translocations involving chromosome 6 are inordinately frequent.

Description and Hematologic Findings

Most patients with B-PLL present in Binet stage C with massive splenomegaly and white counts in excess of 100,000 cells/μl. Invasion of nodes and nonlymphoidal tissues is minimal in B-PLL, and most problems arise as complications of splenomegaly, which often can be dealt with for a time by splenic irradiation. T-PLL is even more aggressive than the B cell counterpart: leukemic cells infiltrate liver, lymph

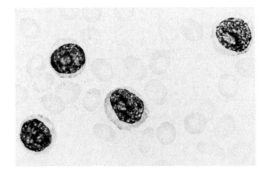

FIGURE 17-15

PLL prolymphocytes (the four large cells) are most notable for their single prominent nucleolus, which serves as a diagnostic medallion. (From Jandl JH: Chapt 25, in Blood: Textbook of Hematology. Boston, Little, Brown and Company,1987.)

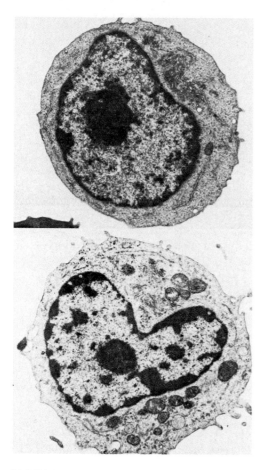

TEM of typical B-PLL cells showing the large central nucleolus and peripheral chromatin condensation. Leukemic prolymphocytes usually have rounded nuclei (above), but indented (below) or even cleft nuclei are frequent. (From Costello C et al: Prolymphocytic leukaemia: an ultrastructural study of 22 cases. Br J Haematol 44:389,1980.)

nodes, and skin, as well as spleen, and unresponsiveness to therapy leads to a very dismal prognosis (median survival: 7 months).

Morphology of Leukemic Prolymphocytes

Prolymphocytes are larger than normal or CLL lymphocytes, cytoplasm is abundant, and nuclear chromatin is moderately condensed; the eye-catching feature on both light- and electron microscopy is the single bold, centroidal, medallionlike nucleolus (Figure 17-15) [15]. This

unmistakable clue can be obscured in cells shrivelled by drying artifact, emphasizing the eternal imprecation in hematology to select well-spread areas for microscopic examination.

The large, central, compact nucleolus is even more notable on transmission electron microscopy (TEM), regardless of variability in cytoplasmic volume and nuclear conformation (Figure 17-16) [16].

B-PLL versus T-PLL morphology   B-PLL and T-PLL cells can appear identical by routine staining, but T-PLL cells reveal strong focal or chunky reaction patterns typical of T cells when stained with α-naphthyl acetate esterase or acid phosphatase. The cytoplasm of T-PLL cells is often scanty and nuclei may appear irregular by light microscopy; the latter distinction is more obvious on TEM (Figure 17-17) [17].

FIGURE 17-17

TEM of a boldly nucleolated prolymphocyte from a patient with T-PLL reveals deep nuclear fissures and grooves, which reflect folding and gnarling of the nucleus. Note the sparse cytoplasm in this small cell variant, the circular profiles of endoplasmic reticulum, and (at the bottom) electron-dense bodies in which the esterases and other lysosomal enzymes reside. (From Matutes E et al: The morphological spectrum of T-prolymphocytic leukaemia. Br J Haematol 64:111,1986.)

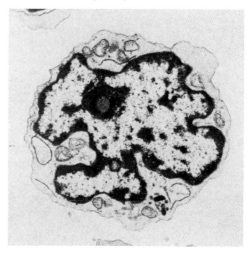

Blood counts and marrow findings In B-PLL white counts at presentation average about 350,000 cells/μl, and counts in T-PLL rise to even higher levels; in both variants, white counts may exceed 1,000,000. Hb levels are moderately depressed at diagnosis, but platelet numbers remain nearly normal until leukemic encroachment smothers all hematopoietic elements.

Prolymphocytoid Transformation Is Sometimes a Finale to CLL

Most PLL arises as a malignancy de novo without a preleukemic prelude. In prolymphocytoid transformation of established B-CLL, the innocuous-looking CLL lymphocytes are replaced by larger, more vigorously proliferative prolymphocytes and occasionally immunoblasts. During this lethal transformation, which begins in splenic or nodal foci, CLL lymphocytes become admixed with large, burly, strongly Ig+ prolymphocytes, creating a striking and ominous lymphoid dimorphism (Figure 17-18). When prolymphocyte numbers exceed about 15,000 cells/μl, the pace of the lymphoid malignancy quickens to match that of de novo PLL [18]. This change to a more aggressive, morphologically and clonally distinct malignancy is analogous to blast crisis in CML and is similarly resistant to conventional therapies.

Management

Diagnosis of PLL calls for urgent and intensive combined modality therapy, but remissions are generally partial and evanescent. Splenectomy plus leukapheresis effectively counters the immediate problems of massive splenomegaly and leukostasis, but improvement is not lasting. Recombinant IFNα—so effective in hairy cell leukemia and myeloma—has had limited trial at this writing, but several impressive longterm remissions have been reported.

HAIRY CELL LEUKEMIA

Hairy cell leukemia (HCL), née leukemic reticuloendotheliosis, is an uncommon chronic lymphoproliferative disease that originates as a lymphoma of splenic B cells (or rarely T cells), progresses to infiltrate spleen and obliterate marrow, and ultimately emerges as a leukemia. Accordingly, the hallmarks of progression are gross splenomegaly, pancytopenia, and appearance in marrow and blood of a monoclonal population of uniquely tasseled lymphocytes described inelegantly as hairy cells. HCL is primarily a disease of middle-aged men; it has a protracted course and is often amenable to judicious therapy.

The Hairy Cell

Exposition of the pathogenesis of HCL must be prefaced by characterization of the peculiar appearance and structure of hairy cells, for these determine most features of the disease and are key to the diagnosis. Leukemic hairy cells project long thin or ruffled cytoplasmic processes that appear shaggy and disheveled on blood smears (Figure 17-19), alarmingly frenetic on TEM (Figure 17-20) [19], and clownishly wiglike on SEMs (Figure 17-21) [20]. Hairy lymphocytes also possess a set of features that together distinguish HCL from other, less mature B cell neoplasms: (1) tartrate-resistant isozyme 5 of acid phosphatase (TRAP), (2) strong expression of IL-2 receptors (CD25 Tac antigens), (3) densely displayed surface receptors for C3bi (but not

FIGURE 17-18

Blood lymphocyte dimorphism during prolymphocytoid transformation in CLL. The two largest cells at center possess abundant cytoplasm, and their transformed nuclei contain one or more prominent nucleoli. Commingling with the prolymphocytes are several smaller lymphocytes having scant, vacuolated cytoplasm and displaying nuclear aberrations typical of CLL cells. (Photo by CT Kapff.)

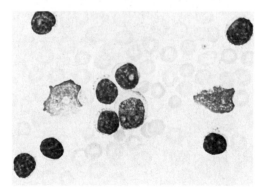

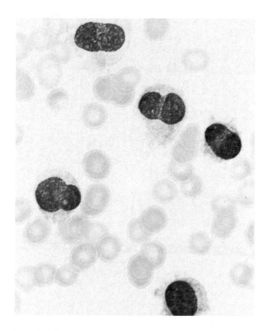

FIGURE 17-19

Representative variations in the appearance of hairy cells in the blood of a man with HCL. All cells display shaggy, wispy, filamentous, or torn cytoplasm. Nuclear shape ranges from ovoid to indented or bisected; most nucleoli are small and indistinct. (Photo by CT Kapff.)

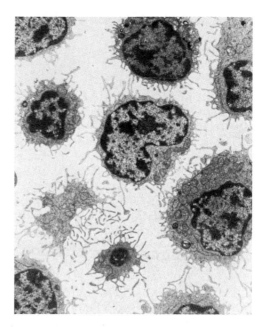

FIGURE 17-20

TEM of hairy cells revealing scores of busy, threadlike, filamentous processes sprouting from the cell surfaces. (From Turner A and Kjeldsberg CR: Hairy cell leukemia: a review. Medicine 57:477,1978. © by Williams & Wilkins, 1978.)

C3d) and for FcγR, and (4) expression of monoclonal sIg, commonly sIgG.

Pathophysiology: Hairy Cells May Be Chimeric Clonal Products

Demonstration of clonally rearranged Ig genes and their corresponding mRNAs within HCL cells indicates conclusively that HCL cells are committed B cells, as was prophesied by most of the surface marker characteristics just cited. The precise cellular origin of the hairy cells has been a topic of lingering debate, for no normal counterpart has been identified, with the possible exception of splenic marginal zone B lymphocytes. The expression of IL-2 receptors suggests T-B hybrid ancestry, while the unique class II antigen decor (DR⁺, DC⁻, and DS⁻) conforms with monocyte membership, as does the propensity of hairy cells to engage in erythrophagocytosis. The broad and conflicting phenotypic polymorphism of HCL cells and "inappropriate" inclusion of T cell and monocyte features suggest that hairy cells are

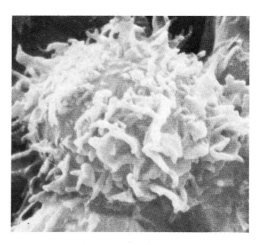

FIGURE 17-21

By SEM the surface of a typical hairy cell is seen to be adorned with a confusion of comic tassels, ruffles, ridges, and crooked villi. (From Golomb HM et al: "Hairy" cell leukaemia (leukaemic reticuloendotheliosis): a scanning electron microscopic study of eight cases. Br J Haematol 29:455,1975.)

mixed lineage, chimeric products of malignant multipotential cells, although their temperament is predominantly that of preplasmacytic B cells.

T cell variant   Rarely the leukemic cells of clinical and morphologically typical HCL have been found to express T lineage markers, CD4 and CD8, in addition to sheep red cell receptors. Notable in this connection is that the human retrovirus HTLV-II (Chapter 13) has been isolated from cell lines derived from two patients with T-HCL. In about half of T cell variants of HCL, leukemic cells have a dual T and B cell phenotype and display both E rosette and sIg positivity; surface markers and gene rearrangements in this subset wax and wane unaccountably. Progression toward the T phenotype is usually auspicious, whereas reversion to classic sIg+ B cell status is predictive of clinical deterioration.

Description

In about 10% of patients, usually elderly men whose spleens are impalpable, the disease sputters and requires no specific therapy. In the remainder, fatigue, weight loss, and weakness are progressive, and the patients present with one or more cytopenias leading to anemia, superficial bleeding, or infection. In one-quarter of cases, patients present with the symptoms of massive splenomegaly, usually unaccompanied by adenopathy.

Splenomegaly

As the spleen appears to be the site of origin of the founding clone in most cases of HCL, splenomegaly is almost invariably prominent and often is sufficiently massive to impinge on other organs and to cause marked pooling of red cells and platelets. Splenic weight at autopsy ranges from 0.5 to 5.0 kg. Splenic histology is distinctive in that sinuses and cords are filled with a uniform population of lymphoid cells whose dark oblong, dented, cleaved, or folded nuclei are kept evenly spaced apart by the long bristly cytoplasmic projections. On fixed sections the nuclear spacing creates a loose polka-dot pattern quite unlike the dark compact packing customarily seen in lymphocytic infiltrates (Figure 17-22)

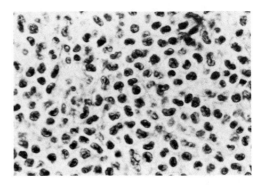

FIGURE 17-22

Section of spleen from a patient with HCL, showing diffuse infiltration of cords and sinuses by a uniformly spaced population of hairy cells. Note the variably indented, cleft, or peanut-shaped nuclei and forceful thinning-out of endothelial cells. H & E stain. (From Turner A and Kjeldsberg CR: Hairy cell leukemia: a review. Medicine 57:477,1978. © by Williams & Wilkins, 1978.)

[19]. Inflation of red pulp sinuses and cords by expanding growth of the sticky and prickly hairy cells causes pressure atrophy of lymphoid follicles, and rents in the vascular compartments allow formation of characteristic blood lakes or "pseudosinuses" lined by the malignant invaders. Lymph nodes, when involved (especially after splenectomy) show a similar diffuse infiltrative pattern of widely spaced lymphocyte nuclei that, on high-power view, resembles a tray of fried eggs.

Hematologic Findings

Most HCL patients are pancytopenic at presentation, and the percentage of hairy cells is low (0 to 20%). As the tumor mass expands, hairy cells eventually spill into the bloodstream in greater numbers, but even in advanced disease white counts seldom climb above 25,000 cells/μl, a more usual figure being 10,000. Marrow replacement by tumor cells almost always leads to thrombocytopenia and eventually to purpura, and neutropenia is a constant feature. Neutropenia is the nemesis of HCL and accounts for infection being the major cause of morbidity and mortality. Host resistance is further undermined by severe monocyte depletion—a peculiar and innate feature of HCL, the morbid impact of which is aggravated further by an 80% reduction in NK activity.

Marrow examination   Dry taps reward most efforts at marrow aspiration, for marrow infiltrated by hairy cells becomes knit together by the interlocking Velcrolike processes of the commingled hairy cell population, forming a fabric reinforced by reticulin fibrosis. As in splenic infiltrates, tumor cells in marrow are held apart by the webbing of their spidery projections, and tumor cells appear less crammed than in other lymphocytic leukemias or lymphomas. Hairy cell nuclei may be ovoid, convoluted, or indented and are devoid of nucleoli or mitotic figures.

Management

Most patients have pancytopenia and splenomegaly, but if neither of these creates problems patients should be spared from meddlesome or aggressive therapy.

Splenectomy Is Palliative Therapy for HCL

In HCL patients with moderately severe pancytopenia, bulky splenomegaly, repeated infections attributable to leukopenia (neutrophil counts less than 1,000/μl), or transfusion dependency, splenectomy is the conventional choice for rapid palliation. Nearly all patients are improved by splenectomy, and in many cases additional therapy is unnecessary; however, about 60% eventually relapse and require additional or alternative measures.

Alpha-2 Interferon (IFNα) and Pentostatin (2'-Deoxycoformycin)

Both recombinant IFNα2a and IFNα2b are highly effective in restoring blood counts to normal and in reducing the hairy cell population of marrow. In longterm studies blood counts remain normal or nearly so with continued therapy, but a complete response (eradication of tumor cells) is rare.

Greater success has been achieved with pentostatin, a high-affinity inhibitor of adenosine deaminase (ADA). Initially assumed to be a specific toxin for T cells, which depend on high intracellular concentrations of this deaminase, pentostatin has proved to be surprisingly effective against tumors of both T cell and B cell provenance, particularly slow-growing neoplasms having low levels of enzyme. Unlike IFNα, pentostatin is capable of inducing complete remission in about 60% of patients, including those who have failed on IFNα [21, 22]. In blocking adenosine deaminase, pentostatin therapy introduces a risk of serious lymphopenia and immunodeficiency analogous to that encountered in congenital ADA deficiency. Severe, sometimes fatal, infections have occurred in a small percentage of patients, and most HCL patients develop symptomless immune dysfunction on maintenance pentostatin, as demonstrated by lymphopenia and depressed T cell function and NK activity. At this writing, nonetheless, the balance of benefit to risk appears favorable, and pentostatin may well become frontline therapy for HCL; time will tell.

REFERENCES

1. Greaves MF et al: Chapt 9, in Atlas of Blood Cells: Function and Pathology, vol. 1, Zucker-Franklin D et al, Eds. Milan, Edi. Ermes s.r.l.,1988

2. Bertoli LF et al: Analysis with antiidiotype antibody of a patient with chronic lymphocytic leukemia and a large cell lymphoma (Richter's syndrome). Blood 70:45,1987

3. Deegan MJ et al: High incidence of monoclonal proteins in the serum and urine of chronic lymphocytic leukemia patients. Blood 64:1207,1984

4. Feliu E et al: Cytoplasmic inclusions in lymphocytes of chronic lymphocytic leukaemia. Scand J Haematol 31:510,1983

5. Kay NE and Perri RT: Evidence that large granular lymphocytes from B-CLL patients with hypogammaglobulinemia down-regulate B-cell immunoglobulin synthesis. Blood 73:1016,1989

6. Montserrat E et al: Lymphocyte doubling time in chronic lymphocytic leukaemia: analysis of its prognostic significance. Br J Haematol 62:567,1986

7. Gunz FW and Henderson ES: Chapt 11, in Leukemia, 4th ed, Gunz FW and Henderson ES, Eds. New York, Grune & Stratton, Inc.,1983

8. Kruskall MS and Harris NL: Chronic lymphocytic leukemia with the recent devel-

opment of hepatosplenomegaly and ascites. Case 31-1983. N Engl J Med 309:297,1983

9. Sweet DL Jr et al: Chronic lymphocytic leukaemia and its relationship to other lymphoproliferative disorders. Clin Haematol 6:141,1977

10. Hoffbrand AV and Pettit JE: Chapt 9, in Clinical Hematology Illustrated. An Integrated Text and Color Atlas. Philadelphia, WB Saunders Company,1987

11. Sheridan W et al: Leukemia of non-T lineage natural killer cells. Blood 72:1701,1988

12. Foroni L et al: T-cell leukemias with rearrangements of the γ but not β T-cell receptor genes. Blood 71:356,1988

13. Binet JL et al: A new prognostic classification of chronic lymphocytic leukemia derived from a multivariate survival analysis. Cancer 48:198,1981

14. French Cooperative Group on Chronic Lymphocytic Leukemia: Prognostic and therapeutic advances in CLL management: the experience of the French Cooperative Group. Semin Hematol 24:275,1987

15. Jandl JH: Chapt 25, in Blood: Textbook of Hematology. Boston, Little, Brown and Company,1987

16. Costello C et al: Prolymphocytic leukaemia: an ultrastructural study of 22 cases. Br J Haematol 44:389,1980

17. Matutes E et al: The morphological spectrum of T-prolymphocytic leukaemia. Br J Haematol 64:111,1986

18. Melo JV et al: The relationship between chronic lymphocytic leukaemia and prolymphocytic leukaemia. IV. Analysis of survival and prognostic features. Br J Haematol 65:23,1987

19. Turner A and Kjeldsberg CR: Hairy cell leukemia: a review. Medicine 57:477,1978

20. Golomb HM et al: "Hairy" cell leukaemia (leukaemic reticuloendotheliosis): a scanning electron microscopic study of eight cases. Br J Haematol 29:455,1975

21. Golomb HM and Ratain MJ: Recent advances in the treatment of hairy-cell leukemia. N Engl J Med 316:870,1987

22. Grem JL et al: Pentostatin in hairy cell leukemia: treatment by the special exception mechanism. JNCI 81:448,1989

18

Multiple Myeloma and Related Plasma Cell Dyscrasias

☐

Multiple myeloma (plasma cell myeloma or plasmacytoma) is a differentiated B cell neoplasm characterized by clonal expansion of malignant plasma cells, which produce monoclonal immunoglobulin (Ig) defined by unique idiotypic determinants. The homogeneous monoclonal immunoglobulins or immunoglobulin fragments ("M components") are composed of a single heavy (H) chain class (IgG, IgA, IgM, IgD, or IgE, in descending order of frequency) and a single light (L) chain class, κ or λ. Most myelomas produce or secrete IgG or IgA, but free light chains are the only gene product in over 10% of cases, attesting to severe secretory imbalance. Rarely, monoclonal proteins consist of isolated heavy chains, or tumor cells may elaborate two or more monoclonal proteins, or, in nonsecretory myeloma, none at all.

Multiple myeloma (MM) is a solid tumor having more in common with lymphoma than leukemia. Although myelomas may originate in nodes or soft tissues, tumor masses usually appear first within marrow and show a decided tropism for marrow during dissemination, cropping up throughout the skeleton to form aggressively expanding multifocal osteolytic lesions. Few tumor cells loiter in the bloodstream during dissemination, plasmacytosis being an unusual feature. Myeloma cells display Ig gene rearrangements that took place after Ig class switching, explaining the variety of Ig classes and subclasses expressed in various individuals afflicted with MM. Pre B and mature B cells are not part of the malignant clone, as was once thought, but may acquire a spurious clonal MM phenotype through passive attachment of myeloma Ig to Fc receptors on blood lymphocytes [1]. The complete clinical expression of MM can be explained by the collective effects of vigorous tumor cell growth in the cordial compartments of the marrow, the self-serving secretion of destructive cytokines that facilitate tumoral aggressions, and the mounting accumulations of useless and harmful M components. The net result is a devastating and dispiriting syndrome of successive calamities that include pathologic fractures, hypercalcemia, renal failure, immunosuppression with recurrent infections, hemorrhagic catastrophies, and spoliation of the marrow.

PATHOPHYSIOLOGY

Malignant plasma cells are a paradigm of monotypic Ig expression and are associated with the final phenotypic vestments of end-stage maturation: cIg$^+$, sIg$^-$, plasma cell associated antigen (PCA-1 and PCA-2)$^+$, and pan-B$^-$ (CDs 19, 20, 21, and 22 negative), HLA-DR$^-$, CALLA$^-$, and TdT$^-$. Coexpression on terminally differentiated MM cells of early B, myeloid, and T cell markers has also been observed, indicating that myeloma cells are in part a product of infidelity in high places, siting some of the oncogenic events in myeloma at early stages of hematopoiesis [2].

Myeloma Cells Must Evade the Immunologic Network to Be Productive

As described in Chapter 12 the sequential activation of heavy and light chain genes and the intricacies of isotype class switching terminating the Ig rearrangement cascade involve multitudinous recombinatorial events, TdT-promoted mutagenic gene movements, and precise exon extirpations, all of which are error prone. In light of the busy movements and rearrangements of genetic elements at the Ig loci, the frequency of B cell neoplasms is not surprising. In the case of myeloma there is ample evidence that monoclonal cell populations are generated frequently in response to public antigens and that damage control mechanisms are implemented through the offices of the immunologic network. Constrained monoclonal plasma cell proliferations are consigned to the awkward category of "monoclonal gammopathy of undetermined significance" (MGUS) when monoclonal Ig levels are held below 3 g/dl and marrow plasmacytosis is less than 10%; individuals with Ig levels greater

than 3 g/dl and plasma cell populations in excess of 10%, but who show no immediate evidence of malignant progression are said to have "smoldering myeloma." By employing immunoisoelectric focusing for detecting M components, over 10% of apparently normal persons over age 45 can be demonstrated to have nascent monoclonal gammopathies. These incipient malignancies—myelomas manqué—are usually held in check by anti-idiotypic antibodies under the hegemony of Id (idiotype)-sensitized suppressor T cells.

Anti-Id Antibodies: An Imperfect Star Wars Defense

In incipient MM, idiotype expression is carried to extremes: clonal expansion of novel plasma cells incites vigorous secretion of specific anti-Id antibodies and causes proliferation of isotypic anti-Id–bearing suppressor T cells, which collaborate in blocking further growth of myeloma cells. Binding of anti-Id antibodies inhibits expression of monoclonal Ig by causing antibody-aggregated Ig secreted by myeloma cells to coalesce into disposable vesicles. Meanwhile Id-specific suppressor T cells downregulate synthesis of monoclonal Ig by blocking expression of light chain mRNA—so-called light chain isotype suppression.

MM Triumphs by Overthrowing Immunity: Malignant Plasma Cells Induce B Cell Suppression

The elaborate immunoregulatory containment of myeloma clones fails in patients with overt MM, for plasma cell tumors attaining sufficient size induce a profound suppression of antibody synthesis with general hypogammaglobulinemia, and production of anti-idiotype antibodies suffers proportionately. Malignant plasma cells exude a 55,000 M_r RNA-containing "PC factor" which stimulates macrophages to secrete a low molecular weight protein that selectively suppresses B cell function but spares helper T cells. Consequently humoral immunity is severely depressed and patients become vulnerable to bacterial infections, whereas cell-mediated immunity is preserved and patients are normally resistant to fungal and most viral infections and display normal delayed-type hypersensitivity reactions to skin test antigens.

Cytokinetics of MM   Whether or not the immunologic network usually collapses acutely as a prelude to typical MM is unknown. In individuals fortuitously discovered to have MGUS, the early clonal trend is slow, and uninvolved (polyclonal) immunoglobulins are moderately diminished in only about 30% of cases; in these patients evolution of MGUS to MM occurs only after long periods of a clonal standoff (Figure 18-1) [3].

In patients presenting with overt disease the doubling time (Td) of the myeloma mass can be calculated from the rate of increase in monoclonal protein in circulation. The median Td is 6 months and the number of cell doublings necessary to accumulate 10^{12} (1 kg) of tumor cells is about 40. As tumor growth appears to be exponential, it can be estimated that a single malignant stem cell would require 15 to 20 years to become clinically evident, perhaps explaining in part the association of this malignancy with aging. It is unlikely, however, that tumor doubling obeys nice log kinetics, for myeloma clones are stalled initially by the immunologic network, growth kinetics accelerate sharply when tumor cells break loose from anti-idiotypic restraints, and kinetic studies have shown that later at diagnosis plasma cell replication tends to slow down again (plateau phase) as signified by a low ^{3}H-TdR labeling index. In those patients presenting with a high labeling index (>3% of tumor cells in S phase) the chance of surviving 12 months is only 50%; patients with a lower labeling index (the majority) have an average

survival of about 3 years. The heterogeneity of MM from patient to patient bears emphasis, for myeloma cells displaying a mixed or chimeric phenotype that includes early B cell markers (pre B and CALLA antigens) forecast very aggressive clinical disease [2, 4].

Myeloma Cells Promote their Own Growth by Secreting Advantageous Cytokines

Myeloma cells secrete multiple self-promoting cytokines in addition to immunoglobulins. Among these are the osteoclast activating factors (OAFs) usually generated by lymphocytes: TNF_β (lymphotoxin) and $IL-1_\beta$. TNF_β of myeloma cell origin is responsible for most of the osteoclastic bone destruction and hypercalcemia that torment patients with MM (Figure 18-2) [5]. Myeloma cells also express receptors for IL-5 (BCGF-II) and IL-6 (BSF-2), and it appears that by secreting IL-4, IL-5, IL-1, and TNF_β these tumor cells set up an autocrine growth-stimulating circuitry that is abetted by IL-6 released by neighboring marrow monocytes. Most of these cytokines are B cells growth factors, which may account for the proliferation of aberrant B cells that accompany myeloma tumors.

Chromosome Abnormalities

As befits any B cell neoplasm, the most consistent structural aberrations in MM involve a marker chromosome 14q+, with the breakpoint in Burkitt's band, 14q32. Reciprocal

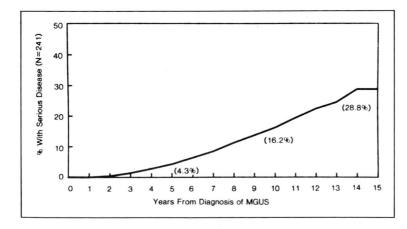

F I G U R E 18-1

Occurrence of MM (and some related disorders) following first recognition of a "benign" monoclonal immunoglobulin spike. Actuarial analysis is given parenthetically for 5, 10, and 15 years. (From Kyle RA: 'Benign' monoclonal gammopathy. A misnomer? JAMA 251:1849,1984. Copyright 1984, American Medical Association.)

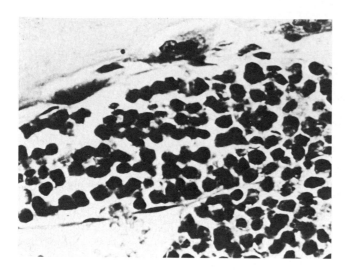

FIGURE 18-2

Histologic section of an osteolytic lesion in a patient with MM. Masses of malignant plasma cells (below) press firmly against the endosteal monolayer of multinucleated osteoclasts (upper left). Stimulated by TNF$_\beta$ released from contiguous myeloma cells, osteoclasts are goaded to proliferate and then demineralize subjacent bone. (From Mundy GR et al: Evidence for the secretion of an osteoclast stimulating factor in myeloma. Reprinted, by permission of The New England Journal of Medicine, 291:1041,1974.)

translocations include t(11;14) and t(8;14)— the latter causing dysregulation of c-*myc* and having a peculiar association with the fact that clonal mutations in myeloma occur after heavy chain class switching. The t(11;14)(q13;q32) rearrangement resembles that in CLL (Chapter 17) and similarly juxtaposes the *bcl*-1 oncogene of chromosome 11 to the Ig enhancer element between the J_H and switch regions of the severed μ gene segment on chromosome 14; the dislocated q13→qter segment appears to propel a more malignant evolution of MM. Virtually all chromosomes have exhibited abnormalities in patients with MM; these tend to become complex during rapid disease progression, and, as dysplastic hyperploidy and bi- or multinuclearity are evinced, aneuploidy is striking. On flow cytometry studies hyperploidy is evident in 80% of patients (Figure 18-3) [6]. Hypodiploidy occurs mainly in patients with Bence Jones (BJ) protein as the only clonal product and is associated with resistance to chemotherapy.

Monoclonal Protein Abnormalities

The most constant, diagnostic, instructive, and stage-related feature of MM is the manufacture and release into serum or urine of a single homogeneous idiotype-specific immunoglobulin or immunoglobulin fragment. Secretion of monoclonal Ig is ordinarily proportional to tumor mass, serves as an index of disease progression or recession, and corresponds quantitatively to the extent to which normal polyclonal Ig synthesis is suppressed. Analysis of serum and urine for monoclonal protein depends upon screening methods for detection and specific assays for identification of heavy chain class and light chain type.

FIGURE 18-3

Direct relationship between DNA index (DNA ploidy by flow cytometry) and karyotype index (modal chromosome number). (From Gould J et al: Plasma cell karyotype in multiple myeloma. Blood 71:453,1988.)

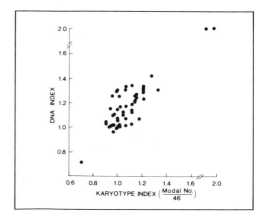

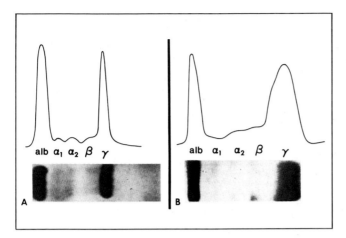

FIGURE 18-4

Appearance of stained patterns of serum proteins after electrophoresis (below), and corresponding densitometric tracing (above). Anode is on the left. (A) Narrow homogeneous band situated in the midst of the γ globulin region signifies a monoclonal M component. (B) Broad polyclonal band representing the summation of thousands of physiologic monoclonal peaks in a patient with hypergammaglobulinemia of chronic infection. (From Kyle RA and Greipp PR: The laboratory investigation of monoclonal gammopathies. Mayo Clin Proc 53:719,1978.)

Electrophoresis for Detection

Serum protein electrophoresis should be performed on all patients in whom MM, Waldenström's macroglobulinemia (WM), or amyloidosis is suspected, and in such patients with proteinuria, concentrated urine should be examined similarly. After electrophoresis on cellulose acetate membrane and protein staining, monoclonal protein having single H chain class and L chain type appears as a narrow peak on the densitometer tracing and as a discrete dense band on the cellulose membrane (Figure 18-4) [7].

Electrophoresis of both serum and urine   Intact tetrameric Ig is trapped in serum, unless there is proteinuria, and migration of monoclonal bands may vary according to the net charge of the malignant protein product. The paraprotein most often found in urine is Bence Jones protein (BJ protein), which represents monoclonal free light chains unassembled by the mutant plasma cells. In about 12% of myelomas H chain synthesis is blocked or faulty and BJ protein in the urine is the only monoclonal marker (although not evident by the "dipstick" reaction). When both monoclonal Ig and isotypic L chains are secreted, as is true in 80% of myelomas, serum contains Ig and no BJ protein (barring renal failure), and urine contains BJ protein and no Ig (barring glomerular leakage). Representative electrophoretic patterns in serum and urine are displayed in Figure 18-5 [8].

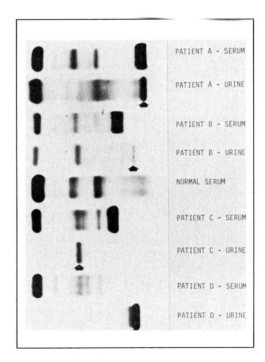

FIGURE 18-5

Serum and urine electrophoresis showing urinary BJ protein (arrows) in the same position as the monoclonal IgG (A), more cathodic (B), more anodic (C), and BJ myeloma with no visible serum paraprotein (D). In the urine of patient B there is a second heavier BJ protein in the $\alpha 2$ region, reflecting polymerization of some L chains. (From Riches PG: Chapt 5, in Multiple Myeloma and Other Paraproteinemias, Delamore IN, Ed. Edinburgh, Churchill Livingstone,1986.)

Immunoelectrophoresis for Identification

In patients with a narrow homogeneous band found on cellulose acetate or high-resolution agar gel electrophoresis, or in individuals in whom such a band is suspected but is small, complexly contoured, or buried within a polyclonal pattern, monospecific antisera to IgG, IgA, IgM, IgD, and IgE, as well as to κ and λ light chains are utilized. In immuno-electrophoresis (IEP), serum specimens are placed in wells on pairs of microscopic slides covered with 1% agarose, and customarily serum from the patient is pipetted into each upper well and normal serum is put in each lower well. After electrophoresis separates the proteins, a trough is cut into the agar between wells and filled with monospecific antisera which then diffuse to form precipitation lines or arcs where antigen and antibody meet. An IEP pattern of an IgGκ monoclonal protein is identified in Figure 18-6 [7].

FIGURE 18-6

Immunoelectrophoretic pattern in IgGκ myeloma. (A) Antiserum to IgG (γ) shows a thickened but brief arc hugging the trough from the patient's serum (upper well) as contrasted with the long sinuous polyclonal arc representing IgG from normal serum (lower well). (B) Antiserum to κ chains creates an arc similar in shape and dimension to the monoclonal IgG arc (upper well) and differs from the long polyclonal arc of normal serum in the lower well. Together these IEP patterns identify the monoclonal protein as IgGκ. (From Kyle RA and Greipp PR: The laboratory investigation of monoclonal gammopathies. Mayo Clin Proc 53:719,1978.)

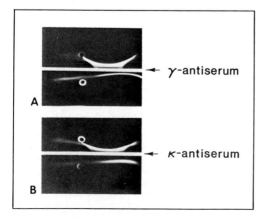

FIGURE 18-7

Routinely stained serum electrophoretic pattern of a patient with myeloma (a) and a conspicuous M component (arrow) is compared with that of a normal serum pattern (b). IF analysis with specific antisera identifies the monoclonal protein as IgA λ (upper portions of third and sixth paired panels) and reveals pathologic absence of IgG, IgM, and κ chains. (From Riches PG: Chapt 5, in Multiple Myeloma and Other Paraproteinemias, Delamore IN, Ed. Edinburgh, Churchill Livingstone, 1986.)

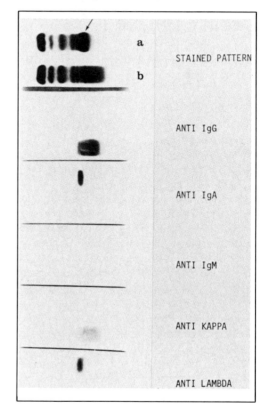

Immunofixation is a sensitive backup for IEP

Immunofixation (IF) is particularly effective in characterizing small blips of monoclonal protein, especially when concealed within a polyclonal increase, and the methodology—while similar to IEP—is simplified by omitting the diffusion stage. Serum (and urine) proteins are first separated by electrophoresis, antiserum is then applied directly to the agarose or cellulose acetate matrix, and background protein is removed by rinsing (Figure 18-7) [8].

Clinical Impact of MM Correlates with the Class and Subclass of Monoclonal Protein

The proportion of monoclonal Ig products found among patients with MM corresponds roughly with the fractional synthetic rates for polyclonal Ig in healthy individuals, suggesting that malignant transformation is a random event. Different types of M components are associated with different clinical syndromes. Patients with light chain disease, for example, have a poorer prognosis because of the high incidence of nephropathy, and patients with λ light chain disease have the poorest prognosis of all. Collectively IgG, IgA, and BJ myelomas account for over 95% of all cases, the percentages being approximately 60%, 25%, and 12%, respectively, in most series. The biochemical, cytokinetic, and clinical characteris-

TABLE 18-1

Clinical features in MM patients grouped according to monoclonal protein

Clinical feature	IgG	IgA	BJ
Mean serum level of M protein (g/dl)	4.3	2.8	Trace
Mean doubling time of M protein (months)	10.1	6.3	3.4
Lytic bone lesions (%)	55	65	78
Hypercalcemia (%)	33	59	62
Serum urea > 79 mg/dl (%)	16	17	33
Normal immunoglobulins < 20% mean normal	68	30	19
Hospital admissions because of infection (%)	60	33	20
Detected amyloidosis (%)	1	7	10

Source: From Hobbs JR: Immunochemical classes of myelomatosis. Including data from a therapeutic trial conducted by a Medical Research Council working party. Br J Haematol 16:599,1969.

tics of these three major categories of MM patients are distinctive in several notable ways (Table 18-1) [9]. In IgG myeloma tumor growth is less rapid than in other forms of MM, but the unusually high levels of myeloma protein cause "hypercatabolic" reductions in normal immunoglobulins—IgG catabolism being directly proportional to total IgG concentration. Consequently failure of humoral immunity and recurrent pyogenic infections are the major cause of morbidity. The only subclass-dependent difference in clinical expression of IgG myeloma devolves from the peculiar propensity of IgG3 molecules to form Fd fragment-linked aggregates that create severe hyperviscosity problems when in concentrations exceeding 3 to 4 g/dl. IgA myeloma proteins are also prone to cause hyperviscosity through formation of elongated polymers, but their most notorious association is with amyloidosis and hypercalcemia—sinister features shared with light chain disease. Light chain nephropathy (usually involving λ chains) exacerbated by hypercalcemia is also characteristic of IgD myeloma, an uncommon and aggressive form of MM of young men which leads to a lethal crescendo of anemia, uremia, hypercalcemia, and death within 14 months after diagnosis. IgE myeloma is exceedingly rare and most renowned for presenting as plasma cell leukemia.

Myeloma Growth Is Driven by Antigen

Initially regarded as nonsense products, many myeloma proteins have been discovered to possess clonal specificity for single commonplace antigens, however useless and harmful this may be to the host. Among antigens most commonly recognized by myeloma Ig are autologous determinants present on cells, cell constituents, plasma proteins, and ubiquitous phospholipids; in these cases the agents provocateur are intrinsic and inescapable and may play an essential role in carcinogenesis. Some antigens recognized by myeloma proteins are heterologous, being present on cell walls or products of ubiquitous organisms, in which case the constancy of stimulation may rival that of autoantigens. A logical sequitur of the "ligand connection" in the pathogenesis of MM is that light chain myelomas may also arise from autoimmune or cross-reactive stimulation, for L chains are components of the antigen combining site and have some capacity to react with specific ligands [10]. A condensed list of antigens (autologous and heterologous) shown to react specifically with monoclonal Ig is presented in Table 18-2 [11].

It is overreaching to define MM as an autoimmune neoplasm, for the revelation that each myeloma protein may have its privy antigen does not explain the fixity of the

TABLE 18-2

Antibody activities of human monoclonal immunoglobulins in plasma cell dyscrasias

Ligand ("antigen")	Possible source
Complex carbohydrates	
Ii, Pr (blood group antigens)	RBC membranes
Pyruvylated galactans	Klebsiella; *Helix pomati*
Sulfated polysaccharides	Agar
Dextran sulfate	
Heparin	Tissues
Chondroitin sulfate	
Proteins	
IgG	
β-lipoprotein	
Fibrin monomer	
Transferrin	Autologous
Albumin	plasma
Factor VIII	
Thyroglobulin	
Streptolysin O	Streptococcus
Hyaluronidase	Streptococcus
Staphylolysin	Staphylococcus
Lipids	
Cardiolipin	Mitochondria
	Membranes
Phosphorylcholine	Myelin
	Pneumococcus
	Lactobacillus
Phosphatidylcholine (lecithin)	
Glycosphingolipid, Forsmann	Membranes

Source: From Osserman EF et al: Multiple myeloma and related plasma cell dyscrasias. JAMA 258:2930, 1987. Copyright 1987, American Medical Association.

response and the failure to progress normally to polyclonal expansion. The role of antigen presumably is to foment proliferation of a preselected mutant clone.

Secretory Imbalance May Be Extreme

The rate of synthesis of L and H chains is balanced in some patients with MM, but in over 80% of cases L chains are produced in mild or moderate excess over H chains. In over 12% of patients complementary H chain production is virtually undetectable (light chain disease). An antithetical imbalance is responsible for formation of heavy chain fragments uncoupled from light chain production, resulting in a unique group of uncommon lymphoid myelomas that secrete as their variant Ig product defective heavy chains.

Heavy Chain Diseases

In heavy chain diseases (HCDs) the anomalous proteins produced are incomplete versions of at least three major heavy chain classes (γ, α, and μ), occurring as a result of internal deletions of the C_H1 genes. Interruptions in the heavy chain structural sequence reflect specific clonal defects in the H chain coding region on chromosome 14 and result in splicing errors. Absence of L chain production results from interruption in the H-to-L sequence of Ig biosynthesis.

γ *HCD*   This uncommon and vague disease is characterized by fever, malaise, anemia, hepatosplenomegaly, and progressive lymphadenopathy. Nodal enlargement vacillates and often involves Waldeyer's ring, causing erythema and swelling of palate and uvula. Blood aberrations include eosinophilia and increased numbers of lymphoid plasma cells ("plymphs"), which may become so numerous as to simulate plasma cell leukemia. A constellation of autoimmune disorders and recurrent infections is the principal cause of morbidity, and diagnosis is made by discovery of monoclonal H chain fragments reactive with antisera to γ heavy chains but not to light chains (Figure 18-8) [12].

α *HCD* α HCD is the commonest form of HCD and unlike other malignancies of Ig-

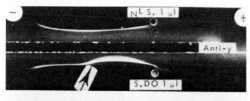

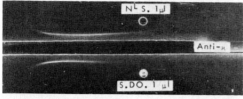

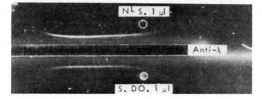

FIGURE 18-8

Immunoelectrophoretic analysis of serum from a patient (S DO) with γ HCD using antisera monospecific for γ, κ, and λ chains. The thick arcuate precipitin line given by HCD protein (upper panel) begins at the point where the long thin line of normal IgG spurs over it (arrow). Note that HCD protein does not form a corresponding arc with antisera to light chains (lower two panels). (From Seligmann M et al: Heavy chain diseases: current findings and concepts. Immunol Rev 48:145,1979. © 1979 Munksgaard International Publishers, Ltd., Copenhagen, Denmark.)

secreting cells occurs in patients between ages 10 and 30. The "intestinal lymphoma," which is endemic in Mediterranean, Middle Eastern, and several tropical regions, is localized to the secretory IgA system of the small intestine. Infiltration by a mixture of plasma cells, lymphocytes, plymphs, and a scattering of immunoblasts begins in the lamina propria of the duodenum and jejunum and their regional mesenteric and retroperitoneal nodes. With time the infiltrates penetrate the gut wall, obliterate and flatten villous structures, and eventually transform to create immunoblastic tumors of the entire mesenteric area. Chemotherapy analogous to that used in conventional MM plus oral tetracycline may bring amelioration or even remission.

Nonsecretory MM: clones without a product

Some disseminated myelomas having cytologic and osteolytic properties indistinguishable from classic MM fail to secrete any M components, although monoclonal Ig accumulates within cytoplasm and endoplasmic reticulum. This uncommon and incompetent variant (accounting for 1 to 2% of MM cases) is less malevolent than most myelomas; absent secretion of useless Ig, there is no washout of normal immunoglobulins, antibody levels are not severely depressed, and infection is less of a problem.

Myeloma Cells

MM ordinarily behaves like an intramedullary lymphoma, only rarely emerging as leukemia. Diagnosis is made by marrow aspiration or biopsy. Geographic distribution of plasma cell infiltrates varies with progression, and early in the disease malignant plasma cells are recognizable not by their sheer numbers but by their penchant for forming morular clusters and sheets, often surrounded by the heavy background staining and rouleaux signifying hypergammaglobulinemia. As usual, the extent and architectural pattern of infiltration is most apparent on histologic sections (Figure 18-9) [13].

Myeloma Cells Are Heterogeneous

Plasma cells of patients with slowly progressive MM appear normal ("mature") but slightly large and have rounded eccentric nuclei possessing one or two small nucleoli. Cytoplasm is abundant, even voluminous, and is stained a murky blue-gray peppered with vacuoles and reddish inclusions. Plasma cells vary considerably from patient to patient and there is rough correspondence between the degree of plasma cell atypia and their biologic belligerence. Immature plasma cells having a diffuse chromatin pattern, a large or duplicated nucleus, and large nucleoli are more aggressive than more normal-appearing cells, and in patients with fulminant disease (median survival: 10 months) the tumor cells are plasmablasts—possessing finely divided chromatin, a centroidally placed nucleus, and comparatively modest amounts of cytoplasm (Fig-

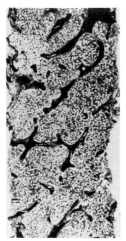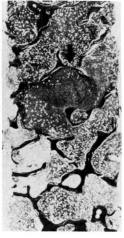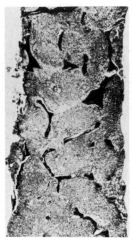

FIGURE 18-9

Histologic patterns of
MM infiltration of mar-
row: left, interstitial;
center, nodular (at ar-
row); right, diffuse.
Gomori stain. (From
Bartl R et al: Histologic
classification and stag-
ing of multiple mye-
loma: a retrospective
and prospective study
of 674 cases. Am J Clin
Pathol 87:342,1987.)

ure 18-10). Prognostic staging is complicated
by the admixture in most patients of varying
proportions of mature and undifferentiated
forms, and the presence of colorful but ominously dysplastic forms creates difficulty in
prognostic scoring on the basis of morphology
alone.

A cytologic bestiary of myeloma cells   MM
engenders a wild assortment of cytologic
forms, among which are giant multinucleated
cells, "flame cells," and plasma cells bearing
crystalloid inclusions known as Russell bodies

FIGURE 18-10

Marrow aspirates from three patients with
MM. Well-differentiated plasma cell morphology (left) is associated with unhurried (albeit remorseless) progression. Immature plasma cells
showing binucleate forms and cytologic atypia
(center) connote a more rapid cytokinetic pace,
and plasmablast predominance (large round
plasma cells with nucleoli) forecasts an explosive course refractory to therapy. (Photo by CT
Kapff.)

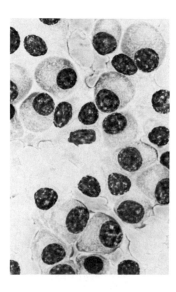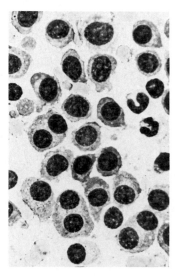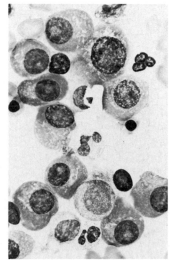

or globular grapelike bodies identifying the cells as "Mott cells." None of these dysplastic deformities is emblematic of malignancy unless the numbers are large and the company congeneric. Among the most dazzling are huge multinucleated plasma cells that stain carmine red on their fiery fringes; these flame cells are glutted with intracisternal plugs of precipitated immunoglobulin which constipate the secretory channels and devitalize cell margins, eventually causing the dying cell to shed hardened fragments of cytoplasm (Figure 18-11). More commonplace than flame cells are plasma cells decorated with pink or blue bodies; these Russell bodies, representing condensed, crystalline, or coacervated proteins synthesized by myeloma cells, are impacted within the distended channels of RER (Figure 18-12) [14]. Agglomeration of scores of Russell bodies within plasma cells, but outside the RER, causes them to form large bunches of bluish grapelike vesicles; two such Mott cells are shown amidst a cluster of myeloma cells of various stages in Figure 18-13 [15].

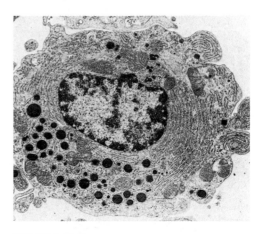

FIGURE 18-12

EM of myeloma cell containing numerous spheroidal electron-dense Russell bodies, most of them trapped within dilated segments of endoplasmic reticulum. Note the busy scrollwork of whorling RER, some of which has budded off into locks and free fragments. (From Weinstein T et al: Electron microscopy study of Mott and Russell bodies in myeloma cells. J Submicrosc Cytol 19:155,1987.)

FIGURE 18-13

Myeloma marrow containing two Mott cells within a mixed field of mature plasma cells, plasmablasts, and plasma cells with two nuclei or multiple vesicular inclusions. (From Jandl JH: Chapt 26, in Blood: Textbook of Hematology. Boston, Little, Brown and Company,1987.)

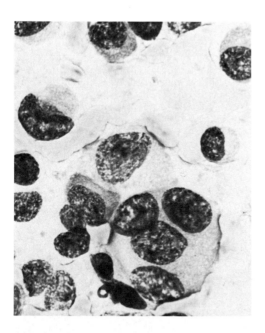

FIGURE 18-11

Giant multinucleated flame cell accompanied by heterogeneous plasmablasts in marrow from a patient with IgG1 myeloma. (Photo by CT Kapff.)

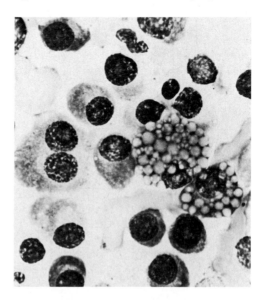

Cytology and histology in prognostic staging

Assessment of marrow morphology (specifying the proportions of mature plasma cells versus undifferentiated plasmablasts) combined with quantitation of total marrow occupancy by plasma cells of all stripes yields a staging system highly predictive of survival. Both cellular maturity and intramedullary plasma cell mass have strong prognostic impact.

DESCRIPTION

MM debilitates the patient system by system. Irruption of myeloma cells throughout the marrow stifles marrow function and erodes cortical and trabecular bone. Myeloma secretory products clog the kidneys, thicken blood viscosity, and cripple antibody synthesis. Infection and renal failure are the most frequent causes of death, but skeletal lesions account for most of the agony and demoralization.

Skeletal Disease

Myeloma cells thrive when lodged in marrow, oozing some cytokines that subdue neighboring cells and others (OAFs) that erode bone and create tumor space (Figure 18-14) [16]. Skeletal tumors initially implant in the centripetal marrow of ribs, sternum, skull, spine, clavicles, shoulders, pelvis, and proximal ends of long bones and are first noted because of localized tender swelling or persistent pain. Often the deadly nature of the disease is proclaimed sharply by the sudden onset of pain from pathologic fracture through a diseased segment of bone, or by abrupt collapse of a vertebra (Figure 18-15) [17].

Radiologic Changes

By radiologic bone surveys the most typical findings are multiple punched-out osteolytic lesions having sharp edges; these are particularly obvious where bone structure is uncomplicated as in the calvarium and shafts of long bones (Figure 18-16) [18, 19]. Periosteal reactions involving osteoblastic hyperactivity are rare in MM, and most myeloma lesions appear "cold" (nonradioactive) by radionuclide imaging, except during reparative responses to obvious fractures.

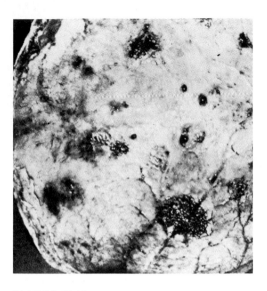

FIGURE 18-14

Focal areas of myeloma tumor growth and bony erosion as seen from the inner aspect of the calvarium of a patient felled by MM. (From Hayhoe FGJ et al: Chapt 6, in Multiple Myeloma and Other Paraproteinemias, Delamore IN, Ed. Edinburgh, Churchill Livingstone,1986.)

FIGURE 18-15

Appearance at autopsy of the vertebral column of a patient with MM showing multiple small tumor nodules and collapse of one vertebra. (Left) Section of vertebral column revealing compression fracture. (Right) Close-up view of site of collapse, displaying numerous pale gelatinous tumor nodules ranging up to 1 cm across. (From Azar HA: Chapt 1, in Multiple Myeloma and Related Disorders, vol. I, Azar HA and Potter M, Eds. New York, Harper & Row, Publishers, Inc.,1973.)

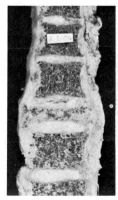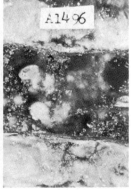

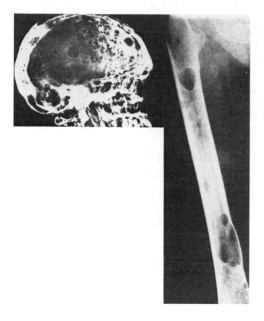

FIGURE 18-16

Radiograms revealing multiple punched-out lesions characteristic of MM. (Left) Skull is riddled with large and small, circular, sharply marginated lesions, many of them perforate. (Right) Discrete and confluent circumscribed osteolytic lesions of the femur, some of them bulging through the thinned-out cortex. (From Snapper I: Medical Clinics on Bone Diseases. New York, Interscience Publishers, Inc., 1943; and Snapper I: Rare Manifestations of Metabolic Bone Disease. Springfield, Charles C. Thomas, Publisher, 1952.)

CT versus MR imaging   In patients suspected of having myeloma, CT scanning permits detection of lesions invisible by routine radiography. The lower thoracic and lumbar spine is the region most frequently involved by MM. CT screening of the entire spine in patients with neurological complaints is seldom feasible, but the field of visualization by magnetic resonance imaging (MRI) is large, normal marrow emits a characteristic signal pattern, and the spinal canal and its contents are delineated sharply. In MRI the images created mirror the magnetic properties of hydrogen atoms during strong magnetic perturbation. The spin-lattice relaxation time (T1) and the spin-spin relaxation time (T2) denote the time taken by tissue nuclei to regain equilibrium after being perturbed by a radiofrequency pulse—unveiling fundamental features of cells and tissues such as molecular motion and free water versus fat content; the captured images yield exquisite textural and structural detail that discriminates between fat, normal marrow, and tumor tissue. Normal marrow has high signal intensity at both T1 and T2 scan sequences due to its fat content. Neoplastic processes that replace marrow fat decrease the T1 signal, but T2-weighted images display intermediate signal enhancement (Figure 18-17) [20]. MR imaging is of surpassing value in surveying for tumors, even very small ones, that have not created extensive bony lesions. CT scanning is unri-

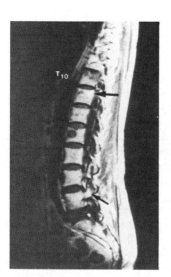
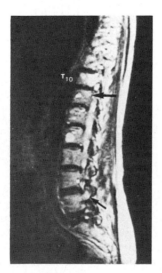

FIGURE 18-17

MR imaging of the spine in MM. (Left) T1-weighted sagittal image of lower thoracic and lumbar spine shows multiple foci of reduced signal intensity, the dark areas (particularly in T10 through L1) indicating myeloma tumors. (Right) T2-weighted imaging demonstrates an increase in signal in tumor areas that were revealed by T1-weighted views. For signal calibration note the luminous fatty areas of marrow in the dorsal aspect of T11 and the pedicle of L4 (arrows). (From Fruehwald FXJ et al: Magnetic resonance imaging of the lower vertebral column in patients with multiple myeloma. Invest Radiol 23:193,1988.)

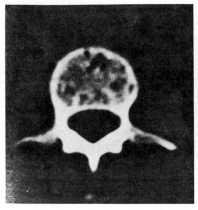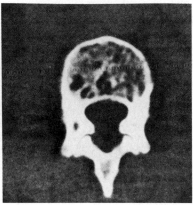

FIGURE 18-18

CT scans through L4 (left) and L5 (right) vertebral bodies in a patient with MM and negative x-rays. Both vertebrae are honeycombed with lytic foci but cortical walls and posterior elements are spared. (From Helms CA and Genant HK. JAMA 248:2886,1982. Copyright 1982, American Medical Association.)

valed for defining the details of osseous destruction in bony structures found to be involved by MRI (or by x-ray) and permits examination of the spongiosa of vertebral bodies to a degree not possible by conventional radiography and linear tomography (Figure 18-18) [21].

Hypercalcemia

In most patients with extensive osteolysis (and in 30% of all MM patients) serum calcium is elevated above 11 mg/dl at diagnosis. Ca^{2+} unbound to albumin is deposited as calcium salts in renal parenchyma, impairing calcium secretion, and setting up a vicious cycle. About half of patients with hypercalcemia develop weakness, nausea, polyuria, drowsiness, disorientation, and even coma. Acute management requires firm support of hydration starting with saline diuresis and judicious use of the parathormone antagonist, calcitonin, given in combination with glucocorticoids, or of nondemineralizing diphosphonates. Longterm control of hypercalcemia requires suppression of OAF-secreting myeloma cells with adequate chemotherapy.

Amyloidosis in MM Is an L Chain Sediment Disease

In about 10% of patients with MM (and less frequently in patients with B cell dyscrasias of other sorts) amyloid deposition is sufficient to cause a severe multisystem disease formerly known as primary amyloidosis. Amyloid deposits are derived from overabundance of monoclonal free light chains—particularly λ chains—which have undergone proteolytic degradation to V_L light chain fragments that collect in the tumor cells, mesenchymal cells, and kidneys, liver, and spleen. Deposits of the fragmented light chains form stable double-stranded fibrils (AL fibrils) which align as antiparallel β-pleated sheets. The lardaceous deposits of AL amyloid stain an amorphous pink with H & E, but under polarized light, Congo red staining of amyloid produces a characteristic apple green birefringence. By EM, amyloid appears as a feltlike fabric composed of rigid fibrils, and these indestructible pleated fibrils are responsible for damage to the cardiac, renal, and other tissues in which they are deposited. In most MM cases the bulk of surplus light chains and light chain fragments is excreted through the kidneys, but damaging amount of λ chains remain trapped within the glomerular basement membranes, often resulting in nephrotic syndrome and renal failure (Figure 18-19) [22]. Deposits of AL amyloid in heart muscle occur in over 80% of patients with amyloidosis secondary to MM, causing cardiac enlargement and stiffening, with refractory pump failure. Amyloid may infiltrate and damage all regions of the gastrointestinal tract from tongue to rectum. Macroglossia is a common, often disturbing manifestation of amyloid deposition, for it may interfere with deglutition and respiration, as

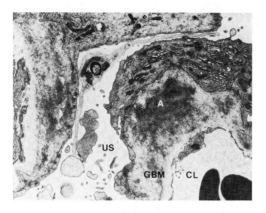

FIGURE 18-19

EM of part of a glomerulus from an MM patient with amyloid nephrosis. The glomerular basement membrane (GBM) is thickened and deformed by feltlike aggregations of amyloid fibrils (A). CL = capillary lumen and US = urinary space. (From Coward RA: Chapt 16, in Multiple Myeloma and Other Paraproteinemias, Delamore IN, Ed. Edinburgh, Churchill Livingstone,1986.)

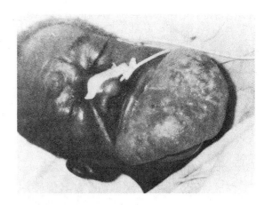

FIGURE 18-20

Monstrous macroglossia in a 74-year-old man with MM and amyloidosis of the tongue. At presentation the patient was unable to retract his immense tongue and could not swallow; airway obstruction necessitated tracheostomy. (From Jacobs P et al: Massive macroglossia, amyloidosis and myeloma. Postgrad Med J 64:969,1988.)

illustrated by the grievous protuberance portrayed in Figure 18-20 [23].

Amyloid has a peculiar tendency to infiltrate volar carpal tunnels and their ligaments, and among the trials besetting MM patients with amyloidosis is the "carpal tunnel" syndrome, with median nerve compression and arterial insufficiency of both hands (Figure 18-21) [24].

Renal Disease

About half of MM patients are persecuted by nephropathies of several distinctive sorts, which can be combined into two basic categories: those related to excretion of light chains; and those resulting from tissue deposition of paraproteins, usually in the form of amyloid or κ chain fragments. The most common renal

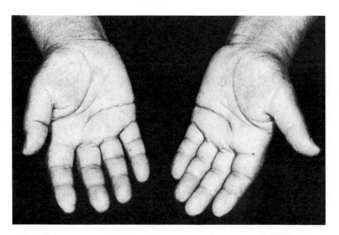

FIGURE 18-21

Carpal tunnel syndrome in a patient with MM and amyloid deposits compressing the median nerve. Wasting of thenar muscles is evident, and the patient complained of weakness and paresthesias of both hands. (From Hoffbrand AV and Pettit JE: Chapt 11, in Clinical Hematology Illustrated. An Integrated Text and Color Atlas. Philadelphia, WB Saunders Company,1987.)

complication is myeloma cast nephropathy provoked by light chain excretion.

Light Chain (BJ) Nephropathy Is Caused by Obstructive Tubular Casts

The load of light chains excreted by patients with MM is commonly in the range of 5 to 10 g/day, and resultant formation of large, hard, tubular casts is the hallmark of BJ nephrosis (Figure 18-22) [17]. Unusually large impacted casts burst tubular basement membranes, stirring up acute and chronic inflammation in the peritubular tissue that can eventuate in interstitial fibrosis and renal failure. Dehydration with poor renal perfusion expedites precipitation of BJ protein in the tubular lumen and protein precipitates may be turned to concrete by the excessive levels of Ca^{2+}. Recovery is nonetheless possible if renal perfusion is restored and loop diuretics are employed to flush out calcium.

Tissue Deposition of Paraproteins

Two types of paraprotein accretion in tissues can be differentiated: amyloid and nonamyloid. Both are derived from light chains, being predominantly λ chains in amyloid and κ chains in nonamyloid deposits. Both light chain isotypes are preferentially and initially deposited in the same renal structures (mesangium, tubular basement membranes, and vessel walls), but κ chains are particularly toxic to tubular basement membranes (Figure 18-23) [25]. The severity of nephrotoxicity in light chain disease has little correlation with the urinary level of free light chains, prompting the view that damage to proximal tubules is determined by the charge (isoelectric point), sialylation, or polymeric size of the light chain fragments; however, none of these properties (including isoelectric point) shows a clear correspondence with the degree of irreversible damage [26].

The shadow of renal failure darkens the prospects of all patients with uncontrolled light chain disease. When a patient is threatened with acute renal failure it becomes imperative to instigate such measures as forced alkaline diuresis and even plasmapheresis to encourage riddance of light chains, calcium, uric acid, and other noxious metabolites. These ministrations,

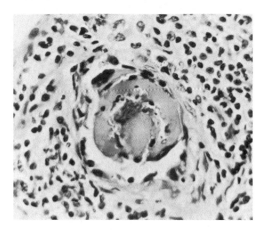

FIGURE 18-22

BJ nephrosis with plugging of the excretory tubule by a dense lamellated cast containing internal fractures. Note epithelial reaction to the protein casts, including (at the top of the field) epithelial giant cells. (From Azar HA: Chapt 1, in Multiple Myeloma and Related Disorders, vol. I, Azar HA and Potter M, Eds. New York, Harper & Row, Publishers, Inc.,1973.)

FIGURE 18-23

Diffuse κ chain nephropathy. Renal medulla in a patient with κ chain myeloma, showing ribbonlike PAS+ thickening of the tubular basement membranes. (From Hill GS et al: Renal lesions in multiple myeloma: their relationship to associated protein abnormalities. Am J Kidney Dis 2:432,1983.)

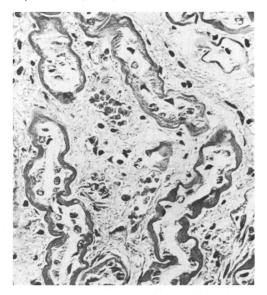

however necessary, are temporizing; lasting effect depends on the degree of success in suppressing growth of secretory myeloma cells.

Neurologic Problems

As may be predicted by the foregoing inventory of complications common in MM—infections, compression fractures, hypercalcemia, amyloidosis—the course of myeloma is savaged by neurologic sequelae, the most calamitous of which is spinal cord compression. Myeloma tumors leading to cord compression arise either in the epidural space or in the vertebral bodies themselves, and crowding of the cord progresses rapidly (within a few weeks of onset of back pain), causing paraplegia, incontinence, and a "sensory level" below the involved dermatome. Plasma cell tumors are highly radiosensitive, and fractional doses of irradiation totalling 30 Gy are well tolerated by the cord. Radiotherapy alone is advisable only when compression is partial and is diagnosed and localized early. Most patients suspected of spinal cord compression should have a myelogram and MRI scan for defining the tumor with sufficient precision to permit decompressive surgery.

Hematologic Findings

The nature of myeloma cells, their growth patterns in marrow, and the sequelae of marrow replacement were described earlier. Most patients with MM present with a moderate, slowly evolving nondescript normocytic anemia, which may precede other aberrations suggestive of myeloma by 1 or 2 years. As anemia worsens, the first clues to diagnosis are often the prosaic findings of prominent rouleaux and heavy background graying in Wright-Giemsa—stained blood smears. Anemia is caused by erythroid hypoplasia as well as by myelomatous replacement, and leukoerythroblastic reactions are present but curiously subdued. Severity of the anemia is exaggerated by plasma volume expansion caused by intravascular trapping of immunoglobulins. Geographic occupancy of the marrow is widespread but stealthy, with inexplicably few plasma cells surfacing in the bloodstream. A comparably mysterious exception to this generalization is the occurrence in 1% of MM

patients of "plasma cell leukemia." Defined by the fiat that plasma cell levels must be in excess of 2,000/μl, plasma cell leukemia (PCL) can occur either as the finale to advanced MM (secondary PCL) or more often as a rampaging primary event, associated with plasma cell concentrations averaging 30,000/μl, massive infiltration of marrow, spleen, liver, and lungs with plasmablasts, and severe anemia and thrombocytopenia. Paraproteinemic problems are usually severe in primary PCL and monoclonal IgE is overrepresented. Primary PCL, unlike the "leukemoid" terminal phase of pervasive MM, sometimes responds well, if briefly, to chemotherapy.

Management

MM runs an erratic but inexorable downhill course with a median survival of 2 to 3 years. For lack of definitive therapy patients are subjected to a biblical crescendo of crippling and debilitating agonies that test the spirit of the patient and the compassion and resourcefulness of physicians and nurses. In patients with highly proliferative myeloma dominated by plasmablasts and associated with hypodiploidy, incongruous phenotypic features such as CALLA-positivity, and a large tumor mass, the outlook is grim, survival seldom exceeding several months. For the past 25 years the standard chemotherapeutic combination used to combat this dogged and deadly neoplasm has been melphelan plus prednisone (MP). Subsequent combinations of alkylating agents with or without adriamycin have not improved survival further, and experience with more intensive chemotherapeutic protocols offers no evidence that MM is chemocurable. The slight gain in quality of life is offset by the inordinate frequency of secondary AML (Chapter 13). In recent years superior results have been obtained with three non-cross-resistant regimens: high-dose melphelan plus total body irradiation; high-dose glucocorticoid therapy intensified by continuous infusion of vincristine, adriamycin, and dexamethasone ("VAD") for hyperproliferative MM; and recombinant alpha interferon (IFNα) for patients with low tumor-mass disease [2]. Complete remissions after marrow ablation and autologous transplant rescue are infrequent, better results being achieved with allogeneic marrow transplantation [27].

Weapons of a different sort may be needed to halt this remorseless growth. The wealth of receptors expressed by myeloma cells can be exploited for targeting immunotoxins, and the possibility that autostimulatory cytokines employed by myeloma cells might be countered with biological modifiers sustains the Panglossian conviction that MM will some day be conquered.

WALDENSTRÖM'S MACROGLOBULINEMIA

Waldenström's macroglobulinemia (WM) is an uncommon indolent secretory B cell malignancy manifested by accumulation of monoclonal IgM in plasma, invasion of marrow by plasmacytoid lymphocytes, and infiltrative enlargement of lymph nodes, spleen, and liver. WM presents with anemia, bleeding, peripheral neuropathy, serum hyperviscosity, and cardiovascular effects of plasma expansion caused by intravascular trapping of IgM paraprotein.

Pathophysiology

WM is a chronic lymphoproliferative disorder manifested by infiltration of marrow and lymph nodes by heterogeneous populations of lymphoid and lymphoplasmacytoid cells that synthesize and secrete IgM having a singular heavy and light chain type and idiotype. The large lymphoid and plasmacytoid cells contain cytoplasmic IgM, and more conventional-appearing lymphocytes in the malignant admixture express sIgM (and sometimes sIgD): both cytoplasmic and surface molecules of IgM in these populations of "plymphs" share the same idiotype as the serum M component. Furthermore, in those cases where the M component has demonstrable antibody activity, surface membrane molecules of lymphoid cells have identical specificity. Hence, despite their cytologic pleomorphism, the lymphs, plymphs, and plasma cells comprising WM infiltrates are members of the same clone, and their clonal IgM class places the point of mutation at a level just prior to the heavy chain class switch. The motley, polymorphic appearance of tumor cell infiltrates of lymph nodes and marrow explains the heavy reliance on the "fudge"

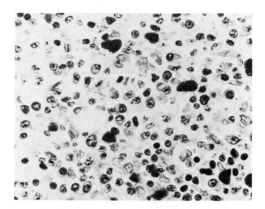

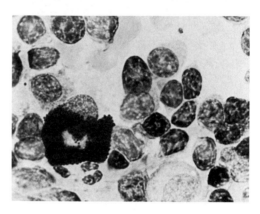

F I G U R E 18-24

Polymorphic appearance of marrow from a patient with WM. (Above) Low-power view of Giemsa-stained marrow biopsy reveals a busy farrago of lymphocytes, plasma cells, and many intermediate forms, plus numerous mast cells. (Below) High-power view of Wright-Giemsa–stained aspirate brings out the lymphoid appearance of most cells and the range of their heterogeneity, encompassing small lymphocytes, large plymphocytes, and a few plasma cells. The eye-catching mast cell—a regular member of the cast in WM marrow—appears squashed. (From Jandl JH: Chapt 26, in Blood: Textbook of Hematology. Boston, Little, Brown and Company, 1987.)

ending "-oid" so prevalent in descriptions of WM cytology (Figure 18-24) [15].

Monoclonal IgM in WM often Reacts with a Defined Antigen

As with MM, in which the M components often have antigenic specificity toward autogenous or exogenous antigens (Table 18-2), monoclonal IgM in WM commonly (in at least 20% of cases) reacts with self-antigens, sometimes with important clinical consequences. IgM paraproteins often show specific affinity for red cell antigens at low temperature. The commonest targets are I antigen alone or in conjunction with H, A, or B determinants. The most frequent known antibody specificity of IgM in WM is for polyclonal IgG molecules; interaction results in mixed-type cryoglobulins. Both cold-active reactions are capable of causing acrocyanosis by obstructing chilled peripheral vessels (Figure 18-25) [28].

Clonal IgM autoantibodies may be encoded by perseverating ancestral genes   There is a suspicious similarity among M components having antigen specificity. Monoclonal IgM antibodies are almost always IgMκ and appear to be focused on a very limited number of autogenous targets, among which are Ii antigens (against which people normally possess autoantibodies) and intermediate filament proteins such as vimentin and myelin-associated glycoproteins, which may explain the mysteriously high incidence of autoimmune neuropathies in WM. In WM—even more plausibly than in MM—the vigorous production of monoclonal autoantibodies appears to reflect a limited breakdown in self-tolerance, particularly for molecules encoded by ancestral germline genes highly conserved in human evolution.

Description

Most clinical features of WM stem from high levels of IgM and the resultant hyperviscosity. The cardiovascular burden of pumping viscous blood is magnified by a concurrent expansion of plasma volume. Because of its great molecular girth, over 90% of IgM remains confined to the plasma compartment, where it exerts an unbalanced transendothelial osmotic force and hence hypervolemia. The expanded plasma volume engenders dilutional anemia, volume overload, vascular distension, and augmented cardiac filling and output. The combined increase in cardiac output and blood viscosity eventually exhausts the laboring myocardium and congestive failure sets in. In a rheologic

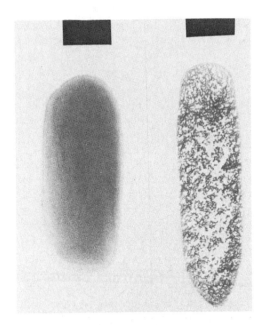

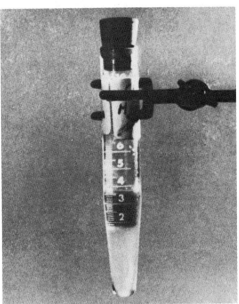

FIGURE 18-25

Cold agglutination and cryoprecipitation caused by monoclonal IgM from patients with WM. (Above) Agglutination at 4°C of autologous red cells (while being smeared) is shown on the right; control is on the left. (Below) Serum cryoprecipitate consisting of monoclonal IgM having anti-IgG activity. (From Greaves MF et al: Chapt 9, in Atlas of Blood Cells: Function and Pathology, vol. 1, 2nd ed. Zucker-Franklin D et al, Eds. Milan, Edi. Ermes s.r.l.,1988.)

sense, WM is an etiolated equivalent of polycythemia vera.

Ocular Manifestation

Macroscopic rouleaux induced by high concentrations of IgM are just as visible in conjunctival vessels and by fundoscopy as in drawn blood. Fundoscopy provides a window for monitoring circulatory aberrations in WM. As IgM levels rise, patients complain of darkened vision, and fundoscopy reveals sausagelike segmentation of the distended, tortuous retinal veins; eventually retinal hemorrhages, exudates, and microaneurysms crop up (Figure 18-26) [29].

Neuropsychiatric Problems

The most common neurologic consequence of macroglobulinemic hyperviscosity is acute cerebral malfunction, starting with headache, slowed mentation, and confusion, progressing to somnolence and coma (coma paraproteinicum). Disturbances in affect and mentation, often accompanied by mysterious neurologic complaints, are often misinterpreted as psychopathic manifestations; patients seen by hematologists prior to psychiatric referral rapidly recover their mental balance following plasmapheresis.

Polyneuropathy The peripheral neuropathy afflicting 10 to 20% of patients with WM is usually unrelated to hyperviscosity effects, and its protean manifestations mirror the multitude of its mechanisms. In some instances lymphoplasmacytoid infiltrates have been found surrounding small vessels that nourish affected nerves; in others amyloid deposits are responsible for nerve damage. The most distinctive lesion involves selective fixation of monoclonal IgM to myelin sheaths; frequently IgM attached to nerves or Schwann cells shows idiotypic identity to plasma IgM, suggesting that the polyneuropathy of WM may be a malignant autoimmune process.

Renal Abnormalities

Although BJ proteinuria occurs in about 70% of WM patients, the quantity of light chains excreted is minimal and cast nephropathy does not occur. When present, renal damage is

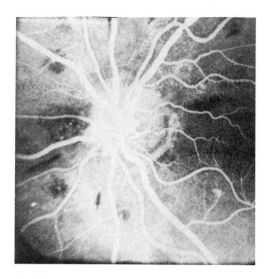

FIGURE 18-26

Retinal appearance in a patient with WM and hyperviscosity syndrome. All vessels are distended, particularly the veins which show bulging and A:V constriction, and the fundus is spattered with white exudates and dark hemorrhages; the fanlike arteriolar expansions are microaneurysms. All aberrations reverted to normal following plasmapheresis. (From Paladini G: Chapt 13, in Multiple Myeloma and Other Paraproteinemias, Delamore IN, Ed. Edinburgh, Churchill Livingstone,1986.)

confined to glomeruli, which become damaged or obstructed by accumulations of IgM that collect on the endothelial side of the basement membrane.

Hematologic Findings

Anemia, which is almost invariable, results from severe hemodilution, usually complicated by recurrent loss of blood from engorged nasal, gingival, intestinal, and other mucosal surfaces. Red cells are either normocytic or hypochromic, and characteristically form striking rouleaux that cause a proportionate increase in sedimentation rate. Leukocytosis is uncommon, lymphocyte counts usually falling below 4,000 cells/μl. With or without mild lymphocytosis, lymphoplasmacytic cells usually can be found, and the monoclonal nature of these B cell variants can be verified by κ/λ analysis of cellular sIg.

Monoclonal IgM Hampers Hemostasis

WM patients are beset with recurrent bleeding problems primarily involving mucosa of the mouth, gums, nose, and gastrointestinal tract. Platelet levels are usually normal, but platelet function is disturbed by nonspecific coating by IgM. The most characteristic coagulation defect is prolongation of the thrombin time as the result of binding of M component to fibrin: this blocks orderly aggregation of fibrin monomers and the un-crosslinked fibrin forms bulky gelatinous clots incapable of retraction. Surplus IgM also gums up factors VIII, V, and VII, thereby impeding activation of the prothrombinase complex.

Marrow and Histologic Staging

The pleomorphism of lymphoplasmacytic infiltrates in marrow makes morphologic quantitations difficult, but a staging system has been advocated for segregating three cytologic patterns having prognostic significance. These are based upon distinguishing lymphocyte predominance (lymphoplasmacytoid pattern),

FIGURE 18-27

Schematic matching of geographic growth patterns in WM marrow sections (left) with cytologic patterns (right). (From Bartl R et al: Bone marrow histology in Waldenström's macroglobulinaemia. Clinical relevance of subtype recognition. Scand J Haematol 31:359,1983. © 1983 Munksgaard International Publishers Ltd., Copenhagen, Denmark.)

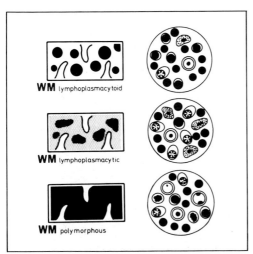

plasma cell plurality (lymphoplasmacytic pattern), and a mixed "polymorphous" pattern in which plasmablasts (as well as lymphocytes and plasma cells) are numerous and accompanied by small numbers of immunoblasts and follicular cells (centrocytes and centroblasts). The merit of this subclassification is that these three cytologic patterns correlate with the geographic magnitude of growth pattern in marrow biopsies (Figure 18-27) [30].

Management

WM is a slow-growing neoplasm that has no cure but requires attentive shepherding to cope with the hazards of anemia, bleeding, and hyperviscosity. Tumor growth is controlled on an ad hoc basis with low-dose oral alkylators such as chlorambucil. Hyperviscosity problems respond quickly to plasmapheresis, which should be repeated as necessary until the relative viscosity of serum falls below 4.

REFERENCES

1. Clofent G et al: No detectable malignant B cells in the peripheral blood of patients with multiple myeloma. Br J Haematol 71:357, 1989

2. Barlogie B et al: Plasma cell myeloma—new biological insights and advances in therapy. Blood 73:865,1989

3. Kyle RA: 'Benign' monoclonal gammopathy: a misnomer? JAMA 251:1849,1984

4. Grogan TM et al: Delineation of a novel pre-B cell component in plasma cell myeloma: immunochemical, immunophenotypic, genotypic, cytologic, cell culture, and kinetic features. Blood 70:932,1987

5. Mundy GR et al: Evidence for the secretion of an osteoclast stimulating factor in myeloma. N Engl J Med 291:1041,1974

6. Gould J et al: Plasma cell karyotype in multiple myeloma. Blood 71:453,1988

7. Kyle RA and Greipp PR: The laboratory investigation of monoclonal gammopathies. Mayo Clin Proc 53:719,1978

8. Riches PG: Chapt 5, in Multiple Myeloma and Other Paraproteinemias, Delamore IN, Ed. Edinburgh, Churchill Livingstone,1986

9. Hobbs JR: Immunochemical classes of myelomatosis. Including data from a thera-

peutic trial conducted by a Medical Research Council working party. Br J Haematol 16:599,1969

10. Merlini G et al: Monoclonal immunoglobulins with antibody activity in myeloma, macroglobulinemia and related plasma cell dyscrasias. Semin Oncol 13:350,1986

11. Osserman EF et al: Multiple myeloma and related plasma cell dyscrasias. JAMA 258: 2930,1987

12. Seligmann M et al: Heavy chain diseases: current findings and concepts. Immunol Rev 48:145,1979

13. Bartl R et al: Histologic classification and staging of multiple myeloma: a retrospective and prospective study of 674 cases. Am J Clin Pathol 87:342,1987

14. Weinstein T et al: Electron microscopy study of Mott and Russell bodies in myeloma cells. J Submicrosc Cytol 19:155,1987

15. Jandl JH: Chapt 26, in Blood: Textbook of Hematology. Boston, Little, Brown and Company,1987

16. Hayhoe FGJ et al: Chapt 6, in Multiple Myeloma and Other Paraproteinemias, Delamore IN, Ed. Edinburgh, Churchill Livingstone,1986

17. Azar HA: Chapt 1, in Multiple Myeloma and Related Disorders, vol. I, Azar HA and Potter M, Eds. New York, Harper & Row, Publishers, Inc.,1973

18. Snapper I: Medical Clinics on Bone Diseases. New York, Interscience Publishers, Inc., 1943

19. Snapper I: Rare Manifestations of Metabolic Bone Disease. Springfield, Charles C. Thomas, Publisher,1952

20. Fruehwald FXJ et al: Magnetic resonance imaging of the lower vertebral column in patients with multiple myeloma. Invest Radiol 23:193,1988

21. Helms CA and Genant HK: Computed tomography in the early detection of skeletal involvement with multiple myeloma. JAMA 248:2886,1982

22. Coward RA: Chapt 16, in Multiple Myeloma and Other Paraproteinemias, Delamore IN, Ed. Edinburgh, Churchill Livingstone, 1986

23. Jacobs P et al: Massive macroglossia, amyloidosis and myeloma. Postgrad Med J 64:969,1988

24. Hoffbrand AV and Pettit JE: Chapt 11, in Clinical Hematology Illustrated. An Integrated Text and Color Atlas. Philadelphia, WB Saunders Company, 1987

25. Hill GS et al: Renal lesions in multiple myeloma: their relationship to associated protein abnormalities. Am J Kidney Dis 2:423,1983

26. Johns EA et al: Isoelectric points of urinary light chains in myelomatosis: analysis in relation to nephrotoxicity. J Clin Pathol 39:833,1986

27. Gahrton G et al: Allogeneic bone marrow transplantation in 24 patients with multiple myeloma reported to the EBMT registry. Hematol Oncol 6:181,1988

28. Greaves MF et al: Chapt 9, in Atlas of Blood Cells: Function and Pathology, vol. 1, Zucker-Franklin D et al, Eds. Milan, Edi. Ermes s.r.l.,1988

29. Paladini G: Chapt 13, in Multiple Myeloma and Other Paraproteinemias, Delamore IN, Ed. Edinburgh, Churchill Livingstone,1986

30. Bartl R et al: Bone marrow histology in Waldenström's macroglobulinaemia. Clinical relevance of subtype recognition. Scand J Haematol 31:359,1983

19

Hodgkin's Disease

☐

Hodgkin's disease (HD) is a solid lymphoid neoplasm originating in lymph nodes and eventually (unless halted by therapy) disseminating at will throughout the lymphatics and neighboring tissues. HD differs from other malignant lymphomas in several remarkable ways. The neoplastic founder cell and talisman of HD—the numinous Reed-Sternberg (RS) cell and its mononuclear companions—generally comprise a very small percentage of tumor cells. In most subtypes of HD these novel giant cells are vastly outnumbered and surrounded by a disorganized polyclonal admixture of normal-appearing lymphocytes, eosinophils, and plasma cells; this rabble ordinarily forms the militia of immune reactions, and the picture conveyed is of guerrilla warfare rather than clonal conformity. Finally, HD is curable in over 70% of cases, whereas most non-Hodgkin's lymphomas are eventually fatal. The rebellious histology of HD, the manifold subforms of the disease, and difficulties in verifying the phenotype and clonality of RS cells have long bred doubts as to whether or not HD is a true neoplasm; indeed, as noted below, HD has some characteristics of an infection. Nevertheless, HD certainly behaves like a neoplasm: it grows without control, infiltrates vital organs, and is only eradicated by tumoricidal weapons. In its comportment, HD qualifies as a malignant disorder, even though we lack the molecular means of calling it one [1].

Incidence and Epidemiology

The annual crude incidence for HD in the United States is 36 per million white men and 26 per million white women, with an average age at diagnosis of 32 years. In 1989 there were 7,400 new cases and 1,600 fatalities, implying an overall mortality of about 20%.

Unlike other malignancies including non-Hodgkin's lymphomas (NHLs), which show a steep rise in frequency with age, HD incidence is bimodal with an initial peak at age 20 to 30 and a separated second summit after age 60, which, while prominent, lacks the magnitude of that of other hematologic neoplasms (Figure 19-1) [2].

Is HD an Infectious Malignancy?

Despite lack of evidence for lateral transmission, the sudden rise in disease frequency in adolescence and early adulthood and bimodality created by resurgence in later life is reminiscent of chronic infections such as tuberculosis, and has nourished the view that HD in young adults is a deranged response to infection, while the disease in older adults (which is far less responsive to therapy) is a conventional malignancy. In economically developed countries, risk of HD is associated with a background of cloistered or sheltered upbringing (small family size, single family housing, high maternal educational level); in the crowded, less ordered environments of underdeveloped countries, the peak onset is shifted toward childhood, particularly in boys. This characteristically soft epidemiologic evidence for an infectious etiology has received firmer support from observations that approximately 20% of patients with HD have Epstein-Barr virus (EBV) DNA within RS cells and that the infected cells are monoclonal [3]. Any further discussion of the pathophysiology of HD requires focus on the central character in HD tumors, the bizarre and beguiling Reed-Sternberg cell.

PATHOPHYSIOLOGY

Central to the diagnosis of HD, RS cells are the exotic insignia of HD. On Wright-Giemsa–stained smears of aspirates, classic RS cells are very large and possess voluminous pale cytoplasm enveloping two or more large oval or lobular nuclei, each of which contains an immense nucleolus (Figure 19-2) [4]. Although RS cells are emblematic of HD, similar cells, often having similar phenotypes, may be encountered in reactive lymph nodes containing activated T cells, in anaplastic large cell lymphoma, and in post-thymic or peripheral T cell lymphoma. Certification as RS cells requires that they be accompanied by malignant-looking variant macrophages (histiocytes or "H cells") or form rosettes with adherent T cells.

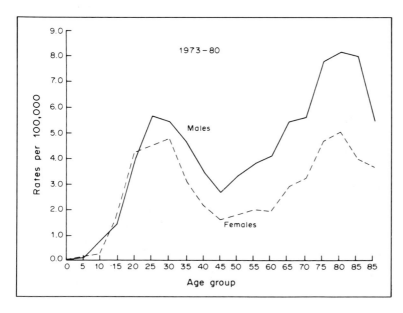

FIGURE 19-1

Average annual age-specific incidence of HD for all SEER regions combined, by sex. SEER = Surveillance, Epidemiology, and End Results program of the National Cancer Institute. (From Glaser SL: Recent incidence and secular trends in Hodgkin's disease and its histologic subtypes. J Chron Dis 39:789,1986.)

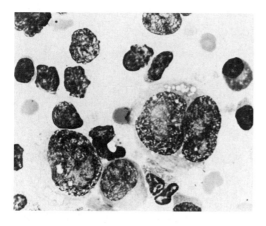

FIGURE 19-2

Marrow smear from a patient with advanced (stage IV) Hodgkin's disease. The classic binucleate RS cell at the right of center stage possesses huge, deformed nucleoli; the twinned nuclei with their nucleolar inclusions create distorted mirror images. The mononuclear variants to the left complete a representative trio and are usually members of the same malignant clone. The three large tumor cells are surrounded by a mélange of lymphocytes, plasma cells, and eosinophils. (From Jandl JH: Chapt 27, in Blood: Textbook of Hematology. Boston, Little, Brown and Company,1987.)

Enigmatic Variations

RS cells have the phenotype of activated lymphoid cells, expressing receptors for IL-2 (CD25), HLA-DR, and Ki-1 (CD30). In most subtypes of HD the RS cells and their "histiocytic" (H cell) colleagues are nonphagocytic, lack Fc receptors, and are strongly immunoreactive for CD15 (Leu M1) and nonreactive for B cell antigens and leukocyte common antigen (CALLA). This phenotypic profile is suggestive of T cell or null cell provenance, and in many cases of nodular sclerosing (NS) HD or mixed cellularity (MC) HD, Southern blot analyses have revealed clonal T cell receptor (TcR) rearrangements. Unfortunately, no canonical clarity has emerged from such probing, for in other clinically similar patients clonal immunoglobulin (Ig) gene rearrangements have also been revealed, and in many instances immature genotype patterns are inappropriately associated with late activation markers (Figure 19-3) [5]. In patients with lymphocyte predominant (LP) type of HD, nodular form, the lymphocytic and histiocytic (L&H) variants of RS cells uniformly exhibit immunoreactivity with the pan B cell marker, L26 [6], and the

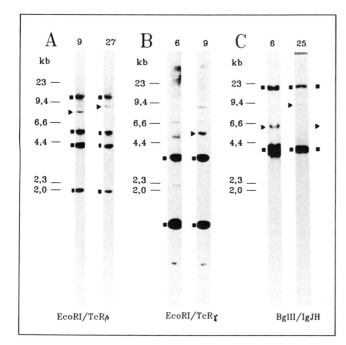

FIGURE 19-3

Southern blot analysis of DNA digests from four patients with HD. Black squares = germline bands; black arrowheads = rearranged bands. Numbers at the top of each lane identify individual patients. In patients 9 and 27, clonal rearrangements were identified by probes for either TcR$_\beta$ or TcR$_\gamma$ or both. In patient 6, no clonal TcR rearrangements were detected, but probing for JH chain genes revealed an Ig rearrangement band, as was true also in patient 25. (Reprinted with permission from Herbst H et al: Immunoglobulin and T-cell receptor gene rearrangements in Hodgkin's disease and Ki-1-positive anaplastic large cell lymphoma: dissociation between phenotype and genotype. Leuk Res 13:103. Copyright 1989, Pergamon Press PLC.)

disease preferentially invades B cell areas of lymph nodes, in contrast to the T zone distribution of most forms of HD. In some patients with nodular sclerosing HD (NS HD), RS cells and H variants contain (and are immortalized by) EBV genomes, as demonstrated by Southern blot analysis and in situ hybridization studies, providing indirect evidence that these tumor cells are of clonal B cell origin [3]. Before leaping to any generalization it should be noted that, as in Burkitt's lymphoma, EBV infection may operate as a cofactor in these immunosuppressed patients, causing polyclonal B cell hyperplasia and predisposing to a second event such as translocation that triggers malignant transformation.

HD Is a Consortium of Lymphomas

At this writing molecular probe technology has not satisfactorily resolved the issues as to the clonality or lineage derivation of RS and H cells. The most prevalent HD subtypes—mixed cellularity (MC) and nodular sclerosing (NS)—have features of activated lymphoid cells, some of B and others of T cell origin, and some are mixed or chimeric. The torrential confusion as to the genetic, antigenic, and clonal makeup of HD tumor cells is best summarized by acknowledging—as has long been suggested by histologic appearances—that HD represents an extended family of distinctive lymphoid neoplasms, analogous in their diversity and mixed lineages to the family of non-Hodgkin's lymphomas. Collectively HD encompasses a consortium or confederacy of clonal lymphocyte populations in which different rearrangement patterns (simple or complex) are associated with different histologic subclasses of HD. In making this politic assertion, the author admittedly is unnerved by the unblinking owlish glare of the imperious RS founder cell itself (Figure 19-4) [7].

Cell-Mediated Immunity Is Defective in HD, Predisposing to Opportunistic Infections

Although antibody responses to soluble antigens are robust in HD and Ig levels are normal or elevated, cell-mediated immunity is enfeebled early in the disease process, as indicated by anergy to recall skin tests, impaired rejection of

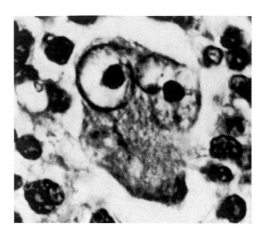

FIGURE 19-4

Glaring visage of an RS cell highly magnified, from a lymph node of a patient with HD, mixed cellularity type. H & E section. (Reproduced by permission from: Cawson RA et al, Eds: Pathology. The Mechanisms of Disease, 2d ed. St. Louis, The CV Mosby Company,1989.)

skin allografts, and increased susceptibility to opportunistic fungal and viral infections. Selective depression of cell-mediated immunity stems from unresponsiveness of the T cell network, as manifest by subnormal production of IL-2 and indecisive display of IL-2 receptors after appropriate stimulation—a defect akin to that in patients with AIDS. In addition HD patients are characteristically lymphopenic, and T cells undergo a T4:T8 inversion that favors immunosuppression.

Histopathologic Classification of HD

The diverse histopathology of HD is subdivided (according to the Rye modification of the Lukes and Butler classification) into morphologically distinctive entities in recognition that HD tumors may manifest lymphocyte predominance (LP) at one extreme and lymphocyte depletion (LD) at the other, with intermediate patterns between, characterized by mixed cellularity (MC) or a picturesque pattern in which RS cells are individually encased by nodular sclerosis (NS). Characteristics of the several histologic types of HD are summarized in Table 19-1 [8].

TABLE 19-1

Summary of histopathologic features and RS cell phenotypes in HD

Subtype	Frequency (%)	RS cell variant	Appearance of RS cell	Histologic pattern	Phenotype
LP	15	Popcorn cell	Wrinkled, twisted nucleus; small nucleoli; RS cells infrequent	Intrafollicular	B; CD30$^+$, CD15$^-$
NS	40	Lacunar cell	Pale retracted cytoplasm; 1 or several nuclei; small, sometimes basophilic nucleoli	Inter- or intrafollicular with sclerosis	T, B, or null; CD30$^+$, CD15$^-$
MC	30	Classical	Binucleate or multinucleate, with huge inclusionlike nucleoli	Interfollicular or diffuse	T, B, or null; CD30$^+$, CD15$^-$
LD	15	Sarcomatous	Pleomorphic hyperchromatic nuclei; nucleoli often indistinct	Diffuse fibrosis	Unknown; CD30$^+$, CD15$^-$

LP = lymphocyte predominance, NS = nodular sclerosis, MC = mixed cellularity, LD = lymphocyte depletion.

Source: Modified and amended from Greenberger J et al: Hodgkin's disease, in Hematology—1988 Education Program. American Society of Hematology, December 1988.

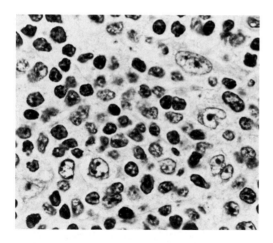

FIGURE 19-5

Lymphocyte predominant HD. Small lymphocytes predominate in this comparatively benign subtype of HD, but scattered about are large typical and atypical H cells, some of which have a puffy, exploded look (lower left) inspiring the term "popcorn cell." Characteristically many fields have to be scrutinized to find the single elusive but demonic binucleate RS cell toward the lower right. (Section stained with Giemsa.) (Photo by CT Kapff.)

Lymphocyte Predominant HD

In the LP subtype of HD, lymph nodes are heavily infiltrated by mature B lymphocytes, often vaguely arrayed in large nodular formations surrounded by ragged clusters of epithelioid H cells, among which are mononuclear cells with knobby or twisted nuclei that sometimes bear a fanciful resemblance to popped corn (Figure 19-5). The LP subtype most commonly occurs in young men and presents as localized high cervical adenopathy. The plenitude of healthy-looking lymphocytes symbolizes strong host resistance, and fewer than 30% of cases progress beyond stage II involvement; response to therapy is usually rapid and durable.

Nodular Sclerosing HD

In NS HD, tumor cell infiltrates are subdivided into nodules by dense collagenous bands. Atypical H cells and RS cells, imprisoned within sclerotic chambers, retract their cytoplasm as an artifact of dehydration and fixation and acquire a larval appearance. The tumor cells

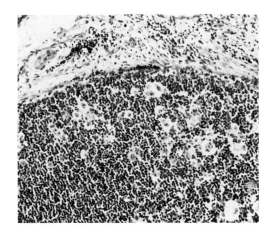

FIGURE 19-6

Lymph node biopsy showing a large lymphoid tumor nodule firmly enveloped by broad bands of collagenous connective tissue. Within the compact masses of lymphocytes are individual lacunar cells trapped like bugs in amber; shrinkage artifact accounts for the capacious caskets. (Section stained with Giemsa.) (Photo by CT Kapff.)

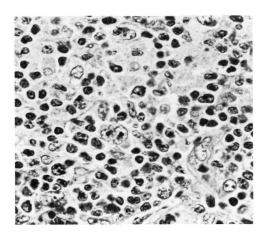

FIGURE 19-7

Mixed cellularity HD. Disorderly mix of macrophages, epithelioid cells, lymphocytes, and eosinophils, mingling freely with RS and H cells, with occasional lacunar cells (top center). Indistinct groupings of cells are vaguely suggestive of a granulomatous reaction. (Section stained with Giemsa.) (Photo by CT Kapff.)

within their cocoons are termed "lacunar cells," and whether or not they resemble classic RS cells, lacunar cells confer the imprimatur of HD (Figure 19-6). NS is the most common histologic subtype of HD, constituting over 40% of cases, and is the only variant more common in women than men. It has a predilection for mediastinal, pulmonary, and supraclavicular involvement, and often appears to arise in the thymus. NS HD spreads only by direct contiguity and prognosis at a given stage of extension is relatively good, possibly because of the host's fibrogenic defense.

Mixed Cellularity HD

Biopsy discloses a polymorphous infiltrate composed of lymphocytes, macrophages, eosinophils, and plasma cells; the histologic pattern is usually disorganized and may contain small foci of necrosis. Loose granulomatous conformations may be found with some fibrosis but no collagen band formation. Classical RS cells and mononuclear variants are numerous (5 to 10 per high-power field), and occasional lacunar cells may be discovered (Figure 19-7).

FIGURE 19-8

Lymphocyte depletion HD. Parenchymal structure of this node has been plundered by large, deviant RS cells and their accomplices. Many tumor cells are clustered, some are hyperchromatic, and much of the sarcomatous infiltrate is enmeshed in diffuse fibrillar connective tissue. Lymphocytes are sparse and appear devitalized. (Section stained with Giemsa.) (Photo by CT Kapff.)

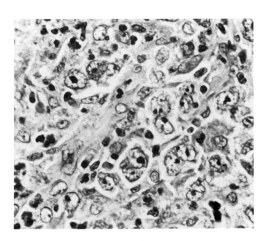

In MC HD the lymphocyte population appears to be outnumbered by tumor cells and nodes display features of inflammation, signifying an intermediate degree of host resistance and a prognosis less sunny than that of NS.

Lymphocyte Depletion HD

In this, the least desirable form of HD, normal cellular elements of affected lymph nodes are replaced by swarms and clusters of large atypical H cells and RS forms, with only a few embattled remnants of lymphocytes remaining (Figure 19-8). Patients with LD HD are generally older than other HD patients and usually present with retroperitoneal adenopathy, fever, and advanced stage disease.

DESCRIPTION

HD arises from a single anatomic focus, starting in lymph nodes in 90% of cases. It usually presents as painless asymmetrical enlargement of nodes above the diaphragm, initially as discrete rubbery adenopathy but spreading by direct contiguity within the lymphatics to form coalescent masses (Figure 19-9) [9]. Diagnosis is made by histologic examination of excised nodes, which on cut section reveal a pale, uniform, fish-flesh appearance (Figure 19-10) [7]. The pattern of spread of HD is characteristically axial, with contiguous progression to mediastinal and paraaortic nodes via lymphatic channels. Lesions first noted in the neck occasionally skip the mediastinum and spread to upper retroperitoneal nodes, possibly by retrograde flow. Primary subdiaphragmatic presentation is uncommon.

Extranodal Involvement

HD spreads to extranodal sites either by direct extension or by hematogenous dissemination. Thoracic duct fluid from patients with extensive paraaortic nodal involvement invariably contains RS cells, and eventual trapping of these bulky stem cells by the spleen is inevitable. A beachhead in the spleen, in turn, favors metastatic dissemination to liver and then to marrow. This "island hopping" mode of dissemination to marrow is relatively common in advanced HD with mixed cellular or lympho-

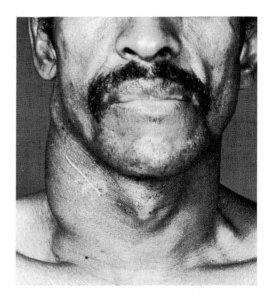

FIGURE 19-9

Clustered right cervical lymphadenopathy in Hodgkin's disease. Note well-healed biopsy incision. (From Hoffbrand AV and Pettit JE: Chapt 10, in Sandoz Atlas of Clinical Hematology, London, Gower Medical Publishing,1988.)

FIGURE 19-10

Coalescing mass of enlarged cervical lymph nodes from a patient with Hodgkin's disease. Observe the uniform fleshy appearance of their cut surfaces and fine lines of demarcation outlining individual nodes. (Reproduced by permission from: Cawson RA et al, Eds: Pathology. The Mechanisms of Disease, 2d ed. St. Louis, The CV Mosby Company,1989.)

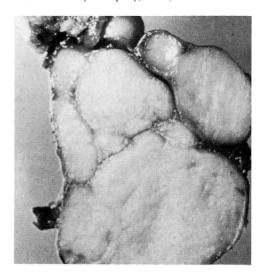

cyte depletion histologies but is rare in patients with nodular sclerosis or any form of early stage disease. By definition, HD in marrow signifies pathologic stage IV disease.

Systemic Symptoms of HD

Systemic symptoms associated with HD are portentous prognostic indicators, and their presence is designated in staging classifications by appending the letter B. The classic B triad consists of fever, sweats, and loss of 10% or more of weight within the prior 6 months. Severe pruritus—not occasional itchiness, but obstinate, formicating, crawling pruritus leading to excoriations—is somehow linked to the biology of aggressiveness of HD and should be included as a B symptom.

Major Syndromes and Organ Involvement

Mediastinal HD

Mediastinal involvement occurs in nearly half of patients with supradiaphragmatic disease, and most cases respond rapidly to therapy. Early occurrence of bulky mediastinal adenopathy, on the contrary, poses a serious threat to adjacent vital structures (trachea, lung, bronchi, and pericardium) and may represent a medical emergency. Mediastinal adenopathy is defined as bulky if the ratio of the width of the mass over maximum thoracic cage diameter (M:T ratio) is in excess of 0.3. No calculator is needed to make this assessment in the patient with nodular sclerosing HD whose chest radiograph is shown in Figure 19-11 [10]. Bulky mediastinal adenopathy mandates prompt and intensive combined modality therapy, and the consequence of misjudging the magnitude of tumor involvement can be catastrophic. Tracheobronchial constriction by paratracheal HD tumors—particularly the leathery noose of nodular sclerosing HD—is quite capable of throttling the patient unless the tumor mass is forced to loosen its grip by appropriate irradiation. CT scanning is unrivalled in defining the size, shape, and malign potential of upper mediastinal, hilar, and paracardiac nodal involvement (Figure 19-12) [11].

Subdiaphragmatic HD

HD patients seldom present with disease limited to nodes below the diaphragm, but

Posteroanterior film shows a huge lobulated mediastinal mass formed by a conglomeration of large lymph nodes in a 17-year-old woman with NS HD. (From Kaplan HS: Hodgkin's Disease, 2d ed. Cambridge, Harvard University Press,1980.)

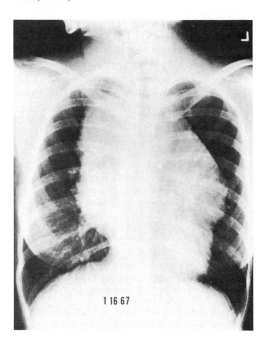

subdiaphragmatic tumors develop in over 40% of patients whose lymphomas originated above the diaphragm. Scouting for subdiaphragmatic involvement is most easily performed by high-resolution CT scanners, which can detect nodal groups (such as celiac axis nodes) invisible by other modalities. If CT (or radiogallium) scans are negative in patients suspected of abdominal or retroperitoneal disease, paraaortic, paracaval, and parailiac nodes can be opacified with bipedal lymphangiography (lymphography)—a procedure in which radioopaque dye is injected into lymphatic channels in both feet. An advantage of lymphography over the easier, noninvasive (but expensive) technique of CT scanning is that it illuminates lymph node architectural patterns, rather than merely recording nodal bulk, which may be minimally enlarged in early widespread disease (Figure 19-13) [10]. CT scanning and lymphography are complementary in coverage, but lymphography is unneces-

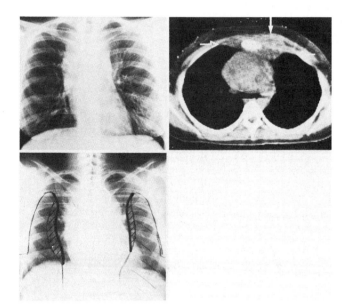

FIGURE 19-12

Bulky anterior mediastinal adenopathy in HD. (Upper left) Posteroanterior chest film shows symmetrical mediastinal widening. (Upper right) CT scan delineates a broad anterior mediastinal mass with subtle lateral extensions (between two lateral arrows) invisible on x-rays; CT also exposes occult parasternal infiltration (upper arrow). (Below) Simulator film outlines on radiograph the proposed irradiation field as determined from CT studies. Hatched parasternal areas indicate additional target tissue to be included in the irradiation portal as tumor shrinkage is ascertained by follow-up CT. (From Meyer JE et al: Impact of thoracic computed tomography on radiation therapy planning in Hodgkin's disease. J Comput Assist Tomogr 8:892, 1984.)

sary even in patients with negative CT scans of the abdomen if their disease is so advanced (B symptoms, involvement of liver or marrow) that choice of therapy would be unaffected.

Neurologic Involvement

HD has a penchant for spreading by direct extension from paravertebral nodes through intervertebral foramina in thoracic or lumbar regions and causing extradural spinal cord compression. Back pain is a prologue to cord transsection, starting with weakness of lower extremities and followed by sensory impairment below the affected dermatome, loss of sphincter control, and paraplegia. Onset of backache and lower body weakness in an HD

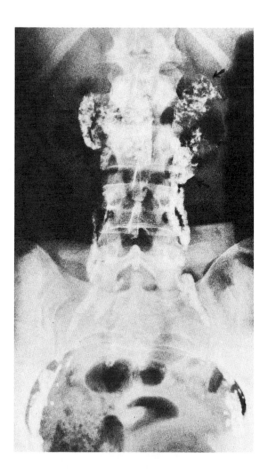

FIGURE 19-13

Bipedal lymphogram revealing lymphomatous infiltration of paraaortic nodes in a 25-year-old patient with NS HD. Note the foamy architecture and filling defects in the bilaterally enlarged upper lumbar paraaortic nodes (arrows). For comparison see the smaller homogeneously opacified normal nodes in the lower lumbar and pelvic lymphatic chains. (From Kaplan HS: Hodgkin's Disease, 2d ed. Cambridge, Harvard University Press, 1980.)

patient should serve as a forewarning of impending cord compression, and mandates an immediate counterattack involving radiography, myelography, and possible surgical decompression plus local irradiation.

Hematologic Findings

Examination of blood and marrow ordinarily provides little essential diagnostic information, abnormalities such as anemia being mild, secondary to disease activity, and late. The most important reason for performing marrow biopsy is in staging disease spread, for the finding of tumor cells in marrow automatically classifies the process as stage IV HD. Marrow involvement by HD is evident in only about 10% of all patients at first examination, but the proportion ranges from about 5% in the favorable subtypes (LP and NS) to over 20% in the unfavorable LD category.

In about 5% of cases, new or relapsing disease activity is accompanied by Coombs-positive autoimmune hemolytic anemia. The autoantibody responsible has been identified in eluates as an IgG anti-I variant selectively reactive with the fetal i antigen as it accompanies ontogenic transition to the adult I determinant. Hence the warm-active autoantibody in HD has been nicknamed "antitransition-" or anti-I^T, a recondite antibody also found in patients with angioimmunoblastic lymphoma. The hemolytic anemia responds well to corticosteroid therapy, but sustained remission and elimination of the antibody requires control of the underlying lymphoma.

Thrombocytopenia may crop up in capricious bouts independent of tumor progression. Usually thrombocytopenic purpura is self-limited, but in some cases severe immune thrombocytopenic purpura is a stubborn complication of HD that may persist despite control of the malignancy. Total white counts in HD are either normal or elevated slightly, and in 10 to 20% of cases eosinophilia may be notable and occasionally is extreme. Lymphopenia is common in HD and contributes to the immunosuppression described earlier.

Staging

Prognosis and choice of therapy depend both on histopathologic classification, described

TABLE 19-2

Hodgkin's disease: Ann Arbor staging classification

Stage	Characteristics
I	Involvement of a single lymph node region (I) or of a single extralymphatic organ or site (I_E).
II	Involvement limited to one side of the diaphragm, either of two or more lymph node regions, or localized involvement of an extralymphatic site (II_E) plus one or more lymph node regions.
III*	Involvement of lymph node regions on both sides of the diaphragm, which may include localized involvement of an extralymphatic site (III_E) or spleen (III_S) or both (III_{SE}).
IV	Diffuse or disseminated involvement of one or more extralymphatic organs or tissues, with or without associated lymph node involvement. The reason for classifying the patient as stage IV should be specified by identifying site with symbols. Hepatic (H) or marrow (M) involvement always indicates stage IV disease.
A	If asymptomatic.
B	If any of the following are present: unexplained loss of more than 10% of body weight in the preceding 6 months; unexplained fever, with temperatures above 38°C; night sweats; severe pruritus.

*Stage III may be divided into: III_1, indicating that disease below the diaphragm is limited to the upper abdomen; and III_2, denoting paraaortic, mesenteric, iliac, or inguinal nodal involvement.

Source: From Jandl JH: Chapt 27 in Blood: Textbook of Hematology. Boston, Little, Brown and Company, 1987.

earlier, and on the geographic extent of disease, as judged by clinical and pathologic staging (CS and PS, respectively). The Ann Arbor classification routinely used in staging of HD includes both clinical and pathologic staging and is presented in Table 19-2 [12]. Until recently radiotherapy was the standard treatment for all stages of HD except stages IV and IIIB. In most centers, combination chemotherapy, which attacks HD throughout the body, has replaced radiotherapy for all patients with B symptoms and for most of those with stage IIIA disease, thus diminishing the need for staging laparotomy. Indeed, some doyens affirm that laparotomy (at $5,000 to $10,000 for inclusive charges) is rarely justified even in stage IA and IIA patients on the grounds that limited-stage disease destined to relapse after radiotherapy can be identified beforehand by use of prognostic indices that take into account age, sex, and presence or absence of mediastinal involvement. Opposing views on "stagecraft" have launched many spirited and rebarbative debates.

MANAGEMENT

Unlike most hematologic malignancies, HD can be eradicated in 60 to 70% of patients. The goal and expectation of therapy is to achieve cure rather than palliation, employing the two most effective weapons at hand: radiation and combination chemotherapy.

Radiation Therapy in HD

The tumoricidal dose level in HD is 35 to 45 Gy delivered in split fractions over a period of about 1 month, and most patients with IA or IIA disease above the diaphragm can be managed with radiotherapy alone. Radiation is best delivered as megavoltage (6–10 MeV) photon beams from a linear accelerator, which permit treatment of large fields at an extended distance and avert damage to the skin. The techniques of field simulation, port-film verification, and tailoring of individually designed contour shielding blocks cut from lead or cast from Lipowitz metal (cerrobend) represent a level of artistry too complex for description here. Suffice it to say that irradiation fields can be designed to encompass nodal regions while sparing uninvolved tissues. Treatment areas may be limited to known involved fields, expanded to include contiguous regions, and later contracted as the tumor mass shrinks. Treatment delivered to all major lymphoid regions above and below the diaphragm is known as total nodal irradiation (TNI). As an illustration of radiotherapeutic strategems, mantle field irradiation is described briefly below.

Mantle Field Irradiation

The mantle field incorporates all of the major lymph node groups above the diaphragm (cervical, supraclavicular, axillary, infraclavicular, mediastinal, and pulmonary hilar nodes) and extends from the inferior portion of the mandible to the insertion of the diaphragm. Among the organs within this field that must be fully or partially shielded are the lungs, heart, and spinal cord. By various deployments of radiopaque blocks, the quantity of radiation delivered to heart and lungs can be modified to suit the pattern of infiltration, and as disease regresses wider blocks may be cut to protect more of the lungs (shrinking field technique). Typical design of a posterior mantle field for a patient with mediastinal disease and right hilar adenopathy is shown in Figure 19-14 [13].

Subdiaphragmatic Irradiation

By analogous contrivance, radiation of subdiaphragmatic HD tumors is achieved and radiosensitive normal tissues are protected by use of an inverted Y field, and in patients whose pelvic nodes are uninvolved the Y field is truncated to create a legless "spade" field. Total nodal irradiation is achieved by combining mantle and inverted Y fields. Careful blocking contours are essential in treatment of the pelvic component of subdiaphragmatic disease to minimize damage to the large volume of encumbent marrow. Usually lumbosacral irradiation totalling no more than 30 to 35 Gy is followed by complete restitution of hematopoietic elements in the area treated within several months or years, but in a large minority of patients regrowth of hematopoietic stem cells remains incomplete or is abrogated, possibly accounting in part for the occurrence of post-therapy AML in patients treated with pelvic irradiation in concert with alkylator chemotherapy. Persistent hematopoietic "sterilization" in an irradiated pelvic area called the "lumboaortic bar"—as well as the steep gradi-

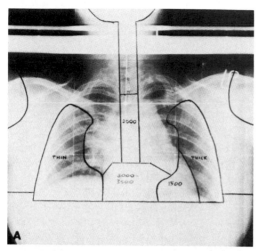

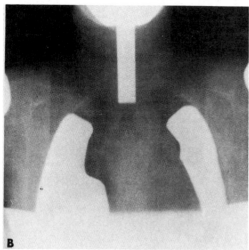

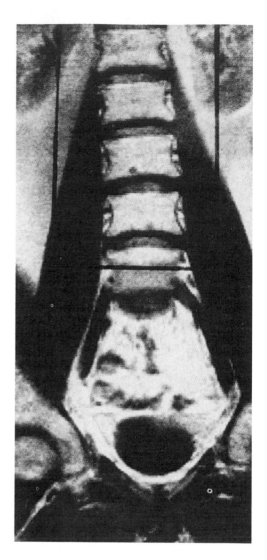

FIGURE 19-14

Posterior mantle field for mediastinal and right hilar HD; the opposing anterior mantle field (not shown) differs somewhat in contour and omits cord blocks. (A) "Setup" film in which regions to be protected and their cumulative radiation dose limits are annotated. A block is placed posteriorily over the thoracic spinal cord after a cumulative dose of 20 Gy. (B) A double-exposure port film confirms correct positioning of the shielding blocks. (From Hoppe RT: Radiation therapy in the treatment of Hodgkin's disease. Semin Oncol 7:144,1980.)

FIGURE 19-15

Coronal MR image demonstrating hematopoietic depletion in a 41-year-old man treated for HD 5 years earlier by lumboaortic bar irradiation (36 Gy). The irradiated area portrayed (outlined by a black rectangle) extends from L1 through the upper half of L5. Note the sharp definition of marrow injury and fatty replacement, which in L5 is limited to the upper half of the vertebral body; below this, L5 is normally cellular. (From Casamassima F et al: Hematopoietic bone marrow recovery after radiation therapy: MRI evaluation. Blood 73: 1677,1989.)

ent at field edges—is illustrated in Figure 19-15 [14].

Chemotherapy and Combined Modality Therapy

Combination chemotherapy with or without adjuvant irradiation (combined modality therapy) is the treatment of choice for patients with stage III and stage IV HD and for patients who relapse after radiotherapy. Drugs are administered in cyclic fashion with periods of rest to permit normal tissue recovery. The largest experience has been with MOPP, but several other non-cross-resistant drug combinations have been equally successful and can be used in alternating fashion (Table 19-3) [14]. The general tactic in most chemotherapy programs is to treat patients until they achieve complete remission and for two cycles thereafter, with a minimum total of six cycles. The current outcome of treatment of HD (radiotherapy, chemotherapy, and combined modality therapy

are reported collectively) is quantitated in Figure 19-16 [14]. It is a triumph over an ugly lapse of nature that the majority of patients diagnosed as having Hodgkin's disease, once a forlorn and irremediable sentence of death, can now be cured.

Footnote to success   A penalty of success in treating HD has been the therapy-induced occurrence of second neoplasms, particularly AML. The cumulative risk of secondary AML increases steadily, starting 1 year after initiation of alkylator therapy, and reaches a peak of 13% at 10 to 12 years, after which there is no further increment. Secondary AML is the bête noir of combination chemotherapy, but there is reason to believe that substituting nonalkylating agents will abolish this fearful reprisal.

For the minority of patients who fail to achieve complete remission or who relapse after two or more remissions, the outlook on conventional salvage regimens is grim. Even in

TABLE 19-3

Drug combinations used in treatment of Hodgkin's disease

Drug combination	Agents	Dose (mg/m²)	Route	Days	Treatment schedule cycle duration (days)
MOPP	Nitrogen mustard	6	IV	1, 8	28
	Vincristine (Oncovin)	1.4*	IV	1, 8	
	Procarbazine	100	PO	1–14	
	Prednisone	40	PO	1–14	
PAVe	Procarbazine	100	PO	1–14	28
	Alkeran	7.5	PO	1, 2, 8, 9	
	Vinblastine	6	IV	1, 8	
ABVD	Adriamycin	25	IV	1, 15	28
	Bleomycin	10	IV	1, 15	
	Vinblastine	6	IV	1, 15	
	Dacarbazine	375	IV	1, 15	
MOPP/ABVD	MOPP	——	——	1–14	56
	ABVD	——	——	29, 43	

Note: IV = intravenous, PO = oral.
*Minimum = 2.0 mg.

Source: From Hoppe RT: The contemporary management of Hodgkin disease. Radiology 169:297,1988.

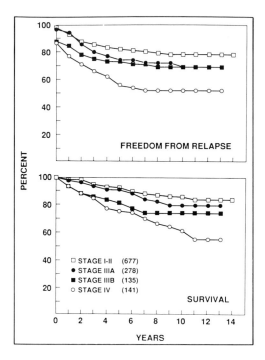

FIGURE 19-16

Actuarial freedom from relapse (above) and survival (below) of 1,321 patients treated for paravertebral HD at Stanford University between 1974 and 1988, reported as a function of stage. The numbers of patients in each of the four stages are shown in parenthesis. (From Hoppe RT: The contemporary management of Hodgkin disease. Radiology 169:297,1988.)

this desperate category of last resort, promising results have been obtained with high-dose hybrid therapy followed by rescue with cryopreserved autologous marrow.

REFERENCES

1. Hagemeister FB: Prognostic factors in decision-making in the clinical management of Hodgkin's disease. Hematol Oncol 6:257, 1988

2. Glaser SL: Recent incidence and secular trends in Hodgkin's disease and its histologic subtypes. J Chron Dis 39:789,1986

3. Weiss LM et al: Detection of Epstein-Barr viral genomes in Reed-Sternberg cells of Hodgkin's disease. N Engl J Med 320:502, 1989

4. Jandl JH: Blood: Chapt 27, in Blood: Textbook of Hematology. Boston, Little, Brown and Company,1987

5. Herbst H et al: Immunoglobulin and T-cell receptor gene rearrangements in Hodgkin's disease and Ki-1-positive anaplastic large cell lymphoma: dissociation between phenotype and genotype. Leuk Res 13:103,1989

6. Pinkus GS and Said JW: Hodgkin's disease, lymphocyte predominance type, nodular—further evidence for a B cell derivation. L & H variants of Reed-Sternberg cells express L26, a pan B cell marker. Am J Pathol 133:211,1988

7. Cawson RA et al, Eds.: Pathology. The Mechanisms of Disease, 2d ed. St. Louis, The CV Mosby Company,1989

8. Greenberger J et al: Hodgkin's disease, in Hematology—1988 Education Program. American Society of Hematology, December 1988

9. Hoffbrand AV and Pettit JE: Chapt 10, in Sandoz Atlas of Clinical Hematology, London, Gower Medical Publishing,1988

10. Kaplan HS: Hodgkin's Disease, 2d ed. Cambridge, Harvard University Press,1980

11. Meyer JE et al: Impact of thoracic computed tomography on radiation therapy planning in Hodgkin's disease. J Comput Assist Tomogr 8:892,1984

12. Hoppe RT: Radiation therapy in the treatment of Hodgkin's disease. Semin Oncol 7:144,1980

13. Casamassima F et al: Hematopoietic bone marrow recovery after radiation therapy: MRI evaluation. Blood 73:1677,1989

14. Hoppe RT: The contemporary management of Hodgkin disease. Radiology 169:297, 1988

20

Non-Hodgkin's Lymphomas

□

Non-Hodgkin's lymphomas (NHLs) constitute a confusing and extended family of malignant solid tumors of lymphoid tissues. The members of this family are distinctive clonal neoplasms representing malignant perversions of the cellular components of normal lymph nodes—primarily of lymph node follicles. Hence NHLs are mainly B cell tumors (80%), 15% are of T cell lineage, and the remainder stem from macrophages and their descendants. The character and behavior of NHL tumors is determined by the level of differentiation and size of the cell of origin, its rate of cycling, and the histologic pattern of growth. Pattern of growth and cell size are the most important determinants of tumor aggressiveness: tumors that grow in follicular (nodular) patterns vaguely recapitulate normal B cell lymphoid follicular structures and are less belligerent than lymphomas having unstructured diffuse or anarchic growth; lymphomas of small lymphocytes often are associated with more indolent (albeit incessant) progression than those of large lymphocytes, which are always of intermediate or high-grade aggressiveness.

The reader should be forewarned that no well-paved avenues guide access to NHLs; there are simply too many disparate entities and too much terminological turmoil. For author and reader alike, NHLs are a complex minefield. It may help to clarify at the outset that in the landmark Rappaport morphologic classification of NHLs, the terms "nodular" and "histiocytic" were introduced; these still enjoy popularity in hematologic argot, but in biologic reality "nodular" alludes to follicular aggregates of malignant B cells and "histiocytic" is a nonce term for large mutant lymphocytes or macrophages.

INCIDENCE, EPIDEMIOLOGY, AND ETIOLOGY

Collectively, NHLs are the most prevalent of hematopoietic neoplasms, with over 35,000 new cases diagnosed in the United States annually (as of 1989), resulting in over 18,000 (3.6%) of cancer deaths. NHL is the seventh most common malignancy, with an annual crude incidence of over 100 per million people, and ranks fourth among cancers in person-years of life lost. The mean age of onset (reflecting actuarial factors) is reached in the early sixties, but age-specific incidence climbs steeply (unlike Hodgkin's disease) beginning in early adulthood (Figure 20-1) [1]. In adults NHLs are 50% more frequent in males than in age-matched females, but the selectively high incidence in males below age 20 cannot be explained by postulated occupational exposures. The cause of most NHLs is unknown.

FIGURE 20-1

Age-specific incidence of NHL by ethnic group and sex. (From Newell GR et al: Incidence of lymphoma in the US classified by the Working Formulation. Cancer 59:857,1987.)

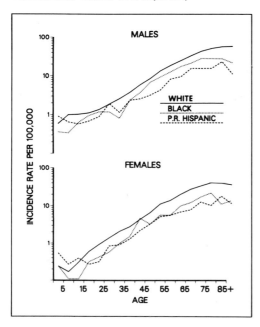

The etiologic role of HTLV-I (and rarely HTLV-II) and of Epstein-Barr virus (EBV) in causing T cell lymphoma in adults and Burkitt's B cell lymphoma in children are described in Chapter 13. In aggregate these two lymphomagenic viruses account for a very small proportion of NHLs, but the increasing prevalence of acquired immunodeficiency syndrome (AIDS) and broadening use of immunosuppressive agents in renal, cardiac, and marrow transplant patients has increased the percentage of secondary NHLs to over 5% of the total.

Most NHLs Following Immune Deficiency or Immunosuppression Are Associated with EBV Reactivation

Malignant lymphoma occurs with high frequency in patients with congenital or acquired immunodeficiency disorders, the most prevalent being AIDS caused by the human immunodeficiency virus (HIV). The Centers for Disease Control now includes occurrence of diffuse aggressive intermediate or high-grade NHL in an individual seropositive for HIV among the diagnostic criteria for AIDS. A disproportionate fraction of AIDS-associated lymphomas arise in unusual extranodal sites including brain, skin, maxilla, lung, anus, and retina. The tumors invariably express monotypic sIg and exhibit clonal Ig heavy chain and light chain rearrangements (but not TcR gene rearrangements), certifying them as B cell NHLs. HIV is not expressed within the neoplastic cells, indicating the tumors evolve as an indirect consequence of the immunodepressed state (Chapter 12). In most AIDS-associated NHLs, DNA extracts contain EBV genomic sequences, and DNA in situ hybridization studies show that the neoplastic B cells harbor EBV [2]. These data suggest that EBV infection either incites opportunistic lymphomas or collaborates by immortalizing the clone.

Appearance of solid lymphoreticular malignancies is especially frequent in organ transplant recipients receiving longterm courses of chemical immunosuppressants such as Imuran and prednisolone. As in AIDS victims, the proliferative process in transplant patients begins as an ambiguous outgrowth of multifocal clusters of large blastic lymphoid cells, some clusters showing κ chain predominance, others showing λ chain predominance ("polymorphic B cell lymphoma"). This clonal ambiguity is followed within several months by a monoclonal takeover evolving into an overt diffuse high-grade B cell lymphoma, a majority being B cell immunoblastic tumors or noncleaved cell lymphomas, and some having Burkittlike features. In both HIV- and drug-induced immunosuppression, several consecutive steps appear to be operative: (1) sabotage of the T cell network; (2) escape of latent EBV (or analogous) particles lurking within B cells, which further depresses immunity and exerts strenuous proliferative pressure on newly infected B cell progenitors; and (3) an eventual clonal chromosomal abnormality—most often at (8;14), with rearrangement and activation of the c-*myc* gene (Chapter 13). Rearrangements of c-*myc* have also been observed in AIDS-associated NHLs lacking EBV sequences (a pattern reminiscent of sporadic Burkitt's lymphoma), indicating that it is the c-*myc* recombination with the switch region of the Ig$_H$ chain locus that triggers lymphomagenesis, whether or not EBV (or a surrogate) is still present [3]. Once this third step has occurred, a mutant founder cell is empowered to spawn a monoclonal dynasty of malignant lymphocytes.

PATHOPHYSIOLOGY

Most NHLs Are of Follicle Center Origin

NHLs are tumors of lymphoid organs and the various neoplastic tumor cell lines correspond to each of the cellular components of reactive lymph follicles. To understand the pathogenesis of B cell NHLs it is necessary to become familiar with the cellular troupe that participates in normal germinal center responses to antigen.

Normal Follicle Center Cell Response to Antigen

Lymph follicles are created during the germinal center response to antigenic stimulation, the purpose being to amplify the numbers of B cells. Within 3 to 4 days after antigen exposure untutored (virgin) B cells divide to form spherical masses of large basophilic blasts. These partly differentiated forms, called centroblasts, have a pale rounded nucleus with two or more nucleoli adherent to the nuclear membrane. Centroblasts of the basal zone of the expanding follicle become admixed with large, pale tingible body macrophages, creating a "starry sky" appearance; meanwhile centroblasts drifting over to the outer zone of the follicle transform en route to become angular cells, large and small, having cleaved nuclei and pale cytoplasm. By the seventh day the parental globular mass of germinal center cells becomes cloaked with a heavy mantle composed of crowds of small B cells (and some T cells), completing the zonal structure of the secondary follicle (Figure 20-2) [4]. Although rarely found in the germinal center, T cells (T4 and T8) represent a minor population within the B cell mantle zone and are the predominant lymphocytes in the loose interfollicular "T cell zone," in which matrix the secondary follicles are embedded.

The dramatis personae of lymph node follicles

Only B cells—both early virgin B cells (not yet seduced by antigen) and antigen-violated cells—home to follicles by adhesion to nodal vascular homing receptors. B cells within normal secondary follicles can be divided into four cytologic types: noncleaved centroblasts, large and small; and cleaved centrocytes, large and small. Centroblasts do not display appreciable sIg but their B cell lineage is affirmed by pan-B cell monoclonal antibodies and by DNA analysis indicating Ig gene rearrangements. In addition to expressing pan-B antigens and Ig gene rearrangements, centrocytes display surface μ chains. Neither centroblasts nor centrocytes possess surface δ chains or TdT, but both flaunt the common acute lymphatic leukemia antigen (CALLA) and the family of HLA-DR antigens. Effector B cells of follicle centers, when educated by exposure to antigen, transform to liberated B immunoblasts (Chapter 12), and offspring of immunoblasts may acquire plasmacytoid features and secrete monoclonal IgM. The cast of cells involved in these

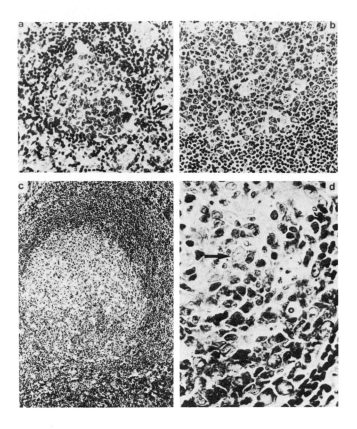

FIGURE 20-2

Germinal center of a lymph follicle. (a) During early response to antigen, the nascent germinal center is composed of pale centroblasts surrounded by a mantle of mature B cells. (b) Later, very large, pale macrophages containing ingested nuclear debris (tingible bodies) wander in, creating the starry sky effect. (c) Zonal spherical structure of a follicle seen at low magnification. The light-staining central area is rich in centroblasts and centrocytes and is bound into a geodesic sphere by the sticky branching processes of dendritic macrophages. The surrounding dense mantle zone is composed predominantly of memory B cells (B_2 lymphocytes). (d) High magnification view of germinal center reveals centroblasts with marginal nucleoli, centrocytes with dark angular or cleaved nuclei, and a dendritic macrophage (arrow). (From Stein H et al: The normal and malignant germinal centre. Clin Haematol 11:531,1982.)

several stages of differentiation and translocation are portrayed diagrammatically in Figure 20-3 [5].

Murphy's Law and NHLs

NHLs arise as clonal transformations occurring at specific stages of normal B cell (and T cell) differentiation during antigenic stimulation, a generalization that serves as the basis for the Kiel histopathologic classification. This is in obedience to Murphy's law, which holds that for every cell type and stage of differentiation there will exist neoplastic counterparts. Malignancies of relatively well-differentiated cells—lymphocytes (B or T), plasmacytoid cells (B), and centrocytes (B)—are low-grade or "good risk" lymphomas; those of poorly differentiated cells—lymphoblasts (B or T), immunoblasts (B or T), centroblasts (B), and macrophages—are high-grade or "bad risk" lymphomas.

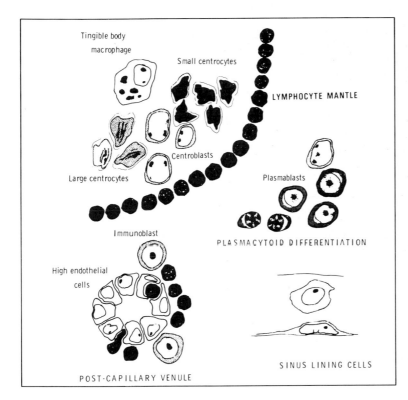

FIGURE 20-3

Cellular constituents of
a normal reactive
lymph node. Cells en-
closed by the lympho-
cyte mantle are germi-
nal center (follicle cen-
ter) cells. Large and
small centroblasts and
centrocytes are termed
in the Lukes and Col-
lins classification of
NHLs small and large
noncleaved and small
and large cleaved cells,
respectively. (From Stu-
art AE et al, Eds.:
Chapt 1, in Lym-
phomas Other Than
Hodgkin's Disease. Ox-
ford, Oxford University
Press,1981.)

Follicular NHLs Are Less Aggressive than Diffuse Lymphomas

Follicular (nodular) lymphomas as a group have a better prognosis than diffuse lympho-mas. All follicular lymphomas, comprising al-most half of NHLs, are of B cell origin (Figure 20-4) [6]. As noted earlier, tumor cell size and pattern of involvement are the cardinal determi-nants in grading NHL tumor cell aggressive-ness. Lymphomas of small lymphocytes are less incursive than those composed of large

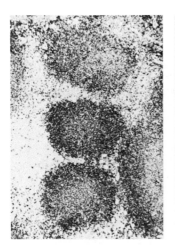
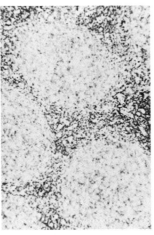

FIGURE 20-4

Strongly nodular conformation of frozen section of this NHL identifies it as
a follicular lymphoma. (Left) The tumor cells stained intensely for κ light
chains by the immunoperoxidase technique, but were entirely negative for λ
light chains, signifying monoclonality. (Right) Staining of the same
specimen with a pan-T monoclonal
antibody (for CD3) shows only a few
T cells trapped within tumor nodules,
but T cells are numerous in the interfollicular (T zone) areas. (From
Jaffe ES: Chapt 9, in Atlas of Blood
Cells: Function and Pathology, vol. 2,
Zucker-Franklin D et al, Eds. Milan,
Edi. Ermes s.r.l.,1988.)

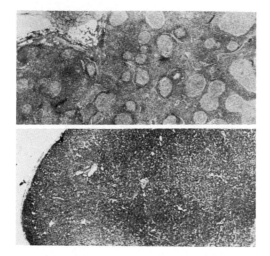

FIGURE 20-5

Follicular versus diffuse growth patterns in small cleaved cell NHL. (Above) Nodular formations in this inguinal node are characteristic of follicular small cleaved cell lymphoma, a low-grade malignancy. (Below) This ultrastructured infiltrative lesion in a cervical node represents a diffuse version of small cleaved cell lymphoma—a higher-grade tumor. (From Tindle BH: Malignant lymphomas. Am J Pathol 116:115,1984.)

lymphocytes (lymphoblasts). The second main feature correlating with tumor growth is architectural rather than cellular: follicular (nodular) NHLs as a group have a distinctly better prognosis than diffuse lymphomas. This difference is most striking during the first 5 years after diagnosis and fulfills the intuitive expectation that tumor growth patterns possessing some resemblance to normal nodal structure are more likely to be indolent than diffuse growths lacking structure and insinuating anaplasia (Figure 20-5) [7].

Chromosome Rearrangements, Oncogenes, and Fragile Sites

The most renowned chromosome rearrangements in NHL are those associated with Burkitt's lymphoma, in which the c-*myc* oncogene is placed into proximity with Ig coding regions, a phenomenon dealt with in Chapter 13. It seems clear that the rearranged and activated c-*myc* gene, when shuffled into

the midst of an Ig coding region, codes for multiple copies of a phosphorylated growth protein, but the nature of B cell growth deregulation is unclear and there is no explanation for why the same or similar t(8;14) rearrangements are also associated with small non-cleaved non-Burkitt's lymphoma, immunoblastic lymphomas, and some large cell lymphomas. The most dramatic and specific correlation between a chromosome change and histopathologic consequence is the high association between the 14;18 translocation and follicular lymphomas.

t(14;18) Is the Hallmark of Follicular NHLs

A t(14;18)(q32.3;q21.3) chromosomal translocation is associated with 85% of lymphomas with follicular morphology, and is also present in about one-third of diffuse large cell lymphomas. Breakpoints on chromosome 14 have been shown by Southern blot and sequence analysis to occur through the 5′ end of the junctional locus, J_H, indicating that the DNA translocation occurs as a mistake made at the pre B stage of differentiation during attempted D-J heavy chain joining. Fracture through any of the six J_H exons permits union of the 5′ end stumps to a breakpoint near a hereditary fragile site located on the long arm of chromosome 18; a putative recombinase joins the separated segments on both chromosomes, resulting in the 14;18 reciprocal translocation. This juxtaposes a new gene from the breakpoint at 18q21, denoted *bcl*-2 (for B cell leukemia-lymphoma-2), within the H chain locus in exchange for the V_H genes which transfer to 18q−, thus creating a unique translocation-specific J_H;18q21 rearrangement that is presumed to be a transforming event (Figure 20-6) [8]. On chromosome 18 the major breakpoint region (mbr) and the minor breakpoint region (mcr) are clustered separately within the center of the 3′ untranslocated portion of the *bcl*-2 transcript. Breakpoints at this site do not alter coding of the *bcl*-2 protein, but J_H;18q21 fusion does result in production of abnormally large *bcl*-2 mRNAs.

False dawn or a step forward? At this writing it is unclear whether the *bcl*-2 gene is a bona fide oncogene, or whether the *bcl*-2 protein

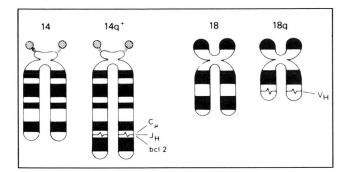

FIGURE 20-6

In follicular lymphomas with the t(14;18) translocation, the *bcl*-2 gene normally situated on band q21 near a fragile site on chromosome 18 translocates to the heavy chain locus on chromosome 14, forming a J_H;18q21 hybrid sequence. (Abridged from Croce CM and Nowell PC: Molecular basis of human B cell neoplasia. Blood 65:1,1985.)

product—a membrane-binding peptide lacking homology with any known protein—participates in propelling uncontrolled manufacture of useless and invasive B cells. That the breakpoint on chromosome 18 underlying translocation of the putative proto-oncogene, *bcl*-2, occurs near a hereditary fragile site supports the possibility of a genetic predisposition to this most prevalent of lymphomas. Unfortunately, no tidy narrative can be construed, for the fragile site is outside of the *bcl*-2 domain and the genetic role of the *bcl*-2 gene and its product is unclear. The most pragmatic byproduct of studies of the 14;18 translocation has been to certify that this lymphoma in all its variant forms is unquestionably of single cell origin. Immunophenotyping is limited by the facts that many NHLs do not express sIg and that normal cell populations frequently dilute out tumor cells, obscuring malignant clones. Analyses of Ig gene rearrangements are extremely useful in establishing clonality, for these generate altered-size restriction fragments which serve as tumor-specific molecular markers in monoclonal expansions of B cells. On the other hand, a given B cell neoplasm may show variation in Ig gene patterns over time or within different lymph node sites, and more mature subclones of the original tumor may mutate, undergo secondary rearrangements, and generate isotype switch variants. Furthermore, routine Southern blot analyses demonstrating gene rearrangements require that tumor cells constitute at least 1% of the cell population biopsied. Despite this potential for confusion and oversight even at this most molecular level, the 14;18 transformation is invariably conserved in follicular lymphomas, indicating that the evolving subpopulations arose from a single common clonal progenitor cell. Even when the tumor population is small, as during clinically effective therapy, it is usually possible to reaffirm the presence of this puzzling but persistent cytogenetic emblem by constructing specific synthetic oligonucleotide primers that flank the J_H;18q21 crossover sites, permitting polymerase chain reaction (PCR)–driven amplification of the t(14;18) hybrid DNA sequence. This technique permits detection of clones of cells carrying the breakpoint even at cell dilutions of 1 in 100,000 and in marrow and blood samples that fail to show any abnormality by morphological examination or conventional Southern blot analysis [9, 10].

T Cell NHLs

In the Western hemisphere about 15% of NHLs are of T cell origin as determined by T cell antigen markers.

NHLs of Thymic Origin

Those lymphomas arising directly from the thymus are termed T lymphoblastic lymphomas, which account for 80% of all lymphoblastic lymphomas and are solid-state versions of T cell ALL. T cell lymphoblastic lymphoma cell populations are frequently pleomorphic and include a mixture of smaller lymphocytes having irregular contorted nuclei and larger blastic cells with round or polylobulated nuclei and abundant water-clear cytoplasm. T cell lymphoblastic lymphomas are TdT$^+$ and have a phenotype approximating midstage or late thymocyte development, displaying a procession of T cell differentiation markers, the most faithful of which is CD7. T lymphoblastic lymphomas share many features with T cell ALL, among them a high male:female ratio, mediastinal presentation, and poor prognosis.

NHLs of Mature T Cell Origin

T cells normally reside in the interfollicular areas of lymph nodes, and T cell lymphomas characteristically arise from the paracortical T cell zones and never possess follicular architecture. Partly differentiated post-thymic lymphoid neoplasms constitute a complex group of neoplasms that includes peripheral T cell lymphomas and the epidermotropic T cell disorders, mycosis fungoides and Sézary syndrome. These latter lesions, collectively designated the cutaneous T cell lymphomas (CTCLs), are indolent but potentially humiliating and deadly disorders to be described later. About 20% of diffuse aggressive lymphomas possess mature T cell markers, almost always including CD4, and despite their heterogeneous morphology and growth habits, are grouped awkwardly as peripheral T cell lymphomas. Histologic features held in common include a heterogeneous inflammatory background, prominent vascularity, and extreme cytologic polymorphism. Often fickle in phenotype, malignant cells of peripheral T cell lymphomas tend to express aberrant or discordant differentiation antigens and frequently betray their lineage markers. The propensity of these cell populations to show phenotypic and cytogenetic transformation, and in some instances to arise as polyclonal growths from which a monoclonal victor emerges can confound diagnosis. With broadened use of DNA probes for TcR it has become evident that almost all T cell NHLs (including CTCLs and "prelymphomas") sooner or later acquire unique rearrangements of one or more chains of this antigen receptor, signifying clonality. Peripheral T cell lymphomas are not to be confused with "adult T cell leukemia/lymphoma," a malignancy endemic in Japan and the Caribbean that is spread by the contagious retrovirus, HTLV-I (Chapter 13).

Classification of NHLs: A Catechism for Clinicians

Classification of lymphomas lacking the logo of Reed-Sternberg cells has long languished in an epistemological dark age, during which all NHLs fell into either of two spectral categories: reticulum cell sarcoma and lymphosarcoma. The entire constellation of NHLs has been classified by what it is not. A footing upon which to build a rational structure was laid by Rappaport and associates, who stress the favorable character of nodular (follicular) varieties and the prognostic impact of level of cytologic differentiation. The Lukes and Collins immunologic classification relates B cell lymphomas to stages of follicular center cell development, and the Kiel classification of Lennert and associates includes T cell lymphomas and sorts all NHLs into low-grade and high-grade groups. In a commendable quest for harmony, the National Cancer Institute called upon a group of lymphoma luminaries to construct a unified systematic classification that would facilitate comparisons of case reports and clinical trials. The product, "A Working Formulation of Non-Hodgkin's Lymphomas for Clinical Usage," or WF, incorporates the compromises and busy wording characteristic of committees, cuts across immunologic lines, and omits cell lineage designations. It is, nevertheless, falling into favor. The Working Formulation, alias New Formulation, is presented in Table 20-1 [11] in the context of immunologic phenotyping and the deplored but durable Rappaport classification.

The Irony of Lymphoma Grading

Separating NHLs into low, intermediate, and high grade (or "risk") categories is pertinent for shortterm (5- to 7-year) prediction, but over a longer period patients encounter a grim paradox. Low-grade follicular lymphomas, for example, are quite amenable to therapy and remain so for years, but these indolent malignancies have an obstinate tendency to recur, and about 40% of patients will transform to a higher-grade histology within 10 years: the disease is remittable but not curable. In contrast, many high-grade lymphomas with unfavorable histology respond promptly and lastingly to in-

T A B L E 20-1

Histopathologic classification of non-Hodgkin's lymphomas

Category	Immunologic pheno-type	New formulation	Rappaport classifi-cation	% of cases
Low grade	Predominantly B	Small lymphocytic (SL)	Diffuse, well differentiated lymphocytic (DWDL)	10–15
	B	Follicular, predominantly small cleaved cell (FSC)	Nodular, poorly differentiated lymphocytic (NPDL)	15–20
	B	Follicular, mixed small cleaved and large cell (FM)	Nodular, mixed, lymphocytic and histiocytic (NM)	5–10
Intermediate grade	B (mature)	Follicular, predominantly large cell (FL)	Nodular, histiocytic (NH)	<5
	B or T (mature)	Diffuse, small cleaved cell (DSC)	Diffuse, poorly differentiated lymphocytic (DPDL)	15–20
	B or T (mature)	Diffuse, mixed small and large cell (DM)	Diffuse, mixed, lymphocytic and histiocytic (DM)	5–10
	B or T	Diffuse, large cell (DL): cleaved or noncleaved cell	Diffuse, histiocytic (DH)	30
High grade	B or T	Immunoblastic (IBL)	Diffuse histiocytic (DH)	5–10
	T (thymocytic)	Lymphoblastic (LL): convoluted or nonconvoluted cell	Diffuse lymphoblastic (LB)	<5
	B	Small noncleaved cell (SNC): Burkitt's or non-Burkitt's	Diffuse undifferentiated (DU)	<5
Miscellaneous	Monocyte-macrophage	Histiocytic		Rare
	T (mature)	Mycosis fungoides		5
	B or T	Composite		Rare
	T	Lennert's lymphoma (epithelioid)		Rare
	B or T	Unclassifiable		<5

Source: Amended from Canellos GP: Section 12, Subsection XI. Malignant Lymphomas, in Scientific American Medicine. Rubenstein E and Federman DD, Eds. New York, Scientific American, Inc.,1988. © 1989 Scientific American Inc. All rights reserved.

tensive and timely chemotherapy, and roughly 50% of such patients appear to be cured.

A Pastiche of Histopathological and Clinical Features

Low-Grade Lymphomas

These lymphomas of middle-aged and elderly patients are usually disseminated at presentation, but patients may feel well and seek attention merely for peripheral adenopathy. Low-grade NHLs are comprised of diffuse small lymphocytic lymphomas with well-differentiated benign-appearing cells, and follicular small cleaved cell and mixed small cleaved and large cell lymphomas.

Small lymphocytic lymphoma Although the growth pattern is ominously diffuse and homogeneous, nodes are infiltrated by seemingly benign collections of small, round, well-differentiated B cells that appear to represent a solid tumor analog to chronic lymphatic leukemia (Figure 20-7). Proliferation of these friendly-looking cells is generally so leisurely and painless that diagnosis may be made during a routine health checkup. This slumbering lymphoma nonetheless has grievous potential and spreads early via the bloodstream to other nodes and marrow. At first easily controlled, small lymphocytic lymphoma is prone eventually to erupt as an immunoblastic sarcoma; during transformation to high-grade NHL the tumor cells continue to bear and secrete the same monoclonal Ig, signifying direct kinetic transformation of the original clone.

Follicular small cleaved cell and mixed small cleaved and large cell lymphomas Collectively these kindred cleaved cell follicular lymphomas constitute 20 to 30% of NHLs and also afflict older adults, who usually present with painless adenopathy without systemic problems. Usually small cleaved cells predominate, but when the cleaved cell population is admixed with comparable numbers of large noncleaved cells the terminology becomes even more wordy. The predominant dark, small cells with irregular or angular nuclei are centrocytes, and the large, chunky, uncleaved pale cells containing one to three bold nucleoli are

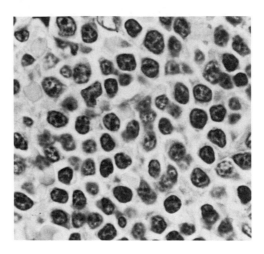

FIGURE 20-7

Small lymphocytic lymphoma. The tumor cells resemble small mature lymphocytes but are slightly larger and indistinguishable from the lymphocytes of CLL. Some nuclei are eccentric, giving those cells a plasmacytoid look, and there may be (as shown here) a faint but counterfeit suggestion of follicular configuration. H & E–stained section. (Photo by CT Kapff.)

FIGURE 20-8

Follicular small cleaved cell lymphoma. The predominant cells are dark and angular, and the nuclei are indented or compressed. Cleavage planes are evident in some nuclei, but the expression "cleaved cell" is hyperbolic. These wizened cells are centrocytes, and the large pale cells with coarse nucleoli scattered among them are centroblasts. H & E–stained section. (Photo by CT Kapff.)

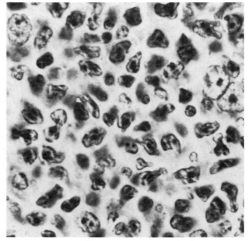

centroblasts (Figure 20-8). In both variants of follicular cleaved cell lymphoma the cells stain brightly for a single light chain type and for CD10 (CALLA), and cytogenetic analysis discloses the t(14;18) signature of follicular lymphomas. The disease is nearly always disseminated presentation, and in about 75% of patients small nodules of paratrabecular (next to a spicule of bone) infiltrates are found on marrow biopsy. Occasionally large numbers of lymphocytes with cleaved nuclei circulate in the blood; this appearance of "lymphosarcoma cell leukemia" invariably attracts an enthusiastic crowd of morphology devotees.

Intermediate-Grade NHLs

The growth pace of these lymphomas of middle age is intermediate at first but often segues swiftly into a runaway, disseminated process. Most patients present with widespread disease and diffuse histology, making staging irrelevant, and when first seen, extranodal involvement (gastrointestinal, Waldeyer's ring, bone, CNS, testes) is commonplace. Diffuse intermediate-grade lymphomas comprise at least 50% of all NHLs, include most T cell lymphomas, and (if untreated) disease progression is very rapid, median survival being measured in months.

Diffuse small cleaved cell lymphoma   Most diffuse small cleaved cell lymphomas evolve from cryptic nests of follicular small cell tumors, and the disease seems to burst forth in metastatic fashion, involving nodes, liver, lungs, and marrow almost simultaneously. The appearance of the dispersed infiltrates responsible for this pervasive disease is monotonous, unrelieved by follicular organization or important numbers of centroblasts (Figure 20-9).

The morphologically heterogeneous postthymic T cell lymphomas encompass several entities, including large cell variants of cleaved cell lymphomas, peripheral T cell lymphomas (described earlier), T zone (Lennert) lymphomas, and polymorphic immunocytoma of the Kiel classification. T cell lymphomas in general usually present with generalized and retroperitoneal lymphadenopathy, often complicated by pleuropulmonary involvement. Nodal proliferation by pleomorphic T cells is distinctively

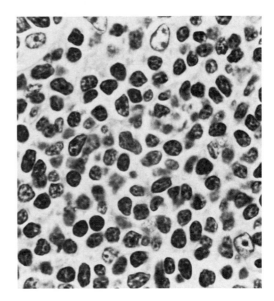

FIGURE 20-9

Diffuse small cleaved cell lymphoma. The teeming cells of this unstructured B cell tumor are uniform in size and random in distribution. Most cells appear rounded, angular, or oatshaped, deeply cleaved forms being uncommon. Centroblasts are few and scattered. H & E–stained section. (Photo by CT Kapff.)

associated with vascular proliferation and an admixture of epithelioid macrophages. Neoplastic T cells are notable for their floral, folded nuclei, but identification of T cell variants of diffuse small or large cell lymphomas requires surface marker analysis or demonstration of clonal rearrangement of TcR genes.

Diffuse large cell lymphoma   Diffuse large cell lymphomas (cleaved or noncleaved cell types) are the commonest of NHLs, and most represent B cell centroblastic proliferations. Spontaneously appearing tumors are prone to form bulky localized masses, and in nearly half of cases initial sites of presentation are extranodal, involving Waldeyer's ring, ocular adnexa, gastrointestinal tract, bone, skin, salivary glands, or CNS. The diffuse cytology of these gross tumors reflects disorderly sheets of large centroblasts, with big potato-shaped nuclei, some of which are notched, folded, or

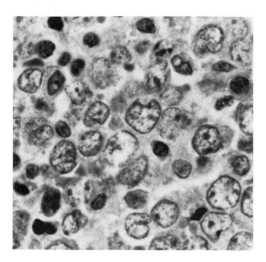

FIGURE 20-10

Diffuse large cell lymphoma. The chaotic mixture of large nucleolated centroblasts, some ovoid and some notched or cleaved, is cluttered further by intermixture of small lymphocytes and several mitotic figures, the latter signifying rapid tumor growth. H & E–stained section. (Photo by CT Kapff.)

cleaved (Figure 20-10). With aggressive combination chemotherapy, even advanced-stage diffuse large cell lymphoma can be brought into longterm remission or even cured in 60 to 70% of cases. Factors associated with poor survival are high proliferative activity of tumor cells, systemic (B) symptoms, and sIg⁺ phenotype.

High-Grade NHLs

Three entirely different diffuse lymphomas, representing about 15% of all NHLs, are grouped together because of their explosive growth kinetics and (with certain exceptions) dismal prognosis. The most common of these malign processes are the large cell immunoblastic lymphomas, most of which (75%) are of B cell origin, the rest being high-grade T cell cancers: neither kind responds well to chemotherapy, with median survivals of under 6 months.

B immunoblastic lymphoma   B immunoblastic lymphoma (or sarcoma) is a high-grade neoplasm of plasma cell precursors (immuno-blasts) and commonly arises in immunocompromised patients with lymphoproliferative processes such as myeloma, chronic lymphatic leukemia, and AIDS [12]. B immunoblast nuclei are highly pleomorphic, and the tumor cell population includes giant Reed-Sternberglike multinucleated or multilobated forms in the company of atypical lymphoid cells of a strongly plasmacytoid cast (Figure 20-11). Most patients with B immunoblastic lymphoma present with extranodal disease and B symptoms; most primary NHLs originating in the CNS are B immunoblastomas.

Lymphoblastic lymphoma   Lymphoblastic lymphoma is a solid tumor counterpart to T cell ALL and occurs similarly in teenage and young adult males. About half of patients present with an anterior mediastinal mass, and lymphoblastic infiltrates disseminate rapidly to marrow and CNS. Tumor cells of medium size flood lymph nodes in a leukemic manner, effacing nodal architecture but often assuming vaguely nodular or pseudofollicular patterns surrounding large vessels and trabeculae. Nuclear membranes are deeply folded in, creating lobulated, cerebriform, and sharply angulated nuclear patterns of the Sézary sort. The pecan-shaped cells are sparse in cytoplasm and some sections appear crowded (Figure 20-12).

Small noncleaved cell lymphomas   Small noncleaved cell lymphomas are high-grade tumors of transformed B cells occurring in children or young adults: the tumor doubling time of 24 to 48 h makes these the fastest growing of human cancers. This category encompasses Burkitt's lymphoma endemic to tropical Africa and New Guinea; sporadic diffuse lymphomas that are similar in morphology, pattern of spread, and response to therapy and hence are known as Burkitt's-like lymphomas; and an assortment of fast-growing, undifferentiated, diffuse lymphomas having dissimilar histology (formerly designated "non-Burkitt's type") and frequently emerging as a terminal eruption of HIV infection.

Burkitt's lymphomas, endemic or sporadic, look alike histologically and are associated with translocations that juxtapose the c-*myc* oncogene of chromosome 8 and Ig gene loci on chromosomes 14, 2, or 22 (Chapter 13).

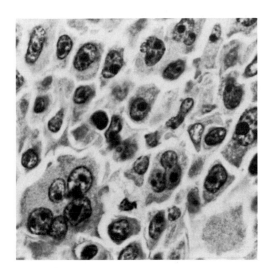

FIGURE 20-11

B immunoblastic lymphoma. In the midst of numerous plasmacytoid cells with muddy cytoplasm and eccentric or comet-shaped nuclei is a scattering of eye-catching multinucleated giant cells possessing similar cytoplasm. All nuclei contain at least one bold nucleolus, as is true also of T immunoblastic lymphoma, but the copious dense cytoplasm of B immunoblasts serves to differentiate them from the pale unfrocked T cell variant. H & E–stained section. (Photo by CT Kapff.)

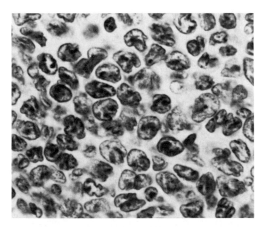

FIGURE 20-12

T lymphoblastic lymphoma. The compact crowd of cells with convoluted pecan-shaped nuclei and sparse cytoplasm are characteristic of T lymphoblastic lymphoma. The extent of cell crowding and nuclear deformation is unrivalled among other lymphomas. H & E–stained section. (Photo by CT Kapff.)

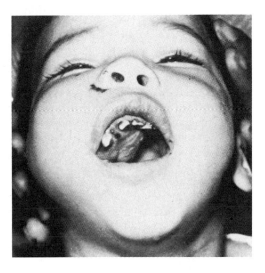

FIGURE 20-13

Massive deforming tumor of the right maxilla with infiltration into the hard palate and loosening of maxillary teeth. Such large jaw tumors are found in over 80% of African Burkitt's lymphoma, but this American child was among the 15% of sporadic cases of Burkitt's lymphomas in which lymphoma presentation was in the jaw rather than the abdomen. (From Kearns DB et al: Burkitt's lymphoma. Int J Pediatr Otorhinolaryngol 12:73,1986.)

Burkitt's and like lymphomas are best known for the starry sky effect (Chapter 12) created by random scattering of large, pale, tingible body macrophages amidst a dark background of crowded, rapidly dividing, malignant lymphocytes. The lymphocytes have small, uniform, rounded nuclei and in fixed sections the chromatin shows a polka-dot pattern overlaid by several small nucleoli. These lymphoma cells look quite different in Wright-Giemsa–stained lymph node imprints or marrow aspirate smears in which size is more variable and cytoplasm is deeply basophilic and punctured by numerous clear, round, fat-filled vacuoles—the morphology of the L3 type of ALL (Chapter 16). Burkitt's lymphoma endemic to tropical Africa is a distinctive syndrome of conspicuous extranodal tumors of the jawbones and abdominal viscera (Figure 20-13) [13]. In contrast non-African Burkitt's lymphomas usually originate in Peyer's patches or mesenteric nodes and then disseminate to abdominal and peripheral nodes and often (20% of cases) to marrow. Onset and relapse of endemic Burkitt's tumors is linked to the presence of EBV DNA, which is found in 95% of cases; the malignant B cells express EBV receptors, which may serve as the Trojan horse, if not the instigator, of malignant transformation. The tumor cells of sporadic Burkitt's lymphoma lack these receptors and EBV particles are found in only a minority of tumors.

Non-Burkitt's (undifferentiated) lymphoma, once a nodal tumor of middle-aged adults, now occurs predominantly in young men and presents in extranodal sites in 90% of cases, originating (in decreasing order) in gastrointestinal tract, CNS, and liver, and often spreading to nodes and marrow. During the past decade this variant of small noncleaved cell lymphomas has occurred increasingly in the setting of immunosuppression caused by HIV infection. The histology often lacks the starry sky gestalt of Burkitt's lymphoma, and the cells show decidedly more nuclear variation and possess a prominent, often single, nucleolus but have a comparable high percentage of cells in cycle (Figure 20-14) [12].

The growth velocity of Burkitt's, Burkitt's-like, and non-Burkitt's lymphomas renders the tumors remarkably responsive to multiagent chemotherapy, treatment that may be abetted (if attempted early) by surgical debulking procedures. Burkitt's lymphomas in younger age groups are among the few NHLs that can be eradicated by timely chemotherapy, the apparent cure rate in children (using high-dose cyclophosphamide, methotrexate, and intrathecal chemoprophylaxis) being over 50%.

Organ Involvement in NHLs

Painless lymphadenopathy is the presenting symptom in over two-thirds of patients with NHL, the remainder complaining of symptoms related to sites of extranodal disease. NHLs can orginate in any organ accessible to lymphocytes, and there is no limit to the patterns of organ involvement. Lymphocytes are denizens of the lymphoreticular system, and it is natural that organs rich in lymphopoietic elements are leading targets of oncogenic opportunity. Marrow, liver, and spleen are infiltrated early, particularly in cases of low-grade small

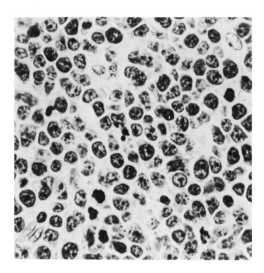

FIGURE 20-14

Non-Burkitt's small noncleaved cell lymphoma occurring as an opportunistic neoplasm in a patient with HIV infection. Note the nuclear variation, the bold and often multiple nucleoli, and the large fraction of cells in active mitosis. (From Knowles DM et al: Clinicopathologic, immunophenotypic, and molecular genetic analysis of AIDS-associated lymphoid neoplasia. Clinical and biologic implications. Pathol Annu 23(part 2):33,1988.)

lymphocytic and follicular small cleaved cell lymphomas. Sensitive flow cytometric methods such as kappa-lambda analysis indicate the presence of monoclonal populations of B cells in the blood of 80% of patients presenting with active NHL, and in low-grade follicular lymphomas, clonal B cells persist in the circulation throughout therapy-induced remission, accounting for the penchant for late relapse. In such patients the numbers of circulating tumor cells may rise to levels between 10,000 and 100,000 cells/μl, in which case the antiquated expression "lymphosarcoma cell leukemia (LSCL)" is used—although lymphoma cell leukemia is a more appropriate appellation. At least 20% of follicular and diffuse small cell lymphomas convert to a leukemic phase and are responsible for the bulk of chronic LSCLs; the lymphoma cells are usually recognizable on blood smears by their large size, copious cytoplasm, and notched, folded, or bisected nuclei (Figure 20-15) [14]. With the freedom of NHL

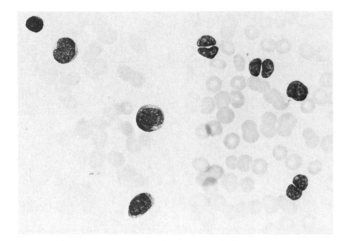

FIGURE 20-15

Lymphoma cell leukemia in a patient with longstanding diffuse small cleaved cell lymphoma. (Left) Large lymphoid cells (compare with normal lymphocyte at top left) with folded or twisted nuclei in the blood of a patient with small cleaved cell lymphoma. (Right) The deeply cleaved or bisected nuclei in malignant lymphoid cells of a patient with small cleaved cell lymphoma correspond to the follicular cleaved cells of centrocyte origin. (From Jandl JH: Chapt 28, in Blood: Textbook of Hematology. Boston, Little, Brown and Company,1987.)

cells to travel, the rapidity of tumoral dissemination is readily understood: both primary and secondary nodal and extranodal tumors are prevalent in NHL and frequently assault vital structures such as the heart, lung, and great vessels (Figure 20-16) [15].

In at least 20% of cases primary tumors arise at extranodal lymphoid sites, the most frequent (in descending order) being Waldeyer's ring, gastrointestinal tract, and skin. In patients immunosuppressed by drugs or HIV infection, extranodal presentations commonly occur in the brain, mucocutaneous sites, and marrow.

FIGURE 20-16 ▼

Advanced confluent infiltration of mediastinal structures by aggregated high-grade NHL tumors. (Left) Posteroanterior chest radiograph demonstrates bilateral hilar and mediastinal lymph node involvement and right pleural effusion. (Right) At autopsy massive confluent nodal involvement is seen to encase all mediastinal structures including the heart and great vessels. Bulky anterior mediastinal presentations in NHL often (as in this case) represent T lymphoblastic lymphoma. (From Schwartz EE et al: Mediastinal involvement in adults with lymphoblastic lymphoma. Acta Radiol 28:403,1987.)

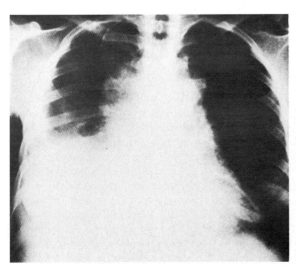

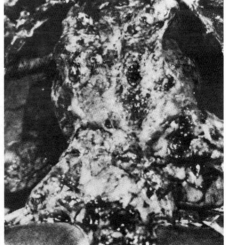

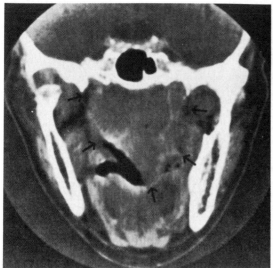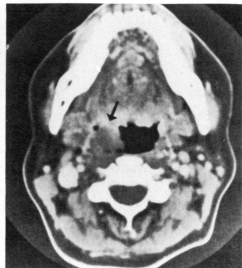

FIGURE 20-17

CT scans of diffuse large cell lymphomas originating in Waldeyer's ring. (Left) Multiple site involvement (arrows) without nodal disease in a
68-year-old woman. (Right) An isolated
lymphoma mass of the right tonsillar fossa (arrow) projects into the oropharynx of this 48-
year-old woman. (From Lee Y-Y et al:
Lymphomas of the head and neck: CT findings
at initial presentation. AJR 149:575,1987.)

NHLs of Head and Neck

If lymphomas arising in Waldeyer's ring, oral
cavity, maxillary sinuses, and nasal cavities are
combined, NHLs of head and neck are the
commonest tumors arising in extranodal sites.
Over half of patients with lymphomas presenting in Waldeyer's ring or nearby lymphoid
structures are stage I or II; they are first
recognized by direct view of the oropharynx
and their inner boundaries can be mapped by
CT scanning (Figure 20-17) [16]. In localized
extranodal NHL of head and neck, disease-free
survival following high-energy electron beam
irradiation averages 50% at 10 years.

NHLs of the Gastrointestinal Tract

Lymphoma originating in the stomach represents over half of gastrointestinal (GI) lymphomas, and its incidence in patients over 50 years

of age appears to be increasing, possibly reflecting more accurate case ascertainment. Most
gastric lymphomas are metastatic growths of
nodal origin, for through proximity the stomach is placed at risk by the tendency of NHLs
to flourish in mesenteric nodes (Figure 20-18)
[17] and to spread or skip along the chains of
paraaortic nodes in the abdominal neighbor-
hood (Figure 20-19) [18].

Primary gastric lymphomas are almost always of the diffuse large cell type. They arise
from lymphoid islands in the lamina propria,
extend along and undermine submucosal
planes, and cause diffuse thickening of mucosal folds and engender nodular submucosal
masses (Figure 20-20) [19].

Patients usually complain of pain, vomiting,
or GI bleeding, and diagnosis is made by
fiberoptic endoscopy and visually directed biopsy. Conventional therapy for early stage
(nonpenetrating) gastric lymphoma is surgical
resection of the tumor-involved region, backed
up in stage II patients (with perforation or
nodal involvement) by 3-port irradiation plus
intensive chemotherapeutic combinations such
as "MACOP-B." Ten-year survival in patients
with early stage primary gastric lymphoma is
70 to 80%, but prognosis is grim in patients
presenting with widespread nodal involvement
or disseminated disease.

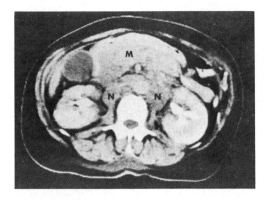

FIGURE 20-18

CT image of the abdomen, revealing a large in-
tramesenteric lymph node mass (M) and
paraaortic adenopathy (N) in a patient with
NHL. (From Golding SJ: Use of imaging in the
management of lymphoma. Br J Hosp Med
41:152,1989.)

FIGURE 20-19

Large-field view of coronal short TI inversion
recovery (STIR) MR scan through abdomen and
pelvis of a patient with suspected dissemination
of NHL discloses left paraaortic and right iliac
lymphomas (arrows). (From Greco A et al: MR
imaging of lymphomas: impact on therapy. J
Comput Assist Tomogr 12:785,1988.)

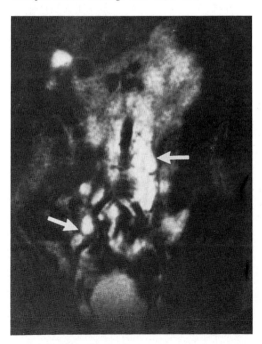

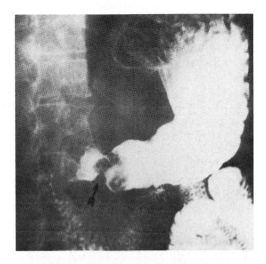

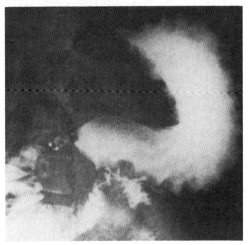

FIGURE 20-20

Contrast radiographic study showing characteristic appearance of primary gastric NHL of diffuse large cell type. (Above) Mass effect in the
antrum (arrow). (Below) The thick wrinkled
mucosal folds create a scalloped pattern evident
on follow-through. (From Haber DA and
Mayer RJ: Primary gastrointestinal lymphoma.
Semin Oncol 15:154,1988).

Other primary gastrointestinal lymphomas   Primary NHL of the small bowel accounts for 20% of GI lymphomas. Patients with coeliac disease, α heavy chain disease, regional enteritis, or various forms of immunodysfunction, including HIV infection, are strongly predisposed to develop intestinal lymphoma. The lymphoma usually originates in follicles in the wall of the terminal ileum and most are of diffuse large cell or small noncleaved cell (Burkitt's-like) histology, although T cell lymphomas have been reported in the upper intestine in patients with underlying coeliac disease. Sporadic Burkitt's lymphoma commonly originates in Peyer's patches and forms polypoid tumors having such prodigious growth potential that patients present with crampy lower abdominal pain and bleeding,

often accompanied by intestinal obstruction. Multiple on-line tumors may protrude from the lamina propria of the ileum or colon, forming large friable polypoid masses that can produce intermittent intussuption as well as bleeding (Figure 20-21) [20].

NHLs of the Central Nervous System

Central nervous system (CNS) involvement usually occurs by metastatic spread of high-grade lymphomas and is so commonplace in Burkitt's lymphoma (endemic or sporadic) that CNS prophylaxis is mandatory. Primary CNS NHLs represent a very small proportion of lymphomas in immunologically competent individuals, but in patients with severe immunosuppression caused by HIV infection or medication primary high-grade neoplasms of B cell origin (small noncleaved cell lymphoma, B immunoblastomas) are comparatively common. In contrast to systemic lymphomas, which are prone to involve the leptomeninges, primary CNS lymphomas present as intraparenchymal tumors. Primary CNS NHLs are often multicentric by the time they are recognized, and the cerebrum is nearly always involved, with later spread to cerebellum or brainstem, or rarely to the spinal cord. Clinical presentation is prompted by global cortical dysfunction (subacute dementia), disorders of gait, or an assortment of more focal neuropathies. Cerebral tumors are usually paraventricular, fungating masses, often possessing merging extensions or satellite tumor nodules, and tend to crop up in the frontal lobes and deep nuclei (Figure 20-22) [21]. Despite confinement to the brain and an inherent radiosensitivity, primary lymphomas of the brain confer a very poor prognosis, obstinately progressing despite valiant combinations of irradiation, systemic high-dose cytosine arabinoside, and intrathecal methotrexate.

Cutaneous T Cell Lymphomas

Cutaneous T cell lymphomas (CTCLs) encompass two closely related indolent but malicious disorders—mycosis fungoides and Sézary syndrome—in which the malignant cells originate in lymph nodes, display a mature helper/inducer T cell phenotype and distinctive mor-

FIGURE 20-21

Left hemicolectomy specimen removed from a 27-year-old man with non-African Burkitt's lymphoma shows polypoid masses of tumor cells growing from the mucosa of the splenic flexure and sigmoid colon. (From Priebe WM: The endoscopic appearance of Burkitt's lymphoma involving the stomach and colon. Gastrointest Endosc 32:352,1986.)

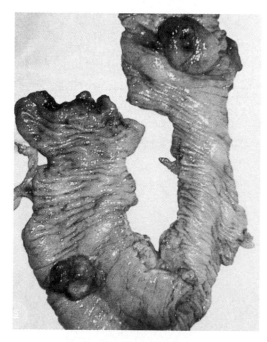

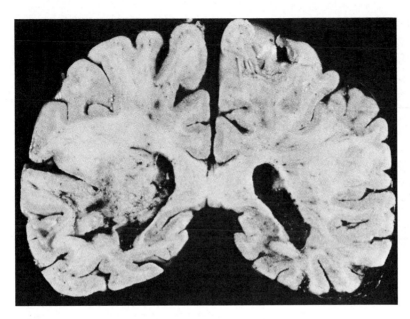

FIGURE 20-22

Gross brain specimen showing large fungating lymphoma in left hemisphere white matter, mushrooming into the ventricle. A smaller granular tumor protrusion is present in the right hemisphere. (From So YT et al: Primary central nervous system lymphoma in acquired immune deficiency syndrome: a clinical and pathological study. Ann Neurol 20:566,1986.)

phology, and possess a singular epidermotropism that causes circulating tumor cells to home in on the upper dermis and epidermis. Tumor cell colonies thrive in the upper dermis, increase their size and deformation, and eventually undergo malignant transformation with clonal rearrangements of the TcR (sometimes accompanied by Ig gene rearrangements), and metastasize to other organs.

Cytology of Sézary cells The malignant cells of CTCL, Sézary cells, are heterogeneous and can be grouped into two principal morphologic categories: large atypical lymphocytes with convoluted nuclei surrounded by clear cytoplasmic vesicles arrayed like a string of pearls; and slightly enlarged lymphocytes having condensed, deeply creased, cerebriform, or lumpy nuclei (Figure 20-23).

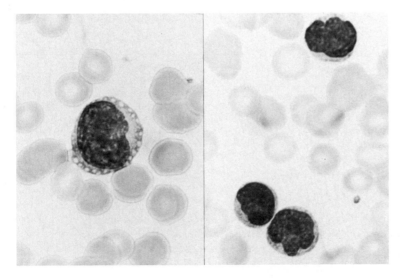

FIGURE 20-23

Malignant T cell variants found in CTCL and known collectively as Sézary cells. (Left) Large hyperdiploid-appearing cell with a cerebriform nucleus surrounded by a pearly necklace of vacuoles. (Right) Three Sézary-type cells (at lower magnification) having grooved, convoluted, or mulberrylike nuclei. Sézary nuclei often resemble a clenched fist. (Photos by CT Kapff.)

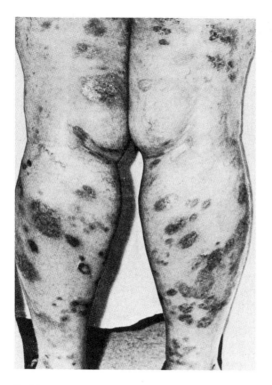

FIGURE 20-24

Plaque-stage mycosis fungoides, showing expanding plaques of various dimensions, with serpiginous margins, central clearing, and psoriatic scaling. (From Winkler CF and Bunn PA Jr: Cutaneous T-cell lymphoma: A review. CRC Crit Rev Oncol Hematol 1:49,1983.)

Cutaneous and extracutaneous lesions Early skin lesions are often evanescent but eventually settle into a staged evolution occurring over a period of 6 to 8 years, known as the Alibert-Bazin progression. Scurfy, itchy, erythematous patches with serpentine margins come and go capriciously but eventually persistent papules appear which coalesce into plaques, and these in turn expand to cover over 10% of the skin surface, signifying the advent of skin tumors and nodal and extranodal tumor cell invasion (Figure 20-24) [22]. Generalized erythroderma often precedes tumor formation, and is associated with exfoliation, denudation, and induration of the entire integument, so that the fixed, dilated vessels of the parched skin are unable to conserve heat and the patient is forced to huddle miserably under layers of blankets.

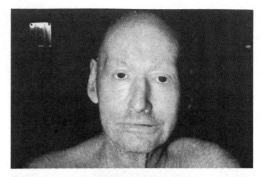

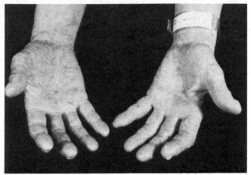

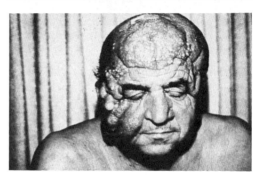

FIGURE 20-25

Progression in CTCL from generalized erythroderma with alopecia and eversion of the eyelids (above) to diffuse induration and leathery fissuring of crease areas such as the palms of the hands (middle). In late-stage disease (below), multiple disfiguring cauliflowerlike tumors cluster around the head and face, creating a leonine appearance. (From Eddy JL et al: Cutaneous T-cell lymphoma. Am J Nursing 84:202,1984.)

Appalling cutaneous tumors appear, particularly on the face (leonine facies) and body folds, further driving the demoralized patient into a state of isolation and self-rejection (Fig-

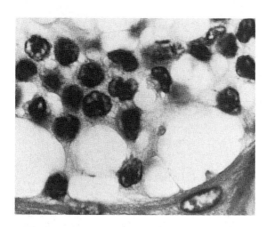

FIGURE 20-26

Skin biopsy of the epidermis in CTCL, showing a Pautrier's microabscess—a disorganized focal infiltrate composed entirely of large atypical lymphocytes having convoluted nuclei. (Reprinted with permission from Winkler CF and Bunn PA Jr. CRC Crit Rev Oncol Hematol 1:49,1983. Copyright CRC Press, Inc., Boca Raton, FL.)

ure 20-25) [23]. Ultimately, in untreated patients, every organ system of the body becomes infiltrated by malignant T cells, and generalized infiltrative adenopathy is invariable. Infection of cutaneous lesions and dissemination of tumor cells to viscera and vital organs are the most common causes of death.

Diagnosis and therapy   Biopsy of an indurated plaque reveals bandlike infiltration of the upper dermis by a polymorphous mixture of inflammatory cells which (as tumor growth advances) become displaced by burrowing nodules of convoluted T4 cells. Infiltrating Sézary cells often collect in chambered clusters called Pautrier's microabscesses—a pathognomonic lesion (Figure 20-26) [22].

Two-thirds of CTCL patients present with limited plaque (Stage I) disease, and "cutaneous treatments" alone are quite effective in subduing the galling symptoms and signs for several years. These skin-deep therapeutic modalities are of three sorts: topical chemotherapy, photochemotherapy with psoralin and ultraviolet A light (PUVA), or whole body electron beam irradiation. For more advanced (Stage II$^+$) disease, combined modality therapy is necessary and grants a reprieve in survival of

70 to 80% of patients at 5 years, although the penalty in side effects may be severe. Therapies still under evaluation include extracorporeal photochemotherapy, IFNα, deoxycoformycin, and monoclonal antibodies such as T101, which is a hybridoma-generated IgG2a directed against CD5, a 60,000 M_r antigen displayed more densely by malignant than by normal T cells. Infusions of T101 have proved disappointing in halting tumor cell progression, but when labelled with ^{111}In and given parenterally, the radioactive antibody targets deep tumor areas with remarkable definition for staging purposes (Figure 20-27) [24]. Meticulous staging as by ^{111}In nodal scintigraphy has revealed extracutaneous dissemination in about 90% of CTCL patients at presentation,

FIGURE 20-27

Anterior and posterior gamma camera images of a 61-year-old woman with erythroderma, palpable adenopathy, and Sézary cells in the blood. The diffuse skin involvement is associated with cervical, submental, axillary, inguinal and femoral node disease. Concentration of isotope in the liver, spleen, and marrow largely represents isotope spillover. (From Carrasquillo JA et al: Radioimmunodetection of cutaneous T-cell lymphoma with ^{111}In-labeled T101 monoclonal antibody. Reprinted, by permission of The New England Journal of Medicine, 315:673,1986.)

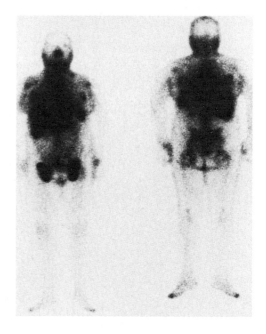

which means that most patients should receive combined modality therapy, despite its punishing side effects; the only alternative possibility for lasting cure is marrow transplantation.

Prelymphomas and Lymphomatoid Disorders

Several uncommon lymphoproliferative processes appear at first to be benign, polyclonal, polymorphic disorders but exhibit a chronic relapsing pattern that often eventuates in overgrowth of homogeneous populations of aggressive diffuse large cell, mixed cell, or immunoblastic lymphomas. Early lesions do not look malignant, for infiltrates are composed of a "reactive" potpourri of lymphocytes, plasma cells, macrophages, and eosinophils. With time this inflammatory melange is joined by increasing numbers of large atypical lymphoid cells or immunoblasts possessing a mature T helper phenotype and exhibiting monoclonality as certified on Southern blot analysis by clonal rearrangement of TcR β and γ chain genes. The issue of whether the staged transformation represents conversion from a prelymphoma to an overt lymphoma is still a matter of dispute, a debate kept alive by the multiple clinical presentations—primarily as lymphomatoid granulomatosis (LG) and angioimmunoblastic lymphadenopathy (AIL), sometimes associated with dysproteinemia (AILD). Nomenclature

has been tortured over the years, but recently this spectrum of post-thymic T cell proliferations has been grouped under the term "angiocentric lymphoma," for a pathologic feature held in common by LG and AIL is that the infiltrates are perivascular, with a strong impetus to invade, occlude, and destroy small blood vessels, resulting in necrosis both of tumor cells and adjacent normal tissue.

Angiocentric Lymphoma

Lesions of angiocentric lymphoma nearly always arise in extranodal sites such as the lungs (lymphomatoid granulomatosis), skin (lymphomatoid vasculitis), and mucosa of the nose and paranasal sinuses (polymorphic reticulosis). Early in the course pulmonary nodules may come and go, but eventually 80% of patients develop bilateral necrotizing pulmonary angitis with multiple poorly marginated nodular densities visible in the lower and middle lobes on radiography. Pulmonary lesions responsible for the patient's dyspnea and chest pain resemble a combination of Wegener's granulomatosis and malignant lymphoma on lung biopsy (Figure 20-28) [25]. The skin is infiltrated by atypical lymphoplasmacytic cells that congregate to cause unsightly erythematous, painful plaques and nodules (Figure 20-29) [26]. Nearly half of patients with early-stage angio-

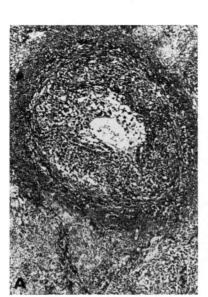
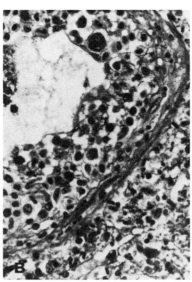

FIGURE 20-28

Angiocentric lymphoma of the lung in a patient with disseminated disease. (A) Section of lung shows vascular infiltration and occlusion by tumor cells, surrounded by extensive necrosis. (B) High-power view reveals the vascular infiltrate to be composed of atypical noncleaved large and small lymphoid cells. (From Lipford EH Jr et al: Angiocentric immunoproliferative lesions: a clinicopathologic spectrum of post-thymic T-cell proliferations. Blood 72:1674,1988.)

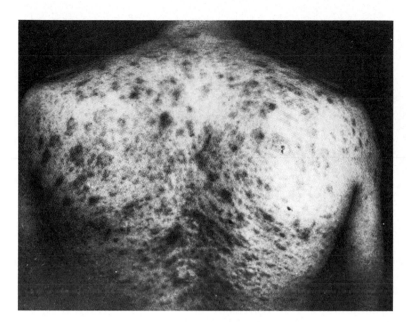

FIGURE 20-29

Erythematous and violaceous plaques of 1 month duration on the back of a 38-year-old man with angiocentric lymphoma. Some of these indurated plaques are annular with central clearing; others show necrosis. (From Jambrosic J et al: Lymphomatoid granulomatosis. J Am Acad Dermatol 17:621,1987.)

centric lymphoma enjoy sustained remission on cyclophosphamide and prednisone, but supervening lymphomas are usually refractory to chemotherapy. The recent therapeutic drift has been toward use of aggressive chemotherapy plus consolidative irradiation in this "prelymphomatous" disorder to avert transformation to an untreatable higher-grade malignancy.

Lymphomatoid papulosis Lymphomatoid papulosis (LP) of the skin is reminiscent of angiocentric lymphoma in its initially benign, fluctuating, and evanescent course (described poetically as "rhythmic paradoxical eruptions"), multifocal expression, and T cell provenance. The characteristic transient papulonodular rashes are caused by fulminant infiltrations of the dermis by a mixture of helper T cells possessing Sézarylike cerebriform nuclei and activated T cells having the multinucleated appearance and Ki-1 antigen ordinarily associated with Reed-Sternberg cells. This malignant eruption can be controlled by local application ad hoc of topical carmustine or by oral methotrexate. In the 10 to 20% of patients whose disease transforms without warning into an aggressive systemic lymphoma, attempts to treat with intensive chemotherapy have proved notably unsuccessful. In its natural history and kinetic caprice, LP is to NHL what preleukemia is to AML.

MANAGEMENT OF NHLs

Management is peculiar to each lymphoma entity, and indications of the kind and success rate of each therapeutic modality have been cited briefly in context with each lymphoma described. Treatment protocols for NHLs are too complex and changeable for the scope of this book. Those readers who are understandably depressed by the grim prognostications applicable to most NHLs may take heart from the successes over high- and medium-grade NHLs using reinforced versions of the "CHOP family" of drugs (e.g., MACOP-B), autologous marrow transplantation (often involving marrow cleanup with complement-fixing monoclonal antibodies), and simultaneous use of recombinant biological response modifiers and tumor-specific antibodies. An example of the last is the joint administration of IFNα with hybridoma-produced anti-idiotype antibodies

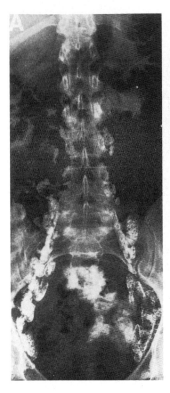
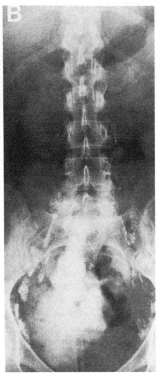

FIGURE 20-30

Lymphangiogram of a 44-year-old woman with disseminated follicular small cleaved cell lymphoma before (A) and after (B) treatment with anti-idiotype antibody and α interferon. Patient also had bulky nodes in the cervical and supraclavicular areas, a mesenteric mass, and marrow infiltration. Tumor regression in all sites was evident within 2.5 weeks after initiation of treatment and was sustained for over 1 year of follow-up. (From Brown SL et al: Treatment of B-cell lymphomas with anti-idiotype antibodies alone and in combination with alpha interferon. Blood 73:651,1989.)

(Figure 20-30) [27]. Means are being developed to prevent escape from such rational therapies. Hybrid anti-idiotypic antibodies are being constructed that are cytolytic for tumor cells in vivo but do not arouse an anti–anti-idiotypic response. It is realistic to surmise that NHLs will go the way of Hodgkin's disease by the year 2000.

REFERENCES

1. Newell GR et al: Incidence of lymphoma in the US classified by the Working Formulation. Cancer 59:857,1987

2. Green TL and Eversole LR: Oral lymphomas in HIV-infected patients: association with Epstein-Barr virus DNA. Oral Surg Oral Med Oral Pathol 67:437,1989

3. Knowles DM et al: Molecular genetic analysis of three AIDS-associated neoplasms of uncertain lineage demonstrates their B-cell derivation and the possible pathogenetic role of the Epstein-Barr virus. Blood 73:792, 1989

4. Stein H et al: The normal and malignant germinal centre. Clin Haematol 11:531, 1982

5. Stuart AE et al, Eds.: Chapt 1, in Lymphomas Other than Hodgkin's Disease. Oxford, Oxford University Press,1981

6. Jaffe ES: Chapt 9, in Atlas of Blood Cells: Function and Pathology, vol. 2, Zucker-Franklin D et al, Eds. Milan, Edi. Ermes s.r.l.,1988

7. Tindle BH: Malignant lymphomas. Am J Pathol 116:115,1984

8. Croce CM and Nowell PC: Molecular basis of human B cell neoplasia. Blood 65:1,1985

9. Lee M-S et al: Detection of minimal residual cells carrying the t(14;18) by DNA sequence amplification. Science 237:175,1987

10. Ngan B-Y et al: Detection of chromosomal translocation t(14;18) within the minor cluster region of bcl-2 by polymerase chain reaction and direction genomic sequencing

of the enzymatically amplified DNA in follicular lymphomas. Blood 73:1759,1989

11. Canellos GP: Section 12, Subsection XI. Malignant Lymphomas, in Scientific American Medicine. Rubenstein E and Federman DD, Eds. New York, Scientific American, Inc.,1988

12. Knowles DM et al: Clinicopathologic, immunophenotypic, and molecular genetic analysis of AIDS-associated lymphoid neoplasia. Clinical and biologic implications. Pathol Annu 23(part 2):33,1988

13. Kearns DB et al: Burkitt's lymphoma. Int J Pediatr Otorhinolaryngol 12:73,1986

14. Jandl JH: Chapt 28, in Blood: Textbook of Hematology. Boston, Little, Brown and Company, 1987

15. Schwartz EE et al: Mediastinal involvement in adults with lymphoblastic lymphoma. Acta Radiol 28:403,1987

16. Lee Y-Y et al: Lymphomas of the head and neck: CT findings at initial presentation. AJR 149.575,1987

17. Golding SJ: Use of imaging in the management of lymphoma. Br J Hosp Med 41:152, 1989

18. Greco A et al: MR imaging of lymphomas: impact on therapy. J Comput Assist Tomogr 12:785,1988

19. Haber DA and Mayer RJ: Primary gastrointestinal lymphoma. Semin Oncol 15:154, 1988

20. Priebe WM: The endoscopic appearance of Burkitt's lymphoma involving the stomach and colon. Gastrointest Endosc 32:352,1986

21. So YT et al: Primary central nervous system lymphoma in acquired immune deficiency syndrome: a clinical and pathological study. Ann Neurol 20:566,1986

22. Winkler CF and Bunn PA Jr: Cutaneous T-cell lymphoma: A review. CRC Crit Rev Oncol Hematol 1:49,1983

23. Eddy JL et al: Cutaneous T-cell lymphoma. Am J Nursing 84:202,1984

24. Carrasquillo JA et al: Radioimmunodetection of cutaneous T-cell lymphoma with ^{111}In-labeled T101 monoclonal antibody. N Engl J Med 315:673,1986

25. Lipford EH Jr et al: Angiocentric immunoproliferative lesions: a clinicopathologic spectrum of post-thymic T-cell proliferations. Blood 72:1674,1988

26. Jambrosic J et al: Lymphomatoid granulomatosis. J Am Acad Dermatol 17:621,1987

27. Brown SL et al: Treatment of B-cell lymphomas with anti-idiotype antibodies alone and in combination with alpha interferon. Blood 73:651,1989

21

Hemostasis

☐

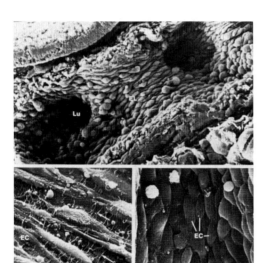

FIGURE 21-1

Scanning EMs of endothelium of small blood vessels. (Top) Capillary endothelium (EL) is composed of flattened ellipsoidal cells aligned along the axis of flow and intimately joined at their margins by fused junctional complexes. Their nuclei cause the cells to bulge at their center into the vessel lumen (Lu). Endothelial cells (EC) of veins (bottom left) are deployed more loosely, being linked corsetlike by lateral fibrillar processes; the intervening exposed subendothelium is potentially thrombogenic and accounts for the prevalence of thrombi in veins. In contrast, endothelial cells of arteries (bottom right) are smooth and tightly joined, their negatively charged surfaces repelling sticky platelets and granulocytes that travel in the marginal stream. (From Tissues and Organs. A Text-Atlas of Scanning Electron Microscopy. By Richard Kessel and Randy Kardon. Copyright (c) 1979 by W.H. Freeman and Company. Reprinted with permission.)

Hemostasis, the arrest of hemorrhage at sites of vascular injury with restored perfusion after damage is mended, is a wondrous achievement of evolution. The system of checks and balances responsible for preventing exsanguination while preserving blood's liquidity is dauntingly complex, involving a symphonic interplay between vascular endothelium, platelets, coagulation, complement, and fibrinolysis. When a blood vessel is severed, an immediate concerted response is achieved by reflex vasoconstriction and formation of a platelet plug (primary hemostasis). This buys time for the slower formation of a tough fibrin meshwork (thrombus) that seals off the defect (secondary hemostasis) and provides a scaffold for angiogenic repair of the vascular wall. The hemostatic sequence is orchestrated and confined to the area of vascular damage by secretions elaborated by vascular endothelium. The miracle of hemostasis is that it usually works: normally blood vessels are capable of self-sealing and yet perfusion is sustained. Failure of the system may lead to bleeding disorders, which are well understood but seldom fatal, or to thrombotic disorders, which are less well understood and represent the commonest of all causes of death.

VASCULAR ENDOTHELIUM IS NONTHROMBOGENIC

Endothelial cells possess numerous kinds of adhesion molecules in their subendothelial (abluminal) surface that anchor them to adventitia, but on the surface facing the bloodstream, endothelium presents a tightly joined nonthrombogenic pavement that separates and shields platelets and coagulation factors of blood from thrombogenic components of the vascular matrix (Figure 21-1) [1].

Synthetic and Secretory Functions of Vascular Endothelium

In addition to providing a smooth, slippery, nonthrombogenic permeability barrier, endothelial cells are busily engaged in active synthesis and secretion both of procoagulants necessary for vascular maintenance and of anticoagulants that forestall or abrogate senseless coagulation. Among coagulants secreted largely from the abluminal surface are collagen, tissue factor (thromboplastin), fibronectin, proteoglycans, and von Willebrand factor (vWF). Among anticoagulants released into the blood are prostaglandin I_2 (PGI_2), thrombomodulin, heparan, and plasminogen activator.

Naturally Occurring Anticoagulant Mechanisms

Several structurally unrelated anticoagulants are produced by endothelium or activated on endothelial surfaces. These factors act in collusion on vessel walls to protect the vasculature from inappropriate activation of the terminal steps of the coagulation cascade: formation of the prothrombinase complex and fibrinogenesis by thrombin. Endothelial cells stimulated by injury or epinephrine synthesize prostaglandin I_2 (PGI_2, or prostacyclin), a potent vasodilator and the most powerful known inhibitor of platelet aggregation. More direct protection of intact endothelium is provided by two distinct anticoagulant mechanisms operative on the endothelial surface: inactivation of thrombin and its cofactors, factors V and VIII, by thrombomodulin and protein C; and neutralization of thrombin, factor X, and several other key coagulation proteases by antithrombin III (AT III), allosteric activation of which depends on heparan sulfate, a glycosaminoglycan activated on the endothelium surface. Finally, should this prophylactic barricade be broken through, endothelium responds by elaborating tissue plasminogen activators (t-PAs), which recruit plasmin—the sole enzyme responsible for liquifying thrombi. The preemptive and anticoagulant arsenal of endothelium is portrayed schematically in Figure 21-2 [2].

Thrombomodulin and activation of protein C

Protein C is a vitamin K–dependent glycoprotein (M_r: 62,000) that circulates as a double chain plasma zymogen (5 μg/ml) and is activated during 1:1 high-affinity binding to thrombin—the pivotal protein of the coagulation cascade. Protein C interaction with thrombin takes place on a thrombin-binding endothelial surface receptor named thrombomodulin. There are 50,000 copies of thrombomodulin situated on each endothelial cell, and when thrombin is seated upon the thrombomodulin receptor the rate at which it activates protein C is accelerated 30,000-fold. Thrombomodulin serves in two ways to contain thrombogenesis: first, it traps circulating free thrombin and alters its substrate affinity so

FIGURE 21-2

Endothelial secretory and surface reactions that prevent or nullify inopportune coagulation. Endothelial cells synthesize PGI_2 (prostacyclin), thrombomodulin, heparan, and plasminogen activators—all of which inhibit thrombosis and help preserve vascular patency. (From Colman RW et al: Chapt 1, in Hemostasis and Thrombosis: Basic Principles and Clinical Practice, 2nd ed., Colman RW et al, Eds. Philadelphia, JB Lippincott Company, 1987.)

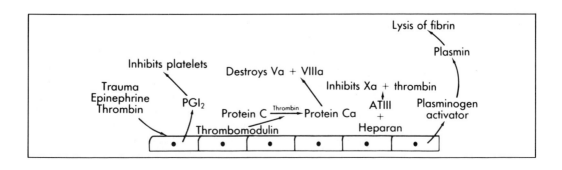

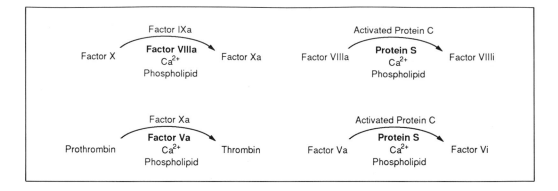

FIGURE 21-3

Role of factor VIIIa and factor Va in blood coagulation (left), and inactivation of these
cofactors to VIIIi and Vi by activated protein C
in the presence of protein S and other cofactors
(right). (From Kane WH and Davie EW: Blood
coagulation factors V and VIII: structural and
functional similarities and their relationship to
hemorrhagic and thrombotic disorders. Blood
71:539,1988.)

that it no longer has coagulant activity; second, it generates a circulating anticoagulant,
protein Ca (activated protein C, or APC).
Protein C in the presence of protein S (another
vitamin K–dependent peptide) has a uniquely
high affinity for platelet surfaces where it is
rapidly converted to APC, which in turn degrades activated cofactors V (factor Va) and
VIII (factor VIIIa) to inactive molecules (Vi
and VIIIi); Vi and VIIIi are incapable of acting
as platelet receptors for the critical enzymes,
factors IXa and Xa, thereby blocking surface
activation of prothrombin to thrombin (Figure
21-3) [3]. Protein C and factor X operate
antithetically: activated protein C destroys essential coagulation cofactors Va and VIIIa but
is held in check by a trace protein named APC
inhibitor; activated factor X is propellant of
the terminal coagulation cascade but is reined
in by antithrombin III.

Antithrombin III (heparin cofactor)   Antithrombin III (AT III), a single chain 58,000 M_r
peptide produced by endothelium, megakaryo-

cytes, and liver and present in plasma at
concentrations of about 150 μg/ml, is the most
important inhibitor of terminal proteases of
the coagulation cascade—notably factor Xa
and thrombin. AT III acting alone is a sluggish
inhibitor of these proteases, but the rate of
binding and inhibition by AT III is accelerated
by over 1,000-fold either by heparin or by
contact with endothelial cells, which secrete
and coat themselves with a monolayer of
heparan sulfate. Heparin and heparan are
highly sulfated, negatively charged glycosa-
minoglycans which bind to lysyl residues on
AT III and induce an allosteric change in its
arginine reactive site that makes AT available
for covalent binding to the active center
(serine) residues of thrombin; 1:1 binding of
thrombin or factor Xa to AT III causes the
inactivated complexes to be washed downstream from the site of injury. When bound to
heparin containing eight or more sulfated
monosaccharide subunits, AT III specifically
inhibits factor Xa, the springboard of the
coagulation waterfall; only with binding of
heparin having additional domains (labelled 2
and 3), does AT III inactivate thrombin, as well
as several other coagulation proteases (XIIa,
XIa, IXa) (Figure 21-4) [4].

Plasminogen activators   Plasmin is the only
enzyme capable of dissolving thrombi and also
acts synergistically with PGI_2 in inhibiting
platelet activation. Conversion of the circulating zymogen, plasminogen, to plasmin is initiated by tissue plasminogen activator (t-PA), a
68,000 M_r serine protease synthesized in re-

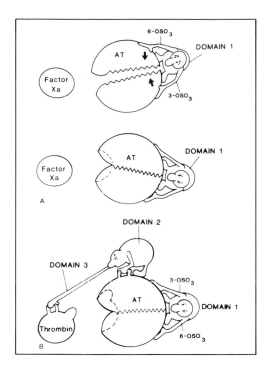

FIGURE 21-4

Specific interactions of heparin with antithrombin (AT) that are required for enzyme activation. (A) Factor Xa—AT III—heparin interactions require participation only of heparin domain 1 containing a total of nine sulfates. (B) Thrombin—AT III—heparin interactions require additional sulfated domains. (From Rosenberg RD: Chapt 5, in The Molecular Basis of Blood Diseases, Stamatoyannopoulos G et al, Eds. Philadelphia, WB Saunders Company,1987.)

sponse to local fibrin deposition, increased shear stress, or vascular occlusion. When complexed with plasminogen bound to fibrin, t-PA undergoes conformational changes causing it to bind fibrin through ligands located on the kringle-2 segment of the activator, yielding a ternary complex. The high affinity of t-PA for plasminogen bound to fibrin surfaces enables efficient generation of plasminogen within a fibrin clot, whereas in plasma, activation of plasminogen by t-PA is virtually nil. Plasmin formed on the fibrin surface has both its lysine-binding sites and the active site serine occupied and thus is protected against proteolysis by α_2-antiplasmin; once released into plasma, free

plasmin is inhibited rapidly by α_2-antiplasmin and by an α_2-macroglobulin (α_2M) secreted by endothelium. Hence the entire fibrinolytic process is triggered by and confined to fibrin.

Synthesis and release of t-PA appears to be regulated by neurochemical signals, and certain drugs (DDAVP, a vasopressin analog, and stanazolol, an impeded anabolic steroid) are potent artificial stimulants of activator release. Expeditious infusion of recombinant t-PA is now an important weapon in reopening acutely thrombosed blood vessels.

Adhesive Secretions of Endothelium: Mechanisms of Cell Adhesion

Adhesion is a universal and primordial feature of such critical processes as embryogenesis, angiogenesis, and cell-mediated immune function and its regulation is of conspicuous importance in hemostasis. Adhesion between cells or between cells and substrates proceeds in orderly stages: recognition; contact; multiple-bond formation; and consolidation. Adhesive interactions are mediated by a family of cell-adhesive molecules (CAMS) that includes intercellular adhesive molecules (ICAMS or IAMS) such as fibrinogen and thrombospondin which link platelets together; and substrate-adhesive molecules (SAMS), such as the vWF, fibronectin, and collagen molecules of the subendothelial matrix which provide solid-state support for anchorage of cells and mediate binding of platelets to subendothelium.

Integrins can read the RGD zip code Almost all adhesion molecules possess a zip code that contains the sequence Arg-Gly-Asp (RGD) and provides them with a recognition site for members of a superfamily of heterodimeric membrane-spanning protein receptors known as "integrins." A fourth residue (usually serine) is often required for firm binding of adhesive proteins to their particular receptors: this is true of the recognition-site domains of vWF, fibronectin, and fibrinogen, and fibrinogen is also equipped with a γ chain peptide that serves as an adhesive pocket for the fibrinogen receptors on platelets. RGD sequences of each of the adhesive proteins are recognized by at least one member of the integrin family of receptors, but some receptors bind to the RGD sequence of a single adhesion protein only, whereas others recognize groups of them. For example, fibrinogen cannot replace fibronectin in mediating adhesion of fibroblasts to the substrate, and fibronectin cannot substitute for fibrinogen in promoting platelet aggregation; on the other hand the platelet integrin, a complex of glycoproteins IIb and IIIa (GP IIb-IIIa), has more relaxed requirements and will bind both fibrinogen and vWF.

RGD adhesives are composed of multiple large subunits held in register by clusters of disulfide bonds. They are designed with inherent elegance, forming long flexible loops capable of retracting into coiled balls. Clearly adhesion to integrin receptors is enhanced if the RGD signal is multiplied by repeating structures (as with collagen) or by multimer formation. The apotheosis of adhesive design is vWF, a critical and complex molecule responsible for stable binding of platelets to exposed subendothelium.

von Willebrand Factor (vWF)

vWF is only one of six components of subendothelium that can potentially bind platelets, but its unique role is attested to by the inability of patients deficient in vWF to form a stable hemostatic plug. Although platelets have their own collagen receptors and adhere to raw collagen fibrils exposed by loss of endothelium (Figure 21-5) [5], stable platelet adhesion following less brutal vascular damage (as occurs daily) requires vWF, which instantly forms a firm bridge between subendothelium and a platelet membrane receptor, glycoprotein Ib (GPIb). This stitch-in-time prevents adhering platelets from being detached by the high shear forces of flowing blood, and additional binding of vWF to the alternative vWF receptor (GP IIb-IIIa) stimulates adherent platelets to spread out like fried eggs.

vWF forms multimeric velcrolike grippers   vWF is synthesized as large precursor polypeptides (pre-pro-vWFs) that undergo posttranslational cleavage to dimers of the mature 220,000 M_r product. These head-to-head dimers serve as the nidus for polymerization to repeating structures ranging up to 20 million M_r; when released into circulation (normal concentration: 10 μg/ml), the zigzag filamentous polymer assumes an accordionated ellipsoidal form approximately 500 nm long but capable of stretching for distances up to 2 μm—a length more than sufficient for binding platelets to damaged vascular surfaces. Each vWF protomer possesses a domain for binding GPIb and an RGD sequence for attachment to the RGD

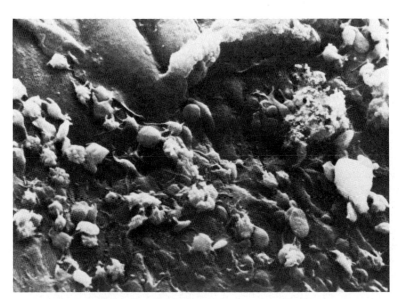

FIGURE 21-5

Scanning EM view of vascular surface after partial deendothelialization. Platelets adhere to exposed connective tissue of subendothelium (below) but not to undisturbed endothelium (above). Note transformation of tightly attached platelets to spiny spheres. (From Stemerman MB et al: Perturbations of the endothelium. Prog Hemost Thromb 7:289,1984.)

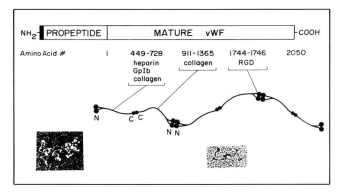

FIGURE 21-6

Organization of the pre-pro-vWF is depicted along with the locations of functional domains. The coiled appearance of the filamentous vWF multimer is shown in a darkfield EM (lower left), and the strung-out structure of a protomeric vWF subunit is shown by rotary shadowed EM (lower right). (From Handin RI and Wagner DD: Molecular and cellular biology of von Willebrand factor. Prog Hemost Thromb 9:273,1989.)

receptor on the IIb-IIIa complex (Figure 21-6) [6]. In addition this multifunctional molecule possesses two sites for binding collagen, one for heparin, and—possibly its most important function—a site for noncovalent binding of factor VIII (antihemophilic factor, AHF) via its 80,000 M_r light chain. vWF is not an enzyme: it is a bridging device—the only plasma factor that mediates platelet adherence to arterial subendothelium—and it is the sole transport protein for factor VIII.

Storage and secretion of vWF   In endothelial cells vWF is synthesized, polymerized, and stored in unique rod-shaped organelles up to 4 μm long, in which vWF molecules become highly polymerized and from which they are released facultatively when endothelium is stimulated by physiologic agonists such as thrombin, histamine, and fibrin or by the vasopressin analog, DDAVP (Figure 21-7) [7]. In the resting state endothelial cells secrete most newly synthesized vWF constitutively, packaging only a portion in Weibel-Palade bodies; most constitutively secreted vWF is in the form of small multimers, unlike the giant multimers discharged by Weibel-Palade bodies as a facultative response to agonist stimulation. The bulk of constitutively secreted vWF circulates in plasma ligated to its passenger,

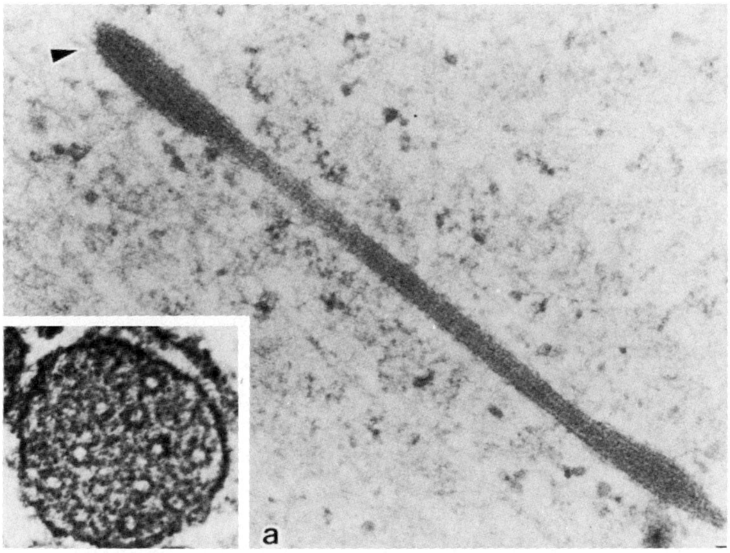

FIGURE 21-7

EMs of Weibel-Palade bodies. (a) A 2-μm-long Weibel-Palade body from an endothelial cell shows longitudinal striations representing sheaths of tubules in which vWF is stored. Note close proximity of a detached microtubule (arrowhead), which may be involved in the vWF transport and release mechanism. Bar = 0.2 μm. Inset: Cross section of a Weibel-Palade body revealing tubular sheaths. (From Wagner DD: Chapt 9, in Coagulation and Bleeding Disorders, Zimmerman TS and Ruggeri ZM, Eds. New York, Marcel Dekker, Inc.,1989. Reprinted by courtesy of Marcel Dekker Inc.)

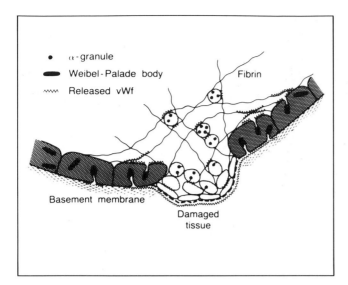

FIGURE 21-8

Schematic representation of the two storage compartments for vWF and their consecutive roles in early repair of vascular injury. vWF released from endothelial Weibel-Palade bodies binds to the exposed matrix and to endothelium; as the coagulation cascade is launched, thrombin activates platelets to discharge vWF from their α granules. Released vWF stabilizes platelet adhesion to the vessel wall, promotes platelet-fibrin interaction, and facilitates movement of endothelial cells over the injured area during wound healing. (From Wagner DD: Chapt 9, in Coagulation and Bleeding Disorders, Zimmerman TS and Ruggeri ZM, Eds. New York, Marcel Dekker, Inc.,1989. Reprinted by courtesy of Marcel Dekker Inc.)

factor VIII, as factor VIII/vWF complexes. As the multimeric size of vWF is directly linked to its adhesive tenacity, it is presumed that facultative secretion is destined primarily for vascular wound healing. About 15 to 20% of vWF is stored in Wiebel-Paladelike tubular structures clustered at the periphery of platelet α granules, making large gluey multimers instantly available during formation of platelet plugs. During hemostasis vWF is required at two levels. At the inner level vWF is used to mend the basement membrane and mediate platelet adhesion. As platelets are activated during incipient phases of coagulation, vWF released from the platelet α granules is needed for trussing platelets to fibrin strands and wounded endothelium (Figure 21-8) [7].

PLATELETS AND FORMATION OF THE HEMOSTATIC PLUG

Platelets are anucleate discoid fragments of highly refined structure, enormous energy, and irreplaceably complex functions. Appearing as a mere furry dot on light microscopy and resembling a doughy pancake on SEM (Figure 21-9) [8], platelets are the most important of the many participants in hemostasis. People may live many years without the kingpin of coagulation, fibrinogen, but can't survive a day

without platelets. Platelets normally circulate for 10 days in numbers ranging from 150,000 to 400,000 "cells"/μl, but fewer than 10% of this number suffice to maintain vascular integrity: the redundancy ensures ample reinforcements should platelet losses be heavy. Platelets are required in each major step of hemostasis, and during their short lives they remain available, confined within the circulation; their comparatively gigantic parents, megakaryocytes, on the contrary, grow and eventually discharge their tiny progeny while imprisoned by their very bulk, pressed against the perforate subendothelial bars of marrow sinuses.

Megakaryocytes and Platelet Production

The megakaryocyte progenitor, CFU-Meg, is aroused from the torpor characteristic of stemhood by IL-3 (Chapter 1), and the megakaryoblastic daughter cells are directed to differentiate and mature by a 30,000 M_r glycoprotein dimer known as thrombopoietin. Stem cell regulation by IL-3 is thought to be mediated by a remote sensor of marrow megakaryocyte mass, but the more stringent control of megakaryocyte manufacture of platelets by thrombopoietin suggests that mature platelets devour their stimulus—a literal feedback mechanism. Acting seriatum, CFU-Meg, IL-3, GM-CSF, and thrombopoietin pro-

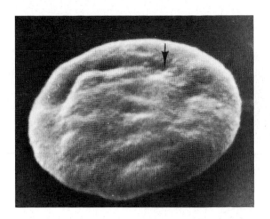

FIGURE 21-9

SEM of resting normal discoid platelet. Indentation (arrow) on the otherwise smoothly contoured surface represents an aperture leading through the cell wall to the cytoplasmic canalicular system. (From White JG: An overview of platelet structural physiology. Scanning Microsc 1:1677,1987.)

FIGURE 21-10

EM view of polar section through mature megakaryocyte cytoplasm reveals a broad gap in the thinned-out marginal zone. Unattached platelets (arrows) appear to be at liberty to escape into the circulation. The lymphocyte (L) can be used for sizing. (From Zucker-Franklin D and Petursson S: Thrombocytopoiesis—analysis by membrane tracer and freeze-fracture studies on fresh human and cultured mouse megakaryocytes. Reproduced from the *Journal of Cell Biology,* 1984, 99:390 by copyright permission of the Rockefeller University Press.)

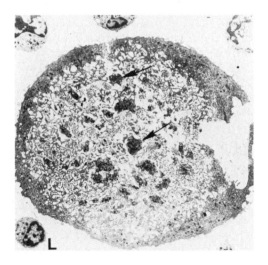

duce three effects on diploid megakaryocyte precursors: increases in their number, size, and ploidy. Unlike other giant cells, megakaryocytes do not replicate by division: ensconced within their paratrabecular marrow niches, megakaryoblasts undergo multiple DNA doublings by the unusual process of endomitosis. The time required for megakaryocytes to complete polyploidization and acquire an 8, 16, 32, or even 64n complement of DNA is about 5 days, during which these bulky cells (average volume: 15,000 fl) acquire a full set of phenotypic markers that are retained by their shed platelets: GP Ib, IIb-IIIa, factor VIII, β-thromboglobulin, and factor V. The most prominent structural acquisitions during early megakaryocyte maturation are the cytoplasmic demarcation system (denoting incipient platelet dimensions), presence of α granules, and expression of a unique "platelet peroxidase" (PPO) activity that serves as a cytochemical EM marker. The stage I megakaryocyte (promegakaryoblast) has a spheroid nucleus and undivided basophilic cytoplasm but as polyploidization continues, nuclear segmentation (or polylobation) occurs, each lobule containing roughly but not exactly a 2n complement of DNA. With maturation toward stage III (adulthood), endomitotic cells display an arborizing demarcation membrane system that divides and subdivides the cytoplasm into granule-containing domains that later define platelet territories. At this stage, the platelet domains acquire individuality, and the granule-rich platelet territories become perforated by small tortuous actin-decorated channels that connect with the open canalicular system and provide access to serotonin, catecholamines, and other storage valuables essential to normal platelet function.

Platelets Are Released by Megakaryocyte Fragmentation

Platelet release as judged by ultrastructural analysis occurs by rapid fragmentation of the ripened megakaryocyte (Figure 21-10) [9]. It is possible that release from fragmenting megakaryocytes (the empty shells of which are later devoured without compunction by macrophages) does not occur explosively, for at least

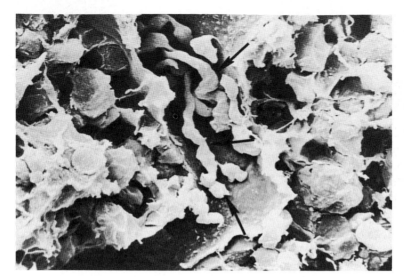

FIGURE 21-11

SEM of marrow sinus into which long platelet chains (arrows) have been extruded by parasinusoidal megakaryocytes. (Modified from Lichtman MA et al: Parasinusoidal location of megakaryocytes in marrow: a determinant of platelet release. Am J Hematol 4:303,1978.)

some platelets are reeled out in connected strands, which dangle into the marrow venous sinuses and develop constrictions, branchings, and finally varicosities that rupture and release individual platelets into the tumult of circulating blood (Figure 21-11) [10].

Platelet Anatomy, Contents, and Responses to Agonists

Platelets are small discoidal pieces of megakaryocyte cytoplasm that have no nucleus and thus no DNA-dependent biosynthetic capability but nonetheless possess a deceptively complex infrastructure that equips them for the multitude of functions the cells subserve. The platelet membrane is a typical trilaminar structure consisting of: an external cloak that contains glycoprotein receptors, which are anchored by their hydrophobic roots; a lipid bilayer to which these receptors are attached; and an underlying submembrane compartment that is composed of actin and myosin microfilaments responsible for platelet shape and shape changes and that contains a complex inventory of platelet granules essential to secretory responses. A singular feature of the platelet cell membrane is that it possesses pores that invaginate deeply to form a surface-connected open canalicular system that allows transport

of agonists inward and discharge of secretions outward ("release reaction"). Platelets have the capacity for directional movement through orderly rearrangements of skeletal components, which direct extension and retraction of pseudopods. While passing through the bloodstream and during shape changes induced by surface activation, platelet integrity is preserved both by ATP-dependent contractile responses of the actin-myosin assembly and by a thick annular bundle of microtubules that underlies the membrane at its greatest circumference and forms an equatorial hoop. In platelets sectioned in an equatorial plane, the peripherally bundled hoops of microtubules are a conspicuous ultrastructural feature and are responsible for the lenticular shape of platelets and the herding together of platelet granules and organelles (Figure 21-12) [11]. For identifying the platelet structures shown in Figure 21-12, a two-dimensional blueprint of platelet design is portrayed in Figure 21-13 [11].

Platelet Shape Changes during Activation

Activation of platelets by exposure to agonists (thrombin, ADP, epinephrine, collagen, and arachidonic acid), subendothelium, or foreign surfaces causes immediate and drastic transformation of shape. In suspension, activated plate-

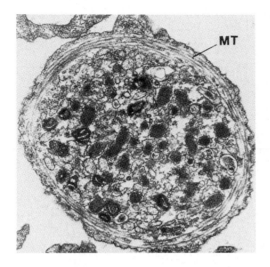

FIGURE 21-12

Equatorial TEM of a normal platelet reveals the thick peripheral hoops of microtubules (MT) that give platelets their lenticular shape. Cytoplasmic organelles and numerous granules heterogeneous in electron density are readily apparent. (From Zucker-Franklin D: Chapt 10, in Atlas of Blood Cells: Function and Pathology, 2nd ed., Zucker-Franklin D et al, Eds. Milan, Edi Ermes s.r.l.,1988.)

lets abruptly transform into spiny spheres, assuming bizarre shapes that actually prepare them to fit together like pieces of a jigsaw puzzle. Platelets exposed to thrombogenic surfaces undergo changes similar to those observed in suspended cells following activation, for the cells become prickly spheres with long spidery pseudopods. Gradually each adherent platelet sinks into the surface, while concentrating its organelles centrally, and extends a broad, smooth lamellar skirt. Removal of the membranes of spread platelets unveils a concentrically woven lacework of cytoskeletal elements, a pattern relieved by lumpy attachment plaques containing actin bundles and microtubules. The sequential shape changes of a platelet ensconced on a carbon grid are displayed in Figure 21-14 [8].

Platelet Adhesion, Aggregation, and Secretory Activity

Adhesion

Within seconds after vascular injury, platelets adhere to the wounded endothelium via the subendothelial bridging molecule, vWF, which

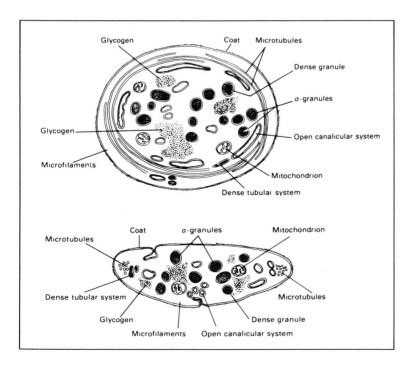

FIGURE 21-13

Schematic representation of platelets cut in the equatorial plane (above) and in cross section (below). (From Zucker-Franklin D: Chapt 10, in Atlas of Blood Cells: Function and Pathology, 2nd ed., Zucker-Franklin D et al, Eds. Milan, Edi Ermes s.r.l.,1988.)

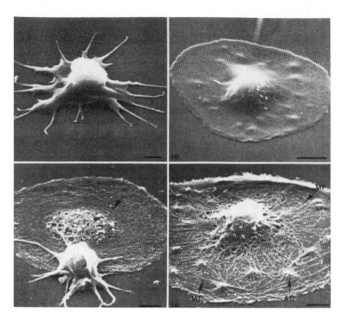

FIGURE 21-14

SEM views of platelet shape changes following contact with a foreign surface (upper panels) and crocheted appearance of the underlying skeletal assembly after the lipid bilayer has been skinned off by detergent extraction (lower two panels). Actin filaments (arrow) at lower left are arranged in a concentric webwork, forcing granules to heap up in a central pile. Actin microfilaments (MF) form the border of this spread fabric (lower right panel), interspersed with microtubules (MT), and as the MTs are constricted into tight rings around the centralized hump of granules, adhesion plaques (AP) glue the platelet to the disputed surface. (From White JG: An overview of platelet structural physiology. Scanning Microsc 1:1677,1987.)

(as described above) has a binding domain for the GPIb receptor seated on the lipid bilayer. Intact GPIb is also the platelet receptor for thrombin, but a peptide fragment of GPIb named glycocalicin is the critical receptor site for native vWF. Platelets respond to activating stimuli with a stereotyped sequence of reactions. After undergoing adhesion and shape changes, platelets aggregate, and finally they secrete prostaglandins and the contents of three different kinds of storage granules in response to a release mechanism initiated by arachidonic acid and implemented by the phosphatidyl inositol–protein kinase C cascade.

Aggregation and the Fibrinogen Receptor

Following adhesion of platelets to the injured vessel wall, the nascent hemostatic plug enlarges by aggregation of platelets to each other. Aggregation is an energetic process stimulated by agonists, the most important of which are ADP, epinephrine, thrombin, and collagen. Aggregation can be quantitated in vitro by use of a modified turbidometer called an aggregometer; the optical principle is identical to that operative when suspended droplets in clouds coalesce to form raindrops, thus clarifying the atmosphere. Aggregation is an immediate consequence of platelet stimulation, as exemplified

by reactions to ADP. After exposure to low concentrations of ADP, the primary or "first wave" aggregatory response is reversible and unassociated with generation of arachidonic acid. After higher concentrations of agonist, a secondary or "second wave" response occurs in which formation of large aggregates is caused by the platelet granule "release reaction," in which platelets are stimulated to secrete their own ADP (causing a chain reaction) and to secrete arachidonic acid, precursor to several potent aggregants (Figure 21-15) [12]. Aggregation in response to all agonists is caused by upregulated expression of platelet receptors for the 34,000 M_r trinodular plasma protein, fibrinogen. The platelet receptor for fibrinogen is a transmembrane glycoprotein dimer, GPIIb-IIIa: the 150,000 M_r GPIIb component binds Ca^{2+}, which acts as an allosteric modifier; the 105,000 M_r GPIIIa part is required for binding of the complex to RGD peptides on the fragment D domain of the fibrinogen γ chains. Normal platelets possess 50,000 GPIIb-IIIa complexes, about 70% of which are located on the platelet membrane, anchored to underlying contractile elements, the remainder being distributed between depots in α granules and the intracellular membranes of the surface-connected canalicular system. Following platelet stimulation by ago-

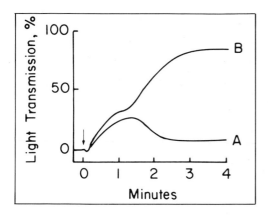

FIGURE 21-15

Platelet aggregation patterns in vitro as monitored by patterns of change in light transmission. (A) At low concentrations of the physiologic agonist ADP, aggregation is limited and reversible. (B) Higher concentrations of agonist induce an amplified "second wave" due to secretion by activated platelets of their own ADP plus byproducts of prostaglandin synthesis. (Reproduced, with permission, from Shattil SJ and Bennett JS: Platelets and their membranes in hemostasis: physiology and pathophysiology. Ann Intern Med 1981;94:108.)

nists, the full complement of membrane receptors (integrins) is bared, and fibrinogen is seized by its RGD and other recognition sites on the Aα chain pair; bound fibrinogen has sufficient reach to form bridges to receptors on adjacent platelets, leading to lattice formation. The GPIIb-IIIa complexes also serve as alternative integrin-type receptors for vWF, thrombospondin, and fibronectin, but fibrinogen in its abundance tends to monopolize the site. As activating stimuli subside, fibrinogen receptors are downregulated and become unavailable to adhesive proteins—a provident feature as platelets normally are immersed in high concentrations (2 to 4 mg/ml) of fibrinogen.

Thrombospondin assists binding of fibrinogen
Binding of fibrinogen to the GPIIb-IIIa receptor of platelets is stabilized by a large (440,000 M_r) bola-shaped multifunctional molecule known as thrombospondin, an α granule protein secreted by activated platelets. Thrombospondin possesses binding domains for heparin, collagen, fibrinogen, and a thrombospondin recep-

tor on platelets, GPIV. During platelet activation, fibrinogen receptors expressed through the agency of protein kinase C or thrombin bind to fibrinogen, and thrombospondin molecules lock the fibrinogen receptor complex to the platelet surface by interacting with fibrinogen at one domain and with the GPIV at another. By fortifying the attachment of fibrinogen to platelet fibrinogen receptors, thrombospondin ensures the second wave of aggregation and makes platelet aggregation irreversible.

Platelet Secretion: Stimulus-Secretion Coupling in Activated Platelets

Platelet secretion (release reaction) commences along with aggregation the moment an agonist binds to its receptor. Secretion is initiated by messenger molecules produced by arachidonic acid and phosphoinositide metabolism and is an ATP-dependent process in which the three major sorts of storage granules are gathered toward the center of the cell by a contracting noose of actin-myosin polymers. Storage granules are of three major sorts: electron-dense (δ) granules contain depot ADP and calcium; α granules are laden with fibrinogen, vWF, fibronectin, and several platelet-specific factors; and a third population (λ granules) contains lysosomal enzymes. A complete inventory is recorded in Table 21-1 [13]. The tightly clustered granule membranes fuse with the platelet surface membrane and within its canaliculi, and the entire contents are discharged by exocytosis.

In its excitable responsiveness to signals by agonists, the platelet is a paradigm of stimulus-response coupling. There are two major, linked pathways by which extracellular agonists (operating via receptors on platelet surfaces) instigate secretion of enzymes, aggregators, and procoagulants.

Prostaglandins   Synthesis of prostaglandins, their endoperoxides, and the powerful aggregator thromboxane A_2 is initiated by liberation of the hairpin-shaped polyunsaturated fatty acid, arachidonic acid (AA). Normally there is no free AA in platelets. Release of AA and its subsequent metabolic conversion to eicosanoid mediators (oxygenated derivatives of AA) requires cleavage by phospholipase C and then by phospholipase A_2 of the ester bonds by

TABLE 21-1

Platelet granule contents

α Granules
   Platelet-specific proteins (low molecular
   weight)
      PF4
      Low-affinity PF4
      β-Thromboglobulin
      Platelet basic protein
   Mitogenic factors (platelet-derived
   growth factor)
   High molecular weight glycoproteins
      Fibrinogen
      von Willebrand factor
      Factor VIII
      Fibronectin
      Thrombospondin
      Factor V
      HMWK
   Albumin

Dense bodies (δ granules)
   ADP
   ATP
   Calcium
   Pyrophosphate

Lysosomal enzymes (λ granules)
   Acid phosphatase
   B-N-Acetylglucosaminidase
   β-Galactosidase
   β-Glycerophosphatase

Granular proteins of uncertain location
   Cathepsins
   Endoglucosidase
   Cyclic-3′,5′-phosphodiesterase
   Collagenase
   Vascular permeability factors
   Proelastase and elastase
   α_1-Protease inhibitor
   α_2-Macroglobulin
   Antiplasmin

Bactericidal protein

Aryl sulfatase

Source: From Coller BS: Chapt 4, in Disorders of
Hemostasis, Ratnoff OD and Forbes CD, Eds.
Orlando, Grune & Stratton, Inc.,1984.

which AA is normally affixed to phospholipids on the inner aspect of the lipid bilayer. Freed AA activates both the cyclooxygenase and lipoxygenase pathways. Little is known of the physiologic role of the lipoxygenase pathway, by which AA is peroxidized to "12-HETE," but in platelets the cyclooxygenase pathway yields thromboxane A_2, the most potent platelet aggregator and vasoconstrictor known, and in endothelium it generates an antithetical eicosanoid, prostacyclin, the most powerful known inhibitor of platelet aggregation and a potent vasodilator (Figure 21-16) [14]. The generating enzyme, cyclooxygenase, is inhibited irreversibly by acetylsalicylic acid and other nonsteroidal anti-inflammatory drugs; inhibition by aspirin is due to covalent acetylation of the enzyme, and platelets once exposed to aspirin are rendered functional cripples for the remainder of their lifespans. By inactivating cyclooxygenase, low doses of aspirin (<80 mg/day) selectively block platelet coagulant activity, and aspirin is a widely used antithrombotic agent.

Phosphoinositide system   Phosphoinositides (PIs) are ubiquitous membrane phospholipids that serve as storage forms for messenger molecules (Chapter 1). Phosphorylated derivatives of PI—PI-4-phosphate (PIP) and PI-4,5-biphosphate (PIP_2)—are formed by sequential phosphorylations and normally are in equilibrium with each other through a futile cycle of kinases and phosphatases. When platelets are activated by coupling of agonists to membrane receptors, phospholipase C is activated by a regulatory guanyl nucleotide (GTP) binding protein, with formation from PIP_2 of two second messengers: inositol 1,4,5-triphosphate (IP_3) and 1,2-diacylglycerol (DG). IP_3 causes Ca^{2+} to be released from intracellular storage depots, and DG both promotes association of protein kinase C (PKC) with the cell membrane and dramatically increases its affinity for Ca^{2+}, which acts as a positive allosteric effector. PKC in turn phosphorylates several proteins, among them the 20,000 M_r myosin light chain and the 40,000 M_r G protein. Hence a single cycle of inositol phospholipid turnover is capable of generating two intracellular messengers at the price of three molecules of ATP. The stimulus-secretion re-

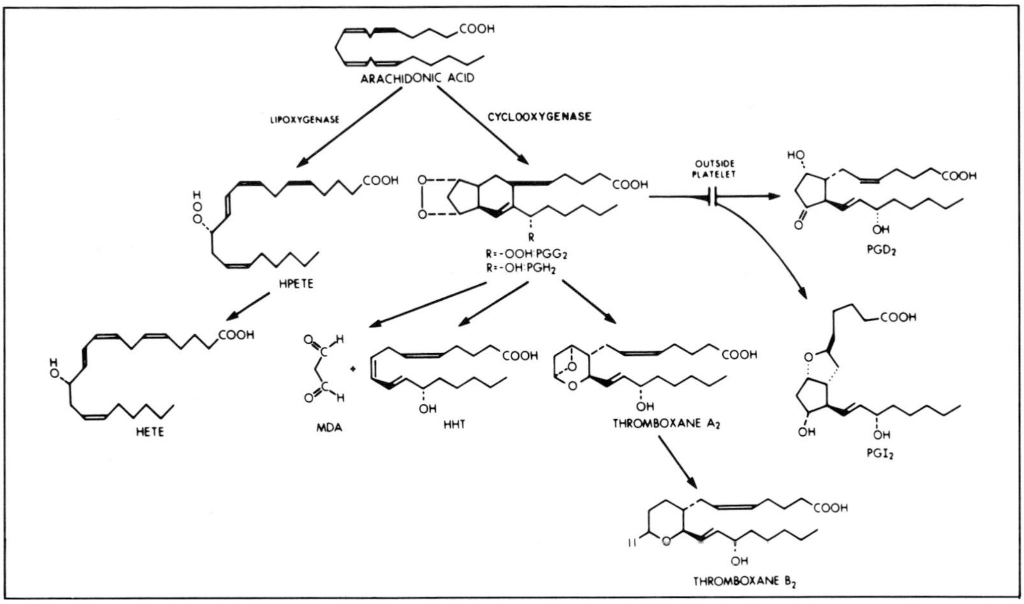

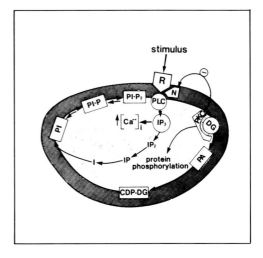

FIGURE 21-16

Arachidonic acid metabolism within platelets
(left center) and outside platelets (right).
Cyclization of arachidonic acid to PGH_2 by
cyclooxygenase leads to formation of PGI_2
(prostacyclin) in endothelium and to thromboxane A_2 in platelets. The various eicosanoids
identified can be divided into those that stimulate platelet aggregation (thromboxane A_2,
PGH_2) and those that inhibit it (PGI_2, PGD_2).
(From Majerus PW: Chapt 19, in The Molecular Basis of Blood Diseases, Stamatoyannopoulos G et al, Eds. Philadelphia, WB Saunders
Company,1987.)

FIGURE 21-17

Role of inositol phospholipid in stimulus-
secretion coupling in platelets. Most abbreviations are identified in the text. R = receptor. N
= guanyl nucleotide binding protein. (From
Marcus AJ: Chapt 38, in Hemostasis and
Thrombosis, 2nd ed., Colman RW et al, Eds.
Philadelphia, JB Lippincott Company,1987.)

sponse subsides when the arachidonyl-stearyl
structure of PI becomes phosphorylated to
phosphatidic acid (PA), which is metabolized
to cytidine-diacylglycerol and then back to PI.
The entire cycle involved during stimulus-
response coupling is recapitulated in Figure
21-17 [15]. The prime purpose of all the busy
cycling involved in PKC activation is mobilization of the actin-myosin contractile mechanism, which moves granules and other secretory factors to the platelet surface for
procoagulant modification or secretion.

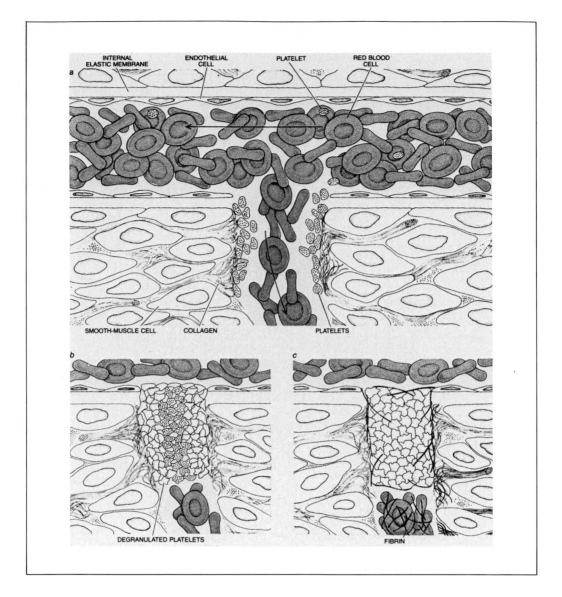

INTERNAL ELASTIC MEMBRANE   ENDOTHELIAL CELL   PLATELET   RED BLOOD CELL

SMOOTH-MUSCLE CELL   COLLAGEN   PLATELETS

DEGRANULATED PLATELETS   FIBRIN

FIGURE 21-18

Schematic review of the role of platelets in hemostasis. Platelets normally circulate in a nonactivated state and do not react with each other or with the vessel wall. As blood begins to flow out through a gap in the vessel wall, however, platelets in the presence of vWF adhere to collagen fibrils in subendothelium (a). This agonist both upregulates fibrinogen receptors and initiates the arachidonic acid and phosphoinositide pathways, which stimulate secretion of ADP and other contents of platelet granules; this causes other passing platelets to adhere to the first layer, building up a loose platelet plug (b). Meanwhile prothrombinase complexes form that convert plasma prothrombin to thrombin, which binds to the surfaces of degranulating platelets. Thrombin in turn converts both plasma and platelet-bound fibrinogen into fibrin strands, which form a meshwork that reinforces the platelet plug and draws the platelets together in a firm, if temporary, seal (c). (From Zucker MB: The functioning of blood platelets. Sci Am 242(6): 86,1980. Copyright © 1990 by Scientific American, Inc. All rights reserved.)

The potentially volatile responses of platelets to commonplace metabolites such as ADP and epinephrine require stern feedback controls. When platelet receptors are occupied, both phospholipases C and A_2 are activated in concert, so that there is usually a single receptor cascade that includes PKC, Ca^{2+}, AA, and stimulatory G protein (GS), which activates adenylate cyclase in the platelet membrane. As the result, the reaction to unsustained activation is accumulation of cAMP, which blocks continued platelet function at a very early stage. In addition platelets possess receptors for PGD_2 and for prostacyclin, which also stimulate formation of cAMP from ATP. Elevation of cAMP by either mechanism inhibits AA release from phospholipids, stops phosphoinositide turnover, and brings secretion to a halt. Normally an equilibrium exists between the proaggregatory activity of thromboxane A_2 and antiaggregatory influence of cAMP: imbalance leads to either thrombotic or bleeding problems.

Platelet Procoagulant Activity

Coagulation proceeds more rapidly when platelets are present than when they are not. When activated by agonists, platelets participate in the generation of thrombin by providing an activity termed platelet factor 3. Activation appears to cause flip-flop rearrangement of membrane phospholipids that exposes phosphatidylserine and creates a negatively charged, phospholipid-rich surface that in the presence of Ca^{2+} furnishes a favorable setting for assembly of coagulation complexes. In the course of activation, platelets project receptors for activated factor V secreted by the platelets themselves or absorbed from plasma; factor V serves as a docking site for factor X, and the seating of X on V in the presence of the phosphatidylserine surface and Ca^{2+} (which holds the complex together) constitutes the "prothrombinase complex." Presence of all components of the complex drive the prothrombin $\rightarrow$ thrombin generation kinetic to rates 20,000 to 500,000 times the rate catalyzed by soluble factor Xa alone.

The basic sequence by which exposure of platelets to a strong agonist (collagen) sets in motion the multiple steps culminating in formation of a fibrin-stabilized hemostatic plug is shown in Figure 21-18 [16].

COAGULATION

Coagulation (clot formation) represents conversion of the soluble, extended, flexible plasma protein, fibrinogen, into an insoluble rigid fibrillar polymer, fibrin. Coagulation is the end result of a complex sequence of reactions in which procoagulant proteins (factors) circulate in plasma as inert precursors until converted to their active forms. Activated coagulation factors are proteolytic enzymes (serine proteases) which in the presence of cofactors cleave other factors in a systematic order. The recurrent theme of activation is limited proteolysis, and the net effect of the clotting cascade is to amplify a small biochemical signal emitted by the damaged vessel into a robust fibrin-generating reaction capable of sealing off the damaged area and arresting hemorrhage.

By international convention most coagulation factors are identified by Roman numerals that signify order of discovery rather than of activation. Originally, most factors were named informally according to their presumed function or as eponymic cognomens immortalizing patients first found to be lacking the factor. A glossary of numbered coagulation factors along with their synonyms and normal plasma concentrations is presented in Table 21-2 [17]. In hematologic parlance, the first four numbered factors are known by their "synonyms" and the remainder by Roman numerals. Numbered factors in their activated state are identified by the letter "a," as in factor Xa.

Why the complexity?   Coagulation cannot occur in one or two simple steps, for any crude and impetuous response to vascular injury would risk instant conversion of the bloodstream into a total body gel. Coagulation occurs as a highly evolved multistep process policed by a series of stop-and-go signals. This permits smooth modulation of coagulation but is hard going for students of hemostasis and has the effect of alienating all but the most motivated reader. The serial interactions between components of the coagulation cascade and the logic of alternative pathways are hard to grasp in one or two readings, but before pursuing coagulation factor-by-factor, a summarized preview may aid in understanding the details to come.

TABLE 21-2

Glossary of coagulation factors

Factor	Synonyms	Normal plasma concentration (mg/dl)
I	Fibrinogen	200–400
II	Prothrombin	10
III	Tissue thromboplastin, tissue factor	0
IV	Calcium ion	4–5
V	Proaccelerin, labile factor	1
VII	Serum prothrombin conversion accelerator, stable factor	0.05
VIII	Antihemophilic factor	1–2
IX	Christmas factor	0.3
X	Stuart-Prower factor	1
XI	Plasma thromboplastin antecedent	0.5
XII	Hageman factor	3
XIII	Fibrin stabilizing factor	1–2
Prekallikrein	Fletcher factor	5
High molecular weight kininogen (HMWK)	Fitzgerald, Flaujeac, Williams factor; contact activation cofactor	6

Source: From Saito H: Chapt 2, in Disorders of Hemostasis, Ratnoff OD and Forbes CD, Eds. Orlando, Grune & Stratton, Inc., 1984.

The Clotting Cascade: A Preview

The cascade consists of a pair of sequences that lead to activation of factor X, a vital crossover reaction uniting these two sequences, and a common final pathway. In every step an inactive clotting factor is converted to an active form by cleavage of one or two particular peptide bonds, a process termed "limited proteolysis." A feature of the clotting cascade is that—as with platelet procoagulant activity—most intermediate steps are carried out by complexes involving two or more factors, Ca^{2+}, and phospholipid surfaces. Clotting factors are far more efficient when cooperating within activation complexes. (In a sense, clotting is conducted by a hierarchy of subcommittees, but these are unlike human committees, in which the quality of the work product is divisible by the number of members.)

1. The intrinsic pathway (triggered by factors intrinsic to plasma) consists of the following sequence:

   XIIa plus kallikrein → XIa → IXa → Xa

2. The extrinsic pathway, launched by exposure of plasma to tissue factor originating extrinsic to plasma, consists of a shorter, parallel sequence:

   VIIa plus tissue factor → Xa

3. The intrinsic and extrinsic pathways are independent activating tracks but are connected by a crossover mechanism, the "alternative" pathway:

   VIIa–tissue factor complex → IXa

4. After the pathways converge, with generation of factor Xa, the cascade is channeled into a final common pathway:

   Xa → IIa → fibrin clot

A noteworthy and simplifying feature of the clotting sequence is that tissue factor activation of factor VII alone is sufficient in promoting both proteolytic cascades leading to thrombin production; factor VIIa activates factor X both directly and indirectly via factor IXa in the presence of cofactor VIII [18]. This unifying collaboration explains why deficiencies of any factors concerned in the intermediate as well as terminal phases of clotting (but not the factor XII–dependent contact phase) lead to severe bleeding disorders.

The Extrinsic Pathway

The extrinsic pathway is sparked by interaction between factor VII and tissue factor, a 30,000 M_r protein present in the surface membranes of many tissue cells including vascular endothelium, adventitial fibroblasts, and monocytes. The initiating molecule, tissue factor (which is linked to phospholipids of the lipid bilayer and often alluded to as thromboplastin), is a high-affinity cell surface receptor and essential cofactor for the serine protease, factor VIIa. The VIIa–tissue factor complex appears to be the first enzyme-cofactor complex formed during blood coagulation in vivo, whereupon it inaugurates coagulation through activation of both factors IX and X. Factors VII, IX, and X are ancestrally related serine proteases that are members of the vitamin K group of clotting factors. Conversion rate of factor VII is swiftly augmented by positive feedback from the first traces of the activation products, IXa and Xa, which through limited proteolysis convert the relatively indolent procoagulant factor VII to a two-chain coagulant having over 100 times the activity of its single-chain precursor. Binding of dual chain factor VIIa to tissue factor severs the Arg-Ile peptide bond in factor X, and release of factor Xa is accelerated 8,000-fold. This dramatic amplification propels the coagulation process and simultaneously engages the alternative pathway in the presence of cofactor VIII, platelets, and Ca^{2+} at the injury site (Figure 21-19) [19]. Containment of the factor VIIa–tissue factor complexes to the site of injury is assured

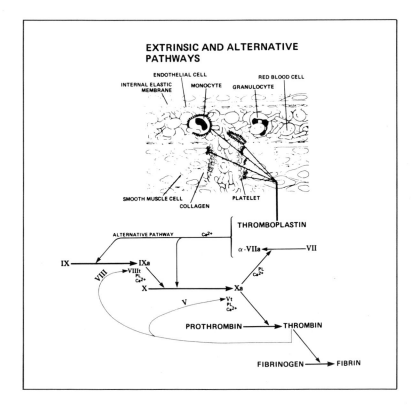

EXTRINSIC AND ALTERNATIVE PATHWAYS

ENDOTHELIAL CELL
INTERNAL ELASTIC MEMBRANE
MONOCYTE
RED BLOOD CELL
GRANULOCYTE

SMOOTH MUSCLE CELL
COLLAGEN
PLATELET

THROMBOPLASTIN

ALTERNATIVE PATHWAY Ca^{2+}

α-VIIa ← VII

IX → IXa
VIII → VIIIt PL Ca^{2+}
X → Xa
PL Ca^{2+}

V → Vt PL Ca^{2+}

PROTHROMBIN → THROMBIN

FIBRINOGEN → FIBRIN

FIGURE 21-19

The extrinsic and alternative pathways of coagulation responding to vessel wall damage. On disruption of the vessel, thromboplastin (tissue factor) of endothelium, subendothelial matrix, smooth muscle, platelets, monocytes, and other damaged cells is exposed and available to act as receptor for both factor VII and VIIa. This launches both the extrinsic (factor VIIa–dependent) and alternative (factor IXa–dependent) pathways for generating factor Xa, propellent of the terminal cascade. (From Osterud B. Scand J Haematol 32:337,1984. © 1984 Munksgaard International Publishers Ltd., Copenhagen, Denmark.)

in part by the limited supply of factor VII; harmful extension or dissemination of coagulation is opposed by a proteinase inhibitor of the complex known provisionally as extrinsic pathway inhibitor (EPI) [20].

The Intrinsic Pathway and Contact Activation

In the intrinsic pathway of coagulation, the zymogen factor XII (Hageman factor) is autoactivated to factor XIIa during contact of blood with a foreign surface such as basement membrane, collagen of damaged vessels, or negatively charged materials such as glass, clay, kaolin, or dextran sulfate. Following binding to such surfaces, factor XIIa, prekallikrein, and high-molecular-weight kininogen (HMWK) form a complex enabling them to engage in a series of mutually reinforcing reactions that eventuates in production of factor XIa, which is capable of tripping the cascade by activating factor IX. These factor XII–dependent interactions probably do not contribute importantly to thrombosis or hemostasis, which is principally the province of factor VII. Patients deficient in factor XII, prekallikrein, and HMWK suffer no bleeding

disorders (unlike patients deficient in factor VII, who are sometimes severe bleeders), and factor XI–deficient patients have only mild and variable bleeding problems. Most evidence suggests that initial components of the intrinsic pathway are of importance mainly in the pathogenesis of complement-mediated inflammatory reactions and local control of blood flow through release of the potent vasodilator, bradykinin, which acts as a counterbalance to the renin-angiotension system in regulation of blood pressure.

The collaboration between intermediate elements of the intrinsic pathway (factor IX and cofactor VIII) and initiators of the extrinsic pathway (factor VII and tissue factor) in activating factor X and completing the cascade is reprised in Figure 21-20 [17]. The final product of the common pathway is fibrin.

Fibrin and Fibrinogen

Clot formation begins with the thrombin-catalyzed conversion of fibrinogen to monomeric fibrin, transforming a solitary and soluble molecule into an insoluble monomer driven to polymerize and then to form a tough

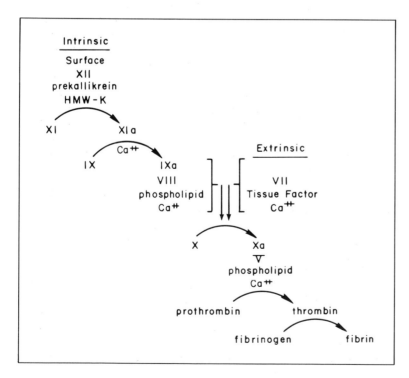

FIGURE 21-20

A scheme of the coagulation cascade. (From Ratnoff OD and Forbes CD: Chapt 2, in Disorders of Hemostasis. Orlando, Grune & Stratton, Inc.,1984.)

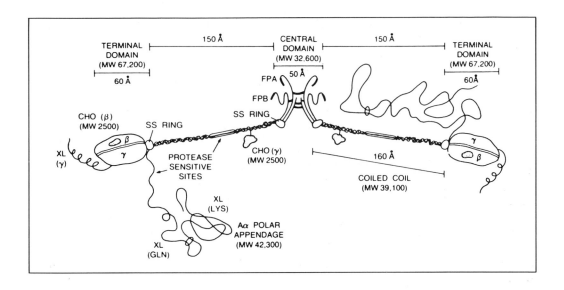

fabric through innumerable zig-zag crosslinkages. Fibrinogen is a long, flexible, elaborately designed trinodular protein (M_r 340,000) composed of three pairs of nonidentical polypeptide chains. The molecule possesses two terminal bilobate domains tethered in linear alignment to a smaller central domain by two triple-stranded supercoiled ropes bound together by a disulfide knot. The central domain is dimeric and contains amino acid terminals of all three pairs of constituent polypeptide chains: these are designated Aα (the chain yielding fibrinopeptide A [FPA] when attacked by thrombin), Bβ (the chain yielding FPB), and γ, which for some reason denotes both of the thrombin-resistant γ chains (Figure 21-21) [21].

Thrombin initiates fibrin formation; factor XIII stabilizes it   Thrombin converts fibrinogen to fibrin by splitting off fibrinopeptides A and B from the center (E) domain, after which the parent molecules—fibrin monomers—polymerize spontaneously into dimers held together by half-staggered overlap binding. Release of the scapular fibrinopeptides exposes charged α and β knobs that link up with sites on the terminal (D) domains of neighboring molecules, enabling the dimer assembly to grow in both directions into two-molecule-thick oligomers arranged like shingles in a half-molecule staggered overlap. The third step in fibrin clot formation requires activated factor XIII (fibrin stabilizing factor), a transglutaminase that crosslinks the growing polymer by forming intermolecular bridges between lysine donors and glutamine receptors on the γ side chains of adjacent polymeric fibrils. As the strands lengthen by γ chain pairing they also thicken into coarse fibers by lateral bridging between α chains. These linkages are further strengthened by factor XIIIa–induced transglutamination that binds fibronectin covalently to distal α chain strands.

Fibrin clotting is a stopgap measure   Fibrin clots are sturdy devices for stanching bleeding and when fibrin is generated during thrombus formation the fibrin plug is buttressed by interactions with other adhesive proteins such as thrombospondin, fibronectin, and platelet fibrinogen released from platelet granules. Fibronectin crosslinked to fibrin forms bridges to the vessel wall via its collagen binding sites, and platelet membrane GPIIb-IIIa joins α granule fibrinogen to intracellular actin, encouraging clot retraction and vessel wall constriction. Clots, however, are designed for planned obsolescence, as final healing requires restoration of endothelium and its supporting connective tissue. Fibrin clots contain the seeds of their own timely dissolution, for during coagulation plasminogen becomes bound to fibrin and eventually splits the crosslinked clot structure into fibrin degradation products (FDPs) or fibrin split products (FSPs), a fibrinolytic process described later in this chapter.

Activation of Prothrombin to Thrombin (the Master Enzyme of Coagulation) Depends upon Enzyme-Cofactor Complexes

Thrombin is the last and most versatile enzyme of the coagulation cascade. It is generated from prothrombin (factor II), a single-chain, 72,000 M_r glycoprotein produced by hepatic parenchymal cells in the presence of vitamin K. Conversion of prothrombin to thrombin is prompted solely by the prothrombin-converting complex (the "prothrombinase" alluded to earlier) composed of factor Xa, cofactor Va, and phospholipid—either as fluid phase complexes or when perched on the surface of endothelium or platelets. Formation of this complex accelerates by several thousandfold the rate of thrombin generation while at the same time shielding factor Xa from inhibition by antithrombin III. Assembly of reactants into complexes for generation of thrombin from prothrombin is illustrative of the subcommittee system by which the cascade is operated (Figure 21-22) [22]. During the initial phase of activation, prothrombin is cleaved at two points to disconnect the "Gla" domain and thereby uncover the serine esterase catalytic domain for proteolytic action. This scission also releases thrombin from the phospholipid surface and dismantles the entire complex by inactivating its linchpin, factor Va; hence thrombin curbs its own formation. Thrombin is an enzyme of many parts: it cleaves not only fibrinogen, but also factors XIII, V, VIII, protein C, and prothrombin itself. Accordingly, nature has sur-

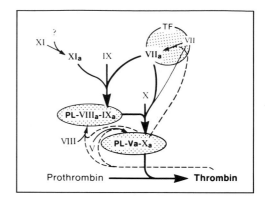

FIGURE 21-22

Generation of thrombin by the prothrombinase complex is exemplary of the major sequential steps in hemostasis, all three of which involve enzyme-cofactor complexes. Interrupted lines signify positive feedback (feedforward) reactions. Note the uncertain status in hemostasis of factor XI of the classical pathway and the lofty position of factor VIIa. PL = phospholipids. (From Rapaport SI: Chapt 23, in Introduction to Hematology, 2nd ed. Philadelphia, JB Lippincott Company,1987.)

rounded thrombin with safeguards, including AT III, α_2-macroglobulin, and protein C.

Vitamin K–dependent enzymes   Vitamin K is required for synthesis of four clotting factors (prothrombin, VII, IX, and X) and at least two anticoagulants (protein C and protein S). Vitamin K is necessary in converting glutamate (Glu) to novel γ-carboxyglutamate (Gla) residues, and each member of this family of factors possesses 10 to 12 of these unusual amino acids clustered near the amino terminus; the strong negative charge of the "Gla" domain bestows the capacity to anchor these molecules in the presence of Ca^{2+} to acidic phospholipids, enabling the free C-terminal end containing the catalytic domain to engage its substrate. The artful structures of four vitamin K–dependent enzymes are portrayed in Figure 21-23 [23].

The vitamin K cycle and its antagonists   In vitamin K–dependent γ-glutamyl carboxylation required for equipping nascent prothrombin and factors VII, IX, and X molecules with a

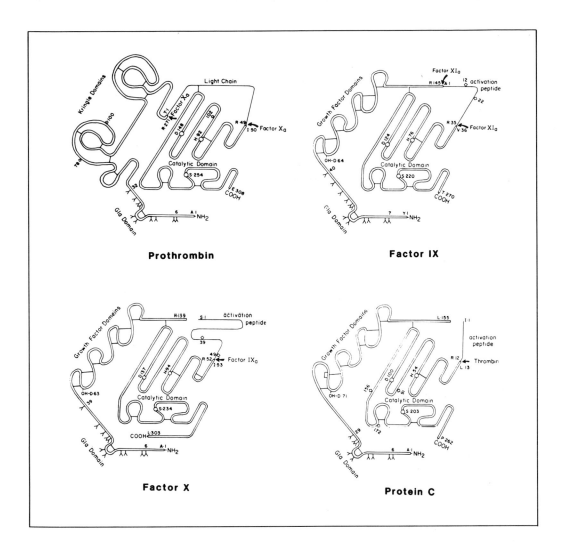

Prothrombin

Factor IX

Factor X

Protein C

FIGURE 21-23

Schematic portraits of the structures of four of the six known vitamin K–dependent coagulant or anticoagulant factors: prothrombin, factor IX, factor X, and protein C. Cleavage sites and enzymes responsible for activating each protein are indicated by heavy black arrows, and amino acids involved in catalysis (H, D, S) are denoted in shorthand. Prothrombin is distinctive in possessing looped "kringle" domains (found also on plasmin), named for their likeness in shape to the paragon of Danish pastries. The Ys identify γ-carboxyglutamate residues of the Gla domain. (From Davie EW: Proteins of blood coagulation: their domains and evolution. Chemica Scripta 26B:241,1986.)

full complement of Gla groups, the vitamin becomes oxidized to the inactive quinone form and must be reduced back to resume its cofactor function. Vitamin K antagonists such as warfarin and other 4-hydroxycoumarin anticoagulants block the first of two serial reductases required for perpetuation of the vitamin K cycle (Figure 21-24) [24]. The four vitamin K–dependent coagulation proteins continue to be synthesized by liver ribosomes during vitamin K deficiency, but they are undercarboxylated and bereft of the densely acidic Gla domains necessary for Ca^{2+}-mediated bridging to phospholipids and cell

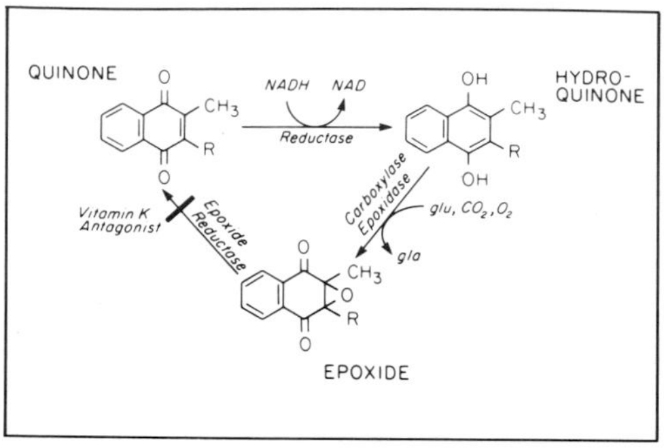

FIGURE 21-24

Vitamin K cycle and site of action of vitamin K antagonists. Reduced (hydroquinone) form of vitamin K is an essential cofactor for carboxylation of glutamate (Glu) to γ-carboxyglutamate (Gla), during which reaction the hydroquinone is oxidized to the quinone epoxide; recovery requires two sequential reductions, the first of which (epoxide $\rightarrow$ quinone) is blocked by coumarin anticoagulants. (From Babior BM and Stossel TP: Chapt 15, in Hematology. A Pathophysiological Approach. New York, Churchill Livingstone Inc.,1984.)

membranes: consequently, the undercarboxylated molecules, which are incapable of activation, interfere with coagulation. Levels of these clotting factors decline at various rates depending on their half-lives in blood, prothrombin persisting longest and requiring several days to fall; hence the anticoagulated state deliberately induced by therapeutic use of vitamin K antagonists is achieved only when all four clotting factors have reached sufficiently low levels. Correction of the vitamin K–deficient state, on the other hand, is rapid, occurring within 1 or 2 days of parenteral administration of the vitamin.

Cofactors of the Clotting Cascade: Factors VIII and V

Factors VIII and V have no enzymatic activity of their own but serve as cofactors in complexes that activate factor X and prothrombin (Figure 21-22). Factor VIII is part of the factor IXa enzyme phospholipid–Ca^{2+} complex, and factor V is a member of the factor

Xa phospholipid–Ca^{2+} complex. Factors VIII and V possess considerable structural homology and appear to have arisen from a common ancestral gene. Each is inert in its native state and requires traces of either thrombin or factor X for conversion to the active cofactor derivative.

Factor VIII is carried by vWF and is essential to factor X activation　Factor VIII is a 285,000 M_r protein product coded and controlled by a gene on the X chromosome near the locus for factor IX, tightly linked to the G6PD locus on band Xq28. Factor VIII molecules are protected from degradation and are transported through plasma by being complexed to polymerized vWF. As vWF is the physiologic carrier of factor VIII, factor VIII levels are low in von Willebrand's disease; in classic hemophilia, factor VIII levels are low because factor VIII itself is deficient or defective. Factor VIII is bound to vWF by hydrophobic and electrostatic forces linking its 80,000 M_r light chain to tetrameric subunits of the relatively huge vWF polymers. When released and then split by factor X or thrombin, the activated cofactor VIIIa bares a lipid binding site on its light chain and exposes a tandem receptor for factors IX and X on the heavy chain. When fully liganded by Ca^{2+}, the ensconced cofactor VIIIa–enzyme complex accelerates the factor X $\rightarrow$ Xa reaction rate 100,000-fold. The primal significance of cofactor VIII in coagulation is underscored by the desperate severity of bleeding problems in patients deficient in this protein: factor VIII deficiency—hemophilia—is the most feared and ruthless of major bleeding disorders.

Factor V provides a seat for factor Xa　Factor V (labile factor), a 330,000 M_r single chain procofactor, is converted to the active cofactor (factor Va) by multistep proteolysis by both factor Xa and thrombin. Proteolytic activation of factor V by factor Xa is a tidy arrangement, for factor Va functions as the seat for factor Xa on the prothrombinase complex. Assembly of the full phospholipid-Va-Xa complex accelerates prothrombin $\rightarrow$ thrombin conversion by 300,000-fold. Deficiency of factor V causes severe bleeding but is mercifully uncommon.

FIBRINOLYSIS AND FIBRIN DEGRADATION

Fibrin clots crosslinked by factor XIIIa are sturdy and effective structures for stemming hemorrhage until endothelium-lined channels are reconstructed, but they are designed to be dismantled rapidly after vascular repair so blood flow can resume. Clot removal—fibrinolysis—is accomplished by a fibrin-splitting serine protease called plasmin.

Plasmin Is Generated Principally by t-PA

Plasmin is converted from its proenzyme form, plasminogen, by enzymes that are either intrinsic components of plasma (comprising a factor XII–dependent cascade of plasminogen activation) or are extrinsic (tissue) plasminogen activators (t-PAs) secreted on demand by injured endothelium and nearby macrophages. The most important activator, t-PA, described earlier in this chapter, binds avidly to fibrin, whereupon it dissociates into two chains having serine protease activity; excited activator molecules somehow seek out plasminogen molecules trapped within the clot and convert them to plasmin by specifically cleaving the Arg 560–Val 561 bonds that hold plasminogen harmlessly together. Conversion of plasminogen to plasmin within or at the surface of fibrin clots transforms the molecule into an endopeptidase that cleaves specifically lysine and arginine peptide bonds that are linked to kringle domains on the heavy chain of plasmin known as lysine binding sites (LBSs). These substrate sites are common among coagulation factors, and thus plasmin is capable of digesting not only fibrin (to which it is attached firmly by LBSs) but also fibrinogen and factors V and VIII.

Plasmin Activity Is Delimited by Protease Inhibitors: α_2-Antiplasmin

Like clot formation, clot dissolution is sternly regulated by a system of checks and balances. Plasma normally contains several antiproteases capable of neutralizing plasmin and preventing runaway fibrinolysis. The most important of these is the fast-reacting plasmin inhibitor, α_2-antiplasmin. Antiplasmin, a 70,000 M_r single-chain glycoprotein, is normally present in plasma at a concentration of 1 μM, assuring confinement of fibrinolysis to the clotsite. α_2-Antiplasmin is also crosslinked to fibrin by factor XIIIa during clot formation, providing a delayed-release mechanism for protecting clots from premature dissolution. This plasmin inhibitor has the unique property of forming 1:1 complexes with plasmin by covalent bonding to the serine active site of the plasmin light chain, a reaction allosterically facilitated by attachment of the inhibitor to LBSs on the heavy chain of plasmin. The inert complexes are then cleared from circulation by macrophages.

Urokinase and streptokinase Urokinase (UK), like t-PA, is a serine kinase that cleaves the Arg 560–Val 561 bond of plasminogen, but unlike t-PA, UK is synthesized by kidney cells and secreted into urine, with the mission of dissolving clots in the extrarenal collecting system. UK and streptokinase (SK)—a structurally different but functionally similar polypeptide produced by β-hemolytic streptococci—are both employed in the treatment of thrombotic disorders, although neither UK nor SK has an affinity for fibrin comparable to that of t-PA.

Fibrin Degradation, Clot Lysis, and "Split Products"

Both plasminogen and t-PA have the advantage over α_2-antiplasmin of binding to specific receptor sites on fibrin. The resultant fibrin-plasmin complex is protected against α_2-antiplasmin attached randomly to other elements of the clot structure: hence clot dissolution commences at the clot surface, and antiplasmin-induced termination of clot lysis is delayed long enough for healing to commence.

Digestion of fibrin monomers by plasmin takes place in an orderly stepwise manner in which 50 to 60 of the 362 lysine and arginine residues are cleaved. Plasmin first releases the outer portions of fibrin α chains, producing an unstable intermediate termed fragment X; this is then split on one side of the disulfide knot into a small fragment D molecule and a large Y fragment consisting of central and terminal domains connected by a coiled coil. A similar later cleavage on the other side of the disulfide knot releases a second D fragment, leaving behind the small piece of central knot called the E moiety. These five degradation products can be separated by column chromatography: fragments X (DED), Y (DE), two Ds, and E. Digestion by plasmin of crosslinked fibrin clots yields more complex degradation complexes that serve as markers for clot lysis as opposed to fibrinolysis.

Digestion of Crosslinked Fibrin

When attacking a crosslinked clot, plasmin cuts the covalently joined fibrin polymers in the same places as with fibrin monomers, but the process of degradation differs in two ways. The rate of digestion is slowed by steric impedance of the closely knit strand structures, and the degradation products are more complex and variable because of superimposed bonding provided by factor XIIIa and fibronectin. A unique fragment, the D-D dimer is derived from adjacent fibrin monomers joined covalently by crosslinks between their γ chain remnants; these telltale covalent complexes are admixed with both fragment E and with noncovalently bound complexes of E and D dimers (DD/E complex). The derivation of more complicated crosslinked fragments is traceable to the double-stranded, half-staggered overlap structure of double-stranded fibrin protofibrils (Figure 21-25) [25]. The most reliable clinical indicator of accelerated or disseminated lysis of crosslinked fibrin is the immunologic demonstration of D dimers.

Fibrin split products act as anticoagulants

Fibrin degradation products, better known as fibrin split products (FSPs), block further coagulation by binding to thrombin at its fibrinogen-receptor site and by forming incoagulable FSP-fibrin complexes that become entrained in the growing fibrin clot, stunting its growth and weakening its structure. Systemic release of FSPs in large quantities contributes to the vascular damage and bleeding problems encountered in patients with disseminated intravascular coagulation (DIC) (Chapter 24).

Measuring fibrinolysis Like other anticoagulants, FSPs cause multiple abnormalities in routine screening tests of hemostasis; prolongation of the thrombin time (TT) indicates interference with the final fibrinogen-to-fibrin step in coagulation and correlates roughly with levels of anticoagulant fibrin degradation products. Several screening tests can be used to demonstrate incoagulable FSPs in serum: these methods include tanned red cell hemagglutination inhibition; antibody-coated latex particle flocculation; and the staphylococcal clumping assay, based on the incidental ability of D dimers to agglutinate *Staphylococcus*

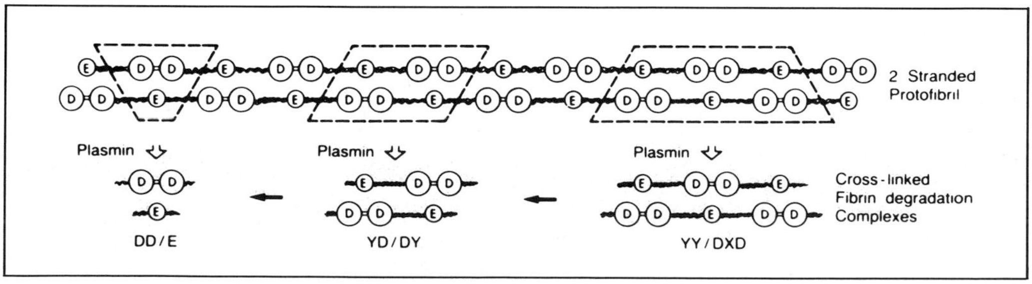

FIGURE 21-25

Plasmin degradation of crosslinked fibrin. Degradation of a double-stranded protofibril generates a mixture of crosslinked complexes, the smallest being the DD/E structure, in which fragment E is joined by noncovalent bonds to the covalently bound DD fragments (note the double bond). The series of larger pieces shown on the right reflects other interdomainal crosslinks between adjacent fibrin strands. (From Francis CW and Marder VJ: Chapt 22, in Hemostasis and Thrombosis: Basic Principles and Clinical Practice, 2nd ed., Colman RW et al, Eds. Philadelphia, JB Lippincott Company,1987.)

aureus. The most definitive measure is to quantitate the level of D dimers (or other FSPs) by immunoassay.

TESTS OF HEMOSTASIS

On the basis of historical and physical data, a judgment can be made as to whether a patient has a severe bleeding disorder, minor or equivocal bleeding, or no hemostatic problem. If history and physical examinations are negative, only two laboratory tests are necessary: a platelet count and an activated partial thromboplastin time (APTT, or simply PTT). If there is evidence or suspicion of a bleeding problem, patients should be examined by a battery of screening procedures that fall into two major groups: tests that screen broadly for defects in primary and secondary hemostasis, and suitable specialized assays of coagulation factors and their inhibitors and of platelet function. Tests for fibrinolysis and defibrination were cited in the foregoing section.

Tests of Primary Hemostasis

Defects in primary hemostasis signify an inadequacy of platelets or defective interaction between platelets and the vessel wall ("capillary fragility"). The visible and historical stigmata of these hemostatic defects are petechiae (multiple small flat bleeding spots the size of freckles), superficial ecchymoses (bruises) occurring promptly after trauma, and spontaneous bleeding from mucous membranes. Petechiae occur initially in dependent areas and any other regions exposed to high hydrostatic pressure (such as the head following vomiting or paroxysms of coughing): numerous petechiae spread over a wide area are known by the term "purpura." Petechiae are the speckled insignia of platelet problems and usually can be distinguished from the palpable purpura of vascular disorders (such as vasculitis) by sight and feel (Chapter 22). The most useful generic tests of defects in primary hemostasis are the platelet count and the bleeding time.

Platelet count   Platelet counts are performed by automated particle-counting machines, but abnormally low counts should be verified by examination of the blood smear to exclude spurious results caused by platelet clumping or partial clotting. Platelet levels above 50,000 cells/μl are seldom associated with bleeding, but any counts below 150,000 warrant monitoring, particularly in patients being prepared for major surgery.

Bleeding time   The bleeding time measures the interaction of platelets with the vessel wall and is prolonged when the level or function of platelets is depressed or when they fail to adhere to damaged vessel walls, as in von Willebrand's disease. Hence the bleeding time corresponds with the rate and quality of platelet plugging and can be assessed by making standardized incisions on the forearm below an inflated blood pressure cuff that holds venous pressure at 40 mm Hg. Automated spring-loaded devices are commercially available for ensuring that the template-guided cut is deep enough (2 mm) to enter the subpapular venous plexus. In patients with platelet counts below 100,000, the bleeding time correlates inversely with the count. Normally bleeding onto applied filter paper blotters stops within 7 minutes, but at platelet counts below 10,000 oozing may continue for 20 to 30 minutes. Bleeding times are unnecessary in patients with frank thrombocytopenia, and patients should be forewarned of the inevitable scar before blade meets flesh.

Tests of Secondary Hemostasis

Defects in secondary hemostasis incriminate the coagulation cascades and are marked by deep ecchymoses, hematomas, hemarthroses, and delayed onset of bleeding after trauma.

Testing the Cascades

Screening tests for the clotting cascades are performed on plasma anticoagulated with citrate, and the speed with which clotting commences after addition of Ca^{2+} is clocked with a stopwatch. Three different activators are used to examine three different portions of the cascade.

Prothrombin time measures the extrinsic pathway and the final common pathway   In this test, tissue factor (thromboplastin) and phos-

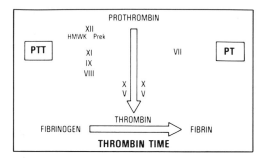

FIGURE 21-26

Coagulation factors tested for by the three standard "coag" screening tests. Note that factors X and V, prothrombin, and fibrinogen affect both the PTT and PT, whereas factors deficient in the two forms of hemophilia (VIII and IX) affect only the PTT. Thrombin time is independent of cascade reactions involved in generation of thrombin. (From Rapaport SI: Introduction to Hematology, 2nd ed. Philadelphia, JB Lippincott Company,1987.)

pholipid are added to citrated plasma, plasma is recalcified, and the clotting time is recorded (normal: 10 to 12 seconds). Prothrombin time (PT) is a good screening test for the sum of the components of the consummated extrinsic pathway: factors VII, V, and X plus prothrombin and fibrinogen.

Partial thromboplastin time tests the intrinsic pathway and the final common pathway   A reagent supplying a phospholipid surrogate for platelet procoagulation activity plus a contact activator of factor XII (usually kaolin powder) is added to citrated plasma, the plasma is recalcified, and the clotting time is noted (normal: 30 to 35 sec). A prolonged partial thromboplastin time (PTT) signifies a defect in plasma clotting factors VIII or IX which are responsible for the two forms of hemophilia (A and B) or of other factors to the left of the arrow in Figure 21-26 [22].

Thrombin time   In this test, dilute thrombin is added to patient's plasma without recalcification, and clot formation is dependent only upon the rate at which the penultimate step in formation of the mature clot (fibrinogen to uncrosslinked fibrin) occurs (normal TT: about

20 s). Causes of a long TT include quantitative and qualitative abnormalities of fibrinogen, increased AT III activity, and presence of FSPs or heparin. TT does not measure the ultimate event, crosslinkage of fibrin by the factor XIIIa transglutaminase reaction. If the TT is prolonged, a reptilase time should be measured, for this is unaffected by heparin.

Specialized Tests of Hemostasis

Factor assays   In patients with abnormal PT or PTT, deficiency of specific clotting factors should be suspected. Deficiencies of the various specific coagulation factors in test plasma can be identified by admixing samples of suspect plasma with equal volumes of plasma from individuals known to be congenitally deficient in the factors of interest. The extent of correction of the recalcified clotting time can be determined by use of standardized calibration curves.

Factor XIII, by covalent crosslinkage of overlapping fibrin filaments, creates thick strands resistant to solubilization by 5 M urea: clot solubility in 5 M urea is indicative of factor XIII deficiency.

Inhibitor screen   If plasma from patients with a prolonged PT or PTT is admixed with normal plasma, the prolonged recalcification time should be corrected, for normally procoagulants are present in excess. Failure of normal plasma to correct the clotting defect signifies presence of an inhibitor (antibody) to one or more coagulation factors.

Aggregation and secretion studies in patients with normal platelet levels   When platelet counts are above 100,000 and yet the patient displays petechiae, a prolonged bleeding time, or other indicators of defective primary hemostasis, platelet malfunction should be suspected. Functional anomalies of platelets are revealed in vitro by turbidometric studies of platelet aggregation following stimulation by natural agonists or by the unique antibiotic ristocetin, or by assaying platelet release (secretory) reactions described earlier. Absence of aggregatory response to agonists identifies the rare anomaly thrombasthenia; primary aggregation with no second wave or subnormal aggregation by colla-

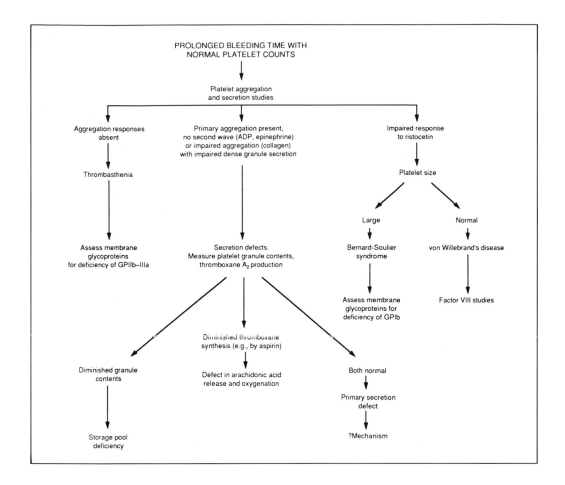

FIGURE 21-27

Algorithm for evaluation of patients having prolonged bleeding times or purpura despite a normal platelet count. (Modified and abridged from Day JH and Rao AK: Evaluation of platelet function. Semin Hematol 23:89,1986.)

gen is characteristic of inborn or acquired secretory defects; an impaired response to ristocetin, which serves as an artificial cofactor in vWF binding to GPIb, is indicative of either von Willebrand's disease or deficiency of GPIb (Bernard-Soulier syndrome).

An algorithm for the diagnosis of patients with defective primary hemostasis and a prolonged bleeding time but normal platelet counts is presented in Figure 21-27 [26].

REFERENCES

1. Kessel RG and Kardon RH: Chapt 4, in Tissues and Organs. A Text-Atlas of Scanning Electron Microscopy. New York, WH Freeman and Company,1979

2. Colman RW et al: Chapt 1, in Hemostasis and Thrombosis: Basic Principles and Clinical Practice, 2nd ed. Colman RW et al, Eds. Philadelphia, JB Lippincott Company,1987

3. Kane WH and Davie EW: Blood coagulation factors V and VIII: structural and functional similarities and their relationship to hemorrhagic and thrombotic disorders. Blood 71: 539,1988

4. Rosenberg RD: Chapt 15, in The Molecular Basis of Blood Diseases, Stamatoyannopoulos G et al, Eds. Philadelphia, WB Saunders Company,1987

5. Stemerman MB et al: Perturbations of the endothelium. Prog Hemost Thromb 7:289, 1984

6. Handin RI and Wagner DD: Molecular and cellular biology of von Willebrand factor. Prog Hemost Thromb 9:233,1989

7. Wagner DD: Chapt 9, in Coagulation and Bleeding Disorders. Zimmerman TS and Ruggeri ZM, Eds. New York, Marcel Dekker, Inc.,1989

8. White JG: An overview of platelet structural physiology. Scanning Microsc 1:1677,1987

9. Zucker-Franklin D and Petursson S: Thrombocytopoiesis—analysis by membrane tracer and freeze-fracture studies on fresh human and cultured mouse megakaryocytes. J Cell Biol 99:390,1984

10. Lichtman MA et al: Parasinusoidal location of megakaryocytes in marrow: a determinant of platelet release. Am J Hematol 4:303, 1978

11. Zucker-Franklin D: Chapt 10, in Atlas of Blood Cells: Function and Pathology, 2nd ed., Zucker-Franklin D et al, Eds. Milan, Edi Ermes s.r.l.,1988

12. Shattil SJ and Bennett JS: Platelets and their membranes in hemostasis: physiology and pathophysiology. Ann Intern Med 94:108, 1981

13. Coller BS: Chapt 4, in Disorders of Hemostasis, Ratnoff OD and Forbes CD, Eds. Orlando, Grune & Stratton, Inc.,1984

14. Majerus PW: Chapt 19, in The Molecular Basis of Blood Diseases, Stamatoyannopoulos G et al, Eds. Philadelphia, WB Saunders Company,1987

15. Marcus AJ: Chapt 38, in Hemostasis and Thrombosis, 2nd ed., Colman RW et al, Eds. Philadelphia, JB Lippincott Company,1987

16. Zucker MB: The functioning of blood platelets. Sci Am 242(6):86,1980

17. Saito H: Chapt 2, in Disorders of Hemostasis, Ratnoff OD and Forbes CD, Eds. Orlando, Grune & Stratton, Inc.,1984

18. Nemerson Y: Tissue factor and hemostasis. Blood 71:1,1988

19. Osterud B: Activation pathways of the coagulation system in normal haemostasis. Scand J Haematol 32:337,1984

20. Rapaport SI: Inhibition of factor VIIa/tissue factor-induced blood coagulation: with particular emphasis upon a factor Xa-dependent inhibitory mechanism. Blood 73:359,1989

21. Doolittle RF: Fibrinogen and fibrin. Annu Rev Biochem 53:195,1984

22. Rapaport SI: Chapt 23, in Introduction to Hematology, 2nd ed. Philadelphia, JB Lippincott Company,1987

23. Davie EW: Proteins of blood coagulation: their domains and evolution. Chemica Scripta 26B:241,1986

24. Babior BM and Stossel TP: Chapt 15, in Hematology. A Pathophysiological Approach. New York, Churchill Livingstone Inc.,1984

25. Francis CW and Marder VJ: Chapt 22, in Hemostasis and Thrombosis: Basic Principles and Clinical Practice, 2nd ed. Philadelphia, JB Lippincott Company,1987

26. Day JH and Rao AK: Evaluation of platelet function. Semin Hematol 23:89,1986

22

Vascular and Thrombocytopenic Purpuras

□

Bleeding disorders caused by vascular aberrations, inability to form an adequate platelet plug, or defective endothelial-platelet interactions represent failures in primary hemostasis, collectively termed the purpuras. Bleeding traceable to a vascular aberration is known as vascular purpura. More commonly purpura is the result of inadequacy in the number or function of platelets.

VASCULAR PURPURAS

Vascular purpuras can be grouped into hereditary disorders of angiogenesis or vascular structure and acquired disorders incurred by vascular damage (Table 22-1).

Hereditary Vascular Purpuras

Vascular purpuras may result from inborn errors of collagen formation or of other elements of vascular support, or from hereditary vascular malformations.

Hereditary Disorders of Connective Tissue

Purpura occurring as an inherited infirmity in connective tissue support is rare and represents

T A B L E 22-1

Classification of vascular purpuras

> I. Hereditary vascular purpuras
>   A. Hereditary connective tissue disorders
>   B. Hereditary vascular malformations
> II. Acquired vascular purpuras
>   A. Mechanical purpuras
>   B. Vasculitis
>   C. Microvascular obstruction
>   D. Other acquired purpuric disorders

439

a group of genetic errors in collagen or elastic tissue metabolism. Connective tissue is so fundamental to form that purpura or other extravasations of blood usually is only one of many concerns to these grievously afflicted individuals, some of whom face a lifetime of irremediable and crippling calamities. Connective tissue disorders include Ehlers-Danlos syndrome, pseudoxanthoma elasticum, osteogenesis imperfecta, and Marfan's syndrome; of these only the first will be described.

Ehlers-Danlos syndrome   Ehlers-Danlos syndrome encompasses a group of ten rare types of collagen abnormalities that are extremely heterogeneous in mode of genetic transmission and clinical severity but share several clinical features: skin fragility, easy bruising, and hypermobile joints. In all patients the skin is velvety like chamois leather and can be stretched for several inches before slowly retracting (Figure 22-1) [1]. Severely affected patients develop a characteristic facies with prominent scars, lop ears, and molluscoid pseudotumors over elbows and knees. Joint laxity and hyperextensibility lead some victims to subject themselves to morbid curiosity as "india rubber men" in sideshows, but the suffering from joint dislocations, prolapse of the mitral valve (floppy mitral valve syndrome), and gaping wounds is not material for comedy. Bleeding problems are particularly severe in the "arterial" type IV disease, in which type III collagen is missing: as type III collagen predominates in large and small vessels, these patients are subject to catastrophic arterial rupture leading to intraabdominal, intrathoracic, or limb-compartmental bleeding, or to sudden death from hemorrhagic stroke. Apart from avoiding trauma and unnecessary surgery, there is no remedy for this wretched disorder.

Hereditary Vascular Malformations

Stimulus-receptor interactions between plasma-derived hydrolytic enzymes such as plasmin and components of the extracellular matrix initiate an angiogenesis cascade that controls growth, construction, and organizational behavior of endothelial cells. Under guidance by angiogenic stimuli, endothelial cells leave their parent venule and release serine pep-

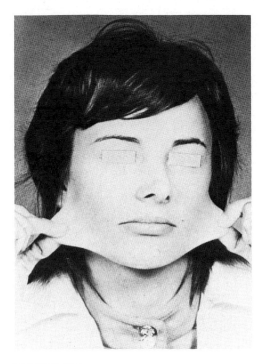

FIGURE 22-1

Pliant laxity of the skin enables this woman with Ehlers-Danlos syndrome to make a seriocomic face that downplays the gravity of her collagen disorder. (Reproduced by permission from: Cawson RA et al, Eds: Chapt 18, in Pathology. The Mechanisms of Disease, 2nd ed. St. Louis, CV Mosby Company,1989.)

tidases that carve holes in the basement membranes that become the site of nascent vessels. Migratory endothelial cells move through these holes to form cylindrical sprouts that elongate in response to proliferative signals, join at their tips, and (under the head of capillary pressure) inflate with flowing blood to become capillary loops. These channels evolve into more complex vascular structures such as arteries, veins, and sinuses during embryogenesis. Hereditary errors in angiogenesis may lead to telangiectasias, benign hemangiomas, or proliferative vascular malformations.

Hereditary hemorrhagic telangiectasia   Hereditary hemorrhagic telangiectasia (Osler-Weber-

Rendu disease) is a dominant genetic disorder of capillary angiogenesis that has been perpetuated because it seldom creates serious problems before adulthood: it is usually recognizable by multiple permanent bright red or red-purple vascular ectasias most visible on the fingers, face, nose, lips, and mucous membranes of palate and tongue (Figure 22-2) [2]. These weakwalled, fragile lesions are easily burst by mechanical force or abrasion, and patients commonly present with recurrent nosebleeds. They pout and enlarge over the years to form nodular vascular tumors the size of split peas, and patients may be plagued by perpetual occult blood loss from gastrointestinal lesions, leading to chronic iron deficiency anemia; in patients without skin or oral lesions, the source

of blood loss may only become evident on endoscopy or mesenteric angiography. In some patients, internal telangiectases may balloon out and unite with other lesions to form arteriovenous fistulas, particularly in the pulmonary circulation, or tangled arteriovenous malformations, especially in the brain. Large pulmonary arteriovenous fistulas that cause massive right-to-left shunting, hypoxia and right heart failure, and cranial arteriovenous malformations causing neurological problems are controlled either surgically or by a vessel-blocking procedure known as "embolotherapy."

Cavernous hemangiomas The most common congenital vascular anomalies are harmless capillary hemangiomas (port wine stains), most of which spontaneously involute and none of which becomes a proliferative lesion. Most cavernous hemangiomas are soft superficial "strawberry" anomalies that are unsightly but nonthreatening. Some cavernous hemangiomas, however, are proliferative structures that may occur at any site and enlarge progressively to impinge on adjacent organs. Cavernous hemangiomas achieving a sufficient size are known as giant hemangiomas; giant hemangiomas are disfiguring, threaten neighboring internal structures, and when very large may cause a syndrome of platelet trapping and "intratumoral" consumption coagulopathy known as the Kasabach-Merritt syndrome (Figure 22-3) [3]. In this syndrome— also occurring in some large hemangioendotheliomas and hemangiosarcomas—localized consumption of platelets and activation of coagulation often lead to both thrombocytopenic purpura and findings indicative of disseminated intravascular coagulation (DIC): microangiopathic hemolytic anemia (Chapter 8), consumption of fibrin, and release of anticoagulant fibrin split products including the pathognomonic D dimer. Recurrent bleeding, hemolytic anemia, and obstruction of vital structures by tumor expansion require intervention by surgical excision. In giant hemangiomas that are unresectable because of location, consumption of platelets and coagulation factors and fragmentation of red cells can often be halted by high doses of the plasmin inhibitor, epsilon amino caproic acid (EACA). By blocking fibrinolysis, EACA stabi-

FIGURE 22-2

Myriads of small (1 to 3 mm across), red, blood-filled ectasias of lips and tongue in hereditary hemorrhagic telangiectasia. The distended thin-walled vessels lack adventitial support, and even when flat the lesions blanch on being pressed by a glass slide. (From Hoffbrand AV and Pettit JE: Chapt 13, in Sandoz Atlas of Clinical Hematology. London, Gower Medical Publishing, 1988.)

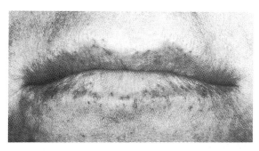

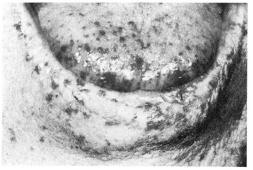

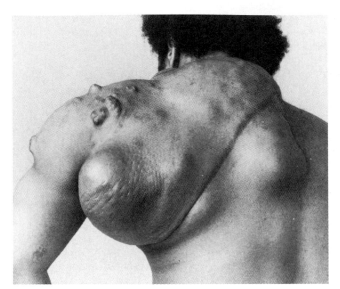

FIGURE 22-3

Giant hemangioma and several smaller proliferative satellites in a 32-year-old man whose lesions had enlarged progressively since childhood. Platelet consumption in the sluggish anastomosing spongiform channels of these Brobdingnagian vascular tumors resulted in repeated episodes of hematochezia, hematuria, hematemesis, and hemoptysis. (The scar across the back represents a prior surgical excision.) (From Ortel TL et al: Antifibrinolytic therapy in the management of the Kasabach Merritt syndrome. Am J Hematol 29:44,1988.)

lizes intratumoral clotting and may seal off blood flow through the troublesome tumor by thrombotic occlusion.

Kaposi's sarcoma   Kaposi's sarcoma is a multicentric hemorrhagic endothelial tumor most often encountered in patients with severe underlying immunosuppression, being particularly common in patients with AIDS (Chapter 12). Kaposi's sarcoma occurring as an opportunistic "marker" neoplasm in AIDS victims is of the highly invasive sort that initially causes warty hemorrhagic skin tumors the size of cranberries or larger (Figure 22-4) [4]. These bloody endothelial tumors metastasize broadly to lymph nodes, salivary glands, mucosal surfaces, and viscera. The endothelial origin of these unsightly and predatory tumors is certified by the emblematic presence of Weibel-Palade bodies and factor VIII antigen.

Acquired Vascular Purpuras

Sufficient mechanical force can produce purpura in anyone, and in patients complaining of easy bruising historical enquiries are the first indicator as to whether the bruises were appropriate to the force or needful of explanation. Many women seem unusually susceptible to bruising of the trunk, legs, and upper arms,

FIGURE 22-4

Hemorrhagic cutaneous tumors, nodules, and plaques on the foot of a patient with Kaposi's sarcoma (A). Biopsy (B) reveals a deceptively bland histology, composed of interwoven groups of spindle cells that form slitlike arcades filled with red cells. (From Murphy GF and Mihm MC Jr: Chapt 27, in Robbins Pathologic Basis of Disease, 4th ed., Cotran RS et al, Eds. Philadelphia, WB Saunders Company,1989.)

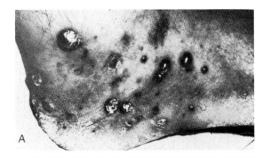

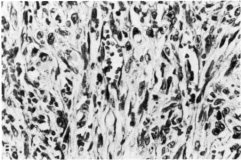

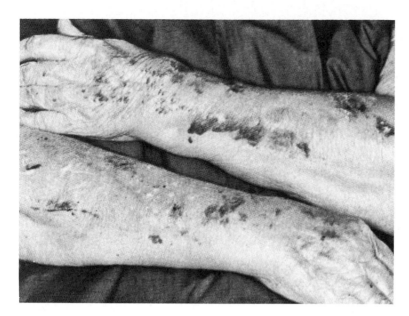

FIGURE 22-5

Sharp-bordered patches of vascular purpura on the extensor surfaces of the hands and arms of an elderly man. (From Fritsch WC: Managing age-related vascular skin lesions. Geriatrics 30(3):45,1975.)

especially during the reproductive period, and no ample explanation has been discovered: hence the ingenuous terms "purpura simplex" and "devil's pinches." Many forms of purpura elicited by the modest, commonplace, quotidian burden of bumps signify weakening of vascular structure, as occurs with wasting or during normal aging. Some are melancholy stigmata of denied battery or secret self-abuse.

Age-Related Vascular Purpura

A variety of colorful and benign vascular lesions serve to remind folks they are growing old. Among these are bright red cherry angiomas, purple papules called venous lakes, and spidery vascular dilations on the face known as senile telangiectasia. More common are the large well-demarcated superficial patches of purple or mahogany found on the backs of the hands, wrists, forearms, and other extensor regions most apt to be bumped, and known by the pejorative expression senile purpura (Figure 22-5) [5]. Senile purpura and identical shallow bruising seen in cachexia is the combined result of thinning and inelasticity of skin, collagen attrition, and loss of adventitial cushioning. A senile purpuric lesion may persist for months, for most of the blood seepage is into cornified epithelium inaccessible to macrophages: the oxidized hemoglobin remains undigested, lend-ing a mahogany hue, whereas deeper bleeding (as in ecchymoses) rapidly undergoes the more familiar blue-mauve-yellow transition as macrophage heme oxygenase splits the heme ring to create bilirubin degradation products. Therapy is unnecessary, but venipunctures in elderly or wasted individuals should be performed with care to avert patient resentment toward iatrogenic discolorations.

Factitial Purpura: Psychogenic Bleeding

Many forms of inexplicable bruising represent abuse or self-abuse and are vivid expressions of domestic pathology or severe psychiatric problems. A deplorable fact of life is that people often batter weaker relatives. Battered wives may seek medical sanctuary from drunk or demented husbands even while denying the source of injury for fear of retaliation. Children subjected to repeated and vicious savaging by their parents may acquire a silent reproachful countenance described as "frozen watchfulness." Invariably the parental account is cloaked in denial to hide the dark underlying patterns of maladjustment, paranoia, or drug abuse that fuel these sickening outbursts of rage against the helpless.

Self-abuse Self-injury with factitial bleeding, although remarkably common, is usually so well-concealed and inventive—and often practiced by individuals with some knowledge of medicine—that the bizarre patterns of bruising or bleeding may sorely tax the physician's acumen. The surreptitious acts of self-injury may be so well shielded by layers of unconscious self-deception that the patient is unaware that he or she is baiting the physician. Factitial purpura signifies a profound emotional disturbance, and if the unconscious hoax is bluntly exposed, the confrontation is very likely to provoke attempted suicide. Deeply disturbed individuals may phlebotomize themselves aggressively or secretly ingest sufficient warfarin to induce serious bleeding; these dangerous ploys are discoverable, respectively, by searching for needle marks or finding a greatly prolonged prothrombin time. The physician's task, once any emergency measures are completed, is to gently motivate the patient to accept nonthreatening psychiatric help.

Most cases of painful bruising attributed to "autoerythrocyte sensitization" and "autosensitivity to DNA" have been traced to furtive self-abuse rather than to occult immunologic processes. The key to management is longterm psychotherapy.

Scurvy

This ancient and fearful scourge, once endemic among mariners and residents of wintry or besieged cities, remains among us in urban centers as an affliction of the impoverished, reclusive, or abandoned, or of those (such as recently widowed men) incapable of or unused to fending for themselves—so-called "bachelor scurvy." Ascorbic acid (vitamin C) is an essential cofactor for hydroxylation of proline and lysine residues in collagen; these residues stabilize the hydrogen bonds responsible for its triple helical structure. In ascorbic acid deficiency unhydroxylated procollagen and collagen are unable to assume this stable conformation, and newly formed collagen types III and IV so essential to vascular structure exist as randomly disoriented coils that are soon degraded. In scurvy, collagen wasting is most damaging to rapidly growing connective tissue structures such as hair follicles, gingival moorings, and healing wounds.

As was once the fate of mariners on prolonged sea voyages, persons isolated in lonely apartments without access to or knowledge regarding the necessity of ascorbate-rich foods such as fresh fruits or vegetables become "chemically" scorbutic within 4 to 6 weeks, and shortly afterward the earliest signs of scurvy appear in the form of scattered petechiae and spontaneous ecchymoses. Within 2 to 3 months of ascorbate deprivation hyperkeratotic papules and perifollicular hemorrhages appear on the hairy surfaces of arms and legs: emergence of coiled and brittle hairs in corkscrew fashion through the congested follicles creates the pathognomonic triad of scurvy—hyperkeratosis, corkscrew hairs, and perifollicular petechiae. In patients with teeth, gingival overgrowth soon becomes

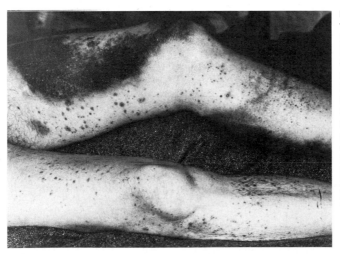

FIGURE 22-6

Massive hemorrhages into the left leg and overlying skin plus showers of spreading perifollicular hemorrhages in a scorbutic man admitted for blood loss anemia and hypotension. The tautly enlarged left thigh and calf contained an estimated 2 quarts of extravasated blood. Hemorrhage into the weight-bearing undersurfaces of the left leg extended into the buttocks (not shown). (From Jandl JH: Chapt 30, in Blood: Textbook of Hematology. Boston, Little, Brown and Co., 1987.)

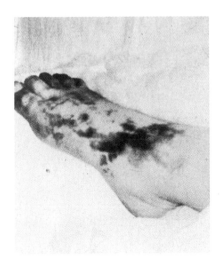 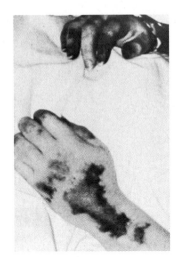

FIGURE 22-7

Necrotizing purpura and gangrene of hands and foot in a 39-year old woman with meningococcal septicemia, shock, and renal tubular necrosis. (From Lazarus JM et al: A 39-year-old woman with Raynaud's phenomenon, hypotension, and acute renal failure. Case 4-1988. Reprinted, by the permission of the New England Journal of Medicine 318:234, 1988.)

apparent, and the increasingly boggy, swollen, friable, dark purple gums become subject to purulent gingivitis and putrefaction.

Hemorrhagic scurvy Active patients with established scurvy may present in orthopedic clinics with hemarthroses or in dental clinics with bleeding gums. More often patients are victims of their own neglect and arrive by ambulance in hypovolemic shock from gross hemorrhage into major muscle groups, visible as "saddle hemorrhages" and tense swellings of thighs and calves, overlaid with broad areas of extravasated blood (Figure 22-6) [6]. All patients with manifest scurvy are in peril of sudden demise through shock, myocardial infarction, or hemorrhagic stroke, and should receive ascorbic acid immediately and several times daily until at least 4 g has been administered. Therapy must not be deferred for measurement of blood or buffy coat ascorbate levels, since diagnosis rests on clinical findings and the price of delay is death.

Vascular Purpura Caused by Infection: Septic Purpura Fulminans

Septicemia or viremia can cause vascular purpura by direct invasion of endothelium (as in rickettsial diseases), release of bacterial toxins damaging to endothelium (as in meningococcemia), or igniting DIC (as in gram-negative shock). In fulminant meningococcemia, febrile and meningeal symptoms are often followed swiftly by peripheral vascular collapse, renal failure, and necrotizing cutaneous hemorrhages. Endotoxins released by *Neisseria meningitides* (predominantly type C) cause an unusually virulent purpura with necrotizing vasculitis very similar to the murderous purpura fulminans of hereditary protein C deficiency (Figure 22-7) [7]. The similarity is more than coincidental, for release of meningococcal endotoxin induces both a consumption coagulopathy with DIC and severe reductions in components of the protein C anticoagulant pathway.

Hypersensitivity (Allergic) Vasculitis

Hypersensitivity vasculitis encompasses a group of syndromes in which small vessel damage and necrosis is caused by vascular deposition of immune complexes and complement as a self-destructive reaction to certain antigens. Most common of the causative agents are drugs, particularly aspirin, coumadin, iodides, penicillin, phenacetin, quinidine, quinine, and sulfonamides. Circulating drug-antibody immune complexes deposit on platelet and vascular surfaces and penetrate to the basement membrane, where they activate the alternative complement sequence; release of chemotactic components lures neutrophils to the vessel wall, where the excited cells congregate in cuffs and discharge lysosmal hydrolases that cause extravasation of blood and "palpable purpura." The resultant "leukocytoclastic" vasculitis

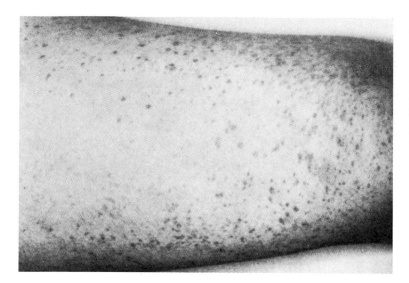

FIGURE 22-8

Purpuric and urticarial rash on the thigh of an 18-year-old woman with Henoch-Schönlein purpura. (From Miyagawa S et al: Anaphylactoid purpura and familial IgA nephropathy. Am J Med 86:340, 1989.)

simulates the Arthus reaction and presents as transient urticaria followed by palpable polymorphic purpuric eruptions ranging in magnitude from pinpoint lesions to large black necrotic patches surrounded by purpura. Purpuric vasculitis syndromes are most often drug-induced, but a spectrum of kindred reactions is associated with serum sickness, mixed cryoglobulinemia, connective tissue disorders, malignancies, and a peculiar anaphylactoid disorder known as Henoch-Schönlein purpura.

Henoch-Schönlein purpura   Henoch-Schönlein purpura is a self-limited allergic or anaphylactoid vasculitis of the skin that often affects joints, kidneys, and the gastrointestinal tract, occurring usually in children or young adults. Allergic purpura commonly commences 1 to 3 weeks after an upper respiratory infection and presents as an acute erythematous or urticarial rash distributed symmetrically over the extensor and lateral aspects of legs, arms and buttocks (Figure 22-8) [8]. Most patients experience transient arthralgias leaving no residual, some suffer temporary but frightening neurologic episodes, and many are subject to recurring bouts of colicky abdominal pain and intestinal bleeding from erosive purpuric infarcts of the alimentary mucosa.

Serum of patients with Henoch-Schönlein purpura invariably contains soluble IgA immune complexes (composed of IgA antibodies to the Fab portion of IgG) during the early phases of illness; as in all immune complex diseases, vessels most jeopardized are those of renal glomeruli. Indeed, it is probable that IgA nephropathy is a limited expression of Henoch-Schönlein purpura, for IgA antibodies eluted from renal tissue of Henoch-Schönlein purpura nephritis and from kidneys of patients with familial or sporadic IgA nephropathy are cross-reactive. Furthermore, immunofluorescent antibodies added to skin biopsies of purpuric lesions in patients with IgA nephropathy reveal IgA deposits in the small vessels of the upper dermis. In purpuric patients destined to develop IgA nephritis, a nephrotic syndrome caused by glomerular deposition of IgA immune complexes develops within 3 months (Figure 22-9) [9]. In most patients the nephropathy is mild and transient, but chronic uremia ensues in over 10% of afflicted adults. In patients facing endstage renal failure, renal allografting is the preferred therapy but should be deferred until all systemic manifestations of this relapsing disorder have ceased.

QUANTITATIVE DISORDERS OF PLATELETS

Once released individually or in reels or strands from the collapsing walls of ripened megakaryocytes (Chapter 20), platelets enter the blood and

FIGURE 22-9

Biopsies of skin and glomerular lesions in a patient with anaphylactoid purpura and IgA nephropathy. (Top) Leukocytoclastic vasculitis of dermal capillaries. (Middle) Light microscopy of a glomerulus from the same patient, showing segmented proliferation of the capillary tuft and (leftward) a large cellular crescent (PAS stain). (Bottom) Immunofluorescent view highlighting mesangeal deposition of IgA. (From Miyagawa S et al: Anaphylactoid purpura and familial IgA nephropathy. Am J Med 86:340,1989.)

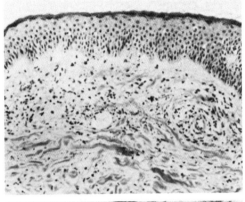

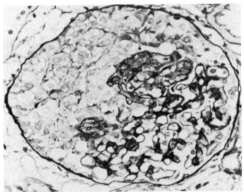

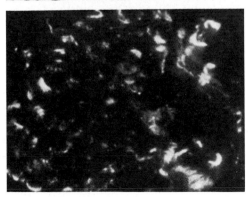

normally remain confined there until their peaceful expiration 8 to 10 days later. The normal daily rate of platelet production is sufficient to add about 35,000 of these tiny "cells" per μl of blood, a number just sufficient to replace losses by attrition. A unique feature of platelets is that their small size enables them to move back and forth between sinuses and cords as they traverse the spleen (Chapter 11). These harmless excursions slow passage through the spleen and create an exchangeable platelet pool amounting to 30% of the total platelet mass in resting individuals. In moments of excitement or in response to blood loss, the normal splenic pool serves a reservoir function, discharging platelet-rich blood into circulation while preventing platelet reentry by adrenergic clamping of the splenic artery. Normally platelets die of old age, and thus a sample of blood platelets labeled randomly with regard to age by ^{51}Cr or ^{111}In disappears after reinfusion by "linear" (arithmetic) decay, with a half-survival of about 5 days.

In patients with vastly enlarged spleens, splenic pooling is increased in proportion to splenic blood flow. With this compartmental shift, as much as 80 to 90% of the platelet mass may be detoured through the expanded cordal compartment, causing partially reversible thrombocytopenia in the general circulation. In contrast, patients splenectomized for splenic rupture sustain a moderate thrombocythemia for lack of a splenic pool. As splenectomy or congenital asplenia do not prolong the actuarial survival of platelets beyond normal, the natural graveyard for exhausted platelets is unknown.

Thrombocytopenic Purpura Due to Diminished Platelet Production

Thrombocytopenia resulting from defective production should be suspected in congenital thrombocytopenic purpuras and in thrombocytopenias associated with generalized marrow failure. Inability of marrow to produce sufficient platelets may occur as an inherited megakaryocytic disorder, often accompanied by skeletal or other anomalies (e.g., Fanconi's syndrome); more often it is the result of drug toxicity or viral infection.

Hereditary Thrombocytopenias

Amegakaryocytic thrombocytopenia and the TAR syndrome

Hereditary amegakaryocytosis (thrombocytopenia with absent radii: TAR syndrome) is an autosomal recessive disorder in which thrombocytopenia caused by near-absence of megakaryocytes is associated with various somatic abnormalities, the most constant of which is bilateral radial aplasia. The first year of life is the most dangerous; during this period mortality from cerebral hemorrhage and other major consequences of numerically and functionally deficient platelets is roughly 40%. In survivors of the first year, hemorrhagic problems, often interspersed with unexplained leukemoid bouts, slowly abate as the platelet levels gradually rise and their malfunctions are corrected spontaneously.

Wiskott-Aldrich syndrome

This X-linked disorder of males is characterized by thrombocytopenia, small platelets, and failure of T cell-mediated immunity that leads to eczema, repetitive infections, and a high risk of early death from fulminant sepsis or opportunistic lymphomas. Platelets are half-normal in volume and deficient in GPIb, the vWF receptor; hence bleeding time is prolonged disproportionate to the thrombocytopenia. The battery of therapies required to contest this multipronged inborn disorder usually fall short, allogeneic marrow transplantation offering the only definitive recourse. A *forme fruste* of this deadly malady, "X-linked amegakaryocytic thrombocytopenia," is caused by a defect in the same gene on the short arm of chromosome X. These afflicted boys are spared the perils of immunodeficiency, but the severity of thrombocytopenia seldom permits them to survive adolescence.

Acquired Megakaryocytic Hypoplasia

Drug-induced megakaryocyte hypoplasia

Megakaryocytes are among the first casualties of any agent causing damage to pluripotential stem cells, and because of the short lifespan of platelets, drugs that block megakaryocyte formation by CFU-Megs can cause life-threatening thrombocytopenic purpura beginning as soon as 2 to 3 weeks. Nearly all myelosuppressive agents used in chemotherapy inhibit megakaryocyte replication as a dose-dependent adverse effect. Phase-specific agents (methotrexate, cytosine arabinoside) cause a prompt but rapidly reversible depression in platelet production, cell cycle–specific drugs such as cyclophosphamide induce myelosuppression intermediate in rate of onset and subsidence, and cycle-nonspecific alkylators (busulfan, nitrosoureas) cause more gradual but longlasting damage to megakaryocytes and other marrow elements. Chlorothiazide and its congeners can cause an idiosyncratic megakaryocytic hypoplasia of moderate severity that remits on discontinuation, but in some idiosyncratic reactions—as to chloramphenicol or carbonic anhydrase inhibitors (used for treating glaucoma)—megakaryocytopoiesis may be shut down completely and ineluctably, resulting in death from massive purpura within a few weeks or months.

Viral infections

Certain viruses (including those that cause measles, varicella, cytomegalovirus syndrome, infectious mononucleosis, dengue, and Thai hemorrhagic fever) are megakaryocytotropic, adsorb to platelets and megakaryocytes during viremia, and undergo endocytosis. Platelet counts are reduced during infection, but bleeding is disproportionately severe because of virus-induced impairment of platelet aggregation and procoagulant activity.

Thrombocytopenic Purpura Caused by Increased Platelet Destruction

Thrombocytopenia due to increased removal of platelets from circulation occurs through either of two major mechanisms: immune thrombocytopenia, in which platelets coated with sufficient immunoglobulin are cleared by phagocytosis or complement-induced lysis; and increased consumption of platelets (destruction by adhesion to damaged endothelium) as occurs in DIC or thrombotic thrombocytopenic purpura (TTP).

Immune Thrombocytopenic Purpura (ITP)

Immunologic destruction of platelets can be caused by antibodies against platelet autoantigens or alloantigens, autologous or heterologous antigens adsorbed to platelet surfaces, or adsorption by platelets of immune (antigen-antibody) complexes (Table 22-2). Evidence

TABLE 22-2

Causes of immune thrombocytopenia

Immune thrombocytopenic purpura (ITP)
  Acute
  Chronic
Alloantibody-induced
  Neonatal
  Posttransfusion
Drug-induced
Disease-associated
  Connective tissue disorders
  Lymphoproliferative disorders
  Solid tumors
  Infections
    Viral
    Bacterial
    Parasitic

Source: From McMillan R: Immune thrombocytopenia. Clin Haematol 12:69,1983.

that immunoglobulins are responsible for platelet destruction, when attached to platelets through any of these mechanisms, is now so complete that the long-cherished nonce term "idiopathic thrombocytopenic purpura" has been superseded, and the initialism ITP is now recognized to stand for immune thrombocytopenic purpura. Patients with ITP may or may not experience petechiae and increased bruising at platelet levels between 20,000 and 50,000 cells/μl, but counts below 10,000 almost always entail generalized bleeding into skin, mucosa, and internal organs; patients with extreme reductions (platelet counts below 2,000/μl) live on the brink of intracranial hemorrhage. In their resolute response to prodding by CFU-Meg, thrombopoietin, and other CSFs, marrow megakaryocytes proliferate (Figure 22-10) and sometimes release their cargo of platelets precipitately while still relatively immature. Because megakaryocyte maturation and platelet release are rushed in compensatory response to brisk platelet destruction, abnormally large blood platelets are detectable on blood smears and by electronic sizing.

Antibody-coated platelets are trapped and destroyed by macrophages　　By direct measure employing radioisotope-labeled monoclonal antibodies, each platelet normally binds less than 100 molecules of IgG to its surface (platelet-associated IgG, or PA IgG), mostly by attachment to GPIIIa, which contains the IgG receptor of platelets. In ITP platelets are coated with increased amounts of IgG, ranging in very rough proportion to the rate of platelet destruction, from 200 to over 10,000 IgG molecules/platelet. As antibody-coated platelets pass through the sinuses of spleen and liver, the protruding Fc fragments are seized by Fc receptors (FcγRs) on monocytes and resident macrophages; the captured platelets are at first imprisoned by elaborate tendrils springing

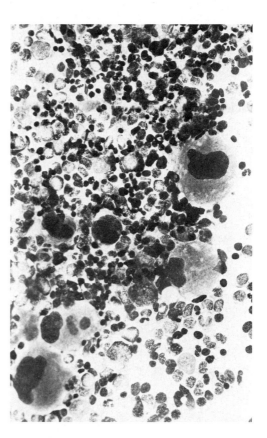

FIGURE 22-10

Clusters of smooth hypolobular "nonbudding" megakaryocytes in marrow of a patient with immune thrombocytopenia. Despite the shift toward immaturity and low ploidy of individual megakaryocytes, net platelet production by the hyperplastic young forms can exceed normal by up to 8-fold. (Photo by CT Kapff.)

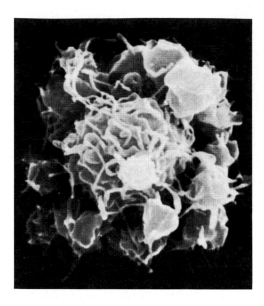

FIGURE 22-11

SEM of a macrophage-platelet rosette created by the grappling of multiple antibody-coated platelets by the long, sticky (FcγR-bearing) fingers of a covetous macrophage. (From Court WS et al: Human monocyte interaction with antibody-coated platelets. I. General characteristics. Am J Hematol 17:225,1984.)

FIGURE 22-12

Anterior view scintigrams obtained after reinfusion of ^{111}In-labeled autologous platelets in three patients exhibiting splenic (left), splenohepatic (middle), and hepatic (right) platelet destruction patterns. (From Schmidt KG and Rasmussen JW: Kinetics and distribution in vivo of ^{111}In-labelled autologous platelets in idiopathic thrombocytopenic purpura. Scand J Haematol 34:47,1985. © 1985 Munksgaard International Publishers Ltd., Copenhagen, Denmark.)

from the macrophage surface (Figure 22-11) [10], and then are either dismembered piecemeal or swallowed in a single gulp. Fc receptor–mediated macrophage trapping of antibody-coated platelets occurs in a manner analogous to that operative in immunohemolytic anemias (Chapter 8). The site of platelet entrapment by macrophages is similarly influenced by the quantity of antibody bound and relative blood flow through the organs of the RES, heavy coating of antibody usually being associated with brisk uptake and destruction in the high-flow hepatic sinuses; slower and more orderly destruction of lightly sensitized cells takes place mainly in the comparatively fastidious, low-velocity sinuses of the spleen (Figure 22-12) [11].

Acute ITP

Acute ITP is a disease of children and young adults that usually occurs abruptly 1 to 2 weeks after onset of a seasonal viral illness. During the immune response to virus, IgG antibody attaches to viral antigens adsorbed on platelet surfaces; when sufficient amounts of PA IgG accrue, platelet levels may plummet to counts below $20,000/\mu l$, leading to petechiae, multiple ecchymoses, and mucosal bleeding. Ordinarily acute ITP is self-terminating, but during the first 2 weeks after onset in severe cases (platelet counts below $10,000/\mu l$), bleeding may be profuse and hemorrhagic bullae may appear. Such imperiled patients should be treated with high doses of prednisone and daily infusions of purified IgG, both of which interfere with clearance of antibody-coated platelets by macrophages. Effi-

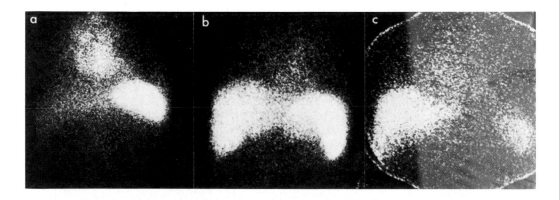

TABLE 22-3

Comparison of acute and chronic ITP

Characteristic features	Acute	Chronic
Peak incidence	2–9 years	20–40 years
Sex ratio	1 to 1	3 females to 1 male
Antecedent infection	Common	Uncommon
Platelet count	$<20,000/\mu l$	$20,000–100,000/\mu l$
Onset of symptoms	Abrupt	Gradual
Hemorrhagic bullae on mucous membranes	Common	Uncommon
Duration	2–6 weeks	Years
Spontaneous remission	>80% of cases	Uncommon
Response to corticosteroids	Uncommon	Common
Response to splenectomy	Variable	Common

Source: Modified from Koller CA: Immune thrombocytopenic purpura. Med Clin North Am 64:761,1980.

cacy of this therapy is hard to evaluate because spontaneous recovery begins within 2 to 4 weeks in over 90% of patients regardless of these therapies. In an unpredictable minority,

mostly young adults, acute ITP pursues a relapsing or unremitting course requiring continued therapy. ITP that fails to clear within 6 months is a disorder with a different natural history and pathogenetic basis: chronic ITP.

Chronic ITP

Chronic ITP, one of the commonest autoimmune hematologic disorder of adults, is characterized by the insidious appearance of unexplained mucocutaneous hemorrhages, petechiae of dependent areas and oral mucosa, and recurrent episodes of spontaneous bruising, epistaxis, and menorrhagia. Chronic ITP differs from the acute form in many ways apart from its chronicity (Table 22-3) [12]. In most patients, bleeding is moderate, but the finding of hemorrhagic bullae (blood blisters) on the tongue or mucous

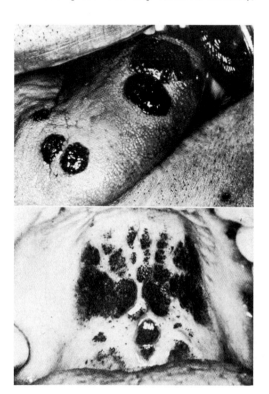

◀ **FIGURE 22-13**

Mucosal bleeding in a young man with severe chronic ITP. (Above) Hemorrhagic bullae (blood blisters) of the tongue are a portent of worse bleeding to come. (Below) Showers of petechiae on the palate of the same patient, with coalescence of some to form bullae. (From Cawson RA: Essentials of Dental Surgery, 3rd ed. Edinburgh, Churchill Livingstone, Inc.,1978.)

membranes mandates intensive platelet transfusion therapy and other emergency measures to forestall intracranial or other deadly bleeding calamities (Figure 22-13) [13].

Chronic ITP is caused by IgG antibodies to platelet glycoproteins   Antibodies responsible for most cases of chronic ITP are of the IgG1 subclass. Eluates of PA IgG bind both autologous and heterologous platelets and thus are not self-specific; most react with epitopes on the GPIIb-IIIa complex, some react with GPIIb or GPIIIa alone, and in a few cases determinants on GPIb represent the target. That specificity is most often for GPIIb-IIIa (the fibrinogen receptor) was inferred from the fact that platelets deficient in this receptor (from patients with Glanzmann's thrombasthenia) are usually unreactive with antibody eluates. The spleen plays a pivotal role in chronic ITP for not only does it house the most exacting filter for capturing antibody-coated platelets, but its plasma cells produce the bulk of platelet-specific antibody. As the spleen is both the primary source of antibody and the major disposal site for antibody-coated cells, the argument for early splenectomy in ITP refractory to frontline prednisone therapy is a rational one. Splenectomy is the most definitive treatment for chronic ITP, raising platelet counts to acceptable levels in over 70% of cases. In the 15 to 30% of patients who fail to sustain an adequate response to prednisone, splenectomy, or both, nearly half will benefit

from intravenous infusion of gamma globulin (purified IgG). Infusions of polyvalent IgG in amounts sufficient to raise plasma IgG levels by 50 to 100% inundate the Fc receptors of splenic and other macrophages; because commercial preparations contain IgG aggregates, the nonpartisan IgG competes to some extent with platelet-bound antibody for occupation of macrophage Fc receptor sites. Hence infusions of "high-dose gamma globulin" concentrates partially blockade the RES. Children with acute ITP respond uniformly and permanently to IgG, and IgG infusion can be lifesaving in desperate cases; in chronic ITP of adults persisting despite splenectomy, repeated infusions of high-dose IgG eventually may produce lasting remission, but only in about one-third of cases (Figure 22-14) [14]. The rest either remain dependent on repetitive (and very costly) infusions or relapse and are candidates for immunosuppressive therapy.

Neonatal ITP and alloimmune thrombocytopenia of the newborn   About 50% of newborn offspring of mothers with chronic ITP become thrombocytopenic predelivery or at birth by transplacental "inheritance" of IgG antiplatelet antibodies. As the antibody is not autogenous, neonatal ITP is a self-limited process, but the risk of intracranial hemorrhage during the compressive tumult of delivery usually can be averted by controlling maternal antibody activity with prednisone plus high-dose IgG infusions begun several days before delivery.

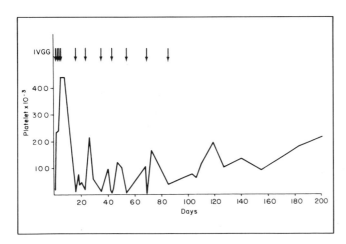

FIGURE 22-14

Temporary and then sustained response to infusions of IgG totaling over 500 g in a 30-year-old woman with chronic ITP refractory to splenectomy and to dangerously prolonged treatment with prednisone. (From Bussel JB et al: Maintenance treatment of adults with chronic refractory immune thrombocytopenic purpura using repeated intravenous infusions of gammaglobulin. Blood 72:121,1988.)

Alloimmune neonatal thrombocytopenia is analogous to erythroblastosis fetalis: it results from formation in the mother of an antibody to a paternally derived antigen in the fetus. There are two allelic forms of the universal Pl^A alloantigen, Pl^{A1} and Pl^{A2}, both of which have been localized to the GPIIIa molecule on platelet surfaces. Since 98% of the population carries the Pl^{A1} antigen, Pl^{A2} homozygous women are at high risk of producing antibodies to paternal Pl^{A1} antigens present on fetal platelets; in a minority of cases, maternal immunization is against Bak^a or other less common platelet antigens such as Pl^{E1} or HLA-A2 antigens. The fetal fatality rate in alloimmune neonatal thrombocytopenic purpura is high, largely as the result of intracranial hemorrhage. Preventive measures in women suspected of being at risk include antenatal platelet typing by fetal blood sampling and transfusion in utero of maternal platelets, which are guaranteed to be compatible regardless of the antigen-antibody system involved.

Posttransfusion Purpura

Posttransfusion purpura (PTP) is a singular and baffling syndrome characterized by fulminant thrombocytopenic purpura and bleeding commencing about 7 days after blood transfusion given for surgery or hemorrhage. The vast majority of PTP cases have been middle-aged or elderly multiparous women who are Pl^{A1}-negative and whose sera contain acute phase high-titer anti-Pl^{A1} alloantibody reactive with an epitope on GPIIIa. The enigma of PTP is that the anti-Pl^{A1} anamnestic response to transfused Pl^{A1}-positive blood somehow brings about massive lysis of the patient's own Pl^{A1}-negative platelets. The intensity and rarity of the process (about 100 case reports) might be attributed to the fact that platelet lysis is mediated by a unique complement-activating IgG3, but the coincident and persisting slaughter of the innocents is unexplained. Several exegetic hypotheses have been advanced, including the ingenious suggestion that Pl^{A1} antigen released from transfused platelets as they are destroyed transfers to the structural deletion site on patients' Pl^{A1}-negative platelets, making them targets for antibody destruction; this and other suggestions have not received experimental support

[15]. While the mystery lingers, the mortally endangered patient warrants immediate intervention to avert massive platelet destruction: best immediate results are achieved with high-dose immunoglobulin infusion, preceded in selected instances by exchange transfusion. In most patients this bizarre but frightening purpuric process terminates spontaneously within 3 to 4 weeks.

Drug-Induced Immune Thrombocytopenia

Many medications promote immunologic destruction of platelets, the most notorious being quinine, quinidine, gold salts, sulfonamide combinations, and heparin. In most instances the soluble drug or drug-protein complexes bind weakly to certain platelet glycoproteins. On rechallenge IgG antibodies are generated that bind via their Fab domains to platelets coated with drug, forming a stable antibody-drug complex on the platelet surface. The platelet receptors for drug dependent antibodies vary from drug to drug and among different patients exposed to the same drug, the principal receptors being components of GPIb, GPIIb, GPIIIa, and GPIX. Depending on continued presence of the guilty drug, accumulation of sufficient numbers of antibody molecules on the platelet surface (Fc domains aimed outward) ensures lysis of the Ig-coated cells either by complement activation or by clearance from circulation by FcγR-equipped macrophages.

The quinine-quinidine pattern Of the scores of drugs known to cause antibody-mediated thrombocytopenia, the stereoisomers, quinidine and quinine, are most renowned. Although purpura occurs uncommonly in persons exposed to these prevalent ingredients of medicinals and fizz-water tonics, ingestion of drug to which a person has been sensitized by prior exposure may be followed within minutes or hours by an explosive sequence of menacing events, starting with anaphylactic or pyrogenic reactions and progressing to generalized purpura and hemorrhages erupting down the corridors of the gastrointestinal tract. Unless the patient succumbs, bleeding ceases within 5 to 10 days, pending the decline of PA IgG as additional antibody binding to platelets is halted by disappearance of the haptenic

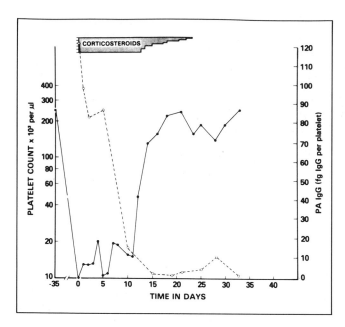

FIGURE 22-15

Platelet counts (uninterrupted line) and PA IgG (interrupted line) in a 56-year-old man who had received quinidine sulfate therapy for 1 month and suddenly experienced the violent onset of generalized thrombocytopenic purpura. Despite corticosteroid therapy and abstinence, bleeding was only partially curbed by multiple transfusions of packed platelets; not until PA IgG levels fell below 10 fg/platelet did counts rise and stabilize. (From Kelton JG et al: Drug-induced thrombocytopenia is associated with increased binding of IgG to platelets both in vivo and in vitro. Blood 58:524,1981.)

culprit (Figure 22-15) [16]. Drug-dependence of antibody binding to platelets can be demonstrated in vitro by incubating normal platelets with patient plasma in the presence versus absence of the suspect drug. As antibody levels are exhausted within 4 weeks of a purpuric reaction, delayed testing for antibody can be performed following a minute (1 μg) booster dose of drug. Drug challenge in vivo in patients with a remote history of possible drug-dependent thrombocytopenic purpura involves a prohibitive risk of incurring runaway purpura, a few mg being capable of inciting catastrophic bleeding.

Platelet Consumption Disorders
Chapter 8 describes these disorders.

Thrombocythemia
The reader is referred to Chapter 15.

Qualitative Disorders of Platelets

Patients with hemorrhagic problems in whom the bleeding time is prolonged and yet platelet counts are normal suffer from platelet malfunction and impairment of primary hemostasis. The impairment may stem from a qualitative abnormality of the platelet itself, or an extrinsic aberration that alters the function of nor-

mal platelets, as in von Willebrand's disease (Chapter 23). Inherited qualitative disorders of platelets are uncommon but instructive, for these genetic errors have revealed much about how platelets work; acquired disorders are more commonly responsible for bleeding, but their molecular mechanisms are less crisply defined.

Hereditary Qualitative Disorders of Platelets

Patients with bleeding problems commencing early in life in whom bleeding time is prolonged but platelet counts are normal (or almost normal) can be presumed to have an inherited qualitative disorder of platelets. Three sorts of genetic dysfunction have been defined: defects of platelet adhesion, failure of primary aggregation in response to physiologic agonists, and abnormalities of platelet secretion.

Inborn Disorders of Platelet Adhesion

Bernard-Soulier (giant platelet) syndrome
Bernard-Soulier syndrome (BSS) is a rare hemorrhagic disorder transmitted by two autosomal recessive genes and marked by very large platelets (Figure 22-16) [17], mild thrombocytopenia, and defective vWF-dependent platelet adhesion. Bleeding occurs because BSS

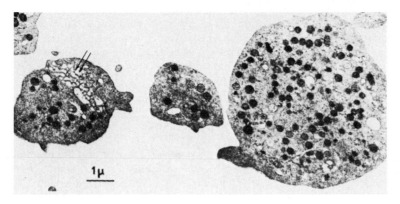

FIGURE 22-16

TEM of BSS platelets demonstrates their great size, which may exceed that of red cells (note 1 μm bar), and the "swiss cheese" appearance created by distension of the open canalicular system (arrows). (From Bellucci S et al: Inherited platelet disorders. Prog Hematol 13:223, 1983.)

platelets lack GPIb, which bears the primary vWF receptor; this prevents vWF-mediated bridging of platelets to wounded subendothelium and predisposes to bleeding from mucosal sites and in response to impact or surgical or dental trauma. BSS must be distinguished from thrombasthenia, which has similar clinical and genetic features but lacks the giant platelets. Diagnosis can be confirmed by immunologic procedures for measuring GPIb, the most artful of which is crossed immunoelectrophoresis, which yields lambent fractal patterns of considerable grace (Figure 22-17)

FIGURE 22-17 ▼

Analysis by two-dimensional crossed immunoelectrophoresis of proteins in normal platelets (above) and in platelets affected by several hereditary qualitative disorders (below). Absence of GPIb (Ib) in Bernard-Soulier platelets (panel 4) is evident when compared with panel 1. Note the peak for the purified fibrinogen receptor, GPIIb–IIIa, in panel 2 and its absence in thrombasthenia platelets (panel 3). TSP = thrombospondin; PF4 = platelet factor 4. (Reprinted, by permission of the New England Journal of Medicine, from George JN et al. 311:1084, 1984.)

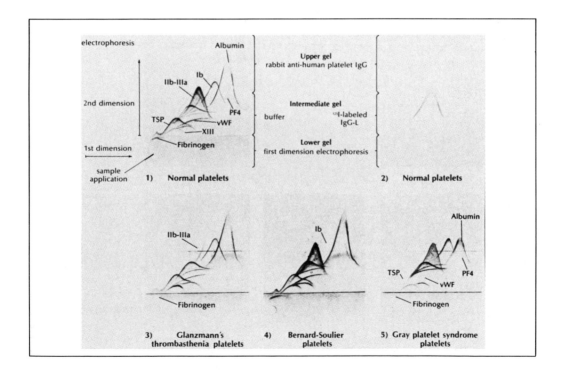

[18]. BSS platelets aggregate normally in response to physiologic agonists but are not agglutinated by ristocetin in the presence of vWF—a presumptive indication that GPIb (the vWF receptor) is missing or deficient. The finding of giant platelets plus a negative ristocetin agglutination test that is not corrected by adding normal plasma distinguishes BSS from all other platelet disorders. Platelet transfusions provide effective replacement therapy but should be reserved for severe bouts of hemorrhage; patients lacking any measurable GPIb are capable of forming IgG alloantibodies (or even autoantibodies) to this glycoprotein receptor, thus blocking vWF-mediated hemostasis and thereby vitiating benefit from platelet transfusion.

von Willebrand's disease   This disorder will be described in Chapter 23.

Inborn Disorders of Primary Aggregation

Glanzmann's thrombasthenia   Thrombasthenia is a rare autosomal recessive disorder, frequently the issue of consanguine marriage, marked by severe mucous membrane and postoperative bleeding, a very long bleeding time, absent clot retraction, and failure of platelets to aggregate in response to all physiologic agonists. Thrombasthenia represents a pure failure of primary platelet aggregation stemming from the lack (type I) or deficiency (type II) of the GPIIb-IIIa fibrinogen receptor (Figure 22-17). This prevents the receptor-mediated fibrinogen crosslinkages and precludes the platelet-platelet aggregation essential to formation of the platelet plug. The clinical manifestations are very similar to those in BSS, and patients lacking any GPIIb-IIIa receptor molecules are similarly at risk following numerous transfusions of developing alloantibodies or occasionally autoantibodies to the receptor complex or to the Pl^{A1} site on GPIIIa. Patients whose alloantibodies render them refractory to transfusions are candidates for allogeneic marrow transplantation.

Inborn Disorders of Platelet Secretion

Hereditary disorders of platelet secretion comprise a group of mild bleeding maladies resulting from either of two basic aberrations: deficiency of storage organelles (storage pool deficiency) or an enzyme defect in the synthesis of thromboxane from arachidonic acid (see Chapter 21).

Dense-body deficiency and other storage pool diseases (SPDs)   SPDs are categorized according to the predominant secretory granule affected, encompassing δ-SPD, α-SPD, and αδ-SPD. The δ-SPD and αδ-SPD group of diseases is characterized by: mild or moderate mucocutaneous, postoperative, and postpartum bleeding; somewhat prolonged bleeding time; impaired to absent aggregation in response to collagen; and no second wave of aggregation at low concentrations of ADP but a robust response to ADP in high concentrations. The last characteristic indicates that δ-SPD platelets can aggregate when exposed to extrinsic ADP but either lack the high concentrations of ADP found in the δ-granular pool of normal cells or are unable to release their δ-granule contents in response to thromboxane A$_2$. The distinction can be made by EM, but this is unnecessary for clinical management. δ-SPD and δα-SPD are often inherited with other disorders, including the Wiskott-Aldrich, TAR, and Chédiak-Higashi syndromes, and a genetic aggregate of tyrosinase-positive oculocutaneous albinism plus SPD known as the Hermansky-Pudlak syndrome.

α-SPD, the "gray platelet syndrome," is a very rare congenital disorder of moderate severity caused by defective packaging of α-granules during megakaryocyte maturation. For lack of membrane containers, α-granules leak their contents (including fibrinogen, vWF, fibronectin, thrombospondin, and the mitogenic platelet-derived growth factor) into the surrounding marrow, often causing local myelofibrosis. The porous platelets lack normal aggregatory responses and look bland and gray on Wright-Giemsa blood smears; on ultramicroscopy the platelets appear riddled with vacuoles (Figure 22-18) [19].

Defects of thromboxane synthesis or responsiveness   A large but uncounted number of patients have mild bleeding problems caused by "aspirinlike" defects in the prostaglandin pathway of thromboxane synthesis (Chapter 21).

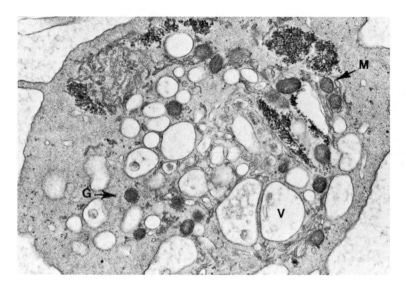

FIGURE 22-18

EM of a platelet in gray platelet syndrome, revealing honeycombed, swollen cell virtually bereft of granules. Numerous vacuoles (V) and chambers left behind after the normally populous α-granules have leaked out are diagnostic of α-SPD. The few granules (G) present are small peroxisomes, mitochondria (M) being the most common organelle remaining. (From White JG: Platelet granule disorders. CRC Crit Rev Oncol Hematol 4:337,1985.)

The best understood of these is cyclooxygenase deficiency, which predisposes to lifelong mucocutaneous bleeding problems through failure to generate the potent platelet aggregator, thromboxane A_2. In some families a similar moderate bleeding propensity is believed to result from genetic lack of a platelet membrane receptor for thromboxane A_2.

Acquired Qualitative Disorders of Platelet Function

Qualitative defects of platelets with bleeding commonly complicate chronic systemic diseases, but the pathogenesis is often obscured by the complexities of general illness, including immunologic and metabolic imbalances, chronic fibrin degradation, and antiplatelet medications. Unless the bleeding time is measured, patients whose platelet counts are normal but who cannot form a sound platelet plug will be overlooked. Often, acquired functional defects of platelets first become recognized when hemostatic mechanisms are subjected to unusual stress, as during surgery, parturition, or preeclampsia.

Uremia

Bleeding manifestations, particularly in mucocutaneous areas, are prevalent in patients with uremia, their incidence and severity correlating well with prolongation of the bleeding time. In uremia, platelets synthesize subnormal amounts of thromboxane A_2, whereas blood vessels elaborate a surplus of the platelet inhibitor, prostacyclin (PGI_2); the two antiaggregatory maladjustments work in synergy to engender bleeding. Uremic patients presenting with serious hemorrhages or faced with importunate surgery cannot await the gradual benefits of dialysis, but can be tided over by platelet transfusions; infusion of cryoprecipitate, or preferably of the vasopressin analog, DDAVP, provides sufficient vWF to override platelet "exhaustion" in uremia, and quickly albeit temporarily shortens the bleeding time sufficiently to permit surgery or renal biopsy. In dialysis-dependent patients who persist in bleeding, renal allografts offer the only durable resolution.

Myeloproliferative and Myelodysplastic Disorders

Acquired platelet malfunctions and bleeding difficulties are prevalent in patients with myelofibrosis, polycythemia vera, or essential thrombocythemia. Among the platelet defects in these chronic myeloproliferative syndromes are loss of α-adrenergic receptors and hence of aggregation by epinephrine, impaired oxidation of arachidonic acid by the lipooxygenase

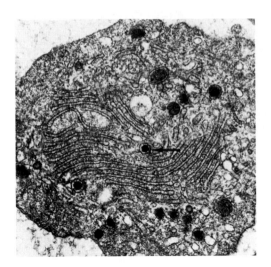

FIGURE 22-19

Dysplastic platelet from a patient with idiopathic myelofibrosis. Note the baroque reduplications and foldings of canalicular membranes, dearth of mitochondria, and the small numbers and size of granules (arrow). (From Zucker-Franklin D: Chapt 10, in Atlas of Blood Cells: Function and Pathology, vol. 1, 2nd ed., Zucker-Franklin D et al, Eds. Milan, Edi. Ermes s.r.l.,1988.)

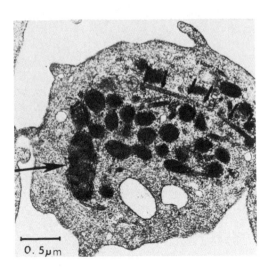

FIGURE 22-20

Granular dysplasia in a patient with myelodysplastic syndrome. Short arrows point to long *en bâtonnet* granules, and the long arrow is aimed at a large mass of fused granules. (From Maldonado JE: The ultrastructure of platelets in refractory anemia ['preleukemia'] and myelomonocytic leukemia. Ser Haematol 8(1):101,1975. © Munksgaard International Publishers Ltd., Copenhagen, Denmark.)

pathway, and an instability of dense granules that leads to depletion of granular ADP as the platelets circulate. Along with their functional peculiarities many of these platelets look peculiar (dysplastic), particularly if viewed by EM (Figure 22-19) [20]. Patients with clonal myelodysplastic syndromes may have severe platelet functional abnormalities, occasionally causing bleeding difficulties that precede evolution to AML by many months. Platelets from patients with myelodysplastic syndromes are often very large, sometimes representing megakaryocyte fragments composed of multiple territories; canalicular systems are rudimentary, and storage granules may be absent, fused into lumpy masses, or aligned to form drumstick-type structures (Figure 22-20) [21].

Drug-Induced Platelet Dysfunction

Any patient presenting with an acquired bleeding disorder and evidence of a qualitative platelet defect should be questioned in detail as to possible exposure to antiplatelet drugs—aspirin and antimicrobial agents being foremost on the list.

Aspirin   Conventional doses of aspirin prolong the bleeding time within minutes of ingestion by inhibiting the second phase of platelet aggregation and secretion. Platelet secretory inhibition results from irreversible acetylation of a portion of cyclooxygenase, blocking synthesis of thromboxane A_2 and inhibiting aggregation for the remainder of the acetylated platelet's lifespan (Chapter 21). In most normal individuals, protraction of bleeding time by conventional doses of aspirin is slight, but even low doses of aspirin can dramatically prolong bleeding time and cause hemorrhages in patients with thrombocytopenia, hemophilia, von Willebrand's disease, or platelet dysfunction accompanying chronic myeloproliferative syndromes. Use of aspirin for analgesia should be avoided in all patients predisposed to bleeding and in those facing hemostatic challenges such as surgery or childbirth; in such cases analgesic agents (e.g., acetaminophen or codeine) which do not disturb platelet function can be substituted with impunity.

Antimicrobial agents   Most of the β-lactam antibiotics, particularly the penicillins when infused in large doses or given to patients with impaired renal or hepatic function, attach to the platelet membrane and block the binding of vWF and of platelet agonists such as ADP and epinephrine to their respective receptors. Platelet dysfunction is maximal 3 to 5 days after start of therapy, and the antiplatelet effect may persist for up to 2 weeks after antibiotic infusions are discontinued. Prolongation of bleeding time and hemorrhage are particularly frequent in patients given ticarcillin, piperacillin, or mezlocillin [22]. Penicillin-induced platelet dysfunction heightens the risk of bleeding in thrombocytopenic patients with marrow aplasia or acute leukemia who require large doses of broad-spectrum penicillins to combat life-threatening infections. In such patients and in uremic patients receiving huge doses of β-lactam antibiotics, the incursion of drug-induced platelet dysfunction can trip the hemostatic balance toward hemorrhage.

REFERENCES

1. Cawson RA et al, Eds: Chapt 19, in Pathology. The Mechanisms of Disease, 2nd ed. St. Louis, CV Mosby Company,1989

2. Hoffbrand AV and Pettit JE: Chapt 13, in Sandoz Atlas of Clinical Hematology. London, Gower Medical Publishing,1988

3. Ortel TL et al: Antifibrinolytic therapy in the management of the Kasabach Merritt syndrome. Am J Hematol 29:44,1988

4. Murphy GF and Mihm MC Jr: Chapt 27, in Robbins Pathologic Basis of Disease, 4th ed., Cotran RS et al, Eds. Philadelphia, WB Saunders Company,1989

5. Fritsch WC: Managing age-related vascular skin lesions. Geriatrics 30(3):45,1975

6. Jandl JH: Chapt 30, in Blood: Textbook of Hematology. Boston, Little, Brown and Co., 1987

7. Lazarus JM et al: A 39-year-old woman with Raynaud's phenomenon, hypotension, and acute renal failure. Case 4-1988. N Engl J Med 318:234,1988

8. Miyagawa S et al: Anaphylactoid purpura and familial IgA nephropathy. Am J Med 86:340,1989

9. McMillan R: Immune thrombocytopenia. Clin Haematol 12:69,1983

10. Court WS et al: Human monocyte interaction with antibody-coated platelets. I. General characteristics. Am J Hematol 17:225,1984

11. Schmidt KG and Rasmussen JW: Kinetics and distribution in vivo of ^{111}In-labelled autologous platelets in idiopathic thrombocytopenic purpura. Scand J Haematol 34:47,1985

12. Koller CA: Immune thrombocytopenic purpura. Med Clin North Am 64:761,1980

13. Cawson RA: Essentials of Dental Surgery, 3rd ed. Edinburgh, Churchill Livingstone, Inc.,1978

14. Bussel JB et al: Maintenance treatment of adults with chronic refractory immune thrombocytopenic purpura using repeated intravenous infusions of gammaglobulin. Blood 72:121,1988

15. Kunicki TJ and Beardsley DS: The alloimmune thrombocytopenias: neonatal alloimmune thrombocytopenic purpura and posttransfusion purpura. Prog Hemost Thromb 9:203,1989

16. Kelton JG et al: Drug-induced thrombocytopenia is associated with increased binding of IgG to platelets both in vivo and in vitro. Blood 58:524,1981

17. Bellucci S et al: Inherited platelet disorders. Prog Hematol 13:223,1983

18. George JN et al: Molecular defects in interactions of platelets with the vessel wall. N Engl J Med 311:1084,1984

19. White JG: Platelet granule disorders. CRC Crit Rev Oncol Hematol 4:337,1985

20. Zucker-Franklin D: Chapt 10, in Atlas of Blood Cells: Function and Pathology, vol. 1, 2nd ed., Zucker-Franklin D et al, Eds. Milan, Edi. Ermes s.r.l.,1988

21. Maldonado JE: The ultrastructure of platelets in refractory anemia ['preleukemia'] and myelomonocytic leukemia. Ser Haematol 8(1):101,1975

22. Fass RJ et al: Platelet-mediated bleeding caused by broad-spectrum penicillins. J Infect Dis 155:1242,1987

23

Disorders of Coagulation

☐

Most hemorrhagic disorders of coagulation stem from hereditary or acquired defects in synthesis of specific clotting factors. Hereditary bleeding disorders represent either of two kinds of genetic defects: mutations that diminish synthesis of a clotting factor, or mutations causing production of a structurally abnormal clotting protein that is dysfunctional or unstable. Inheritance of a single deranged autosomal gene coding for a clotting factor seldom leads to serious bleeding problems because the paired normal allele maintains factor levels at about half-normal; the uncommon event of homozygosity as from consanguine marriage is required for full clinical expression. If the coding gene is located on the X chromosome, on the other hand, a male inheriting the unpaired defective gene may be tormented by a lifetime of hemorrhagic persecution; hence, deficiencies of the X-linked factors, VIII and IX, are the commonest serious hereditary bleeding disorders. Acquired defects in synthesis of clotting factors are less predictable, albeit dangerous, and usually reflect either suppressed production of vitamin K–dependent coagulation proteins or acquisition of antibodies ("inhibitors") that block the action of coagulation proteins.

COMMON HEREDITARY DISORDERS OF COAGULATION

Most prevalent of the hereditary disorders of coagulation are the hemophilias, which have an incidence at birth of about 200 per million males, and von Willebrand's disease (vWD), which represents an extended family of defects in the production of the adhesive polymer, von Willebrand's factor (vWF). About 85% of hemophilia is caused by an X-linked genetic defect in synthesis of functional procoagulant, factor VIII (antihemophilic factor or AHF), and

T A B L E 23-1

Classic inheritance patterns of hemophilia

Parents		Offspring	
Male	Female	Males	Females
Hemophilic	+ Normal	100% normal	100% carrier
Normal	+ Carrier	50% hemophilic 50% normal	50% carrier 50% normal
Hemophilic	+ Carrier	50% hemophilic 50% normal	50% hemophilic 50% carrier

Source: From Levine PH: Chapt 6, in Hemostasis and Thrombosis: Basic Principles and Clinical Practice, 2nd ed, Colman RW et al, Eds. Philadelphia, JB Lippincott Company,1987.

is termed hemophilia A; unqualified, the term "hemophilia" denotes hemophilia A. The balance of hemophilia cases results from deficient manufacture of functional factor IX (hemophilia B); as the factor IX gene is also located on the X chromosome and since factor VIII acts as cofactor to factor IXa in activating factor X, it is understandable that hemophilia A and hemophilia B are clinically indistinguishable. Although the prevalence of worrisome bleeding from vWD is only half that of hemophilia, the combined frequency of all variants of vWD, latent and minimally expressed sorts included, approaches 1% of the general population.

Hemophilia A

Hemophilia A (classic hemophilia, factor VIII deficiency) is a lifelong bleeding disability transmitted by inherited deletions or point mutations in the factor VIII locus of the X chromosome. Hemophilia is transmitted as a classic X-linked recessive disorder: accordingly all males endowed with the defective gene have hemophilia, all sons of hemophilic men are normal, all daughters are obligatory carriers, and daughters of carriers have a 50% chance of being carriers (Table 23-1) [1]. The severity of the coagulation defect in hemophilic males (and the rare female issue of a hemophilic father and carrier mother) varies from family to family but runs true within families. Bleeding is proportional to the de-

gree of reduction in residual factor VIII levels. In patients with factor VIII coagulant (VIII:C) levels below 2 units/dl, spontaneous bleeding into tissues is severe and frequent, and in untreated victims the suffering is malign beyond measure. Plasma concentrations between 2 and 10 units/dl (normal range: 50 to 200) are associated with more moderate bouts of spontaneous hemorrhage, and with levels between 10 and 30 units/dl hemophilic patients bleed seriously only in response to trauma, surgery, or vigorous dental procedures. The different degrees of factor VIII deficiency and clinical severity between kindreds and the constancy within a given pedigree are explained by the fact that many different gene defects can give rise to hemophilia A.

Pathophysiology

The gene for factor VIII is situated at the tip of the long arm of the X chromosome in the $Xq28 \rightarrow Xqter$ region, closely linked to loci for G6PD and deutan color blindness but removed from the Xq locus harboring the hemophilia B gene. The large size of the protein product (M_r = 330,000 after glycosylation) is reflected in the size of the gene: it spans 186,000 base pairs (bps) and consists of 26 exons separated by 25 noncoding introns. At its center the gene contains an unusually large (3,100 bp) exon that encodes the entire midsection of the protein, known as the B domain, which is extirpated during thrombin activation.

Factor VIII mutations and hemophilia Several hundred cloned factor VIII genes have been analyzed by cDNA probes that hybridize with restriction fragments from hemophilia DNA, revealing considerable heterogeneity in the mutations responsible for hemophilia. About two-thirds of hemophilia genes are rendered unproductive by any of an assortment of unique (familial) gene deletions. Only deletions of greater than about 100 bp can be detected by routine Southern blot analysis of genomic DNA, but restriction enzymes such as *Taq*I that contain CG in their recognition sequence have proved capable of detecting small deletions and single-base (nonsense and missense) mutations that are readily evident by blotting, particularly with the aid of polymerase chain reaction technology. Most point mutations detected by *Taq*I are C-to-T or G-to-A substitutions occurring in CG dinucleotide, which is a hotspot of mutagenesis. This dinucleotide is the major site of methylation in human DNA, and deamination of the methyl cytosine can predispose to C → T substitution. In the first surveys of hemophilia DNAs, six different nonsense mutations were found; hybridization data from one family are shown as an example of the procedure in Figure 23-1 [2]. The diversity characteristic of mutations responsi-ble for hemophilia A is illustrated in Figure 23-2 [3].

Because of the low reproductive fitness associated with inadequately treated hemophilia, almost one-third of mutant alleles were lost per generation prior to the modern era. As correctly predicted by Haldane, conservation of the harmful gene can only be explained by an exceptionally high rate of de novo mutations, many of them in the CG dinucleotides. Most of these mutations arise in parental or grandparental germline, and as almost all of these mutations are different, families affected with hemophilia carry their own private mutant allele [4]. It is estimated that 20 to 30% of all new cases of hemophilia are the consequence of recent sporadic mutations.

Laboratory and molecular diagnosis: use of RFLPs in prenatal detection Because the sequence of clotting reactions triggered in vitro by contact activation of plasma requires both factors VIII and IX, the partial thromboplastin time (PTT) is prolonged in both forms of hemophilia. This finding is the diagnostic cachet of hemophilia, all other screening tests being normal. Severity of the defect can be scored by quantitative assays based upon the ability or inability of diluted patient's plasma

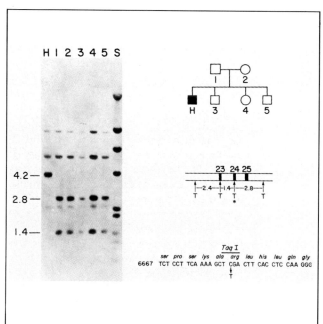

FIGURE 23-1

Analysis of the factor VIII gene of a severe hemophilic patient and his family. A Southern blot of DNA from patient H and his family was probed with a radioactive cDNA fragment that includes exons 23–25 and parts of neighboring exons. Lanes H, 1, 2, 3, 4, and 5 correspond to family members in the accompanying pedigree shown at the upper right. Lane S contains DNA size standards. The diagram below the pedigree signifies with an asterisk the location of the missing *Taq*I site in exon 24. Below this is displayed the pertinent sequence of normal DNA and the single base change in H DNA (arrow) that led to the loss of the *Taq*I site and occurrence of an in-frame stop codon TGA. (Rearranged from Gitschier J et al: Detection and sequence of mutations in the factor VIII gene of haemophiliacs. Reprinted by permission from Nature 315:427,1985. Copyright ©1985 Macmillan Magazines Ltd.)

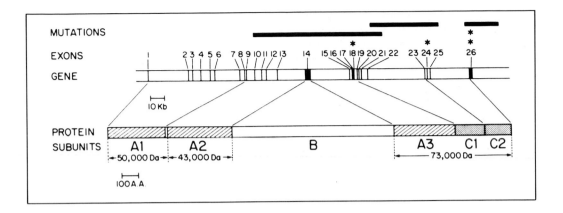

F I G U R E   23-2

Human factor VIII gene, its encoded protein, and 7 of the 20 to 30 mutations known to be responsible for hemophilia. The size and location of gene deletions are signified by black bars, and point mutations (nonsense and missense) are denoted by asterisks. As noted in the text, the large B subunit of the protein (below) is ablated during activation by thrombin. (From Lawn RM et al: Cloned factor VIII and the molecular genetics of hemophilia. Cold Spring Harbor Symp Quant Biol 51:365,1986.)

T A B L E   23-2

Factor VIII nomenclature

Symbol	Meaning
VIII	Factor VIII protein
VIII:Ag	Antigenic expression of factor VIII protein
VIII:C	Factor VIII procoagulant activity
vWF	vWF protein
vWF:Ag	Antigenic expression of vWF protein
VIII/vWF	Noncovalent complex of VIII and vWF, the form in which these two proteins circulate in plasma

to correct the prolonged PTT of known hemophilia A and hemophilia B plasmas. If factor VIII is found deficient, the plasma level of vWF antigen (vWF:Ag) must be measured, for factor VIII:C circulates in plasma complexed to the comparatively huge multimers of vWF, which transport and stabilize the antihemophilia factor; accordingly, factor VIII levels may be low in vWD for lack of adequate carriage, rather than from defective production. (A brief glossary of factor VIII and vWF abbreviations is given in Table 23-2.) About 15% of patients who have been transfused with factor VIII concentrates will develop antibodies (inhibitors) to AHF. This portentous development can be demonstrated by mixing equal parts of patient plasma and normal plasma: failure of admixed normal plasma to appropriately shorten the prolonged PTT signifies presence of a factor VIII inhibitor.

Female carriers of hemophilia have on average 50% of the normal plasma level of factor VIII:C, but there may be considerable overlap (about 15%) with normal due to extreme lyonization with preferential inactivation of the guilty chromosome. At the other extreme, predominant inactivation of the normal X chromosome is responsible for some of the rare cases of hemophilia in heterozygous women. Carrier detection should be based both on measurement of factor VIII:C and on pedigree analysis; the latter has been enormously expedited by the utility of restriction fragment length polymorphisms (RFLPs) associated with the factor VIII gene.

DNA sequence polymorphisms in (intra-genic) or near (extragenic) the factor VIII locus permit tracking of alleles in affected families and can be used for timely prenatal diagnosis [4]. These polymorphisms are detected as RFLPs by Southern blot hybridizations employ-ing DNA probes either from the gene itself or from neighboring ("anonymous") genomic fragments shown by linkage analysis to lie within several recombination units of the factor VIII gene. Analysis requires that the mother be heterozygous (informative) for the RFLP and that DNA be available from a sufficient num-ber of family members to assign one of the RFLP alleles to the flawed chromosome. The first informative RFLP within the factor VIII gene was detected using the restriction enzyme *BclI* which recognizes a polymorphic site just 3' to exon 18. Presence of this site is signified by restriction fragments 879 bp long that hybrid-ize to full-length factor VIII cDNA; absence of the site is indicated by a much larger (1,165 bp) DNA fragment. Provided the mother is heterozygous for this RFLP (exhibiting both fragments), the fetal DNA obtained at 8 weeks by chorion biopsy can predict presence or absence of the hemophilia gene. DNA-based di-agnosis of hemophilia is not only definitive but (in women) is unaffected by lyonization. If the carrier mother is homozygous for the RFLP, ab-sence of the hemophilia gene can be predicted only by exclusion based on family studies (Fig-ure 23-3) (5).

Dysfunctional factor VIII   The qualitative het-erogeneity of hemophilia is compounded by the existence of two classes of patients with severe hemophilia. About 75% lack both fac-tor VIII activity (VIII:C) and factor VIII anti-gen (VIII:Ag) and are defined (rather primi-tively) by the term cross-reacting material negative (CRM⁻); this implies simple failure or deletion of gene expression. The remainder also have decreased or absent activity but produce an immunologically recognizable but functionless protein and are termed CRM⁺; in these cases the mutant gene encodes a faulty, often truncated, protein product that lacks cofactor function.

Bleeding is delayed in hemophilia   Hemophilia patients seldom bleed from small wounds, and

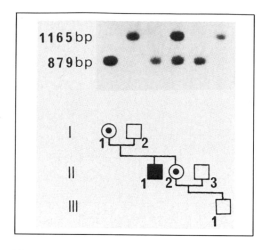

FIGURE 23-3

Utility of RFLP analysis for antenatal diagnosis and carrier detection of hemophilia A gene. At the top, DNA from family members was di-gested with *BclI*, electrophoresed, blotted on fil-ter paper, and hybridized with a radiolabeled fragment of factor VIII gene. The two polymor-phic fragments released measure 1,165 and 879 bp. Each DNA track is aligned vertically with the membership of the kindred, as diagrammed below. DNA was obtained by chorion biopsy taken at 8 weeks from the fetus (III-1). In this family the 879 bp allele segregates both with the hemophilia gene (family members I-1, II-1, and II-2) and with the unaffected gene, the mother being homozygous for the fragment. Nevertheless, the procedure correctly predicted birth of a normal boy, who had inherited the 1,165 bp allele from his unaffected grandfather (I-2). (From Geschier J et al: Antenatal diagno-sis and carrier detection of haemophilia A using factor VIII gene probe. Lancet 1:1093,1985.)

ordinarily the bleeding time is not prolonged. After more extensive vascular damage the pri-mary hemostatic plug forms promptly, but fibrin formation is limited to laying down of thin, frayed strands at the wound periphery, with only a mushy core of platelets to stanch bleeding. Failure of secondary hemostasis in the depths of wounds remote from tissue factor is the problem in hemophilia and a direct conse-quence of impaired factor VIII–dependent acti-vation of the intrinsic pathway of coagulation. Hemostasis is dependent entirely on the frail outer layer of fibrin strands generated by the extrinsic pathway, and as the result bleeding characteristically erupts or restarts afresh several hours after trauma has occurred. The deep bleeding of hemophilia has a satanical tendency to extend and dissect its way relentlessly into compartments and along channels or fascial planes—compressing, undermining, eroding, and eventually tunneling through pressure-necrosed flesh to create ragged fistulas or expanding hematomatous tumors.

Description

Because primary hemostasis is normal, bleeding in hemophilia is characteristically deep or internal and occurs in episodes that are often so frequent and so diabolically unpredictable that the patient and his entire family become demoralized. The impact of these bewildering bouts of bleeding and musculoskeletal pain can lead to severe psychological and social dysfunction. In the solipsistic mind of the embattled victim, painful hemorrhagic crises can only be understood as a form of punishment for which parents, family members, and nurses or physicians are responsible. This leads to regressive behavior in the child, who uses his travails— and often deliberately invites them by defiant and reckless behavior—as a perverse means for manipulating attention. The mother in turn feels guilty for transmitting the disease, siblings become resentful, and the entire family is gripped by a sense of helpless fear and martyrdom. The family of a child with hemophilia faces a stern challenge but is in a position through physician-guided education and open discussion to provide him with the supportive environment needed for coping with the recurrent physical and emotional trials.

Hemarthroses Hemarthroses are the cardinal lesions of hemophilia, occurring in over 90% of severely affected patients. Joints that bear weight and are most subject to impact are at particular risk, and thus knees, elbows, ankles, shoulders, wrists, and hips (in descending order of frequency) are the usual sites of bleeding. Acute bleeding into a joint space is heralded by pain and paresthesias, an early stage that can be aborted by prompt administration of factor VIII preparations; if untreated, the joint becomes swollen and tense, restricting movement and leading to a reflexly fixed

flexion that minimizes the volume of the joint space (Figure 23-4) [6]. Bleeding originates in the highly vascular synovial plexus, and once a joint has been bled into it becomes the target of recurrent hemorrhage; with each recurrence the synovia thickens further, grows increasingly hyperemic, and forms spaghettilike villi and folds that become trapped and crushed during joint action, causing more bleeding. Eventually joint cartilage is exposed, eroded, fragmented, and pitted; as cartilage is torn and dislodged, underlying bone is resorbed and

FIGURE 23-4

Acute hemarthrosis of left knee in a 10-year-old boy with severe hemophilia. Note flexed posture of left knee, bruises and hematomas of right leg, and tense swelling of right calf. (From Willert H-G et al: Orthopaedic surgery in hemophilic patients. Arch Orthop Trauma Surg 101:121,1983.)

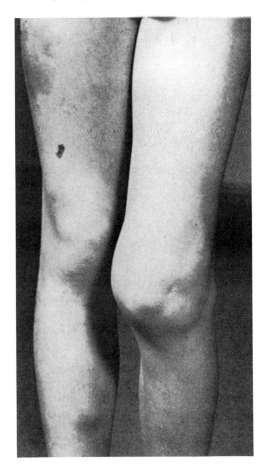

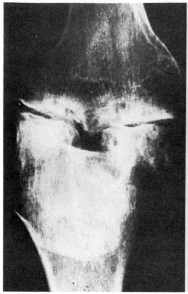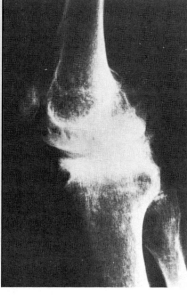

FIGURE 23-5

Radiographic appear-
ance of the knee in
chronic hemophilic
arthropathy, showing
narrowing of joint
space, erosion of articu-
lar surfaces, small subjacent cystic areas, and enlargement of the in-
tercondylar fossa.
(From Bloom AL:
Chapt 20, in Haemo-
stasis and Thrombosis,
Bloom AL and Thomas
DP, Eds. Edinburgh,
Churchill Livingstone
Medical Division of
Longman Group Lim-
ited,1981.)

subchondral cysts develop that are typical of chronic hemophilic arthropathy (Figure 23-5) [7].

Muscle bleeding and hematomas　　If not atten-tively safeguarded by adequate replacement therapy, the life of a hemophiliac with factor VIII levels below 1% of normal is punctuated by an appalling panoply of painful, deforming, and life-threatening tissue hemorrhages and hematomas. The most common sites are the large flexor muscle groups, the iliac muscle, the calf, and the anterior compartment of the forearm. If bleeding into large deep mus-

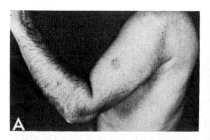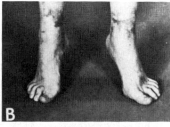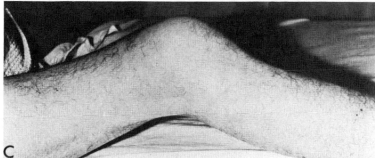

FIGURE 23-6

The most common
hemophilic joint con-
tractures. (A) Fixed flexion deformity at the el-
bow. (B) Equinus defor-
mity of the ankles. (C)
Flexion fixation of the
knee, with characteristic
posterior subluxation of
the tibia. (From Atkins
RM et al: Joint con-
tractures in the hemo-
philias. Clin Orthop
Relat Res 219:87,
1987.)

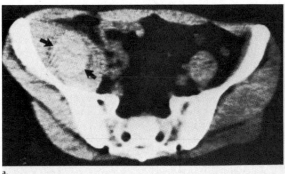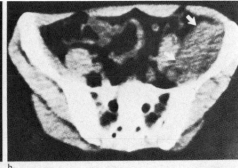

a.   b.

FIGURE 23-7

Iliopsoas hemorrhage in hemophilia. (a) In a patient presenting with right groin pain and weakness of the right thigh, CT scan shows heightened density within the right psoas due to recent bleeding (arrows) within swollen iliacus muscles. (b) Patient later returned with similar complaints on the left side: CT scan showed bleeding into the left iliacus (arrows) and medial displacement of the psoas. (From Shirkhoda A et al: Soft-tissue hemorrhage in hemophiliac patients. Radiology 147:811,1983.)

cles remains untreated, tensely distended hematomas may compress adjacent nerves and vessels, resulting in ischemia and pressure atrophy, and bleeding into tight fascial compartments or tissues that impinge on vital structures may endanger life and limb. Gradual fibrous replacement of inflamed or necrotic muscle in a position of shortening accounts for the high incidence of joint contractures in the distal arm (Volkmann's contracture) or more often in elbows, ankles, and knees (Figure 23-6) [8].

Hemorrhage within the iliopsoas sheath is the commonest site of major muscle bleeding in hemophilia. Iliopsoas hematoma can be initiated by strenuous coughing or (in Boston) tumultuous passage through potholed streets. Resultant bleeding into the iliopsoas causes reflex flexion of the hip and, as the femoral nerve is compressed against the inguinal ligament, sensory loss over the patella and weakness of the quadriceps. The expanding hematoma may burst into the retroperitoneum,

creating shock and general havoc, or it may point into the right iliac fossa, where it can be visualized and monitored following factor VIII therapy by MR or CT scanning (Figure 23-7) [9].

Blood cysts and pseudotumors   Hemophilic blood cysts occur within the substance of a muscle (usually in thighs, buttocks, or pelvis) when the volume of trapped blood is too large for digestion and elimination by macrophages. The dark brown porridge of half-clotted blood slowly becomes walled off by a tough fibrous capsule that may point inward or outward through the skin (Figure 23-8) [7]. Cysts arising from subperiosteal hematomas pry up periosteum and cause ischemic necrosis of cortical bone as they expand. Some of these bony pseudotumors continue to enlarge, becoming huge, honeycombed, and brittle; if not removed early, pseudotumors may rupture, become infected, and compel amputation.

Other sites of hemorrhage   Nearly 90% of severe hemophiliacs experience at least one episode of spontaneous hematuria in their lifetime. Usually renal bleeding is painless and nonrepetitive, but in patients with recurrent hematuria renal pathology should be suspected and sought out. Intracranial bleeding is the most common cause of death (25%) in hemophilia, and despite factor VIII replacement therapy, patients presenting with evidence by MR scanning of intracerebral or subdural bleeding have a mortality rate of 40%, and 50% of survivors show residual mental impair-

FIGURE 23-8

Large hemophilic cyst of the gluteal region that had tunneled through the corrupted skin and formed fistulae. The cyst later was removed surgically. (From Bloom AL: Chapt 20, in Haematostasis and Thrombosis, Bloom AL and Thomas DP, Eds. Edinburgh, Churchill Livingstone Medical Division of Longman Group Limited, 1981.)

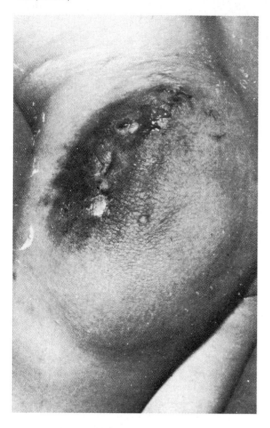

ment. As a history of head trauma can be elicited in nearly half of these patients, hemophiliacs and their parents must be instructed early on to seek medical attention following any important blow to the head.

Epistaxes and bleeding from other mucous membranes are common in hemophilia and can constitute a medical emergency. Intraoral trauma is particularly dangerous, for sublingual or peritonsillar hematomas can speedily expand into shiny blue hemorrhagic swellings that displace the tongue, dissect into the neck, and menace the airway.

Replacement Therapy and its Complications

Patients with hemophilia depend throughout their lives on factor VIII replacement infusions to prevent and control bleeding. As factor VIII has a biologic intravascular half-life of about 10 h, protection against hemorrhage is unachievable without use of preparations enriched in AHF. For the past 30 years, two plasma-derived kinds of replacement therapy have been available: cryoprecipitate and lyophilized concentrates. Cryoprecipitate is prepared by a simple closed-bag technique for separating the last ice crystals from slowly thawing fresh-frozen plasma. The cold-insoluble products in the last crystals to melt contain most of the factor VIII (plus vWF, fibrinogen, and factor XIII), and this can be stored frozen in small bags containing 80 to 100 U of VIII:C and vWF in a volume of 10 to 20 ml. Cryoprecipitates from single donors or small pools of donors are the treatment of choice for managing mild hemophilia. Commercial lyophilized factor VIII concentrates are prepared in lots made by pooling the plasma of 2,000 to 30,000 donors. The lyophilized powder is packaged in bottles supplying up to 1,000 factor VIII units each, which can be dissolved in 10 to 100 ml of diluent just prior to infusion. One unit of VIII:C per kg is infused for every increase in 2 U/dl (2 percentage points) desired. In a 70-kg man with a baseline level less than 1% of normal, elevation to half-normal (50 U/dl) requires infusion of 1,750 VIII:C units. This would require over 20 bags of cryoprecipitate or several vials of concentrate, with repetition of the dose every 8 to 12 hours.

Patients with severe hemophilia A suffer an average of 30 episodes of spontaneous hemorrhage annually, and the availability of lyophilized concentrates has revolutionized the care of these perpetually threatened individuals by making possible self-therapy through home infusion. Home therapy translates into independence, freedom to travel, and opportunity to assume responsible, even stressful employment.

Unfortunately replacement therapy—particularly use of commercial concentrates—is accursed by hazards that can be more dangerous than the disease itself: formation of antibodies to factor VIII; impairment of cellular immunity; and inevitable exposure to hepatitis, AIDS, and other bloodborne infections. Plasma replacement therapy with infusions of concentrate is virtually certain to transmit hepatitis B and the more elusive and hardy agent believed to be responsible for non-A, non-B (NANB) hepatitis, now known as hepatitis C. It appears likely that both of these feared agents can be destroyed by pasteurization with little loss of procoagulant activity. The human immunodeficiency virus (HIV) responsible for AIDS caused almost 700 cases of that dread complication of replacement therapy by the year 1985, and about 70% of hemophilic patients treated with concentrate before that date have become seropositive for HIV by western blot assay as of 1990. Fortunately HIV is inactivated by both dry heat and wet heat (pasteurization), but to assure absence of this loathsome agent in plasma concentrates, systematic procedures are now in use involving successive donor screening, heat-treatment of concentrates, and purification of highly concentrated materials with monoclonal antibody affinity chromatography; these arduous precautions appear to have eliminated all viral activity from concentrates now in use. This assertion is still subject to longterm follow-up, however, and the possibility of procedural error can never be entirely eradicated.

The happy prospects raised by cloning of the factor VIII (and IX) genes have come to fruition, for it has been demonstrated recently that recombinant factor VIII expressed by hamster-derived cell lines provides a pure, safe, and effective reagent for therapy and maintenance of hemophilic patients without risk of HIV or other viral contamination. Indeed, the successful expression of the factor VIII gene in mammalian cells justifies hope for the eventual development of gene-insertion therapy for permanent cure of hemophilia [10]. A very different, more limited avenue of lasting cure that has succeeded in several selected patients has been the perilous procedure of liver transplantation, a daring maneuver applicable to patients with endstage cirrhosis caused by chronic hepatitis. Because hepatocytes are the synthetic source of factor VIII, liver transplantation can both cure the coagulation defect and replace the defunct organ.

Hemophilia B

Hemophilia B (Christmas disease) is an X-linked hemorrhagic disorder caused by hereditary deficiency in factor IX activity. About 15% as prevalent as "classic hemophilia," hemophilia B is clinically identical to hemophilia A and engenders the same physical, psychological, and social woes, including the Faustian price of therapy. That hemophilia B closely mimics classic hemophilia—even in the quantitative demands for replacement therapy—is unsurprising, for factor VIII is the cofactor for activating factor IX and neither works without the other.

Pathophysiology: Factor IX Protein May Be Absent or Structurally Abnormal

The mode of inheritance of hemophilia B is similar to that of hemophilia A. Factor IX gene is located near the tip of the long arm of chromosome X between bands q26 and q27 and consists of eight exons separated by seven introns, most of which exceed the largest exon. Roughly 40% of patients have less than 3% factor IX activity and no detectable antigen and are designated CRM$^-$ or B$^-$, about 30% have similarly low factor IX activity but normal amounts of antigen (CRM$^+$ or B$^+$), and the remainder have only partial reductions in levels of both activity and antigen. DNA probe analysis has revealed that most CRM$^-$ hemophilia B patients have large deletions in the factor IX coding region which either block synthesis of the coagulant or engender truncated, dysfunctional variants that are very unstable and often so diminutive that the mutant gene product is lost into the urine. The incidence of alloantibody inhibitors is much lower in hemophilia B than in classic hemophilia, and the majority of antibodies found (but only in 2 to 3% of cases) occur in individuals with CRM$^-$ hemophilia. Most CRM$^+$ variants result from heterogeneous point mutations leading to production of an excess of factor IX antigen that is functionally defective. Several of the multitudes of point mutations leading to CRM$^+$ variants have been characterized fully. The molecular defect in factor IX$_{Chapel Hill}$ is substitution of His for Arg at position 145 so that only the Arg^{180}-Val^{181}

bond is cleaved by factor XIa. This genetic error can be attributed to a G to A transition within the corresponding Arg codon, changing it from CGT to CAT. The G → A substitution gives rise to a factor IXaα variant of the molecule in which the activation peptide remains bound to the light chain and the false protein has only 8% of normal coagulant activity.

Carrier detection and genetic screening: genotype assignment by DNA hybridization   Isolation of the factor IX gene has made it possible to construct DNA probes capable of detecting partial gene deletions through DNA hybridization methodology. In cases arising from small deletions or point mutations, identification of the mutant sequences is enormously enhanced by amplification via polymerase chain reaction technology. Of more general (and complementary) use in genotype assignment are RFLPs that enable tracking of polymorphisms in families at risk. A polymorphic *Taq*I restriction site has been exploited as a marker for the segregation of abnormal factor IX alleles. The polymorphic intragenic *Taq*I site occurs near exon IV in the factor IX gene and is present in about 30% of X chromosomes. Using a probe that includes exon IV, blotting of DNA digested with *Taq*I reveals a fast band if the polymorphic site is present or a slow band if it is not. Provided the mother is heterozygous for this RFLP, analysis of an affected male will establish whether the mutant gene is associated with the fast or slow band. Once this association is determined, the *Taq*I pattern observed in all female relatives can be used to identify or exclude the carrier state.

Replacement Therapy in Hemophilia B

Factor IX is much more stable than factor VIII and has a biological half-life of about 24 h. Hence in mild hemophilia B, single-donor fresh-frozen plasma alone often provides adequate protection and control of minor bleeding. Management of severe bleeders requires use of a factor IX–rich preparation capable of maintaining coagulant levels at 10 to 20% of normal, with higher levels needed for surgery or in patients with head injuries. The usual replacement therapy for hemophilia B is infu-

sion of prothrombin complex concentrates (PCCs) derived from the supernatant harvested during production of cryoprecipitate. PCC is a mixture of vitamin K–dependent factors (principally factors II, IX, and X) and thus its value in replacing the deficient procoagulant is partly offset by its risk of triggering thrombotic complications caused by trace amounts of preactivated factors IX and X. PCCs are also bedeviled by the potential for transmitting both hepatitis and AIDS virus, although the hazard is greatly diminished by heat treatment. Production of factor IX courtesy of recombinant DNA technology has been delayed somewhat by the requirement that the synthetic factor IX be equipped with the posttranslational 12 γ-carboxyglutamic acid residues in the amino terminal Gla domain.

von Willebrand's Disease

von Willebrand's disease (vWD) is the commonest and most heterogeneous of hereditary disorders of coagulation, with a worldwide prevalence estimated to be as high as 1%. vWD should be the prime suspect in any patient with a history of lifelong or recurrent mucocutaneous bleeding, a prolonged bleeding time, and normal platelet counts. In a given patient the symptoms vary with time and not all affected members of the family necessarily experience bleeding of comparable severity. vWD results from deficiency of the adhesive glycoprotein, vWF, a multifunctional secretory product of endothelium and megakaryocytes that has two essential purposes: promotion of platelet adhesion to wounded endothelium via vWF bridgings, and transport and stabilization of factor VIII. vWD is usually transmitted by a defective autosomal dominant gene located on chromosome 12. In 70% of cases (type I vWD), plasma is deficient in all multimeric forms of vWF, and the gene product (vWF:Ag) is quantitatively reduced to levels 15 to 60% of normal. In most forms of type II vWD, the larger, more adhesive multimers of vWF are disproportionately diminished, signifying production of qualitatively (structurally) abnormal protomers of vWF. In either case, vWD is primarily associated with a breakdown in primary hemostasis, although in severe cases the intrinsic pathway of secondary hemostasis also may be compromised for lack of adequate factor VIII transport.

Pathophysiology and Classification

Molecular defect   vWD is a bleeding disorder caused by either quantitative or qualitative abnormalities in vWF-mediated formation of platelet plugs, aggravated variably by reduced VIII:C activity affecting fibrin formation. Southern blotting studies using vWF cDNA probes that hybridize to the 150 kb vWF gene locus on the long arm of chromosome 12 have only revealed gene deletions in rare patients with the very severe, homozygous (type III) form of vWF: in these severe bleeders, complete deletion or large partial deletions in both alleles, or complete deletion in one allele and an undefined defect in the other, have been reported. As DNA hybridization does not reveal small deletions or point mutations, more sensitive techniques have had to be mobilized in seeking to explain the defect in the prevalent type I and type II patients. Given the large size and multiple introns present in the vWF gene DNA, sequence analysis has been focused on the much smaller, 8.7 kb mRNA. Using vWF mRNA as template and the polymerase chain reaction for amplification, sequence studies of the amplified transcript in several instances reported to date have revealed various silent (missense) mutations in the vWF alleles, resulting in a cis defect in vWF mRNA transcription or processing. Depending upon their locus, point mutations appear to account for failure to transcribe (type I vWD) or for encoding structurally defective vWF protein that is highly susceptible to proteolysis (type II vWD). In the first instance the quantity of vWF synthesized is drastically diminished but multimer structure and size distribution are normal; in the second, vWF synthetic rate is normal or only modestly diminished, but multimer structure and size distribution are skewed toward low M_r forms, with absence of the large, most functional multimers.

Classification   Most classification schemes divide vWD into two broad categories based principally on vWF multimer patterns ob-

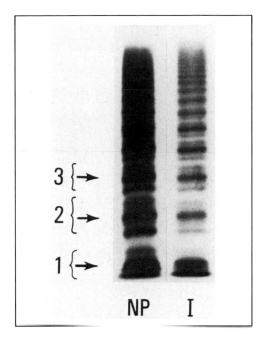

FIGURE 23-9

Multimer analysis of plasma vWF from a normal person (NP) compared with that from a patient with type I vWD, as revealed by SDS-agarose electrophoresis. Both in normal and patient plasma the oligomers travel in a triplet pattern, with the predominant band in the middle (arrows). The three smallest and most visible oligomers are indicated by brackets. Type I vWD is characterized by a proportional reduction in quantity of all sized mutimers. (From Berkowitz SD et al: Chapt 12, in Coagulation and Bleeding Disorders: The Role of Factor VIII and von Willebrand Factor, Zimmerman TS and Ruggeri ZM, Eds. New York, Marcel Dekker, Inc.,1989. Reprinted by courtesy of Marcel Dekker Inc.)

served in plasma. In the common type I disease all normal multimer species are present in a normal pattern but are reduced in quantity, reflecting a simple quantitative deficiency (Figure 23-9) [11]. Patients with the common, classic heterozygous type I vWD usually have moderate to severe bleeding problems, but rarely are they as pronounced or treacherous as in the homozygous or doubly heterozygous type III patients, who are assaulted by episodic hemorrhages, both superficial and deep. Type I

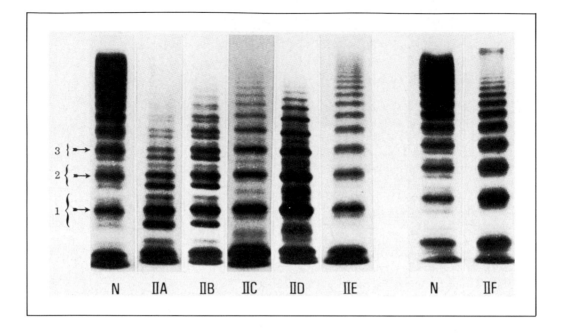

FIGURE 23-10

Multimer patterns in plasma of six known variants of type II vWD and in normal (N), as revealed by SDS-agarose electrophoresis. The three smallest oligomer triplets are indicated by brackets. In all variants high M_r multimers are missing, but triplet repeating patterns and the proportions of intermediate-sized multimers differ. In type IIB, intermediate-sized bands responsible for ristocetin-induced platelet agglutination are disproportionately heavy. In types IIC, IID, IIE, and IIF, individual multimers possessing intrinsic structural abnormalities have formed various abnormal bands or replaced all normal ones. (From Berkowitz SD et al: Chapt 12, in Coagulation and Bleeding Disorders: The Role of Factor VIII and von Willebrand Factor, Zimmerman TS and Ruggeri ZM, Eds. New York, Marcel Dekker, Inc.,1989. Reprinted by courtesy of Marcel Dekker Inc.)

vWD is a highly heterogeneous disorder, but in general there are concordant reductions in plasma vWF, ristocetin cofactor (RCo) activity (a measure of vWF binding to platelet glycoprotein I), and factor VIII.

The principal distinction between the various subsets of type II vWD and type I disease is that larger multimers are selectively lacking in the former variants. The term "type II vWD" encompasses at least six variants having in common a plasma deficit in large sticky multimers, but differing in multimer pattern and platelet agglutination in the presence of ristocetin, which reflects differences in the quantity of intermediate-sized multimers (Figure 23-10) [11]. The pathogenetic properties of the major variants of vWD are summarized in Table 23-3 [12]. The relatively common vWD variants, IIA and IIB, can be differentiated most readily in vitro by the platelet responses to the antibiotic ristocetin. By the semiquantitative ristocetin cofactor assay employing patient's plasma and washed allogeneic (normal) platelets, cofactor activity (as indicated by ristocetin-induced platelet aggregation) is decreased in both variants; by the ristocetin-induced platelet agglutination (RIPA) test employing platelet-rich plasma from the patient, agglutination is paradoxically increased about 3-fold in the IIB variant. The defective aggregation of platelets in type IIA disease stems from diminished ability of endothelial cells to synthesize multimers of any size. The hyperresponsiveness of platelet-rich plasma to ristocetin in patients with type IIB vWD reflects the fact that endothelium releases plentiful quantities of multimers, but the largest molecules are cleared from circulation with abnormal rapidity, some of them binding to the platelet GPI receptor; hence the plasma is left rich in medium-sized multimers, accounting for the strong agglutinative response to ristocetin, and platelet multimer composition is normal. If type IIB patients are infused by the vasopressin analog, 1-deamino-8-D-arginine vasopressin (DDAVP), an endothelial secretogogue, unusu-

ally large multimers are released transiently in such abundance that platelets agglutinate in circulation, and their rapid clearance may precipitate potentially dangerous thrombocytopenia. This adverse response to DDAVP, widely used in type I vWD and mild forms of hemophilia, underscores the need to differentiate variant forms of vWD.

Patients with the rare homozygous disorder type III or "severe" vWD have very little (<1%) detectable vWF or RCo activity in the

TABLE 23-3

Classification of von Willebrand's disease

Variant type	Genetics	Factor VIII	vWF antigen	Ristocetin cofactor activity	RIPA*	Multimer structure
Type I	Dominant	Decreased	Decreased	Decreased	Decreased or normal	Normal in plasma and platelets
Type IIA	Dominant	Decreased or normal	Decreased or normal	Markedly decreased	Absent or decreased	Large and intermediate multimers absent from plasma and platelets
Type IIB	Dominant usually	Decreased or normal	Decreased or normal	Decreased or normal	Increased	Large multimers absent from plasma; normal in platelets
Type IIC	Recessive	Decreased or normal	Decreased or normal	Decreased	Decreased	Large multimers absent from plasma and platelets; increased smallest multimer; characteristic abnormality of multimers and satellite bands
Type IID	Dominant	Normal	Normal	Decreased	Decreased	Large multimers absent from plasma and platelets; characteristic abnormality of multimers and satellite bands
Type IIE	Dominant	Normal	Decreased	Decreased	Decreased	Large multimers absent from plasma and platelets; characteristic abnormality of multimers and satellite bands
Type III	Recessive	Markedly decreased	Absent or markedly decreased	Absent	Absent	None visualized

*RIPA = ristocetin-induced platelet agglutination in platelet-rich plasma.

Source: From Sadler JE: Chapt 87, in The Metabolic Basis of Inherited Disease, 6th ed, Scriver CR et al, Eds. New York, McGraw-Hill, Inc.,1989.

plasma, and for lack of carrier protein, factor VIII levels are less than 10% (usually 2 to 3%) of normal. Unlike patients with heterozygous types I and II vWD, parents of the afflicted children have no bleeding problems, and bleeding times and factor VIII levels are normal. Bereft of both vWF and factor VIII, children receiving a double dose of the defective vWF-coding gene experience hemophilialike bouts of bleeding from mucous membranes and into joints and muscles throughout their lives.

Description

vWD is marked by epistaxes, gingival bleeding, easy bruising, and menorrhagia. Epistaxis is the most frequent and troublesome form of bleeding, and often is the first sign that the patient is a bleeder. In children traumatic bleeding of the mouth and oral cavity is characteristic and can be dangerous if underestimated. Other sorts of potentially hazardous hemorrhage include immediate and prolonged bleeding after dental extraction, tonsillectomy, and various other surgical challenges to hemostasis. Death from bleeding is rare in vWD, the uncommon exception being massive and uncontrollable gastrointestinal hemorrhage.

Management and Replacement Therapy

Cryoprecipitate, preferably of single-donor source, is the cornerstone of replacement therapy, for it contains all molecular forms of VIII/vWF found in fresh normal plasma. Most commercial concentrates used in treating hemophilia A are unsuitable in vWD, for they lack the essential high-molecular-weight multimers, but recently a virus-inactivated, high-purity factor VIII concentrate has become available that possesses a normal multimeric pattern and is highly efficacious in severe forms of vWD [13]. Among the salutary components of fresh plasma and cryoprecipitate is an uncharacterized but welcome lagniappe known as VIII:C stimulating factor, which inspires a delayed increase in plasma levels of factor VIII that exceeds the amount that was passively infused. That factor VIII levels continue to rise for 24 to 36 h after transfusion, whereas the intravascular half-lives of the infused factor VIII and vWF are 10 h and 18 h, respectively, indicates induction of new endogenous synthesis of AHF (Figure 23-11) [14]. To correct both bleeding time and the factor VIII debt, cryoprecipitate should be given twice daily, and in cases of major surgery may need to be continued for 7 to 10 days. Dosage must be determined empirically, for correction of the platelet adhesion abnormality is (for obscure reasons) unpredictable and capricious.

DDAVP provides temporary benefit in Type I vWD DDAVP somehow stimulates endothelium to release vWF. Predictably, this agent is

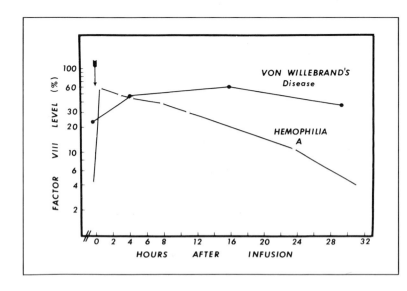

FIGURE 23-11

Logarithmic plot showing continued rise in factor VIII levels in a vWD patient following infusion of cryoprecipitate (arrow); in contrast, factor VIII activity fell steadily after infusion into a patient with hemophilia A. (From Rapaport SI: Introduction to Hematology, 2nd ed. Philadelphia, JB Lippincott Company, 1987.)

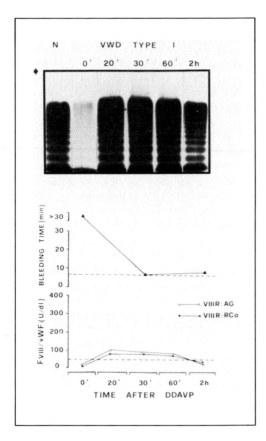

FIGURE 23-12

Prompt increase in plasma vWF, improvement in bleeding time, and rise in factor VIII concentration following infusion of DDAVP into a patient with type I vWD. (Above) Swift release into patient's plasma of abundant vWF multimers including a high proportion of unusually high-molecular-weight forms as shown by SDS-sepharose electrophoresis, normal plasma (N) serving as control. (Below) Simplate bleeding time fell to normal and remained normal for several hours. vWF:Ag (VIIIR:Ag) levels and ristocetin-cofactor activity (VIIIR:RCo) rose and remained elevated for over 2 h. (From Ruggeri ZM et al: Multimeric composition of factor VIII/von Willebrand factor following administration of DDAVP. Implications for pathophysiology and therapy of von Willebrand's disease subtypes. Blood 59:1272,1982.)

most effective in patients having a simple quantitative impairment in vWF synthesis, and in most cases of type I vWD, bleeding can be controlled or ameliorated by intravenous, subcutaneous, or intranasal administration of DDAVP (Figure 23-12) [15]. DDAVP is given initially every 8 to 12 h and is most effective in managing limited acute hemorrhages and minor surgery. More expansive and protracted bleeding requires repeated infusion, which soon exhausts endothelial stores and leads to a form of tachyphylaxis. Type I patients with severe bleeding or major surgery require replacement therapy. Most type II variants cannot respond well or predictably to DDAVP, for the endothelium can only generate defective multimers, and use of this vasopressin analog in type IIB disease is probably hazardous and may actually exacerbate bleeding by inducing thrombocytopenia. Patients with type III disease lack the secretory capability to respond to DDAVP.

RARE HEREDITARY DISORDERS OF COAGULATION

Apart from hemophilia and vWD, hereditary deficiencies or disturbances of coagulant factors are rare, accounting collectively for fewer than 1,500 reported cases.

Disorders of Fibrinogen and Fibrin Stabilization

Afibrinogenemia

In this rare autosomal recessive disorder (often the penance for consanguine mating), blood fails to clot in all coagulation screening tests and the TT, PTT, and PT are infinitely prolonged. No fibrinogen is discernable in plasma by radioimmune assay, and only trace amounts are found in platelet α-granules, accounting for the unpredicted finding in some patients of a prolonged bleeding time. Afibrinogenemia represents a biosynthetic block attributed to large deletions in the fibrinogen gene clusters located on chromosome band 4q2.

Afibrinogenemia often presents in the neonate as umbilical bleeding, and gastrointestinal or genitourinary bleeding are common mishaps in the early years. Thereafter spontaneous hemorrhage is astonishingly infrequent, although patients do bleed heavily after surgery. Through some mysterious hemostatic adjustment—possibly involving alternative adhesives such as fibronectin—bleeding bouts tend to diminish in number and severity with age in surviving patients. Despite absence of fibrinogen, the kingpin of secondary hemostasis, bleeding in childhood is not generally as serious as in severe hemophilia, and mature women seldom are troubled by menorrhagia. When hemorrhage occurs, cryoprecipitate is the replacement therapy of choice.

Dysfibrinogenemias

Hereditary dysfibrinogenemias are a remarkably heterogeneous group of rare autosomal dominant disorders resulting from point mutations of the fibrinogen gene cluster. In nearly every kindred studied, a different single amino acid substitution and thus a different fibrinogen variant (over 70 to date) has been reported. The nondominant allele continues to code for normal fibrinogen, although expression is dampened, and both abnormal and normal fibrinogen coexist in plasma; in some instances the anomalous protein interferes with fibrinopeptide release or fibrin polymerization, thus prolonging the TT and thereby providing a laboratory clue to diagnosis.

About 60% of reported families are symptomless, and most dysfibrinogenemic bleeders have mild mucocutaneous hemorrhages (primarily epistaxis) and bleed excessively only during surgery or menstruation. Patients inheriting fast-clotting fibrinogen variants are paradoxically subject to thromboses. Therapy is tailored to the eccentricities of the variant, ranging from cryoprecipitate in bleeders to anticoagulant prophylaxis in "thrombosers."

Hereditary Deficiency of Factor XIII

Factor XIII (fibrin stabilizing factor), when activated to XIIIa by thrombin, acts as a glutaminase that crosslinks the α chains and then the γ chains of fibrin monomers to form a firm vascular patch of covalently bonded fibrin polymers. In addition, factor XIIIa crosslinks fibrin to strands of fibronectin and collagen, weaving the fibrin polymers into a tough

wound-healing fabric. Consequently, patients homozygous for the rare autosomal recessive gene for factor XIII deficiency present with a characteristic form of delayed bleeding commencing 24 to 36 h after trauma, and commonly wound healing is also delayed and may lead to unusual or expanded or distended scars (Figure 23-13) [16]. Patients experience repeated episodes of subcutaneous and intramuscular bleeding, give a history of hemorrhage from the umbilical stump, and have an unusually high incidence of lethal intracranial hemorrhage. In addition pregnancy in women deficient in factor XIII commonly terminates in spontaneous abortion.

Screening coagulation tests are normal, but a provisional diagnosis can be made by observing dissolution of the recalcified plasma clot on incubation overnight in 5M urea. Replacement therapy and preoperative prophylaxis are quite successful because of the unusually long intravascular half-life of factor XIII (about 1 wk) and the small and infrequent amounts of plasma or cryoprecipitate needed to raise plasma glutaminase activity to safe levels.

Factor XI Deficiency

Deficiency of factor XI (plasma thromboplastin antecedent: PTA) is an uncommon, highly variable bleeding state occurring principally but not exclusively in people of Ashkenazic descent. The disease is transmitted by an incompletely recessive autosomal gene that has been conserved remarkably in Jews of eastern European origin, and in Israel it is estimated that 1 of 1,000 Ashkenazy Jews are homozygous for factor XI deficiency. The persistence of the gene is accounted for by the fact that the bleeding propensity is rarely lethal. The defect can be screened for by demonstrating prolongation of the PTT, which (as in hemophilia screening) reflects malfunction of the intrinsic pathway of coagulation; diagnosis is confirmed by measuring factor XI activity in a quantitative assay.

Factor XI deficiency is the simple consequence of inadequate synthesis, and thus far no structural variants have been reported. In homozygotes the level of factor XI is only 3 to 5% of normal, but there is virtually no correspondence between the measured deficit in this

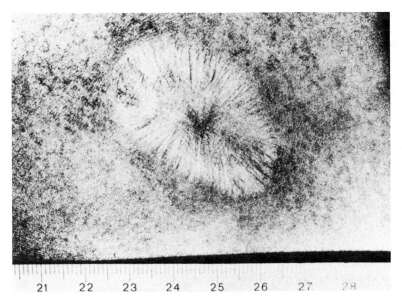

F I G U R E 23-13

Distended scar follow-
ing a puncture wound
in a boy with factor
XIII deficiency. Scale is
in centimeters. (From
Beck EA: Chapt 15, in
Hemostasis and Throm-
bosis: Basic Principles
and Practice, Colman
RW et al, Eds. Philadel-
phia, JB Lippincott
Company,1982.)

protein (the only protein of the contact activation system, deficiency of which may cause
bleeding) and the risk of bleeding. Indeed fewer
than half of deficient individuals experience
spontaneous bleeding, and some patients (unaware of their imperfect inheritance) have
sailed through major surgery without mishap.
In patients who do bleed spontaneously, the
most common problems are epistaxis, menorrhagia, and moderate hemorrhage following
tooth extraction: serious musculoskeletal bleeding and hemarthroses do not occur. Bleeding in
this strangely capricious disorder can be halted
by infusing fresh-frozen plasma, fortified if
necessary by judicious exhibition of EACA.

Hereditary Disorders Prolonging the Prothrombin Time

The hemophilias and factor XI deficiency are
detected on screening test profile by a long
PTT but a normal PT. Hereditary deficiencies
of all other procoagulants necessary for
thrombin generation—factors VII, X, V, and
prothrombin—prolong the PT, and in factor
VII deficiency only the PT is lengthened.

Factor VII Deficiency

Hereditary deficiency of factor VII (proconver-
tin) or synthesis of incompetent factor VII

proteins (dysproconvertinemias) is transmitted
by autosomal recessive genes with intermediate
expression. Homozygotes may have a relatively subdued bleeding propensity, despite factor VII levels as low as 3 to 20% of normal,
but patients with levels falling below this range
suffer the full murderous gamut of bleeding
tribulations encountered in hemophilia A, attesting to the importance of the tissue factor
pathway in normal hemostasis. Heterozygotes
may have mild bleeding difficulties despite
factor levels as high as 50% of normal.

Although quite stable, factor VII has a very
brief intravascular half-life (3–6 h), and so
replacement therapy in hemorrhaging patients
necessitates multiple infusions daily of either
fresh plasma or prothrombin complex concentrates. The thromboembolic risk incurred by
overloading the patient with vitamin K–
dependent factors should be circumvented
when possible by use of purified factor VII
preparations.

ACQUIRED DISORDERS OF COAGULATION

Coagulation disorders can be acquired through
either of two major disturbances: faulty synthesis of coagulation factors or acquisition of
antibodies that inhibit coagulant function.

Bleeding as a consequence of heightened consumption of coagulation factors is discussed in Chapter 24. In practice, acquired coagulation disorders are encountered more often than inherited disorders, but deficiency states usually involve multiple factors and complex associations, and autoimmune processes as usual are veiled in mystery. Most frequent of the acquired maladies are bleeding episodes caused by vitamin K deficiency, severe liver disease, or oral anticoagulants.

Vitamin K Deficiency

The term "vitamin K" encompasses two groups of fat-soluble naphthoquinone derivatives: vitamin K_1 produced by plants and vitamin K_2 manufactured by microorganisms. Thus vitamin K comes from two sources: dietary vegetables and intestinal flora. Once absorbed it is stored in hepatocytes wherein vitamin K is metabolized to the hydroquinone form and acts as cofactor for γ-glutamyl carboxylations of factors II, VII, IX, and X and proteins C, S, and Z. If vitamin K is deficient or is incompletely metabolized by the liver, undercarboxylated versions of these proteins accumulate in plasma and act as competitors to coagulant proteins. Procoagulant activity of vitamin K–dependent clotting factors declines when the alimentary supply of vitamin K is inadequate, when absorption is impaired, or when metabolism of coagulant proteins to their functional carboxylated forms is frustrated by coumarin anticoagulants.

Dietary Deficiency of Vitamin K

The normal daily requirement for vitamin K_1 is in the range of only 0.1 to 0.5 μg/kg, and the diet must be extremely deficient in fat-soluble vitamins for vitamin K deficiency to ensue in malnourished adults. Nevertheless prothrombin levels may plummet in patients maintained on intravenous fluids (depriving them of dietary sources) and given bowel-sterilizing, broad-spectrum antibiotics that eliminate bacterial sources of the vitamin. Postsurgical patients in intensive care units or debilitated patients on fat-free diets may develop bleeding problems within 7 to 10 days if not given supplemental vitamin K.

Hemorrhagic disease of the newborn
In normal newborn infants vitamin K malnutrition occurs as a physiologic oversight, for the placenta transmits lipids poorly, breast milk is a poor source of the vitamin, and the gut is sterile during the first days of life. Infants with hemorrhagic disease of the newborn have very protracted PTs (the badge of vitamin K deficiency) and marked reductions of all vitamin K–dependent proteins. In the United States, newborn infants are routinely given 100 μg to 1 mg of vitamin K to obviate this potentially lethal deficiency. In neglected infants exhibiting dangerous prolongation of the PT or overt hemorrhagic disease, bleeding is arrested by as little as 0.1 mg vitamin K_1 given parenterally.

Vitamin K Malabsorption

Bleeding as the result of malabsorption of this fat-soluble vitamin is an uncommon but hazardous complication of nontropical sprue or regional enteritis, particularly when deficient dietary intake, intestinal malabsorption, and oral antibiotics act in collusion. Severe vitamin K deficiency with bleeding also complicates the course of chronic biliary obstruction, in which bile salts necessary for fat absorption fail to reach the gut. The prolonged PT in patients with obstructive jaundice is shortened by vitamin K therapy; this is not the case in patients with parenchymal liver disease.

Vitamin K Deficiency in Liver Disease

In any form of parenchymal liver disease, levels of all vitamin K–dependent clotting factors are depressed as part of a general failure of protein synthesis that includes factor V but spares factor VIII, which can also be synthesized by endothelial cells of hepatic sinuses. Concomitant deficiency of vitamin K–dependent factors and of factor V is responsible for the long PT characteristic of liver disease. It is only partially improved, if at all, by vitamin replacement because the impaired synthesis of protein precursors is unaffected and utilization by hepatocytes of vitamin K for posttranslational carboxylation may be defective and capable only of generating small quantities of incompetent coagulant proteins. Apart from failure to synthesize coagulant factors, liver disease in-

FIGURE 23-14

Subcutaneous hemorrhage of the upper arm following trivial trauma in a patient with liver disease. Laboratory tests revealed deficiencies of factors II, VII, IX, and X, plus dysfibrinogenemia. (From Hoffbrand AV and Pettit JE: Chapt 14, in Sandoz Atlas of Clinical Hematology. London, Gower Medical Publishing,1988.)

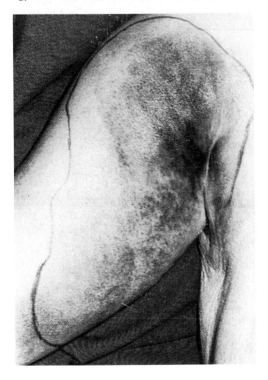

cites baffling and shifting permutations of other hemostatic defects including thrombocytopenia, disseminated intravascular coagulation (Chapter 24), increased fibrinolysis, and dysfibrinogenemia (Figure 23-14) [17]. In liver disease with bleeding unresponsive to vitamin K, transfusion of fresh-frozen plasma can provide partial, temporary amelioration of the deficits in vitamin K–dependent factors and of factor V; correction of thrombocytopenia by transfusing packed platelets and infusion of cryoprecipitate to bolster fibrinogen levels may also be necessary in dealing with the complex hemostatic onslaughts afflicting patients with liver disease.

Drug-Induced Vitamin K Deficiency

Warfarin alias coumadin (4-hydroxycoumarin) and other members of the coumarin family of anticoagulants inhibit synthesis of prothrombin and other vitamin K–dependent factors by blocking vitamin K epoxide reductases, thereby indirectly curtailing γ-glutamyl carboxylation. In patients presenting with mysterious bleeding and a vastly prolonged PT, surreptitious abuse of warfarin (coumadin) should be suspected, a self-destructive behavioral anomaly strangely frequent among covertly depressed medical and paramedical personnel. In patients receiving warfarin for anticoagulant prophylaxis, treacherous interactions between the anticoagulant and other prescribed or proprietary drugs that alter warfarin metabolism or action may precipitate bleeding crises ranging from bruising and painful tissue bleeding to fatal intracranial hemorrhage; indeed, oral anticoagulants used to prevent thromboembolic disease are responsible for 20 to 30% of all subdural hematomas.

Autoantibodies to hemostatic factors Antibodies ("inhibitors") that block coagulant factors may appear in individuals who do not have hereditary disorders of coagulation and who have never received factor replacement therapy. Most antibodies to clotting factors are IgG molecules that act as circulating anticoagulants identifiable in vitro by mixing patient's plasma with a normal source of clotting factor and showing its inhibition. Some antibodies, however, are unusual in that they bind to a given clotting factor without neutralizing its coagulant activity; deficiency in vivo is incurred because of rapid clearance by macrophages of the antibody-coagulant immune complexes.

Factor VIII Inhibitors in Patients without Hemophilia

Autoantibodies to factor VIII may appear inexplicably in postpartum women immediately or shortly after delivery, as an arcane event in patients with underlying autoimmune disorders such as systemic lupus erythematosus, in lymphoproliferative disorders, or rarely as a spontaneous process in otherwise healthy elderly persons. IgG antibodies to factor VIII cause severe, potentially fatal bleeding simulating that of hemophilia A. As in hemophilia A, screening tests reveal a protracted PTT, but PT and TT are normal; unlike hemophilia A, admixing normal plasma fails to correct the prolonged PTT.

Postpartum factor VIII antibodies generally disappear (as mysteriously as they appeared) within 12 to 18 months of delivery, never to return again despite additional pregnancies. In patients with extremely high-titer concentrations of antibody, bleeding can be as vicious and tissue-destructive as the worst cases of classic hemophilia. In these women, life and limbs can be spared by administering immunosuppressive agents along with intensive factor VIII therapy. Unlike the factor VIII anticoagulant antibodies of hemophilic patients, which do not respond to immunosuppression, factor VIII antibodies in nonhemophilic patients usually yield to the combination of prednisone and cyclophosphamide. In patients refractory to immunosuppression and replacement therapy, or in whom the process is fast escalating out of control, plasmapheresis and infusions of prothrombin complex concentrates may tide the patient over until the deadly autoimmune assault subsides.

REFERENCES

1. Levine PH: Chapt 6, in Hemostasis and Thrombosis: Basic Principles and Clinical Practice, 2nd ed, Colman RW et al, Eds. Philadelphia, JB Lippincott Company,1987

2. Gitschier J et al: Detection and sequence of mutations in the factor VIII gene of haemophiliacs. Nature 315,427,1985

3. Lawn RM et al: Cloned factor VIII and the molecular genetics of hemophilia. Cold Spring Harbor Symp Quant Biol 51:365, 1986

4. Vehar GA et al: Chapt 86, in The Metabolic Basis of Inherited Disease, 6th ed, Scriver CR et al, Eds. New York, McGraw-Hill, Inc.,1989

5. Gitschier J et al: Antenatal diagnosis and carrier detection of haemophilia A using factor VIII gene probe. Lancet 1:1093,1985

6. Willert H-G et al: Orthopaedic surgery in hemophilic patients. Arch Orthop Trauma Surg 101:121,1983

7. Bloom AL: Chapt 20, in Haemostasis and Thrombosis, Bloom AL and Thomas DP, Eds. Edinburgh, Churchill Livingstone Medical Division of Longman Group Limited,1981

8. Atkins, RM et al: Joint contractures in the hemophilias. Clin Orthop Relat Res 219:97, 1987

9. Shirkhoda A et al: Soft-tissue hemorrhage in hemophiliac patients. Radiology 147:811, 1983

10. White GC II et al: Use of recombinant antihemophilic factor in the treatment of two patients with classic hemophilia. N Engl J Med 320:166,1989

11. Berkowitz SD et al: Chapt 12, in Coagulation and Bleeding Disorders: The Role of Factor VIII and von Willebrand Factor, Zimmerman TS and Ruggeri ZM, Eds. New York, Marcel Dekker, Inc.,1989

12. Sadler JE: Chapt 87, in The Metabolic Basis of Inherited Disease, 6th ed, Scriver CR et al, Eds. New York, McGraw-Hill, Inc.,1989

13. Berntorp E and Nilsson IM: Use of a high-purity factor VIII concentrate (Hemate P) in von Willebrand's disease. Vox Sang 56:212, 1989

14. Rapaport SI: Chapt 26, in Introduction to Hematology, 2nd ed. Philadelphia, JB Lippincott Company,1987

15. Ruggeri ZM et al: Multimeric composition of factor VIII/von Willebrand factor following administration of DDAVP. Implications for pathophysiology and therapy of von Willebrand's disease subtypes. Blood 59:1272, 1982

16. Beck EA: Chapt 15, in Hemostasis and Thrombosis: Basic Principles and Practice, Colman RW et al, Eds. Philadelphia, JB Lippincott Company, 1982

17. Hoffbrand AV and Pettit JE: Chapt 14, in Sandoz Atlas of Clinical Hematology, London, Gower Medical Publishing,1988

24

Thrombotic Disorders

☐

Thrombotic disorders are the scourge of modern times, responsible collectively for the demise of over half of the members of otherwise advantaged populations. Disabling or fatal thrombotic disease may stem from formation of thrombi within arteries at sites of arterial endothelial damage or in veins as a consequence of venous stasis and increased systemic coagulability. In more particular circumstances thrombi may form within the chambers or on damaged or prosthetic valves of the heart, or within the microcirculation as the result of disseminated intravascular coagulation (DIC). It should be emphasized that most thrombi formed in blood flowing through vessels differ from the homogeneously red rubbery clots observed when shed blood coagulates peacefully in test tubes or postmortem. Thrombi generated in the high-shear arterial side of the circulation have a large platelet component held together by fibrin strands and are pale, dry, and friable. Some large venous thrombi generated in dilated stagnant veins are evenly red and can resemble test-tube clots in their homogeneity and durability, but most venous thrombi that are propagated in regions of slow to moderate flow acquire a small platelet-rich white head and a long red tail dangling downstream. The fibrin strands in these "mixed thrombi" are split up and weakened by siltlike sediments and corralline accretions of fused platelets, predisposing them to fracture and embolization, and the surfaces of these friable red masses are mottled with a faintly ridged or rippled fretwork of gray fibrin, creating a pattern known as the lines of Zahn (Figure 24-1) [1].

PATHOGENESIS OF ARTERIAL AND VENOUS THROMBOSES

Two major mechanisms underlie thrombosis. Arterial thrombi occur where vascular endothe-

FIGURE 24-1

Pulmonary emboli consisting of mixed thrombi that originated in leg veins. Note the nonhomogeneity and the pale surface coating with its rippled pattern (lines of Zahn). (From Freiman DG: Chapt 71, in Hemostasis and Thrombosis. Basic Principles and Clinical Practice, 2nd ed, Colman RW et al, Eds. Philadelphia, JB Lippincott Company, 1987.)

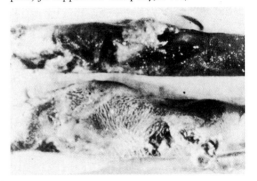

lium has been disrupted, exposing subendothelial adhesives. In venous thrombosis the vessel wall is usually intact: thrombi are generated through the complicity of stasis, disturbed rheology, and imbalance between coagulant and anticoagulant factors.

Arterial Thrombosis

Arterial thrombi form only at sites of underlying arterial wall disease, most commonly caused by arteriosclerosis. Characteristically, rupture of an arteriosclerotic plaque exposes blood to subendothelial adhesives and tissue factor, setting off a complex chain of events involving formation of a platelet nidus that anchors the incipient thrombus to the vessel wall. Subsequent events depend upon the diameter of the vessel and the extent to which the arterial thrombus propagates beyond the site of endothelial damage. In medium-sized arteries, such as the coronary artery, rupture of an arterial plaque and subsequent thrombosis may suffice to cause vascular occlusion. In larger vessels, the comparatively small platelet masses,

trussed together by fibrin strands, may be launched as emboli that occlude smaller distal arteries, with serious ischemic consequences downstream. Thrombotic plugging often provides the *coup de grace,* but the molecular sequence responsible for initiating atherosclerotic vascular disease is both obscure and outside the scope of this presentation.

Venous Thrombosis and Thromboembolism

Venous thrombosis differs mechanistically from arterial thrombosis in that underlying damage to vascular walls is not required for its pathogenesis. Although often difficult to prove or measure, it is clear from circumstantial evidence that increased systemic coagulability plays a key pathogenetic role in the instigation of deep vein thrombosis (DVT). As an illustration, hemophilic patients infused with large amounts of prothrombin complex concentrate containing activated clotting factors often develop venous thrombosis in previously normal, youthful veins. Postoperative DVT, the bugbear of major surgery, is initiated by exposure

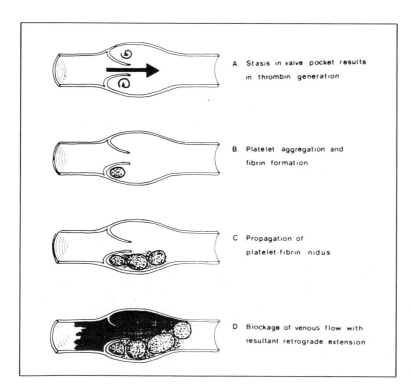

A. Stasis in valve pocket results in thrombin generation

B. Platelet aggregation and fibrin formation

C. Propagation of platelet-fibrin nidus

D. Blockage of venous flow with resultant retrograde extension

FIGURE 24-2

Schematic representation showing development of thrombus in a venous valve cusp subjected to stasis. (From Thomas DP: Chapt 36, in Haemostasis and Thrombosis, Bloom AL and Thomas DP, Eds. New York, Churchill Livingstone,1981.)

of blood to tissue coagulants that issue forth from the wound site. In postoperative, pregnant, immobilized, or inactive elderly patients who are most subject to DVT, thrombi are prone to occur initially in regions of stasis such as dilated sinuses of soleal veins and pockets of large venous valves. In valve pockets or blood stagnating in the arcades of the deep veins of the calf, platelet-rich plasma is separated from circulating and vessel wall anticoagulant factors (Chapter 21) and thrombin is generated; this stimulates platelet aggregation and secretion, with further release of thrombin and establishment of a vicious cycle leading to deposition of fibrin. If laid down in the stagnant sanctuary of a dilated valve cusp, a propagating platelet-fibrin nidus becomes the head of a thrombus, which eventually occludes venous flow (Figure 24-2) [2].

Propagation of Thrombi

As fresh venous blood bathes the valve-anchored thrombus, more platelets accumulate on its growing tail, where they degranulate and (by supplying procoagulant phospholipid) trigger further thrombin production and fibrin deposition; viewed by contrast venography (phlebography), the growing thrombus may acquire the shape of a lamprey eel (Figure 24-3) [3].

Protective Mechanisms for Dissolving Thrombi and Their Failure in Prethrombotic (Hypercoagulable) States

Normally propagation of thrombi is contained or thwarted by the coordination of several defensive mechanisms that include inhibition of activated coagulation factors and activation of the sole enzyme charged with lysing fibrin—plasmin. The first line of defense is preventive inactivation of any surplus of the coagulant amplifiers, factors IXa, Xa, and IIa (thrombin), by antithrombin III and lysis of cofactors Va and VIIIa by activated anticoagulant, protein C. Once fibrin has been laid down or thrombotic occlusion has occurred, the only apparatus capable of resolving the problem is the fibrinolytic system through the offices of the masterful enzyme, plasmin.

Plasmin, plasminogen activators, and their inhibitors Timely activation of plasmin and dissolution of fibrin depends mainly on mobilization of tissue plasminogen activator (t-PA) (Chapter 21), a secretory product of endothelium that is released locally during venous stasis and is the counterpart to urokinaselike plasminogen activator (u-PA). t-PA is released during venous stasis (or when fibrin is deposited on endothelium) from an inactive complex in which it is bound to a 50,000 M_r single-chain polypeptide known as plasminogen activator inhibitor (PAI). Increases in inhibition of t-PA by PAI in its various coigns of vantage (PAI-1 in

FIGURE 24-3

Venographic demonstration of multiple filling defects in the right femoral vein of a patient with DVT. The blunt black head of the long eely thrombus (to the left) is attached to the upper cusp surface of a dilated valve, as its slender sinuous tail undulates in the streaming blood. (From Kakkar VV and Sasahara AA: Chapt 37, in Haemostasis and Thrombosis, Bloom AL and Thomas DP, Eds. New York, Churchill Livingstone,1981.)

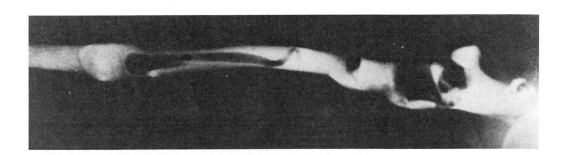

endothelium, PAI-2 in placenta and macrophages, and PAI-3, a u-PA inhibitor of kidney origin) may play an important role in the causation of DVT, although the issue is presently unsettled. The t-PA activity of vein walls and venous blood during stasis is ordinarily lower in the legs than arms, possibly explaining the high frequency of lower leg thrombosis. In postoperative patients, fibrinolytic activity is reduced because of a fall-off in t-PA release during a period of 7 to 10 days following surgery known as the fibrinolytic shutdown. Other malfunctions of the fibrinolytic apparatus that predispose to thrombosis include deficient synthesis or activation of plasminogen and increases in the primary plasmin inhibitor, α_2-antiplasmin.

Evaluation of Increased Thrombotic Risk

The penalty for ignoring historical, physical, or laboratory signs indicative of predisposition to thromboembolic disease is all too often catastrophic, as when a "silent" thrombus of the leg vein breaks loose and lodges in the pulmonary circulation (Figure 24-4) [4]. Evaluation of a patient presenting with thrombosis at an early age or an unusual site or giving a history of recurrent unexplained episodes of venous thrombosis requires a careful personal and family medical history and performance of physical and laboratory examinations selected for their value in identifying inherited or acquired risk associations. A useful classification of disorders associated with thrombosis or thromboembolic disease is presented in Table 24-1 [5].

DESCRIPTION AND DIAGNOSIS OF VENOUS THROMBOSIS AND PULMONARY EMBOLISM

DVT of the lower limbs is commonplace, having an annual incidence in the United States of nearly 3 million cases, and early diagnosis is of pressing concern, so that preventive measures can be initiated to forestall thromboembolic calamities such as that shown in Figure 24-4. Regrettably, early localized thrombosis is diagnosable in only about half of cases, as judged by venography (Figure 24-3) and the classic signs of ankle swelling, calf tenderness, and local warmth with delayed cooling are found in only about one-third of patients. In advanced DVT, on the contrary, the patient usually experiences some form of pain and tenderness that may extend into the groin, accompanied by dependent edema when proximal veins are obstructed. Skin temperature may be elevated because venous return has been rerouted through dilated superficial veins. When iliofemoral vein thrombosis is associated with arterial spasm, pulses may become weak and the leg cold and white—"milk leg," alias phlegmasia alba dolens. With complete ileo-

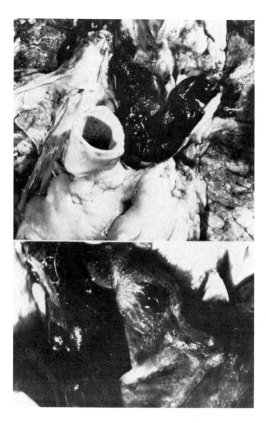

FIGURE 24-4

Postmortem views of large pulmonary embolus that had detached from a leg vein thrombus. (Above) Dark saddle embolus is impacted in the pulmonary artery and extends into both main branches. (Below) Closer view reveals inhomogeneous structure of the embolus, with the wavy fibrinous lines of Zahn embossed on its surface. (Reproduced by permission from: Marchesi VI: Chapt 4, in Pathology, vol. 1, Anderson WAD and Kissane JM, Eds. St. Louis, The CV Mosby Company,1977.)

TABLE 24-1

Disorders associated with increased risk of thrombosis

Abnormality	Mechanism
Hereditary	
1. Antithrombin III deficiency	Impaired neutralization of serine proteases: thrombin, Xa, IXa
2. Protein C deficiency or protein S deficiency	Failure of proteolytic inhibition of the cofactors VIIIa and Va. Impaired activation of fibrinolysis?
3. Homocystinuria	Damage to endothelium of arteries and veins by deposits of homocystine, causing "premature atherosclerosis"
4. Rare disorders of fibrinogen and fibrinolysis	
a. Certain dysfibrinogenemias	Unknown, possible impaired neutralization of thrombin by adsorption to fibrin, impaired binding to plasminogen
b. Abnormal plasminogen	Impaired formation of plasmin
Acquired	
1. Surgery, trauma, and the puerperium	Multiple thrombogenic risk factors
2. Carcinoma	Exposure of blood to tumor cells or tumor products with tissue factor activity
3. Hematologic proliferative disorders	
a. Acute promyelocytic leukemia	Release of tissue factor from primary granules
b. Myeloproliferative disorders (polycythemia, essential thrombocythemia)	Elevated blood viscosity, thrombocytosis, altered platelet membrane receptors and platelet responses
c. Paroxysmal nocturnal hemoglobinuria (PNH)	Unknown, possibly defective (leaky) platelets
4. Lupus anticoagulant	Unknown, related to antibodies reacting with membrane phospholipids
5. Nephrosis	Multiple factors: markedly elevated fibrinogen, factor VIII; low antithrombin III from urinary loss; effects of hyperlipidemia on platelet function
6. Complications of therapy	
a. Oral contraceptives	Unknown, related to estrogen effects upon vessel wall and hemostatic factors
b. Infusion of prothrombin complex concentrates	Infusion of activated clotting intermediates
c. Heparin-induced thrombocytopenia	Unknown, related to intravascular aggregation of platelets

Source: Modified and amended from Rapaport SI: Introduction to Hematology, 2nd ed. Philadelphia, JB Lippincott Company,1987.

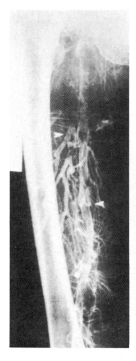
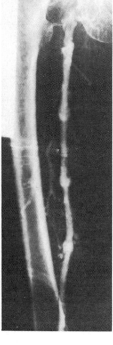

FIGURE 24-5

Venogram of iliofemoral system before (left) and after (right) fibrinolytic therapy with urokinase. Thrombotic occlusion of the entire deep venous system prior to therapy is apparent, including filling defects in the valves of the femoral veins (second arrowhead from top) and opening of numerous collaterals. After therapy, thrombi were lysed completely, as shown by unimpeded filling with contrast medium of the entire vascular system including valve pockets. (From Marder VJ and Bell WR: Chapt 92, in Hemostasis and Thrombosis. Basic Principles and Clinical Practice, 2nd ed, Colman RW et al, Eds. Philadelphia, JB Lippincott Company,1987.)

femoral obstruction, the leg may become painful, cyanotic, and swollen ("blue leg," or phlegmasia cerulea dolens), with occasional progression to gangrene necessitating amputation; when venous occlusion and edema threaten to shut off arterial flow, it is essential to intercede swiftly to prevent this morbid sequence.

Methods for Imaging and Staging Thrombi

During recent years a profusion of mildly invasive or variably "noninvasive" diagnostic maneuvers have been devised that permit accurate diagnosis, staging, and evaluation of therapy. Among these are contrast venography (the reference standard by which newer techniques for detecting thrombi are judged), serial impedance plethysmography, thermography, and an assortment of imaging techniques that includes ultrasonography, CT scanning, MR imaging, and various innovative radioisotope scanning ploys that specifically illuminate thrombi.

Contrast venography   Venography is performed by infusing radioopaque contrast medium into a vein on the dorsum of the foot, monitoring venous filling, and taking x-ray exposures at various intervals thereafter. Venography, like other forms of angiography, is a difficult and invasive procedure, and it can be painful both physically and fiscally; it is nevertheless unexcelled in evaluating the architecture of accessible venous structures and in evaluating the efficacy of fibrinolytic therapy (Figure 24-5) [6].

CT scanning   CT scanning is the most widely available imaging technique for searching out and defining thrombi in comparatively inaccessible locations. It is particularly useful in localizing intracranial, pelvic, renal, and intraabdominal thromboses.

MR imaging   High-field MR imaging is superior to all other noninvasive techniques for demonstrating head and neck thrombi. Projective imaging of pulsatile flow by phase contrast and subtraction is analogous to digital subtraction angiography and eliminates velocity-dependent structures; three-dimensional holograms of the occluded vascular tree emerge that provide remarkably detailed visualization of jugular and cerebral venous thromboses (Figure 24-6) [7].

Imaging with thrombus-avid radiopharmaceuticals   Several radioisotope scanning techniques have been devised that are particularly suitable for imaging and staging thrombi of the legs, arms, and lungs; among them are ^{111}In-labeled platelet and ^{99m}Tc-plasmin scintigraphy. The most sensitive and definitive of these techniques in the diagnosis of DVT is immunoscintigraphy employing radiolabeled monoclonal

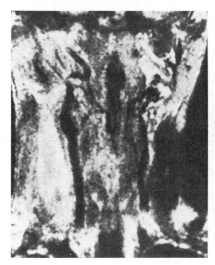
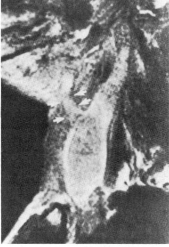

FIGURE 24-6

Coronal (left) and parasagittal (right) MR images reveal intraluminal hyperintensity throughout the right jugular venous system. Note extension of the thrombus into the facial vein on the right (arrows). Poor definition of the soft tissue planes on the right side of the neck is caused by interstitial edema surrounding the thrombosis. (From Braun IF et al: Jugular venous thrombosis: MR imaging. Radiology 157:357,1985.)

antibodies specific for fibrin; radioactive antifibrin monoclonal antibodies generate images of thrombi at all stages of maturation and are not influenced by ongoing anticoagulant (heparin) therapy (Figure 24-7) [8].

Diagnosis of Pulmonary Embolism

For validating the clinical diagnosis of pulmonary embolism (PE) and localizing the site of obstruction, perfusion lung scanning after infusion of radioactive particulate colloid (usually ^{99m}Tc-macroaggregated albumin) is a mandatory initial, but necessarily nonspecific, screening examination. If the perfusion lung scan is positive, specificity can be enhanced by adding a ventilation scan obtained following inhalation of radioactive xenon (^{133}Xe) or ^{99m}Tc aerosol. Used in conjunction, perfusion scans and ventilation scans reveal the presence and extent of ventilation:perfusion (V:P) mismatch, the signature of pulmonary embolism.

Pulmonary angiography is the only definitive method for identifying pulmonary embolism, for it provides direct visualization of the filling defect. Abnormalities such as oligemia, vessel pruning, or nonfilling of small vessels are inconclusive, but presence of a constant intraluminal filling defect or sharp cutoffs in

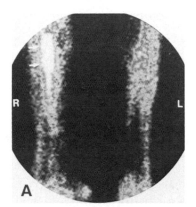
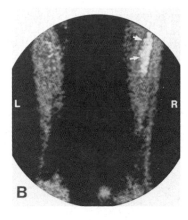

FIGURE 24-7

Anterior (A) and posterior (B) images of a DVT (arrows) in the right midcalf, obtained by infusing ^{99m}Tc-antifibrin monoclonal antibody. (From Koblik PD et al: Current status of immunoscintigraphy in the detection of thrombosis and thromboembolism. Semin Nucl Med 19:221, 1989.)

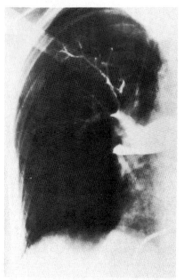
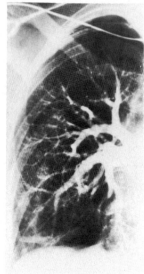

FIGURE 24-8

Pulmonary angiography performed before (left) and after (right) fibrinolytic therapy. Pretreatment angiography demonstrates filling defects of the right main pulmonary artery and occlusion of lobar branches. After therapy, there is no demonstrable embolic material, and small-radical perfusion is restored. (From Marder VJ and Bell WR: Chapt 92, in Hemostasis and Thrombosis. Basic Principles and Clinical Practice, 2nd ed, Colman RW et al, Eds. Philadelphia, JB Lippincott Company,1987.)

vessels greater than 2.5 mm in diameter is diagnostic (Figure 24-8) [6].

HEREDITARY PRETHROMBOTIC DISORDERS

Antithrombin III Deficiency

Antithrombin III (AT III), a member of the serpin family of plasma protease inhibitors, is a key regulator of activated vitamin K–dependent coagulation factors and is especially obsessed with the task of inactivating surplus thrombin. Normally AT III (the activity of which is enhanced by 2 to 3 logs in the presence of heparin or endothelial heparan sulfate) accounts for 75% of all thrombin-inhibitory activity in plasma; however, the concentration of AT III becomes rate limiting for inactivation of thrombin when the plasma level falls below 50%. Deficiency of AT III is transmitted as an autosomal dominant defect, with a gene prevalence of about 1 in 2,000, and affected patients have antithrombin levels that fluctuate in the critical range of 40 to 60% of normal. Severe thromboembolic problems usually do not commence until late adolescence or early adulthood, and it is estimated that 2 to 3% of patients hospital-

ized for recurrent thrombosis have underlying AT III deficiency. About half of AT III deficient patients experience their first episode of thrombosis as a spontaneous event; in the remainder thrombosis first occurs during pregnancy, shortly after delivery, or following surgery or trauma. Among the 65% of AT III deficient patients who have thromboembolic problems, 90% have recurrent DVT, complicated in 40% of cases by pulmonary embolism. Thrombosis of the vena cava or the mesenteric or upper extremity veins is less common, and arterial thrombosis is rare.

Pathophysiology and Diagnosis

AT III is distributed by exchange equilibrium between plasma and endothelial receptors. AT III functions best in the presence of heparan sulfate on the endothelial surface, explaining the poor correspondence between plasma levels of AT III and AT III anticoagulant activity. Mole-for-mole, heparin provides considerably more cofactor activity than heparan sulfate, which may explain why a mere 50% reduction in plasma AT III is sufficient to incur mortal risk of serious thrombotic difficulties.

Two principal categories of AT III deficiency have been defined on the basis of antigen levels in plasma. About 80% of AT III kindreds (classified as type I) have a quantitative abnormality in which both antigen and cofactor activity are reduced to about 50% of normal. Type I deficiency is caused by small deletions, insertions, or nucleotide substitutions in the AT III gene. In the type II category occurring in 20% of families, affected individuals produce normal quantities of AT III antigen but the AT III molecules are dysfunctional and have reduced heparin cofactor activity. The familial variants are highly heterogeneous in terms of inhibitor potency, affinity for heparin, and patterns on crossed immunoelectrophoresis (Figure 24-9) [9]. In the several type II phenotypic variants studied, DNA sequencing has uncovered various single nucleotide substitutions. In the most useful clinical assay for AT III deficiency, patient plasma is mixed with thrombin in the presence of heparin, and residual thrombin is quantified with a fluorogenic or chromogenic substrate.

Management

Affected individuals should be counselled about risk factors such as obesity, immobility, surgery, pregnancy, and the hazard of oral contraceptives, which lower AT III levels. For acute venous thrombotic events or during parturition or surgery, heparin plus the androgenic steroid, stanozolol (which induces sustained rises in functional AT III) is the therapy of choice, given alone or, when necessary, in combination with fresh plasma or AT III concentrate.

Protein C Deficiency

Protein C deficiency, a hereditary thromboembolic disorder with a prevalence of 1 in 7,500, is transmitted by an autosomal dominant gene mapped to chromosome 2. Heterozygous individuals have less than 60% of normal plasma concentrations of protein C, and most of them develop recurrent thromboses in early adulthood, generally before the age of 30, and have a clinical course similar to that of AT III deficiency. Infants born with the uncommon homozygous deficiency have almost no detectable protein C in their plasma (<1% of normal) and within 12 to 24 h of birth are savaged by a brutal and usually lethal syndrome dominated by large necrotizing thromboses of skin known as neonatal purpura fulminans.

Pathophysiology and Description

Protein C circulates in blood as a zymogen that, when activated by a complex of α-thrombin and its endothelial receptor, thrombomodulin, functions as an anticoagulant by proteolytically degrading cofactors VIIIa and Va (Chapter 21). This vitamin K–dependent serine protease is critical to the control of thrombin generation and also participates in fibrinolysis. Deficiency

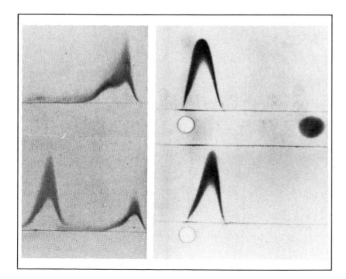

FIGURE 24-9

Two-dimensional immunoelectrophoresis of normal AT III (above) and a dysfunctional variant (below), in the presence (left) or absence (right) of heparin. In the absence of heparin both plasma specimens contain a single AT III peak, but in its presence the variant molecule displays an additional, more anodal peak. (From de Moerloose PA et al: Antithrombin III Geneva: a hereditary abnormal AT III with defective heparin cofactor activity. Thromb Haemost 57:154,1987.)

of protein C—hereditary, or acquired as the consequence of hepatocellular disease, malignancy, or warfarin therapy—predisposes to three syndromes: recurrent venous thrombosis, warfarin-induced skin necrosis, and (in homozygous newborns or heterozygous infants with DIC-induced consumption of all remnants of protein C) purpura fulminans.

Venous thrombosis   Affected heterozygotes have 30 to 60% of the normal level of protein C as measured by chromogenic assay. Recurrent attacks of superficial thrombophlebitis, punctuated by episodes of DVT and pulmonary embolism, begin to harass the patient at age 16 to 20, but as in AT III deficiency arterial occlusions are rare. In most kindreds the mutant gene has sustained a nonsense mutation causing premature termination of protein C synthesis, but missense mutations with production of dysfunctional protein have also been detected by sequencing the cloned gene. As the apparent result of genetic heterogeneity and the presence in some patients of inhibitors to activated protein C, severity of thromboembolic complications varies widely.

Warfarin-induced skin necrosis   Following initiation of anticoagulant therapy with warfarin (or other coumarin derivatives), the level of protein C falls sooner than that of other vitamin K–dependent factors because of its shorter (6 to 8 h) half-life. This creates a temporary imbalance during which activation by factors VIIIa and Va of procoagulant forces (factors IX, X, and II) are unopposed by protein C and activation of thrombin is transiently unbridled. In patients with hereditary or acquired deficiency of protein C, warfarin necrosis over fatty tissue occurs during the first week of anticoagulant therapy. The first evidence is pain caused by diffuse capillary thrombosis in patches of skin. Within hours edema and petechiae coalesce to form purple ecchymotic lesions with sharply defined geographic borders; this occurs just as other vitamin K–dependent factors begin to fall and the prothrombin time becomes prolonged. Consequently, hemorrhagic blisters are characteristic and herald the onset of deep hemorrhagic infarcts and skin necrosis over fatty tissue extending to but not including muscle, followed by black eschars that slough and leave craters or other lesions requiring skin grafts or even amputation (Figure 24-10) [10]. During the first weeks of warfarin therapy in patients with hereditary (heterozygous) or acquired protein C deficiency, the risk of skin necrosis can be averted by bolus infusions of heparin.

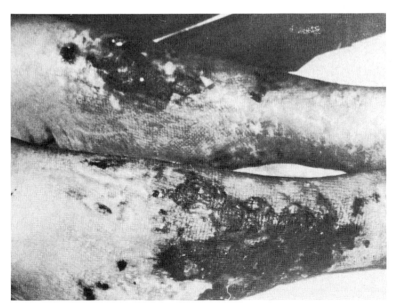

FIGURE 24-10

Warfarin-induced skin necrosis in a 57-year-old woman with functionally defective protein C. Shins and calves show confluent ecchymoses and hemorrhagic bullae. (From Teepe RGC et al: Recurrent coumarin-induced skin necrosis in a patient with an acquired functional protein C deficiency. Arch Dermatol 122:1408,1986. Copyright 1986, American Medical Association.)

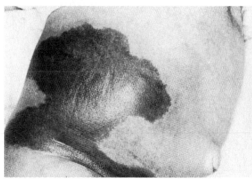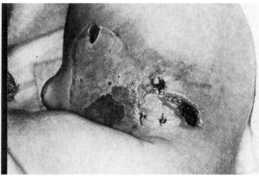

FIGURE 24-11

Typical appearance of thrombohemorrhagic skin lesions in purpura fulminans 24 h (left) and 10 days (right) after birth. Initial lesions on right abdominal wall are deeply demarcated, the central sunken purpuric zone being surrounded by an erythematous halo. At 10 days (right) a large symmetrical lesion on the left flank had become an eschar; epidermal sloughing from a later superimposed area of necrosis is seen in the right part of the infarcted region. (From Auletta MJ and Headington JT: Purpura fulminans. A cutaneous manifestation of severe protein C deficiency. Arch Dermatol 124:1387,1988. Copyright 1988, American Medical Association.)

Neonatal purpura fulminans Neonates homozygous for protein C deficiency present within 24 to 48 h of life with explosive and terrifying thrombohemorrhagic lesions that spread swiftly over large areas of the scalp, chest, abdomen, buttocks, and extremities, frequently accompanied by calamitous intracerebral thromboses and infarcts. The invariable occurrence of skin thrombosis and secondary DIC is unexplained but implies that protein C is foremost an anticoagulant of venules and microvasculature. Skin lesions begin as highly defined ecchymoses rimmed by erythematous haloes and are the result of pervasive microthrombosis of all capillaries and small vessels in the involved regions; they culminate in eschar formation with full thickness ulceration and sloughing (Figure 24-11) [11].

The life and flesh of victims of this most cruel and obstinate of hypercoagulable diseases can only be preserved by repetitious infusions of fresh-frozen plasma, PCC, or pro-

tein C concentrates. Severely deficient patients who do not benefit from warfarin prophylaxis and who require unacceptably frequent administration of plasma products are candidates for orthotopic hepatic transplantation; as hepatocytes are the source of protein C, liver transplantation is a rational recourse in imperiled children, and several longterm successes have been reported.

Protein S Deficiency

Protein S, a 69,000 M_r vitamin K–dependent glycoprotein, is the cofactor to protein C, and the two proteins act sequentially to maintain the nonthrombogenic properties of vascular endothelium: it follows that deficiency of protein S simulates protein C deficiency in predisposing to thromboembolic diseases. Unlike all other vitamin K–dependent hemostatic factors, which when activated function as serine proteases, protein S acts by binding to phospholipids on endothelial and platelet surfaces, thereby providing a docking site for activated protein C. Inactivation of factor Va by protein C is accelerated at least 100-fold when this activated anticoagulant is anchored to vascular and platelet membranes by protein S. About 60% of protein S in plasma is complexed to a spidery molecule known as C4b-binding protein (C4bP), a regulatory component of the complement cascade concerned principally with blocking conversion of C3 to C3b. Although it does not influence C4bP function directly, protein S through its affinity for surface phospholipids serves as a landing site for C4bP and facilitates its localization in regions of vascular damage. During inflamma-

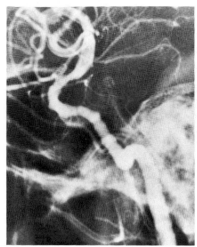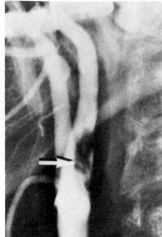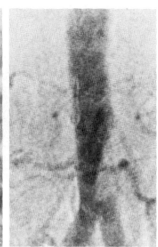

FIGURE 24-12

Angiograms revealing extensive arterial narrowing and thrombotic defects in a 14-year-old boy with homocystinuria. (Left) Arterial phase of left carotid angiogram reveals narrowing of the intracavernous segment of the internal carotid artery and beaded stenosis and irregularity of the ophthalmic artery. (Center) Lateral view of left common carotid arteriogram reveals an intraluminal thrombus (arrow) in proximal internal carotid artery. (Right) Digital IV subtraction angiogram showing a large thrombus in the distal abdominal aorta just above the bifurcation, and focal narrowing of the left iliac artery. (From Zimmerman R et al: Vascular thrombosis and homocystinuria. AJR 148:953,1987.)

tory reactions C4bP preempts protein S and in doing so interferes with the anticoagulant protein S–protein C pathway. Normally this friendly collaboration—one of many ways in which the coagulation and complement cascades interact—minimizes vascular damage, but in individuals deficient in protein S, usurpation by C4bP complexes of the small amount of protein S synthesized heightens the risk of thromboembolic misfortunes.

Description, diagnosis, and management   Protein S deficiency is inherited as a codominant autosomal disorder in which about 80% of heterozygotes are subject to recurrent venous thrombosis, thrombophlebitis, and thromboembolic events beginning in late adolescence or early childhood—a pattern similar to that encountered in protein C deficiency and AT III deficiency. For this reason, screening of patients with hypercoagulable disorders should include immunologic techniques capable of detecting free (uncomplexed) protein S as well as protein C and AT III. In homozygotes the first episodes of DVT occur at an earlier age and with much greater frequency. The incidence and severity of thromboembolic disease in heterozygotes and homozygotes correlates poorly with protein S levels as assayed by routine immunologic methods but can be predicted by special functional assays, or techniques such as crossed immunoelectrophoresis that discriminate between free and bound protein S.

Thromboembolic problems generally yield to anticoagulation with either warfarin or subcutaneous heparin.

Homocystinuria

Hereditary homocystinuria is a highly lethal metabolic disorder caused by homozygous deficiency of the enzyme cystathionine β-synthase, which catalyzes the conjugation of homocysteine with serine. Homocystinuria expresses itself gradually during early life as an assortment of worsening developmental anomalies (commonest of which is ectopia lentis), but the most damaging effect of systemic accumulations of homocystine is on endothelium. Unlike most prethrombotic states, homocystinuria is responsible for arterial as well as venous thrombosis (Figure 24-12) [12]; over half of homozygotes die of arterial occlusion or massive thromboembolism before the age of 20, and three-quarters of these ill-starred individuals succumb before age 30. The incidence of heterozygotes bearing the defective gene has been estimated to be as high as 1 in 70 as indicated by L-methionine loading. In some studies of large groups of patients presenting with peripheral and cerebral arterial occlusive disease before age 50, nearly 30% exhibited pathologic responses to methionine loading, implicating heterozygosity for homocystinuria as a major predisposing factor in cerebrovascular disorders.

More than half of patients with homozygous homocystinuria respond to pharmacologic doses of pyridoxine HCl by concomitant reductions in serum levels of homocystine and in the rate of occurrence of thromboembolic events. Responsiveness appears to require the presence of residual enzyme activity for which pyridoxal phosphate is the cofactor; nonresponders lack detectable cystathionine β-synthase activity.

ACQUIRED PRETHROMBOTIC DISORDERS

Commonplace settings that predispose to thromboembolic problems include major surgery, trauma, childbirth, and malignancy. Numerous thrombogenic risk factors are responsible for these associations, including increased blood coagulability due to release into circulation of tissue thromboplastin, prolonged immobilization, venous stasis, and reduced fibrinolytic activity. These are also risk factors for DIC, and local and disseminated formation of fibrin deposits may be coexistent responses to tissue damage. Unfortunately clearcut exegesis of pathogenetic mechanisms is confounded by the sheer complexity of such global disturbances in hemostasis as occur during and after major surgery or delivery. Specific risk factors are hard to isolate, and in many situations "known" to predispose to DVTs and pulmonary embolism—the postpartum period, advanced age, and congestive failure—statistical analysis of increased thrombotic risk has shown less than meets the eye.

Surgery, Trauma, and the Postpartum Period

Risk of thromboembolism after surgery or deep trauma is determined by the site and extent of tissue damage and by the duration of postoperative immobilization. Orthopedic procedures such as hip surgery and trauma to the pelvis are particularly apt to provoke thromboses, most of which are localized to iliac or femoral veins close to the site of injury. More than 90% of femoral vein thrombi occur on the side of operation, whereas the incidence of remote thrombi of calf veins is evenly distributed between both legs—attesting to the greater role of local vascular trauma, compression, and manipulation as compared to general immobilization. The complicit and potentiative thrombogenic effect of combining surgical trauma and immobilization is illustrated by comparing the incidence of thrombosis after abdominal hysterectomy with that after the transvaginal procedure, and by comparing suprapublic prostatectomy with transurethral excision: the risk of thrombosis is considerably greater when these procedures are performed via an abdominal approach.

The Postpartum Period, Not Pregnancy, Is Thrombogenic

Many physiologic alterations occur during pregnancy that collectively should increase the risk of thrombosis: decrease in fibrinolytic activity, deep venous stasis and dilation caused by uterine pressure, and increases in levels of fibrinogen and several key procoagulants should suffice to foment a hypercoagulable state, particularly in the third trimester. Surprisingly, vast compilations comparing the rates of venous thrombosis in the antepartum period, in the postpartum period, and in nonpregnant females of childbearing age have revealed that the antepartum is not associated with increased risk of venous thrombosis, but the relative risk in the postpartum period is in excess of 20-fold. This startling difference underscores the importance of traumatic and surgical components in the pathogenesis of thromboembolic disease attributed to pregnancy.

Use of oral contraceptive pills rich in estrogens induces many of the physiologic changes once thought to be thrombogenic in pregnancy: decreased fibrinolytic activity, venous dilation, and diminished levels of AT III. Voluminous reports involving legions of women have issued forth indicting oral contraceptives as predisposing to venous thromboembolism, but most hemostasis grandees still await decisive epidemiologic evidence free of methodologic flaws and bias.

Outside the world of surgical, obstetrical, and drug-induced mayhem, there is a mysterious and malevolent autoimmune process that is responsible for a broad repertoire of thrombotic disasters: it is known paradoxically as the lupus anticoagulant syndrome.

The Lupus Anticoagulant

Although originally identified in the laboratory by its heparinlike activity, the lupus anticoagulant antibody is responsible for induction of repeated episodes of venous and arterial thromboses. The tally of misfortunes includes recurrent DVT, cerebrovascular occlusion, pulmonary embolism, and thrombosis of the renal vasculature.

Pathophysiology and Diagnosis

Presence of lupus anticoagulant is defined operationally by prolongation of phospholipid-dependent coagulation tests such as PTT and correction by addition of platelets but poor correction by admixture of platelet-poor plasma. Lupus anticoagulants are a heterogeneous groups of spontaneously occurring IgG (and rarely IgM) antibodies that in vitro react specifically with anionic phospholipids, thereby blocking Ca^{2+}-mediated binding of vitamin K–dependent coagulation factors to activating phospholipid surfaces. Through an analogous reaction, lupus anticoagulant antibodies have high affinity for cardiolipin, and both lupus anticoagulant and anticardiolipin activities are mediated by the F $(ab')_2$ portion of the antibody. The term "lupus anticoagulant" is a contradiction á trois, because the anticoagulant does not inhibit hemostasis in vivo, most patients with lupus anticoagulant do not have SLE, and fewer than 10% of patients with SLE have the anticoagulant. The thrombogenic activity of lupus anticoagulant in vivo is explained by its reactivity with platelet phospholipids, which enhances platelet adhesiveness, and its direct binding to endothelial phospholipids, with suppression of

synthesis and release of prostacyclin (PGI_2) by vascular endothelium; the combined actions cause platelets to adhere to endothelium, leading to noninflammatory vascular obstruction and finally thrombosis.

Description

In nonlupus patients with lupus anticoagulant, leg veins are affected in 65% of thrombotic episodes, cerebral arteries in 25%, and peripheral arteries in 10%. No organ is exempt from the ravages of thrombotic angiopathy, and the range of vascular afflictions is boundless, including as it does both arterial and venous occlusions. In that most visible of organs, the skin, thrombophlebitis, ulceration, and ischemic or hemorrhagic gangrene are about equally frequent, and in all cases the histologic features are similar, showing occlu-

FIGURE 24-13

Skin ulcers in patients with circulating lupus anticoagulant. (Above) Stellate ulceration. (Below) Multiple full-thickness ulcers plus gangrene of the third toe. (From Alegre VA et al: Skin lesions associated with circulating lupus anticoagulant. Br J Dermatol 120:419,1989.)

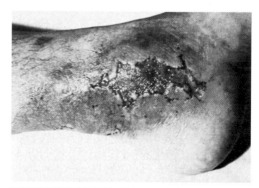

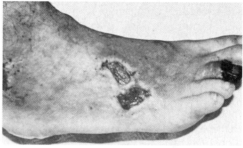

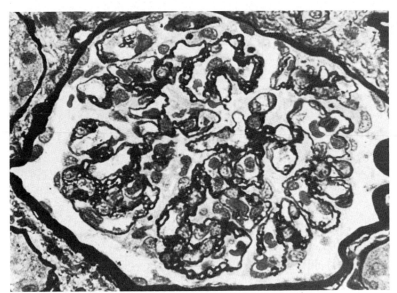

FIGURE 24-14

Renal biopsy from a pregnant patient with lupus anticoagulant. Sclerosis caused by fibrin thrombi creates double contours in glomerular capillaries, conferring a chainlike appearance. (From Kincaid-Smith P et al: Lupus anticoagulant associated with renal thrombotic microangiopathy and pregnancy-related renal failure. Q J Med [New Series] 69(258):795, 1988.)

sive thrombi in dermal vessels without cellular infiltration or signs of inflammation (Figure 24-13) [13]. Pregnant women are particularly vulnerable to the thrombotic problems associated with lupus anticoagulant. Diffuse thrombosis and thrombotic lesions in the renal microcirculation, originally thought to represent "lupus vasculitis," are a characteristic and threatening feature of pregnancy complicated by the presence of lupus anticoagulant antibodies. Thrombotic microangiopathy of the kidneys exhibits a characteristic pattern of fibrin deposition, which in glomerular arterioles and arteries eventuates in chainlike "double contour" sclerosis of glomerular capillaries (Figure 24-14) [14]. Renal function is impaired acutely during pregnancy, and impairment is permanent in some. Women with lupus anticoagulant have a very high incidence of habitual abortion and fetal wastage; placentas in pregnancies doomed by this arcane process exhibit characteristic pathologic patterns of progressive infarctions. The plasmas of nearly half of women plagued by unexplained recurrent miscarriage have been found to contain lupus anticoagulant, and this malign factor should be searched for in all patients with repeated fetal loss or any other unexplained thrombotic problems. Circumstantial suspicion should be aroused in all patients with thromboembolic disease who

also have high-titer anticardiolipin antibodies or antinuclear (anti-DNA) antibodies.

Suppression of antibody level with prednisone combined with aspirin inhibition of platelet cyclooxygenase appears to diminish thrombotic episodes and, if started early in pregnancy, to inhibit fetal wastage in women with lupus anticoagulant.

Prophylaxis and Treatment of Thrombotic Disorders

The purpose of this book is to describe pathologic processes affecting blood and marrow and to explain their molecular or physiologic mechanisms. Where, as is spectacularly the case in marrow transplantation, unique biologic insights are provided by the therapy itself, treatment is described in general terms. In the case of that eternal enemy of our species, thromboembolic disease, this presentation would be incomplete—and the reader might feel unrequited—if some allusion is not made to the major rational remedies (however imperfect) that have become available.

Prophylaxis of Thrombotic Disorders

Several classes of agents are capable of preventing or appeasing the occurrence or recurrence of thrombotic occlusions: drugs that alter platelet function, oral anticoagulants, and heparin given subcutaneously in low doses.

Antiplatelet drugs: aspirin   Antiplatelet prophylaxis has been used primarily in arterial thromboembolic disease. Acting on the presumption that platelet activation at sites of endothelial damage is instrumental in formation of arterial thrombi, major clinical trials have been conducted to evaluate the efficacy of drugs that interfere with platelet function. Of these, aspirin, which blocks cyclooxygenase, the key enzyme in production of the vasoactive prostaglandins (thromboxane A_2 and prostacyclin), has been most exhaustively studied. Aspirin has been used most widely in attempting to prevent new infarction or sudden death in patients who have survived an initial myocardial infarction. In this setting, aspirin is statistically beneficial, although its effect is exerted primarily during the first 6 months. With discovery that aspirin in low doses selectively inhibits cyclooxygenase activity in platelets and not in endothelium, large-scale evaluations have been made of 60 to 80 mg doses of "baby aspirin;" such doses suppress synthesis of platelet thromboxane A_2 (a potent vasoconstrictor and platelet aggregator) but not of endothelial prostacyclin, PGI_2 (an antithetical arachidonate metabolite that is an equally potent vasodilator and antiaggregant). Low doses of aspirin taken daily or on alternate days have been shown to reduce substantially the risk of both new and secondary infarctions in men over the age of 50.

Oral anticoagulants   Oral anticoagulants, specifically warfarin and other members of the coumarin family, are the most effective and well-documented agents for preventing venous thrombosis and pulmonary embolism. The major, seemingly irreducible drawback is the appreciable risk (about 5% per course of therapy) of severe hemorrhage.

Heparin prophylaxis   Heparin is a naturally occurring sulfated glycosaminoglycan originally purified from liver (thus its name), but for commercial preparation it is extracted from bovine and porcine lung or intestine. Heparin contains a large number of repeating

tetrasaccharide sequences having the correct structure and highly negative charge that make it suitable for binding as cofactor to AT III; this converts AT III from a slow inactivator of thrombin, factor Xa, and factor IXa to a fast-acting heparin:AT III complex that neutralizes all of these serine proteases with expedition. AT III complexed with endogenous heparan on the endothelial surface provides a protective shield that wards off thrombin and its coagulant allies; exogenous heparin binds to AT III in the circulating plasma, exerting an immediate anticoagulant effect within the bloodstream itself. Commercial heparin is a nonhomogeneous polydispersed mixture of sulfated polysaccharides having M_rs ranging from 2,000 to 40,000. Most anticoagulant activity resides in low-molecular-weight molecules of heparin averaging about 5,000 M_r, and use of semisynthetic facsimiles of molecules this size or smaller is particularly effective in blocking factor Xa, while skirting the platelet-agglutinating and thrombocytopenic effects of conventional mixtures containing high-molecular-weight heparins. Until the advantages and disadvantages of low-molecular-weight heparins are established, polydisperse heparin preparations remain the standard in prophylaxis and therapy of thromboembolic diseases. All heparin preparations are ineffective orally and must be given subcutaneously or intravenously—but never intramuscularly for fear of inducing large hematomas at the injection site.

Anticoagulant therapy represents a compromise between prevention of thrombosis and impairment of hemostasis. Not unexpectedly the principal complication is hemorrhage. The most informative (but impractical) test in guiding control of heparin dosage during prophylaxis or therapy is the activated clotting time; more widely used is the activated PTT using citrated blood and standardized thromboplastin reagents. Heparin overdose can be countered by infusing its antidote, protamine, which through its strong basic charge binds to and neutralizes the highly sulfated molecules of heparin. The best screen for detecting residual traces of the anticoagulant in blood is the thrombin time, which is exquisitely sensitive to heparin.

Surgical Prevention of Pulmonary Embolism:
Caval Umbrellas and Filters

In patients with partial or total occlusion of the vena cava, possible migration of large emboli that could cause fatal pulmonary artery obstruction can be deterred by the audacious surgical insertion via the internal jugular vein of intracaval filters. Several derring-do devices have been devised, the most popular being the Mobin-Uddin umbrella and the more recent wire cone designed by Greenfield and associates. These appliances are so effective in holding caval thrombi in place that they have largely replaced operative interruption of the vena cava; dislodgement of the filter is uncommon but can lead to spectacular embolization of the device to the heart or lungs. The Green-

FIGURE 24-15

Kim-Ray-Greenfield filter implanted in the inferior vena cava. One spoke of the wire cone appears to lie in a gonadal vein. (From Salzman EW: Chapt 94, in Hemostasis and Thrombosis. Basic Principles and Clinical Practice, 2nd ed, Colman RW et al, Eds. Philadelphia, JB Lippincott Company, 1987.)

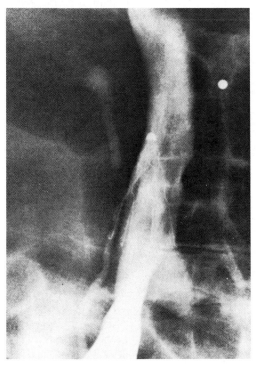

field filter is less subject to complications and far superior in preserving caval patency, allowing for its placement as high up as above the renal veins; the positioning of its spokes after they are unfolded at the catheter tip is intended to force retained emboli to the center of the cone (Figure 24-15) [15].

Thrombolytic Therapy

All thrombolytic agents currently in use act directly or indirectly as plasminogen activators. The crucial plasminogen molecules are those that become bound to fibrin during thrombus formation, and thus when activated to the proteolytic enzyme, plasmin, are perfectly positioned to dissolve the fibrin clot. Tissue plasminogen activator (t-PA) in either its single-chain or double-chain version, and whether of natural or recombinant (rt-PA) provenance, is fibrin-selective: t-PA requires fibrin as a cofactor for plasminogen activation and therefore it induces selective thrombolysis at the clotsite with minimal systemic fibrinolysis. Streptokinase (SK), an antigenic product of β-hemolytic streptococci, activates both free and bound plasminogen indirectly by forming a transient equimolar complex (SK: plasminogen) that liberates plasmin; urokinase (UK) is a two-chain serine protease which activates plasminogen directly. Both SK and UK create an untargeted systemic fibrinolytic state, and for either agent to dissolve a single thrombus at a single site requires indiscriminate systemic fibrinolysis unless the agents are delivered directly and dangerously to the clotsite via catheters. Acetylated plasminogen-streptokinase-activator complex (APSAC) is a derivative compound rendered temporarily inactive by acylation of the serine active site on the plasminogen light chain; deacylation occurs spontaneously in vivo and results in sustained proteolysis of fibrin and fibrinogen (termed the "lytic state"). Recombinant single-chain urokinase (rscu-PA), like rt-PA, induces fibrin-specific thrombolysis as the result of its affinity for fibrin-bound plasminogen, and in the presence of plasmin it is converted to UK on the fibrin surface. A summarizing scheme that portrays the direct or indirect reactions by which these several

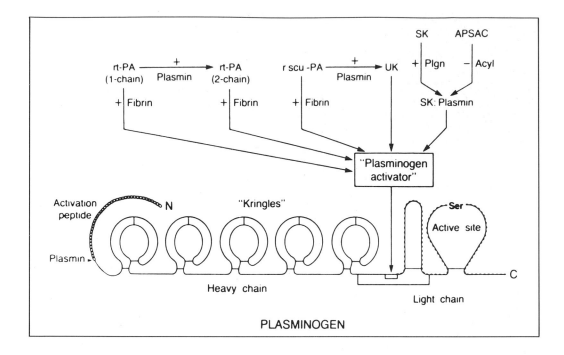

F I G U R E 24-16

All six clinically useful plasminogen activators possess a common property: ability to sever the arginine$_{560}$–valine$_{561}$ bond, a reaction that releases the light chain containing the proteolytic serine active site of plasmin from the heavy chain containing the looped fibrin-binding sites known as kringles. Abbreviations are defined in the text. (From Marder VJ and Sherry S: Thrombolytic therapy: current status (first of two parts). Reprinted, by permission of the New England Journal of Medicine 318:1512, 1988.)

plasminogen activators convert plasminogen to plasmin is shown in Figure 24-16 [16].

The fateful first four hours Significant comparative results for all the thrombolytic agents described above are available only for thrombolytic therapy in patients with coronary artery thrombosis. When treatment is started within 2 to 3 h of onset of chest pain, a similar incidence of reperfusion is achieved by all six thrombolytic agents, but in patients given 100 mg of recombinant t-PA within 4 to 6 h, thrombosed coronary arteries are recanalized in 70% of cases (demonstrated by pre- and posttreatment arteriography), as compared to 30 to 50% reperfusion rates in patients receiving SK or UK (Figure 24-17). Success in inducing reperfusion of freshly occluded coronary arteries by t-PA is an urgent function of timing and medical readiness: given within the first 4 h, t-PA and to a lesser extent SK are remarkably effective in restoring perfusion; after 4 to 6 h the recanalization rate, and hence survival, plummets. Intravenous t-PA therapy represents the most profound victory to date over humanity's worst enemy, but there are hazards. No thrombolytic agent, including t-PA, can discriminate between a coronary thrombus and a safeguarding hemostatic plug at another site. Thus, the major complication of the use of t-PA (and other thrombolytic agents) is hemorrhage into vital organs such as the brain, for which there is no safe antidote. The principal shortcoming of t-PA and SK thrombolytic therapy of coronary thrombosis is reocclusion, which occurs in roughly 20% of treated patients, although this complication may possibly be minimized by adjunctive use of antiplatelet therapy, timed judiciously [7].

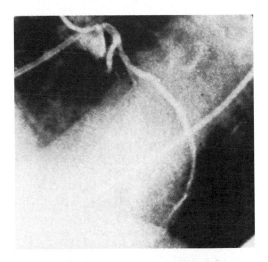

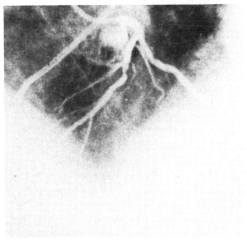

FIGURE 24-17

Complete lysis of coronary artery thrombus by infusion of recombinant t-PA, as documented by coronary angiography. (Above) Before therapy, the left descending artery (and all its branches) are occluded by a thrombus near the origin. (Below) Within 45 minutes after the start of rt-PA infusion, patency of the artery is fully restored. (Courtesy Dr. Eric Topol.)

DISSEMINATED INTRAVASCULAR COAGULATION

Disseminated intravascular coagulation (DIC) is a common and often final complication of disorders that trigger release of fibrin into the bloodstream and its indiscriminate deposition in small vessels and large. The causes of DIC are legion, for it may result from any disease process that generates thrombin in excess of its inhibitors. The most prevalent pathogenetic processes are endothelial injury or tissue damage with systemic release of tissue factor; the most common initiating disorders are septicemia with septic shock, malignancy, surgery, liver disease, and obstetric trauma. Although the initial pathologic events are thrombotic, the presenting clinical manifestation is paradoxical bleeding resulting from consumption of fibrinogen and procoagulants and release of anticoagulant fragments of degraded fibrin—fibrinogen degradation products (FDPs).

Pathophysiology

In DIC, thrombin and factor XIIIa convert fibrinogen into circulating crosslinked fibrin polymers which plate out on vascular walls and create myriads of small thrombi that obstruct the microcirculation of organs, any or all of which are threatened by occlusive shutdown. Plasmin cleaves circulating fibrinogen, fibrin, and microvascular thrombi, releasing both fibrinogen and fibrin degradation products that are harmful to the patient, but useful in gauging the extent of fibrinolysis. The plasmin-degraded products of fibrinogen and non-crosslinked fibrin are simple and similar (Chapter 21); a plasmin digest of fully crosslinked fibrin is considerably more complex and is characterized by dimers, plus an assortment of crosslinked dual- or triple-unit FDPs known collectively as high-molecular-weight (HMW) fragments. D dimers, being neoantigenic fragments released in excess only during extensive plasmin-induced lysis of crosslinked fibrin, are specific markers of DIC and can be detected by an enzyme-linked immunoassay employing monoclonal antibodies (Figure 24-18) [18]. Simplified latex agglutination assays for D dimers have been

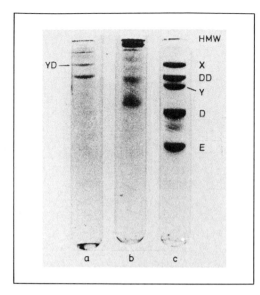

FIGURE 24-18

DD and YD dimers in the sera of two patients with acute DIC (left and center), as revealed by immmunoassay patterns on SDS PAGE and calibrated by a marker gel (right) containing DD and a mixture of non-crosslinked fragments. D-reactive HMW fragments have accumulated at top of gel. (From Elms MJ et al: Measurement of crosslinked fibrin degradation products—an immunoassay using monoclonal antibodies. Thromb Haemost 50:591,1983.)

developed for diagnosis of DIC in routine clinical laboratories: normally dimer levels are below 200 ng/ml, but during DIC, elevations in D dimer concentrations average over 2,000 ng/ml, far exceeding the subtle rises associated with DVT and other localized forms of fibrin deposition [19].

Diagnosis of DIC Laboratory diagnosis of DIC is based on the triad of prolonged PT, high titers of FDPs (if confirmed by an overabundance of D dimers), and microangiopathic deformities of red cells (See Figure 8-14). Most patients also have moderate (and occasionally severe) thrombocytopenia, prolongation of PTT and TT, and low levels of fibrinogen.

DIC Syndromes are Thrombohemorrhagic Disorders

Thrombotic occlusive events occur first as microthrombi that form in the general circulation and then cause broadcast obstruction of the microvasculature, or fibrin-platelet thrombi may be generated in situ within small vessels of any or all organs. Obstruction is then aggravated by hemorrhagic assault stemming from consumption of coagulation factors and platelets and release from fibrin deposits of anticoagulant FDPs; the deadly combination is known by the oxymoron "consumptive thrombohemorrhagic disorder." Activation of coagulation factors and platelets by rampaging thrombin molecules depletes the plasma of fibrinogen, thrombin itself, and factors V, VIII, and XIII (consumption coagulopathy). Free thrombin also stimulates platelets to aggregate and secrete and causes them to be swept from circulation by macrophages. Indeed, the first line of natural defense against particulate fragments of fibrin and clumps of sticky platelets is the macrophage system, but this is a saturable mechanism soon overwhelmed during severe and protracted DIC, setting the stage for platelet thromboembolic complications. Thrombocytopenia with dysfunctional platelets is characteristic of DIC, and its presence distinguishes thrombohemorrhagic processes from the comparatively rare syndrome of direct (primary) fibrinolysis. Also consumed as hemostatic mechanisms cave in are those mortal opponents of free thrombin, AT III and protein C, consumption of which promotes additional fibrin deposition. The swing toward hemorrhage in DIC is accelerated secondarily by the potent anticoagulant actions of fibrin split products: these fragments, particularly D dimers, YD fragments, and the D dimer–E complex, bind abnormally to nascent microthrombi, disrupting fibrin periodicity, and blocking polymerization of fibrin monofibrils at sites of vascular necrosis and hemorrhage.

Description

A list of disorders associated with acute, subacute, and chronic DIC is long and melancholy (Table 24-2) [20]. The most common causes of DIC are sepsis, malignancy, and

T A B L E 24-2

Disorders associated with DIC

Acute	Acute anoxia (e.g., after cardiac arrest)
Shock	Heat stroke
Hemorrhagic, posttraumatic, cardiogenic	Bites of certain poisonous snakes
Anaphylactic, acute allergic reaction to	Severe head injury
drugs or other causes	Following extracorporeal circulation
Septicemia due to meningococci,	Renal disease (glomerulonephritis, trans-
pneumococci, streptococci,	plant rejection)
pseudomonads, or most gram-negative	Necrotizing enterocolitis
bacteria	
Acute intravascular hemolysis	*Subacute*
Incompatible blood transfusion	Malignant disease
Severe hemoglobinemia due to other	Disseminated carcinoma
causes (e.g., malaria, drowning in fresh	Acute promyelocytic leukemia and other
water, ingestion of strong acids)	types of acute myelogenous leukemia, dis-
Purpura fulminans	seminated rhabdomyosarcoma
Acute viral, rickettsial, and protozoal infec-	Obstetric
tions	Retained dead fetus syndrome
Obstetric	Thrombosis at local site (e.g., aortic aneu-
Abruptio placentae, amniotic fluid embo-	rysm)
lism, septic abortion	
Acute pulmonary embolism, dissecting aneu-	*Chronic*
rysm	Liver disease
Burns	Localized neoplasms
Surgical operations, especially thoracic	Systemic lupus erythematosus

Source: From Merskey C: DIC: identification and management. Hosp Pract 17(12):83,1982.

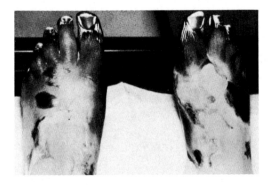

F I G U R E 24-19

Purpura, hemorrhagic bullae, and peripheral gangrene in a woman with sepsis and fulminant DIC. (From Molos MA and Hall JC: Symmetrical peripheral gangrene and disseminated intravascular coagulation. Arch Dermatol 121:1057,1985. Copyright 1985, American Medical Association.)

surgical shock, but DIC may develop in any shock syndrome including cardiogenic and anaphylactic shock and posthemorrhagic hypovolemia. In acute DIC the patient generally presents with sudden multisite bleeding problems, starting often with ominously persistent oozing from venipuncture sites. Thrombohemorrhagic progression may rapidly wreak havoc on skin, lungs, gastrointestinal tract, and central nervous system, leading to catastrophic hemorrhages and life-threatening hypovolemic shock; in moribund patients the denouement is often anticipated by the morbid march of acral cyanosis, bullous hemorrhages, and peripheral gangrene (Figure 24-19) [21].

During DIC and shock, fibrin thrombi appear more frequently in the kidney (68%) than in any other organ, because the glomeruli serve as high-flow sieves for fibrin and its degrada-

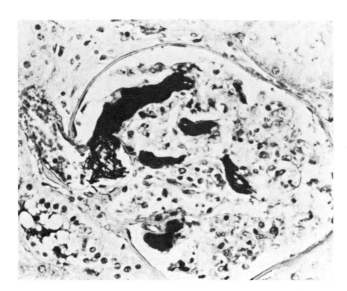

FIGURE 24-20

Multiple fibrin thrombi in glomerulus of a patient with DIC. Fibrin in the distal afferent arteriole (hilus of glomerulus) is composed of loose strands of fibrin; in fibrin aggregates forced into the smaller vessels and capillaries of the tuft, red cells are squeezed out and fibrin is compacted. (Phosphotungstic acid–hematoxylin stain.) (From Minna JD et al: Chapt 10, in Disseminated Intravascular Coagulation in Man. Springfield, Charles C. Thomas,1974.)

tion products (Figure 24-20) [22]. Microthrombotic occlusion of cerebral and pulmonary vessels is a major cause of death in DIC, and most patients in agonal septic shock suffer multiple pulmonary vascular occlusions and interstitial hemorrhages, which produce a clinical picture simulating respiratory distress syndrome. Acute DIC is a feared consequence of traumatic and surgical shock, and following penetrating brain injury, entry of thromboplastic brain tissue into circulation ignites massive intravascular coagulation by activating the extrinsic pathway: the unusually violent DIC following penetrating head injuries has a mortality of over 80%, antithrombotic ministrations notwithstanding.

Obstetric trauma   Mild transitory DIC occurs in most women during labor, but in third trimester patients with preeclampsia, smoldering DIC can erupt suddenly into the life-threatening "HELLP" syndrome (Chapter 8), which may be recognized by hemolysis resulting from microangiopathic fragmentation of red cells and which mandates obstetrical intervention for the sake of mother and child. Premature separation of the placenta (abruptio placentae) is the commonest cause of acute DIC in obstetric practice, and severity of the process and level of FDPs correlate well with the extent of separation and volume of

retroplacental hemorrhage. Placental tissue is rich in thromboplastin (and other uncharacterized coagulants), and its release into circulation may so deplete blood of fibrinogen, factors V and VIII, and platelets as to render it incoagulable. Fibrinogen replacement is inadvisable in this setting for it simply fuels further fibrin deposition and adds to the damage to renal vasculature. The situation demands attention to life support measures and emptying of the uterus—a sad solution that saves the mother at the price of her child. Amniotic fluid embolism is a far less common but even more violent obstetric complication, occurring during unusually tumultuous deliveries in older multiparous women. Hydraulic pressure on a weakened uterine wall is responsible for the forced entry of amniotic fluid into the maternal bloodstream. During delivery the patient experiences the abrupt onset of respiratory distress, shock, and cyanosis caused by occlusion of the pulmonary vessels by amniotic fluid emboli cloaked in fibrin, fetal epithelial cells, and assorted detritus (Figure 24-21) [23]. Amniotic coagulants cause massive, random deposition of fibrin on vascular walls, consuming fibrinogen and generating sufficient anticoagulant FDPs to plunge the patient into a hemorrhagic state having the potential for causing exsanguination from the uterus. Despite the most valiant therapeutic measures, the mortality

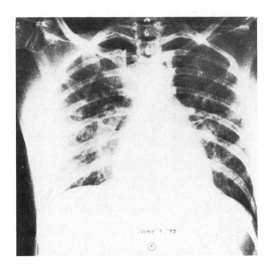

FIGURE 24-21

Chest film 1.5 h after onset of acute respiratory distress in a woman with amniotic fluid embolism and severe DIC. Note pulmonary artery enlargement and increased lung markings over the right lower lung field. (From Ballas S et al: Amniotic fluid embolism and disseminated intravascular coagulation complicating hypertonic saline-induced abortion. Postgrad Med J 59:127,1983.)

FIGURE 24-22

Parotid or venom gland of a viper lies behind the eye and is connected by a duct along the upper gum to an opening at the top of the canalized fang, which is long, mobile, and impressive when erected. (From Reid HA: Chapt 17, in Disorders of Hemostasis, Ratnoff OD and Forbes CD, Eds. Orlando, Grune & Stratton, Inc.,1984.)

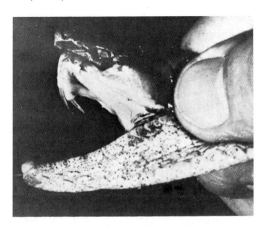

rate exceeds 80%, making this uncommon complication the principal cause of death during active childbirth.

Neoplasia and DIC Thromboembolic complications are commonplace in patients with solid tumors, for venous thromboses antecede or accompany clinical onset of roughly half of malignant tumors. Solid tumors menace the patient in many other ways that may upstage hemostatic problems. In acute promyelocytic leukemia (APL), however, DIC is an inevitable and life-threatening aspect of the malignancy. The dysplastic primary granules of APL promyelocytes—hypergranular or microgranular—are loaded with procoagulants and tissue factor. In APL patients (and to a lesser extent in patients with other variants of AML) having a large tumor burden, the leakage of coagulant materials into the bloodstream sooner or later ushers in a severe systemic DIC, best managed by intensive use of fresh-frozen plasma and platelet support.

Envenomation by snakes Venomous snakes have venom glands connected by ducts to hollow fangs well-suited for hypodermic purposes. Unlike elapid land snakes (cobras and coral snakes) which have short, fixed fangs and glands that secrete mainly neurotoxins, vipers possess retractable fangs 10 to 30 mm long, and their venoms are a virulent but varied brew of defibrinating coagulants, purpura-producing hemorrhagins, and hemolysins (Figure 24-22) [24]. The kind of clotting disorder and the accompanying symptoms caused by viper bites varies among the species in reflection of the specific enzyme content. In the case of the eastern diamondback rattlesnake (*Crotalus adamanteus*), coagulation abnormalities are traceable to a single thrombinlike enzyme, crotalase, which causes specific and direct conversion of fibrinogen to fibrin, without activating other procoagulants. Clotting results from cleavage of fibrinopeptide A from the α chain of fibrinogen, resulting in des-AA fibrin which forms a mutually destructive complex with plasmin, limiting the disruption of hemostasis. Inoculation of venom from the western diamondback (*C. atrox*), on the contrary, indirectly releases sufficient FDPs to render the blood incoagulable. Even so, frank hemorrhage may not ensue despite severe defibrination because vasculature remote from the wound is left intact. The only evidence of purpura may be the appearance of harmless discoid ecchymoses and mild scattered petechiae. What truly grips the attention of the bitee is the sudden onset of agonizing pain, edema, and ecchymoses, followed by spreading hemorrhagic vesicles, bullae, and necrosis reflecting diffusion of hemorrhagins from the puncture site. Patients bitten by a large adult *C. atrox* aroused from its winter's sleep fully stocked with venom are at risk of fatal fibrinolysis, best dealt with by infusing antivenom plus human t-PA to clear away damaging fibrin fragments.

REFERENCES

1. Freiman DG: Chapt 71, in Hemostasis and Thrombosis. Basic Principles and Clinical Practice, 2nd ed, Colman RW et al, Eds. Philadelphia, JB Lippincott Company,1987

2. Thomas DP: Chapt 36, in Haemostasis and Thrombosis, Bloom AL and Thomas DP, Eds. New York, Churchill Livingstone,1981

3. Kakkar VV and Sasahara AA: Chapt 37, in Haemostasis and Thrombosis, Bloom AL and Thomas DP, Eds. New York, Churchill Livingstone,1981

4. Marchesi VI: Chapt 4, in Pathology, vol. 1, Anderson WAD and Kissane JM, Eds. St. Louis, The CV Mosby Company,1977

5. Rapaport SI: Introduction to Hematology, 2nd ed, Philadelphia, JB Lippincott Company,1987

6. Marder VJ and Bell WR: Chapt 92, in Hemostasis and Thrombosis. Basic Principles and Clinical Practice, 2nd ed, Colman RW et al, Eds. Philadelphia, JB Lippincott Company,1987

7. Braun IF et al: Jugular venous thrombosis: MR imaging. Radiology 157:357,1985

8. Koblik PD et al: Current status of immunoscintigraphy in the detection of thrombosis and thromboembolism. Semin Nucl Med 19:221,1989

9. de Moerloose PA et al: Antithrombin III Geneva: a hereditary abnormal AT III with defective heparin cofactor activity. Thromb Haemost 57:154,1987

10. Teepe RGC et al: Recurrent coumarin-induced skin necrosis in a patient with an acquired functional protein C deficiency. Arch Dermatol 122:1408,1986

11. Auletta MJ and Headington JT: Purpura fulminans. A cutaneous manifestation of severe protein C deficiency. Arch Dermatol 124:1387,1988

12. Zimmerman R et al: Vascular thrombosis and homocystinuria. AJR 148:953,1987

13. Alegre VA et al: Skin lesions associated with circulating lupus anticoagulant. Br J Dermatol 120:419,1989

14. Kincaid-Smith P et al: Lupus anticoagulant associated with renal thrombotic microangiopathy and pregnancy-related renal failure. Q J Med [New Series] 69(258):795,1988

15. Salzman EW: Chapt 94, in Hemostasis and Thrombosis. Basic Principles and Clinical Practice, 2nd ed, Colman RW et al, Eds. Philadelphia, JB Lippincott Company,1987

16. Marder VJ and Sherry S: Thrombolytic therapy: current status (first of two parts). N Engl J Med 318:1512,1988

17. Loscalzo J and Braunwald E: Tissue plasminogen activator. N Engl J Med 319:925,1988

18. Elms MJ et al: Measurement of crosslinked fibrin degradation products—an immunoassay using monoclonal antibodies. Thromb Haemost 50:591,1983

19. Bick RL: Disseminated intravascular coagulation and related syndromes: a clinical review. Semin Thromb Hemost 14:299,1988

20. Merskey C: DIC: identification and management. Hosp Pract 17(12):83,1982

21. Molos MA and Hall JC: Symmetrical peripheral gangrene and disseminated intravascular coagulation. Arch Dermatol 121:1057,1985

22. Minna JD et al: Chapt 10, in Disseminated Intravascular Coagulation in Man. Springfield, Charles C. Thomas,1974

23. Ballas S et al: Amniotic fluid embolism and disseminated intravascular coagulation complicating hypertonic saline-induced abortion. Postgrad Med J 59:127,1983

24. Reid HA: Chapt 17, in Disorders of Hemostasis, Ratnoff OD and Forbes CD, Eds. Orlando, Grune & Stratton, Inc.,1984

Index